616.85 8445.
nol.

D1549627

Suicide

Global Perspectives from the WHO World Mental Health Surveys

Suicide

Global Perspectives from the WHO World Mental Health Surveys

Edited by

Matthew K. Nock
Department of Psychology, Harvard University, Cambridge, MA, U.S.A

Guilherme Borges
National Institute of Psychiatry and Metropolitan Autonomous University, Mexico City, Mexico

Yutaka Ono
Keio University, Yokohama City, Kanagawa, Japan

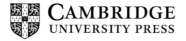

CAMBRIDGE
UNIVERSITY PRESS

CAMBRIDGE UNIVERSITY PRESS
Cambridge, New York, Melbourne, Madrid, Cape Town,
Singapore, São Paulo, Delhi, Mexico City

Cambridge University Press
The Edinburgh Building, Cambridge CB2 8RU, UK

Published in the United States of America by
Cambridge University Press, New York

www.cambridge.org
Information on this title: www.cambridge.org/
9780521765008

First published 2012

Printed in the United Kingdom
at the University Press, Cambridge

A catalogue record for this publication is available from the
British Library

Library of Congress Cataloguing in Publication data
Suicide : global perspectives from the WHO World Mental
Health Surveys / edited by
Matthew K. Nock, Guilherme Borges, Yutaka Ono.
     p. ; cm.
Includes bibliographical references and index.
ISBN 978-0-521-76500-8 (hardback)
I. Nock, Matthew.   II. Borges, Guilherme.   III. Ono, Y.
(Yutaka), 1950–   IV. Title.
[DNLM: 1. Suicide – psychology.   2. Health
Surveys.   3. Self-Injurious Behavior – epidemiology.
4. World Health. WM 165]
LC classification not assigned
362.28–dc23
2011033573

ISBN 978-0-521-76500-8 Hardback

Contents

Color plate section between pp. 84 and 85.

Acknowledgements

The editors would like to acknowledge the amazing efforts of all of the investigators, staff members, and others who help with all aspects of the WHO World Mental Health Surveys. Only a fraction of those involved in this work are listed as authors of the chapters included in this volume, and we are merely representatives of the many people who made this important project a reality. We would like to express our gratitude also to those who helped with the preparation of this volume. Alison Hoffnagle was invaluable in coordinating the work and communication among all of the WMH researchers. Charlene Deming, Christine Cha, Victoria Choate, Sara Slama, Jeff Glenn, Meghan Brady, and Lauren St. Germain put in countless hours of work reviewing and formatting the many, many tables and figures that appear in this volume. At Cambridge University Press, Joanna Chamberlin and Richard Marley provided wonderful guidance (and patience!) throughout the course of this project and we are extremely grateful for their help and support.

This project was carried out in conjunction with the World Health Organization World Mental Health (WMH) Survey Initiative. We thank the WMH staff for assistance with instrumentation, fieldwork, and data analysis. These activities were supported by the United States National Institute of Mental Health (R01MH070884, R01MH077883), the John D. and Catherine T. MacArthur Foundation, the Pfizer Foundation, the U.S. Public Health Service (R13-MH066849, R01 MH069864 and R01 DA016558), the Fogarty International Center (FIRCA R03-TW006481), the Pan American Health Organization, the Eli Lilly & Company Foundation, Ortho-McNeil Pharmaceutical, GlaxoSmithKline, and Bristol-Myers Squibb. A complete list of WMH publications can be found at http://www.hcp.med.harvard.edu/wmh/. The São Paulo Megacity Mental Health Survey is supported by the State of São Paulo Research Foundation (FAPESP) Thematic Project Grant 03/00204-3. The Bulgarian Epidemiological Study of common mental disorders EPIBUL is supported by the Ministry of Health and the National Center for Public Health Protection. The Chinese World Mental Health Survey Initiative is supported by the Pfizer Foundation. The Shenzhen Mental Health Survey is supported by the Shenzhen Bureau of Health and the Shenzhen Bureau of Science, Technology, and Information. The Colombian National Study of Mental Health (NSMH) is supported by the Ministry of Social Protection. The ESEMeD project is funded by the European Commission (Contracts QLG5-1999-01042; SANCO 2004123), the Piedmont Region (Italy), Fondo de Investigación Sanitaria, Instituto de Salud Carlos III, Spain (FIS 00/0028), Ministerio de Ciencia y Tecnología, Spain (SAF2000-158-CE), Departament de Salut, Generalitat de Catalunya, Spain, Instituto de Salud Carlos III (CIBER CB06/02/0046, RETICS RD06/0011 REM-TAP), and other local agencies and by an unrestricted educational grant from GlaxoSmithKline. The Epidemiological Study on Mental Disorders in India was funded jointly by the Government of India and WHO. The Israel National Health Survey is funded by the Ministry of Health with support from the Israel National Institute for Health Policy and Health Services Research and the National Insurance Institute of Israel. The World Mental Health Japan (WMHJ) Survey is supported by the Grant for Research on Psychiatric and Neurological Diseases and Mental Health (H13-SHOGAI-023, H14-TOKUBETSU-026 and H16-KOKORO-013) from the Japan Ministry of Health, Labour, and Welfare. The Lebanese National Mental Health Survey (LEBANON) is supported by the Lebanese Ministry of Public Health, the WHO (Lebanon), Fogarty International, Act for Lebanon, anonymous private donations to IDRAAC, Lebanon, and unrestricted grants from Janssen Cilag, Eli Lilly, GlaxoSmithKline, Roche, and Novartis. The Mexican National Comorbidity Survey (MNCS) is supported by The National Institute of Psychiatry Ramon de la

Fuente (INPRFMDIES 4280) and by the National Council on Science and Technology (CONACyT-G30544- H), with supplemental support from the PanAmerican Health Organization (PAHO). Te Rau Hinengaro: The New Zealand Mental Health Survey (NZMHS) is supported by the New Zealand Ministry of Health, Alcohol Advisory Council and the Health Research Council. The Nigerian Survey of Mental Health and Wellbeing (NSMHW) is supported by the WHO (Geneva), the WHO (Nigeria), and the Federal Ministry of Health, Abuja, Nigeria. The Romania WMH study projects "Policies in Mental Health Area" and "National Study regarding Mental Health and Services Use" were carried out by the National School of Public Health & Health Services Management (former National Institute for Research & Development in Health), with technical support of Metro Media Transilvania, the National Institute of Statistics-National Center for Training in Statistics, SC, Cheyenne Services SRL, Statistics Netherlands, and were funded by the Ministry of Public Health (former Ministry of Health) with supplemental support of Eli Lilly Romania SRL. The South Africa Stress and Health Study (SASH) is supported by the U.S. National Institute of Mental Health (R01-MH059575) and National Institute of Drug Abuse with supplemental funding from the South African Department of Health and the University of Michigan. The Ukraine Comorbid Mental Disorders during Periods of Social Disruption (CMDPSD) study is funded by the U.S. National Institute of Mental Health (RO1-MH61905). The U.S. National Comorbidity Survey Replication (NCS-R) is supported by the National Institute of Mental Health (NIMH; U01-MH60220) with supplemental support from the National Institute of Drug Abuse (NIDA), the Substance Abuse and Mental Health Services Administration (SAMHSA), the Robert Wood Johnson Foundation (RWJF; Grant 044708), and the John W. Alden Trust.

List of contributors

Sergio Aguilar-Gaxiola, MD, PhD
Center for Reducing Health Disparities, University of California, Davis School of Medicine, Sacramento, CA, U.S.A

Jordi Alonso, MD, PhD
Health Services Research Unit,
Institut Municipal d'Investigació Mèdica
(IMIM-Hospital del Mar), Barcelona, Spain;
CIBER en Epidemiología y Salud Pública
(CIBERESP), Barcelona, Spain

Laura Helena Andrade, MD, PhD
Section of Psychiatric Epidemiology, Department and Institute of Psychiatry, School of Medicine, University of São Paulo, São Paulo, Brazil

Matthias Angermeyer, MD
Centre for Public Mental Health, Gösing am Wagram, Austria

Annette Beautrais, PhD
Department of Emergency Medicine,
Yale University School of Medicine,
New Haven, CT, U.S.A

Guilherme Borges, ScD
Department of Epidemiological Research,
Division of Epidemiological and Psychosocial
Research, National Institute of Psychiatry (Mexico)
and Metropolitan Autonomous University,
Mexico City, Mexico

Evelyn J. Bromet, PhD
Department of Psychiatry and Behavioral Science,
State University of New York, Stony Brook, New York,
NY, U.S.A

Ronny Bruffaerts, PhD
Universitair Psychiatrisch Centrum – Katholieke
Universiteit Leuven (UPC-KUL), campus
Gasthuisberg, Belgium

Christine B. Cha, MA
Department of Psychology, Harvard University, Cambridge, MA, U.S.A

Somnath Chatterji, MD
World Health Organization, Geneva, Switzerland

Wai Tat Chiu, MA
Department of Health Care Policy, Harvard Medical School, Boston, MA, U.S.A

Giovanni de Girolamo, MD
IRCCS Centro S. Giovanni di Dio Fatebenefratelli, Brescia, Italy

Ron de Graaf, PhD, MSc
Netherlands Institute of Mental Health and Addiction, Utrecht, Netherlands

Charlene A. Deming, EdM
Department of Psychology, Harvard University, Cambridge, MA, U.S.A

Koen Demyttenaere, MD, PhD
Department of Psychiatry, University Hospital Gasthuisberg, Leuven, Belgium

John Fayyad, MD
Saint George Hospital University Medical Center, Balamand University, Faculty of Medicine, Institute for Development, Research, Advocacy and Applied Care (IDRAAC), Medical Institute for Neuropsychological Disorders, Beirut, Lebanon

Silvia Florescu, MD, PhD
Public Health Research and Evidence Based Medicine Department, National School of Public Health and Health Services Management, Bucharest, Romania

Oye Gureje, PhD, DSc, FRCPsych
Department of Psychiatry, University College Hospital, Ibadan, Nigeria

Janet Harkness, PhD
University of Nebraska–Lincoln, NE, U.S.A; ZUMA, Mannheim, Germany

Josep Maria Haro, MD, MPH, PhD
Parc Sanitari Sant Joan de Déu-SSM, CIBERSAM, Barcelona, Spain

Yanling He, MD
Shanghai Mental Health Center, Shanghai, P. R. China

Steven G. Heeringa, PhD
Institute for Social Research, University of Michigan, Ann Arbor, MI, U.S.A

Hristo Hinkov, MD
Department of Global Mental Health, National Center for Public Health Protection, Sofia, Bulgaria

Yueqin Huang, MD, MPH, PhD
Institute of Mental Health, Peking University, Beijing, P. R. China

Irving Hwang, MA
Department of Health Care Policy, Harvard Medical School, Boston, MA, U.S.A

Elie G. Karam, MD
Saint George Hospital University Medical Center, Balamand University, Faculty of Medicine, Institute for Development, Research, Advocacy and Applied Care (IDRAAC), Medical Institute for Neuropsychological Disorders, Beirut, Lebanon

Norito Kawakami, MD
Department of Mental Health, University of Tokyo Graduate School of Medicine, Tokyo, Japan

Ronald C. Kessler, PhD
Department of Health Care Policy, Harvard Medical School, Boston, MA, U.S.A

Viviane Kovess-Masféty, MD, PhD
EA 4069 Université Paris Descartes, Paris, France; EHESP School for Public Health Department of Epidemiology, Paris, France

Carmen Lara, M. D. PhD
Autonomous University of Puebla, Puebla, Mexico

Sing Lee, MB, BS, FRCPsyc
Department of Psychiatry, The Chinese University of Hong Kong, Prince of Wales Hospital, Shatin, Hong Kong, P. R. China

Jean-Pierre Lépine, MD, HDR
Hôpital Lariboisière Fernand Widal, Assistance Publique Hôpitaux de Paris INSERM U 705, CNRS UMR 7157 University Paris Diderot and Paris Descartes, Paris, France

Daphna Levinson, PhD
Department of Research and Planning, Mental Health Services, Ministry of Health, Jerusalem, Israel

Herbert Matschinger, PhD
Clinic of Psychiatry, University of Leipzig, Leipzig, Germany

Maria Elena Medina-Mora, PhD
National Institute of Psychiatry Ramón de la Fuente, Mexico City, Mexico

Matthew K. Nock, PhD
Department of Psychology, Harvard University, Cambridge, MA, U.S.A

Mark Oakley Browne, PhD
Discipline of Psychiatry, University of Tasmania and Tasmanian Government Department of Health and Human Services, Tasmania, Australia

Bibilola Oladeji, MBBS
Department of Psychiatry, University College Hospital, Ibadan, Nigeria

Yutaka Ono, MD, PhD
Health Center, Keio University, Yokohama City, Kanagawa, Japan

Johan Ormel, PhD
Interdisciplinary Center for Psychiatric Epidemiology, Department of Psychiatry, University Medical Center Groningen, University of Groningen, Groningen, the Netherlands

Bharat N. Panchal, MBBS, MD
Government Medical College, Bhavnagar, Gujarat, India

Beth-Ellen Pennell, MA
Institute for Social Research, University of Michigan,
Ann Arbor, MI, U.S.A

José Posada-Villa, MD
Instituto Colombiano del Sistema Nervioso, Bogotá
D. C., Colombia

Nancy A. Sampson, BA
Department of Health Care Policy, Harvard Medical
School, Boston, MA, U.S.A

Kate M. Scott, PhD
Department of Psychological Medicine,
University of Otago, Dunedin,
New Zealand

Dan J. Stein, MD, PhD
Department of Psychiatry, University of Cape Town,
Cape Town, South Africa

Thatikonda Padma Sudhakar, MD
Department of Psychiatry,
S. V. Medical College, Tirupati,
Andhra Pradesh, India

Maria Carmen Viana, MD, PhD
Section of Psychiatric Epidemiology,
Institute of Psychiatry, School of Medicine,
University of São Paulo, São Paulo SP,
Brazil

David R. Williams, PhD, MPH
Department of Society, Human Development,
and Health, Harvard School of Public Health,
Boston, MA, U.S.A

Alan M. Zaslavsky, PhD
Department of Health Care Policy, Harvard
Medical School, Boston, MA, U.S.A

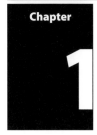

Chapter

1

Global perspectives on suicidal behavior

Matthew K. Nock, Guilherme Borges, and Yutaka Ono

The question of why people behave in ways that are harmful to themselves has puzzled us for thousands of years. The decision of whether to live or die has been called the "fundamental question of philosophy" (Camus, 1955) and has been the focus of scholarly work by most major philosophers throughout history (e.g., Kant, Sartre, Locke, Hume). In the sciences, the existence of self-harm has presented a fundamental challenge to the belief that human and animal behavior is motivated by an innate and ever-present drive for self-preservation and gene survival (Dawkins, 1976; Lorenz, 1963; Wilson, 1978). Clinicians and clinical researchers also have been baffled by the problem of suicide and have struggled to understand why people kill themselves and how to prevent them from doing so (Durkheim, 1897; Freud, 1923; Menninger, 1938; Shneidman, 1998).

Despite centuries of scholarly consideration and scientific investigation, key questions about suicide remain surprisingly unanswered, and it continues to be one of the leading causes of death worldwide. Indeed, suicide accounts for more deaths each year than all wars and other forms of interpersonal violence combined – meaning that we each are more likely to die by our own hand than by someone else's (World Health Organization, 2009). More alarming is that suicide is projected to be an even greater contributor to the global burden of disease in the coming decades (Mathers & Loncar, 2006). Despite these alarming statistics, we know relatively little about suicide. The purpose of this volume is to provide previously unavailable information about the occurrence of suicidal behavior around the globe – from a broad array of countries and cultures including those in the Americas, Europe, Africa, Asia and the Pacific, and the Middle East – in an effort to answer fundamental, and previously unaddressed, questions about this devastating problem.

Prior research on suicidal behavior

An impressive body of research currently exists that provides important information about suicidal behavior. However, despite the fact that thousands of studies have been conducted on this problem over the years, many basic questions remain. For instance, we know that the rate of suicidal behavior and suicide death skyrocket during adolescence, but we do not know why. We know that suicide runs in families, but we do not know how it is transmitted across generations. We know that people who try to kill themselves most often do so in the context of a mental disorder and stressful life events; however, we do not know which disorders or events convey the highest risk, how they might interact to increase risk, or why they sometimes lead to suicide.

Much of what we already know about suicide death and non-lethal suicidal behavior (i.e., suicide ideation, suicide plans, and suicide attempts) is reviewed in Chapter 2 of this volume. The rest of this book is focused on advancing our understanding of suicidal behavior in ways that overcome several of the long-standing limitations that have hindered progress in suicide research to date. Indeed, our inability to answer some of the basic questions about suicidal behavior is due not to a lack of effort, but to the existence of several serious challenges to studying suicidal behavior.

First, although suicide is a leading cause of death, suicide and suicidal behavior occur at fairly low base-rates in the general population. For instance, as discussed in Chapter 13, approximately 0.5% of adults report making a suicide attempt each year. This means that to obtain a sample of just 100 suicide attempters for study would require recruiting 20,000 participants from the general population.

Even more participants would be needed to study suicide attempts in greater detail. Unfortunately, most prior studies have used relatively small, selected samples (e.g., several hundred hospital patients who have attempted suicide), raising concerns about the generality of the obtained results (Ioannidis, 2005). Even in cases in which larger samples have been used, they often have been restricted to people of a particular catchment area or clinical samples from only one region (e.g., Bertolote et al., 2005; Weissman et al., 1999). One could try combining data from across studies to achieve a large sample size; however, different studies typically use very different methods and measures of both suicidal behavior and the risk and protective factors being studied, making such combinations impossible.

Second, suicidal behavior is the result of a combination of a wide range of factors, and most studies lack the time and resources to carefully assess a very broad array of factors. As such, most prior studies of suicidal behavior have focused on a narrow range of potential predictors or treatment for such behavior. Moreover, most studies have examined predictors of the presence of suicidal behavior, but have not yet investigated what factors predict the transition from suicide ideation to suicide attempts, or what factors predict treatment receipt or barriers to obtaining treatment. These types of investigations are among those that require the larger sample sizes mentioned above, and their absence has left major questions about how suicidal behavior develops.

Third, perhaps because of the difficulty of recruiting and interviewing people who experience suicidal behavior, very few studies of suicidal behavior are replicated. The lack of attention to replication is, of course, a problem across many areas of science; however, it is particularly concerning for suicide research given the stakes at hand. Although many potential risk factors for suicidal behavior have been identified, the extent to which they are robust predictors in the general population, and across different parts of the world, remains unknown.

Overall, as a result of these limitations, progress toward understanding and preventing suicidal behavior has been slow. Indeed, one recent epidemiological study documented that although there has been a significant increase in the percentage of people with suicide ideation and behaviors receiving treatment, the rates of such behaviors have not changed as a result (Kessler et al., 2005).

WHO World Mental Health Survey Initiative study of suicidal behavior

This volume presents new data on suicidal behavior obtained from the World Health Organization (WHO) World Mental Health Survey Initiative (WMH). This study, described in great detail in Chapter 3, is a coordinated series of epidemiological surveys conducted in 28 different countries on six continents around the world (data from the first 21 WMH countries are included in this volume). The unique nature and design of this project provides an unprecedented opportunity to overcome each of the limitations of prior suicide research mentioned above.

One of the most important features of the WMH Surveys for suicide research is the size and representativeness of the sample. As outlined in Chapter 3, this study provides data from more than 100,000 participants who, in most cases, are from nationally representative samples. The nature of the study sample allows us, for the first time, to really examine suicidal behavior in a fine-grained way. On balance, it is important to note that although this study provides a unique opportunity to study non-lethal suicidal behavior (e.g., suicide ideation, suicide plans, and suicide attempts), because the WMH Surveys include only living respondents, we are not able to study suicide death per se. Although suicide ideation, plans, and attempts are the steps that lead up to suicide death (i.e., you cannot die by suicide without making a suicide attempt), prior research has revealed that there are important differences between those who make non-lethal suicide attempts and those who die by suicide (e.g., women are more likely to make suicide attempts, whereas men are more likely to die by suicide). This distinction should be borne in mind when reading and using the data presented in this volume.

Another valuable feature of the WMH Surveys is that they carefully assessed a wide range of suicidal behavior, including the: age-of-onset, age-of-offset, and persistence of suicide ideation, suicide plans, and suicide attempts, as well as the probability and timing of transitioning from one of these behaviors to the next. Chapters 4 and 5 of this volume carefully describe these aspects of suicidal behavior in greater detail than ever before possible. These are aspects of suicidal behavior that have not been widely reported in the literature, and studies of the persistence of suicidal behavior are almost completely absent from the field. As such, the data presented in these chapters are valuable not only for scientists who study suicidal behavior, but for clinicians and policy-makers interested in learning more about its occurrence in our communities.

Much of this volume, Chapters 6–12, presents data on a wide range of risk factors for suicidal behavior, including: sociodemographic factors (Chapter 6), parental psychopathology (Chapter 7), childhood adversities (Chapter 8), traumatic experiences during adulthood (Chapter 9), mental disorders (Chapter 10), and chronic physical conditions (Chapter 11). The last chapter in this section, Chapter 12, tests an integrative model of suicidal behavior that includes all of these risk factor domains. Many studies have tested risk factors that appear in each of these chapters; however, the large and representative sample size of the WMH Survey, the careful assessment of each risk factor domain and each suicidal behavior, and the comprehensive nature of the analyses conducted allow this study to provide more definitive findings on the nature of these risk factors than has been possible in prior studies. In a way, we view this effort as a "mapping" of the risk factors for suicidal behavior from a broad range of domains. Each chapter tests the bivariate and multivariate (i.e., unique) effects of each risk factor. We start with temporally prior risk factor domains in earlier chapters (e.g., sociodemographics, parental history) and add risk factor domains in later chapters while controlling for earlier results. At each step, we test the extent to which each risk factor predicts the onset of each suicidal behavior, the transition across suicidal behavior, and the persistence of suicidal behavior over time. We also examine how these effects differ across the lifespan, and across different countries around the world (i.e., high-income countries vs. middle-income countries vs. low-income countries). In this way, these chapters provide a more detailed picture of the nature and risk factors for suicidal behavior than has been possible in prior studies, including earlier studies using the WMH Survey data – as the publication of these findings in book form allows us to present the findings in a more expanded way than is possible in scientific journals.

The final section of this book is focused especially on providing clinically relevant information on suicidal behavior. Chapter 13 reports on the short-term (i.e., 12-month) risk factors for suicidal behavior; such information may be especially useful for clinicians working with suicidal individuals. This chapter also includes risk factor indices that synthesize the results of Chapters 6–12 into useable indices that can aid clinical decision-making about a patient's current level of risk. Chapter 14 describes what the treatment of suicidal behavior looks like around the world in terms of the rates and types of treatment receipt by suicidal people, the barriers to treatment, and the predictors of treatment receipt and barriers. The findings of this chapter are somewhat discouraging and paint a sobering picture of the long road that lies ahead for improving the treatment of suicidal people around the globe.

This volume concludes with a discussion of the scientific, clinical, and policy implications of the findings presented in this book, and offers recommendations for future efforts in each of these areas. The findings presented in this book are extremely comprehensive and detailed in nature, with dozens and dozens of tables of data in each section of the book. Our reason for including this level of detail is that the WMH Surveys provide a richer source of data on suicidal behavior than have ever been available, and so represent a veritable gold-mine of findings. We wanted to make these data maximally useful for current and future researchers, clinicians, and policy-makers, and providing a high level of detail achieves this end. However, these data are useless if they do not have impact beyond this book, and the last section of this volume provides concrete suggestions for ensuring such impact.

Global perspectives

The completion of the WMH Surveys and the preparation of this volume was truly a global effort, involving extensive interviews with more than 100,000 people living in 21 countries on six continents, as well as countless hours of work by first-rate research teams in each of these countries. This volume presents the collective efforts, and perspectives, of all of these respondents, and researchers. It is our hope that the information presented here will bring us just a little closer to understanding, and preventing, suicidal behavior around the globe.

References

Bertolote, J. M., Fleischmann, A., De Leo, D., et al. (2005). Suicide attempts, plans, and ideation in culturally diverse sites: the WHO SUPRE-MISS community survey. *Psychological Medicine*, **35**(10), 1457–1465.

Camus, A. (1955). *The myth of Sisyphus* (J. O'Brien, Trans.). New York, NY: Alfred A. Knopf, Inc. (Original work published 1942).

Dawkins, R. (1976). *The selfish gene*. New York, NY: Oxford University Press.

Durkheim, E. (1897). *Suicide: A study in sociology* (ed. G. Simpson. Translated by J. A. Spaulding, G. Simpson). New York, NY: Free Press, 1951.

Freud, S. (1923). The ego and the id. In *The standard edition of the complete psychological works of Sigmund Freud* (Volume XIX, 1923–1925).

Ioannidis, J. P. (2005). Why most published research findings are false. *PLoS Medicine*, 2(8), e124.

Kessler, R. C., Berglund, P., Borges, G., Nock, M. K., & Wang, P. S. (2005). Trends in suicide ideation, plans, gestures, and attempts in the United States, 1990–1992 to 2001–2003. *Journal of the American Medical Association*, **293**(20), 2487–2495.

Lorenz, K. (1963). *On aggression.* San Diego, CA: Harcourt Brace.

Mathers, C. D., & Loncar, D. (2006). Projections of global mortality and burden of disease from 2002 to 2030. *PLoS Medicine*, 3(11), e442.

Menninger, K. (1938). *Man against himself.* New York, NY: Harcourt Brace World.

Shneidman, E. S. (1998). *The suicidal mind.* New York, NY: Oxford University Press.

Weissman, M. M., Bland, R. C., Canino, G. J., et al. (1999). Prevalence of suicide ideation and suicide attempts in nine countries. *Psychological Medicine*, **29**(1), 9–17.

Wilson, E. O. (1978). *On human nature.* Cambridge, MA: Harvard University Press.

World Health Organization. (2009). Data and statistics: Causes of death. http://www.who.int/healthinfo/statistics/bodgbddeathdalyestimates.xls. Accessed Oct. 4, 2009.

Chapter 2

The epidemiology of suicide and suicidal behavior

Matthew K. Nock, Guilherme Borges, Evelyn J. Bromet, Christine B. Cha, Ronald C. Kessler, and Sing Lee

Abstract

Suicidal behaviors are a leading cause of injury and death worldwide and information about the epidemiology of such behaviors is important for policy-making and prevention efforts. We reviewed government data on suicide and suicidal behaviors and conducted a systematic review of studies on the epidemiology of suicidal behaviors published from 1997 to 2007. Our aims were to examine the prevalence, trends, and risk and protective factors of suicidal behaviors in the U.S. and cross-nationally. The data revealed significant cross-national variability in the prevalence of suicidal behaviors, but consistency in the age-of-onset (AOO), transition probabilities, and the presence of key risk factors. Suicide is more prevalent among men, whereas nonfatal suicidal behaviors are more prevalent among women and among those who are young, unmarried, and have a psychiatric disorder. Despite an increase in the treatment of suicidal individuals over the past decade, incidence rates of suicidal behaviors have remained largely unchanged. Most epidemiological research on suicidal behaviors has focused on patterns and correlates of prevalence. The next generation of studies must examine synergistic effects among modifiable risk factors and protective factors. New studies must incorporate recent methodological advances in survey methodology and clinical assessment and results should guide ongoing efforts to decrease the significant loss of life caused by suicidal behaviors.

Introduction

Suicide is an enormous public health problem in the United States (U.S.) and around the world. Each year over 30,000 people in the U.S. and approximately 1 million people worldwide die by suicide, making it one of the leading causes of death (Department of Health and Human Services. Healthy People 2010, 2000; U.S. Public Health Service, 1999; WHO, 1996). A recent report from the Institute of Medicine estimated that the value of lost productivity due to suicide is $11.8 billion per year in the U.S. (Goldsmith et al., 2002), and reports from the World Health Organization (WHO) indicate that suicide accounts for the largest share of intentional injury burden in developed countries (Mathers et al., 2003), and that suicide is projected to become an even greater contributor to the global burden of disease over the coming decades (Mathers & Loncar, 2006; Murray & Lopez, 1996). The seriousness and scope of suicide has led both the WHO (WHO, 2007) and the U.S. government (Department of Health and Human Services. Health People 2010, 2000; U.S. Public Health Service, 1999) to call for an expansion of data collection on the prevalence and risk factors for suicide and nonfatal suicidal behaviors to aid in planning public health responses and healthcare policy and for monitoring the rate of suicidal behaviors in response to policy changes and prevention efforts.

Addressing these calls, this paper provides a review of the epidemiology of suicidal behaviors and extends earlier reviews in this area (Borges et al., 1995; Bridge et al., 2006; Cantor, 2000; Cantor et al., 1996; Cheng & Lee, 2000; Kerkhof, 2000; Kessler & McRae, 1983; Levi et al., 2003; Monk, 1987; Moscicki, 1999; Spirito & Esposito-Smythers, 2006; Weissman, 1974; Wexler et al., 1978) in two important ways. First, this paper provides an update on the prevalence of suicidal behaviors over the past decade. The socioeconomic and cultural factors in which suicidal behaviors are embedded, such as the quality and quantity of mental health services, have changed dramatically (Kessler et al., 2005a; Kessler et al., 2005b), making it important to examine if and how the prevalence of suicidal behaviors have changed over time. Second, most prior reviews have focused on a specific country (e.g., U.S.), sub-group (e.g., adolescents), or behavior (e.g., suicide attempt). We review data from multiple countries, all age groups, and on different forms of suicidal behavior, providing a comprehensive picture of the epidemiology of suicidal behaviors. Moreover, given recent technological developments in injury surveillance systems (Horan & Mallonee, 2003), as well as the recent completion of several large-scale epidemiological studies examining the cross-national prevalence of suicidal behaviors (Bertolote et al., 2005; Nock et al., 2008a; Platt et al., 1992; Weissman et al., 1999), an updated review of this area is especially warranted at this time.

Terminology and definitions in suicide research

We use the terminology and definitions for suicidal behaviors outlined in recent consensus papers on this topic (O'Carroll et al., 1996; Posner et al., 2007; Silverman et al., 2007a, 2007b). We define *suicide* as the act of intentionally ending one's own life. Nonfatal suicidal thoughts and behaviors (hereafter "suicidal behaviors") are classified more specifically into three categories: *suicide ideation*, which refers to thoughts of engaging in behavior intended to end one's own life; *suicide plan*, which refers to the formulation of a specific method through which one intends to die; and *suicide attempt*, which refers to engagement in potentially self-injurious behavior in which there is at least some intent to die. Most researchers and clinicians distinguish suicidal behaviors from non-suicidal self-injury (NSSI; e.g., self-cutting), which refers to self-injury in which a person has no intent to die and is not the focus of this review (Nock et al., 2006; Nock & Kessler, 2006; Nock & Prinstein, 2005).

We first review data on the current rates and recent trends for suicide and suicidal behaviors in the U.S. and cross-nationally. Next we review data on the onset, course, and risk and protective factors for suicide and suicidal behaviors. Finally, we summarize data from recent suicide prevention efforts and conclude with suggestions for future research.

Method
Main data sources
Suicide

Data on annual suicide mortality in the U.S. are maintained by the National Vital Statistics System of the Centers for Disease Control (CDC) and were retrieved for this review using the Web-based Injury Statistics Query and Reporting System (WISQARS) (CDC, 2008a). In examining recent time trends, we examined rates of suicide in the U.S. from 1990 to 2005, the most recent data currently available. Suicide data for many other countries are maintained by the WHO (WHO, 2007). We included information in this review from a wide range of countries and for those with the highest reported rates of suicide, but we did not include data for every country because of space constraints. Cross-national variability in the most recent year for which suicide data are available precluded an analysis of recent trends at the same level of detail as that for the U.S.

Suicidal behaviors

The CDC also maintains data on the estimated rate of nonfatal self-injury based on a national surveillance system of injuries treated in U.S. hospital emergency departments (National Electronic Injury Surveillance System) (CDC, 2008b). These data were reviewed to estimate the rate of nonfatal self-injury in the U.S. Although these data provide valuable information about the scope of this problem, there are three notable limitations of these data: they lack precision in that they do not distinguish between suicidal and non-suicidal self-injury; they do not provide data on characteristics or risk and protective factors, and they fail to capture self-injury not treated in U.S. hospital emergency departments. In order to address these limitations, data on the prevalence and characteristics of nonfatal suicidal behaviors in the U.S. and other countries also were obtained via a systematic, electronic search of the recent peer-reviewed literature (1997–2007). We searched the U.S. National Library of Medicine's PubMed electronic database using the title and abstract search terms "suicide," "suicidal behavior," or "suicide attempt," and requiring the term "epidemiology" or "prevalence." This search yielded 1052 abstracts, which we reviewed individually and used to inform the review if they reported: the prevalence of suicide (n=28) or suicidal behaviors

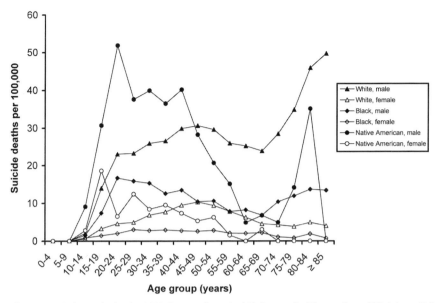

Figure 2.1. U.S. suicide deaths, 2005. Data are from the U.S. Centers for Disease Control Web-based Injury Statistics Query and Reporting System (CDC, 2008a). Data points based on less than 20 deaths per cell may be unreliable. These include: those for ages 0–9 years for all groups, 80–85+ years for black males, 10–14 and 55–85+ years for black females, 10–14 and 45–85+ years for Native American/Alaskan Native males, and all data points except ages 10–14 years for Native American/Alaskan Native females.

(n=65) within some well-defined population, risk/protective factors or prevention programs (n=132), or review of the above (n=102). Excluded were studies: with small sample sizes (<100; n=73), for which the full article was not available in English (n=108); of narrowly defined sub-populations (e.g., specific clinical samples) or irrelevant topic (e.g., cellular suicide) (n=493), and those that did not provide a specific measure of one of the suicidal behaviors outlined above (n=51). When multiple studies were identified reporting on the same data source (e.g., CDC Youth Risk Behavior Survey [YRBS]), only the primary or summary report was used to avoid redundancy.

Results

Suicide in the United States

Current

Suicide occurs among 10.8 per 100,000 persons, is the 11th leading cause of death, and accounts for 1.4% of all U.S. deaths (CDC, 2008a). A more detailed examination of gender, age, and ethnic/racial groups reveals significant sociodemographic variation in the suicide rate. As presented in Figure 2.1, there are no group differences until mid-adolescence (15–19 years), at which time the rate among males increases dramatically relative to

the rate among females. The rise for males is greatest among Native Americans/Alaskan Natives, increasing more than five-fold during adolescence from 9.1/100,000 (10–14 years) to 51.9/100,000 (20–24 years). The rate for Native American/Alaskan Native males declines during middle adulthood before peaking again during older age. Non-Hispanic white males also have a sharp increase during adolescence and young adulthood (from 2.0/100,000 at ages 10–14 years to 23.0/100,000 at ages 20–24 years) and a second one from age 65–69 years (23.9/100,000) to 85+ years (49.7/100,000). The rate for women is lower and virtually non-overlapping with those of men, with the two exceptions being for suicide among Native American/Alaskan Native women during adolescence (10–19 years), and for white women during middle-age (55–59 years). Suicide rates for people of Hispanic and Asian race/ethnicity, not presented in Figure 2.1 due to space constraints, are generally similar to those for black males and females.

Trends

Recent U.S. suicide trends (1990–2005) are displayed in Figure 2.2, with separate lines plotted by gender (male, female) and age (10–24, 25–44, 45–64, 65+ years). Suicide rates stratified by race/ethnicity have not changed over this period and so were not included

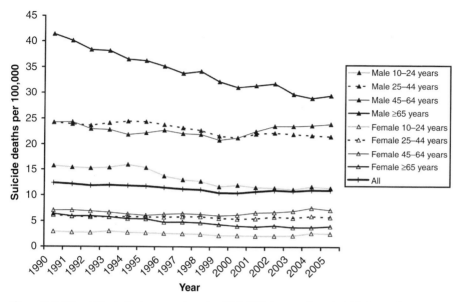

Figure 2.2. U.S. suicide deaths by age and gender, 1990–2005. Data are from the U.S. Centers for Disease Control Web-based Injury Statistics Query and Reporting System (CDC, 2008a).

for ease of presentation. As shown in Figure 2.2, the suicide rate is consistently higher for males than females. Substantive decreases have occurred for elderly males (65+ years), who show a decrease from 41.4 to 29.5/100,000 and for young males (10–24 years), who show a decrease from 15.7 to 11.4/100,000. The overall U.S. suicide rate has decreased from 12.4 to 11.0/100,000 (11.1% decrease) during this time.

Cross-national suicide rates

Current

Data from the WHO indicate that suicide occurs in approximately 16.7 per 100,000 persons per year, is the 14th leading cause of death worldwide, and accounts for 1.5% of all deaths (WHO, 2007). As presented in Figure 2.3, suicide rates vary significantly cross-nationally. In general, rates are highest in Eastern European countries and lowest in Central and South American countries, with the U.S., Western Europe, and Asian countries falling in the middle. Despite the wide variability in rates, there is a consistently higher rate among men than women, with men dying by suicide more than women at a ratio of between 3:1 and 7.5:1. Two notable exceptions are India and China, where there are no clear gender differences. The male-to-female ratio is 1.3:1 in India, 0.9:1 in mainland China, and 2.0:1 in Hong Kong. The reason for the absence of a gender difference in India and

mainland China is not known, but it has been suggested that the lower social status of females in the context of disempowering circumstances and the more lethal methods used, such as self-burning in India (Kumar, 2003) and ingestion of pesticides in China (Lee & Kleinman, 2003), may account for this pattern. Given that India and China alone constitute nearly half of the world's population, this "atypical" ratio may well represent a typical pattern when considered based on the global population.

Trends

Definitive data do not exist on worldwide suicide mortality trends due to cross-national differences in reporting procedures and availability of data. The WHO has maintained cross-national data on suicide mortality since 1950; however, there are inconsistencies in reporting by individual countries, with only 11 countries providing data in 1950, 74 countries in 1985, and 50 in 1998. Moreover, the fact that some governments have treated suicide as a social or political issue rather than a health problem may have diminished the validity of earlier data and resulting estimates. Given these inconsistencies, it is difficult to generate an accurate cross-national estimate of trends. Nevertheless, the data maintained by the WHO suggest that the global rate of suicide has increased from 1950 to 2004, especially for men (Bertolote & Fleischmann, 2002), and data-based projections suggest the number

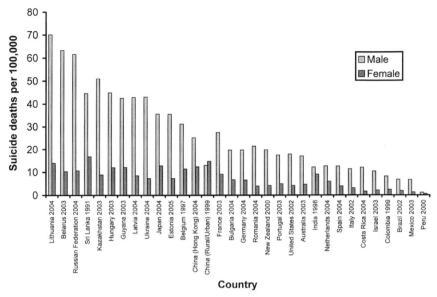

Figure 2.3. Cross-national suicide deaths – most recent year available. Data are from the World Health Organization (WHO, 2007).

of self-inflicted deaths will increase by as much as 50% from 2002 to 2030 (Mathers & Loncar, 2006). Given the inconsistencies in data sources both within and across countries (Bertolote & Fleischmann, 2002; Jenkins, 2002; Pescosolido & Mendelsohn, 1986), though, a definitive picture of the long-term trends in global suicide deaths remains unclear.

Suicidal behaviors in the United States

Current

Data from the CDC (CDC, 2008b) on nonfatal self-injury for 2006 are presented in Figure 2.4. As shown, there is a significant increase in risk of nonfatal self-injury (both suicidal and non-suicidal in nature) during adolescence and young adulthood, which decreases monotonically throughout adulthood. In contrast to suicide mortality, rates of nonfatal self-injury are consistently higher among females. Data from our systematic review suggest that for U.S. adults (18+ years), the lifetime prevalence of suicide ideation is between 5.6% and 14.3% with an interquartile range (IQR) of 7.9%–13.9%, for suicide plans is 3.9%, and for suicide attempts is 1.9%–8.7% (IQR=3.0%–5.1%) (see Table 2.1 for studies). Twelve-month prevalence estimates are in the range of 2.1%–10.0% (IQR=2.4%–6.7%) for suicide ideation, 0.7%–7.0% (IQR=0.7%–5.5%) for suicide plan, and 0.2%–2.0%

(IQR=0.3%–1.3%) for suicide attempt, with higher rates for younger adults and females (see Table 2.1). Some of the variation in rates is likely due to sample selection (e.g., high rate of attempt in the study including only Native Americans) and variability in the items used to assess suicidal behaviors. For instance, questions asking about "thoughts of death" generate higher prevalence estimates for suicide ideation than questions asking about "seriously considering suicide" (Scocco & De Leo, 2002), and responses requiring endorsement of intent to die from self-injury yield lower estimates of suicide attempts than simply asking if one has made a "suicide attempt" (Nock & Kessler, 2006).

Studies on adolescents (12–17 years) suggest that the lifetime prevalence is in the range of 19.8%–24.0% (IQR=19.8%–24.0%) for suicide ideation and 3.1%–8.8% (IQR=3.1%–8.8%) for a suicide attempt (there are no data on lifetime suicide plan). Twelve-month prevalence estimates are in the range of 15.0%–29.0% (IQR=16.9%–24.1%) for suicide ideation, 12.6%–19.0% (IQR=13.8%–18.2%) for plans, and 7.3%–10.6% (IQR=8.0%–8.8%) for suicide attempt (see Table 2.1).

A comparison of the prevalence estimates for suicidal behaviors between adults and adolescents raises the question of how it is possible that adults have a *lower* lifetime prevalence than that of adolescents. In fact, the lifetime prevalence for each suicidal behavior among adults is lower than the 12-month prevalence among adolescents. One possible explanation is that

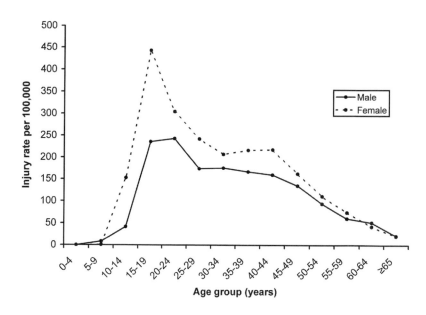

Figure 2.4. U.S. nonfatal self-injury rates – 2006. Data are from the U.S. Centers for Disease Control Web-based Injury Statistics Query and Reporting System (CDC, 2008b). Data points from ages 0–9 years are based on relatively few cases and may be unreliable.

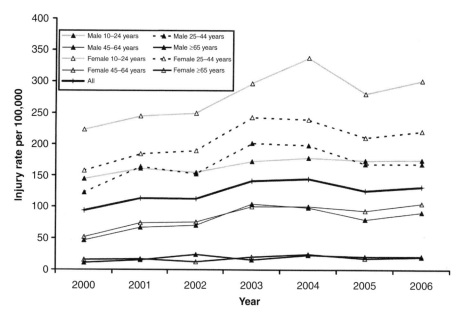

Figure 2.5. U.S. nonfatal self-injury rates by age and gender, 2001–2006. Data are from the U.S. Centers for Disease Control Web-based Injury Statistics Query and Reporting System (CDC, 2008b).

the rates of suicidal behavior in the U.S. are increasing dramatically among adolescents, but this is inconsistent with data on trends in adolescent suicide (reviewed above) and suicidal behaviors (reviewed below). A more likely explanation is that adults underreport lifetime suicidal behaviors. Evidence of such a bias was reported in a study by Goldney et al. (1991) in which 40% of adolescents who initially reported suicide ideation at one time point denied any lifetime

history of suicide ideation when interviewed four years later as young adults.

Trends

Data from the CDC (CDC, 2008b) are available for comparison from 2001 to 2006. As shown in Figure 2.5, the rate of nonfatal self-injury (both suicidal and non-suicidal in nature) shows an increasing trend over this period. Each age and gender group

Table 2.1. Key studies on the prevalence of suicidal behaviors (1997–2007)

Study	Location, design	Sample	Prevalence estimate
U.S. studies – adults (11)			
Kessler et al. (1999)	U.S., nationally representative	5877 adults (15–54 years)	LT ideation = 13.5% LT plan = 3.9% LT attempt = 4.6%
Dube et al. (2001)	U.S., primary care clinic (San Diego, CA)	17,337 adults (mean age = 57 years; SD = 15.3)	LT attempt = 3.8%
Kuo et al. (2001)	U.S., community population (Baltimore, MD)	1920 adults for this follow-up study (at baseline, 18+ years)	LT ideation = 5.6% LT attempt = 1.9%
Ialongo et al. (2002)	U.S., metropolitan area (Baltimore, MD)	1157 African Americans (19–22 years)	LT ideation = 14.3% LT attempt = 5.3% 6 m ideation = 1.9%[a] 6 m attempt = 0.4%[a]
Garroutte et al. (2003)	U.S., Northern Plains reservations	1456 American Indian tribal members (15–57 years)	LT attempt = 8.7%
Joe et al. (2006)	U.S., nationally representative	5181 African Americans (18+ years)	LT ideation = 11.7% LT attempt = 4.1% 12 m ideation = 2.1% 12 m attempt = 0.2%
Nock & Kessler (2006)	U.S., nationally representative	5877 adults (15–54 years)	LT gesture (no intent) = 1.9%[a] LT attempt (with intent) = 2.7% LT total attempt = 4.6%
Fortuna et al. (2007)	U.S., Latino ethnic subgroups	2554 Spanish- and English-speaking members of Latino ethnic subgroups	LT ideation = 10.1% LT attempts = 4.4%
Brener et al. (1999)	U.S., college student population	4609 undergraduate and graduate students (18+ years)	12 m ideation = approx. 10% 12 m plan = approx. 7% 12 m attempt = approx. 2%
Kessler et al. (2005a)	U.S., nationally representative	9708 adults (18–54 years), surveyed either between 1990–1992 (T1; n=5388) or 2001–2003 (T2; n=4320)	12 m ideation (T1) = 2.8% 12 m ideation (T2) = 3.3% 12 m plans (T1) = 0.7% 12 m plans (T2) = 1.0% 12 m gestures (T1) = 0.3% 12 m gestures (T2) = 0.2% 12 m attempts (T1) = 0.4% 12 m attempts (T2) = 0.6%
Borges et al. (2006)	U.S., nationally representative	5692 adults (18+ years)	12 m ideation = 2.6% 12 m plan = 0.7% 12 m attempt = 0.4%
U.S. studies – adolescents (6)			
Alaimo et al. (2002)	U.S., nationally representative	754 adolescents (15–16 years)	LT ideation = 19.8% LT attempt = 4.6%

Table 2.1. (cont.)

Study	Location, design	Sample	Prevalence estimate
Eisenberg et al. (2003)	U.S., metropolitan area (Minneapolis/St. Paul)	4746 adolescents (grades 7–12)	LT ideation = 24.0% LT attempt = 8.8%
Waldrop et al. (2007)	U.S., household probability sample	3906 adolescents (12–17 years)	LT ideation = 23.3% LT attempts = 3.1%
O'Donnell et al. (2004)	U.S., economically disadvantaged neighborhoods (Brooklyn, NY)	879 urban adolescents (16–17 years)	12 m ideation = 15.0% 12 m plan = 12.6% 12 m attempt = 10.6% 12 m multiple attempts = 4.3%
CDC (2007b)	U.S., nationally representative (biannually 1991–2005, Youth Risk Behavior Survey)	Adolescents (grades 9–12), from whom data were biannually collected between 1991 (n=12,272) and 2005 (n=13,953)	12 m ideation (1991) = 29.0% 12 m ideation (1993) = 24.1% 12 m ideation (1995) = 24.1% 12 m ideation (1997) = 20.5% 12 m ideation (1999) = 19.3% 12 m ideation (2001) = 19.0% 12 m ideation (2003) = 16.9% 12 m ideation (2005) = 16.9% 12 m plan (1991) = 18.6% 12 m plan (1993) = 19.0% 12 m plan (1995) = 17.7% 12 m plan (1997) = 15.7% 12 m plan (1999) = 14.5% 12 m plan (2001) = 14.8% 12 m plan (2003) = 16.5% 12 m plan (2005) = 13.0% 12 m attempt (1991) = 7.3% 12 m attempt (1993) = 8.6% 12 m attempt (1995) = 8.7% 12 m attempt (1997) = 7.7% 12 m attempt (1999) = 8.3% 12 m attempt (2001) = 8.8% 12 m attempt (2003) = 8.5% 12 m attempt (2005) = 8.4%
King et al. (2001)	U.S., four geographically and ethnically diverse regions (CT, GA, NY, Puerto Rico)	1285 adolescents (9–17 years)	6 m ideation (among those with no LT attempt) = 5.2%[a] 6 m attempt = 3.3%[a]
International studies – adults (26)			
Statham et al. (1998)	Australia, community (twin) sample	Adult twins from Australian twin panel first surveyed in 1980–82 (n=5995) (females [F], 27–89 years; males [M], 28–85 years)	LT ideation (M) = 23.8% LT ideation (F) = 22.2% LT plans (M) = 5.7% LT plans (F) = 6.2% LT attempts (M) = 1.7% LT attempts (F) = 3.0%
Kebede & Alem (1999)	Addis Ababa, Ethiopia, nationally representative	10,203 adults (15+ years)	LT attempt = 0.9% Current ideation = 2.7%[a]

Table 2.1. (cont.)

Study	Location, design	Sample	Prevalence estimate
Akyuz et al. (2005)	Central Turkey, nationally representative	628 women (18–65 years)	LT attempt = 4.5%
Kjoller & Helweg-Larsen (2000)	Denmark, nationally representative	1362 adults (16+ years)	LT attempt = 3.4% 12 m ideation = 6.9% 12 m attempt = 0.5%
Ramberg & Wasserman (2000)	Stockholm, Sweden, general population and mental healthcare staff	1010 mental healthcare staff (MHCS) (19–64 years); 8171 general population (GP) (20–64 years)	LT ideation (MHCS) = 42.8%[a] LT ideation (GP) = 20.3% LT attempt (MHCS) = 4.8%[a] LT attempt (GP) = 3.6% 12 m ideation (MHCS) = 7.7%[a] 12 m ideation (GP) = 7.3% 12 m attempt (MHCS) = 0.2%[a] 12 m attempt (GP) = 0.4%
Renberg (2001)	Northern Sweden, general population	521 adults (18–65 years) from 1986; 636 adults (18–65 years) from 1996	LT ideation (1986) = 33.3% LT ideation (1996) = 21.1% LT plans(1986) = 10.4% LT plans (1996) = 13.1% LT attempts (1986) = 2.6% LT attempts (1996) = 2.7% 12 m ideation (1986) = 12.5% 12 m ideation (1996) = 8.6% 12 m plans (1986) = 4.2% 12 m plans (1996) = 4.1% 12 m attempt (1986) = 0.6% 12 m attempt (1996) = 0.2%
Rancans et al. (2003)	Latvia, general population	667 adults (18+ years)	LT ideation = 33.0% LT plans = 19.5% LT attempt = 5.1% 12 m ideation = 21.3% 12 m plan = 12.2% 12 m attempt = 1.8%
Crawford et al. (2005)	England	4171 adults (16–74 years) among representative samples of white, Irish, black Caribbean, Bangladeshi, Indian, and Pakistani ethnic groups	LT ideation = 10% LT attempt = 3%
De Leo et al. (2005)	Queensland, Australia, nationally representative	11,572 adults (18+ years)	LT ideation = 10.4% LT plan = 4.4% LT attempt = 4.2% 12 m attempt = 0.4%
Mohammadi et al. (2005)	Iran, general population	25,180 adults (26–55 years)	LT attempt = 1.4%
Agoub et al. (2006)	Casablanca, Morocco, representative of urban general population	800 adults (15+ years)	LT attempt = 2.1% 1 m plan = 1.0%[a] 1 m attempt = 0.8%[a]

Table 2.1. (cont.)

Study	Location, design	Sample	Prevalence estimate
Beautrais et al. (2006)	New Zealand, nationally representative	12,992 adults (16+ years)	LT ideation = 15.7% LT plan = 5.5% LT attempt = 4.5% 12 m ideation = 3.2% 12 m plan = 1.0% 12 m attempt = 0.4%
Liu et al. (2006)	Hong Kong, territory-specific representation	2015 adults (20–59 years)	LT ideation = 28.1% 12 m ideation = 6.0% 12 m plans = 1.9% 12 m attempts = 1.4%
Ovuga et al. (2006)	Makerere University, Uganda	101 older students (OS) (mean age=23.5 years; SD=5.0) and 253 younger students (YS) (mean age=21.3 years; SD=2.4)	LT ideation (OS) = 8.9% LT ideation (YS) = 56.0%
Tran Thi Thanh et al. (2006)	Dongda district, Hanoi, Vietnam, general population	2260 adults (14+ years)	LT ideation = 8.9% LT plan = 1.1% LT attempt = 0.4% 12 m ideation = 3.3% 12 m plan = 0.5% 12 m attempt = 0.1%
Bernal et al. (2007)	Six European countries (Belgium, France, Germany, Italy, Netherlands, and Spain), all nationally representative	8796 adults (18+ years)	LT ideation = 7.8% LT attempts = 1.3%
Bromet et al. (2007)	Ukraine, nationally representative	4719 adults (18+ years)	LT ideation = 8.2% LT plan = 2.7% LT attempt = 1.8% 12 m ideation = 1.8%
Gureje et al. (2007)	21 out of 36 states of Nigeria	6752 adults (18+ years)	LT ideation = 3.2% LT plan = 1.0% LT attempt = 0.7%
Lee et al. (2007)	Beijing and Shanghai, China, general population	5201 adults (18+ years)	LT ideation = 3.1% LT plans = 0.9% LT attempts = 1.0%
Nojomi et al. (2007)	Karaj City, Tehran Province, Iran	2300 adults (including as early as 15 years), attempt rate from pilot study	LT attempt = 1.2%
Borges et al. (2008)	Mexico, nationally representative sample	5782 adults	LT ideation = 8.1% LT plans = 3.2% LT attempt = 2.7%
Hintikka et al. (1998)	Finland, general population	4868 adults	12 m ideation (F) = 2.4% 12 m ideation (M) = 2.3%
Scocco & De Leo (2002)	Padua, Italy, community-dwelling elderly population	611 older adults (65+ years)	12 m ideation = 9.5% 12 m attempt = 3.8%

Table 2.1. (cont.)

Study	Location, design	Sample	Prevalence estimate
Gunnell et al. (2004)	United Kingdom, nationally representative	2404 adults (16–74 years)	12 m ideation = 2.3%
Fairweather et al. (2007)	Australia	7485 adults (20–24, 40–44, 60–64 year cohorts)	12 m ideation = 8.2%
De Leo et al. (2001)	Sweden, France, United Kingdom, Denmark, Italy, Norway, Finland, the Netherlands, Germany, Switzerland, Austria, Spain, and Hungary	1518 people over the age of 65 years	3–5-year monitoring period, at least one attempt = 0.06%[a]
International studies – adolescents (20)			
Olsson & von Knorring (1999)	Sweden (1 town)	2300 adolescents (16–17 years)	LT attempts = 2.4%
Elklit (2002)	Denmark, nationally representative	390 eighth graders (mean age = 14.5 years)	LT attempts = 6.2%
Blum et al. (2003)	Antigua, Bahamas, Barbados, British Virgin Islands, Dominica, Grenada, Guyana, Jamaica, St. Lucia	15,695 adolescents (10–18 years)	LT attempts = 12.1%
Gmitrowicz et al. (2003)	Lodz, Poland, community population	1663 adolescents (14–21 years)	LT ideation = 30.8% LT attempts = 7.9%
Toros et al. (2004)	Turkey	4143 children and adolescents (10–20 years)	LT attempt = 1.9%
Zemaitiene & Zaborskis (2005)	Lithuania, nationally representative	15,586 children (ages 11, 13, and 15 years)	LT plans = 3.0% LT attempts = 1.5%
Young et al. (2006)	Central Clydeside Conurbation, Scotland, community population	1258 older adolescents (19 years)	LT attempts = 6.4%
Sidhartha & Jena (2006)	New Delhi, India, student population	1205 adolescents (12–19 years)	LT ideation = 21.7% LT attempt = 8.0% 12 m ideation = 11.7% 12 m attempt = 3.5%
Dervic et al. (2007)	Vienna, Austria, student population	214 adolescents (mean age=15.6 years; SD=1.4)	LT ideation = 37.9%
Silviken & Kvernmo (2007)	Arctic Norway, representative samples of different ethnic groups	591 indigenous Sami adolescents and 2100 majority adolescents (16–18 years)	LT attempt =9.5% 6 m ideation = 15.1%[a]
Rey Gex et al. (1998)	Switzerland, nationally representative	9268 adolescents (15–20 years)	12 m ideation = 26% 12 m plans = 15% 12 m attempt = 3%
Tousignant et al. (1999)	Canadian sample of refugees from 35 countries	203 adolescents (13–19 years)	12 m attempt = 3.4%

Table 2.1. (cont.)

Study	Location, design	Sample	Prevalence estimate
Miauton et al. (2003)	Switzerland, nationally representative	9268 adolescents (15–19 years)	12 m attempt = 3.0%
Yip et al. (2004)	Hong Kong, territory-specific representation	2586 adolescents (13–21 years)	12 m ideation = 17.8% 12 m plan = 5.4% 12 m attempt = 8.4%
Rodriguez et al. (2006)	Nicaragua, general population	278 adolescents (15–24 years)	12 m ideation = 19.8% 12 m plan = 5.0% 12 m attempt = 1.8%
Rudatsikira et al. (2007)	Guyana, student population	1197 adolescents (<14–16+ years)	12 m ideation = 18.4%
Kaltiala-Heino et al. (1999)	Two regions of Finland, student population	16,410 adolescents (14–16 years)	Current ideation = 2.2%[a]
Khokher & Khan (2005)	Karachi, Pakistan, medical student population	217 medical students (19–22 years)	Recent ideation = 31.3%[a]
Liu et al. (2005)	Shandong, China (5 high schools)	1362 adolescents (12–18 years)	6 m ideation = 19.3%[a] 6 m attempt = 7.0%[a]
Ponizovsky et al. (1999)	Israel, immigrant population	406 Russian-born Jewish immigrants to Israel (11–18 years); 203 indigenous Jewish adolescents in Russia; 104 indigenous Jewish adolescents in Israel	6 m ideation (immigrants) = 10.9%[a] 6 m ideation (Russian natives) = 3.5%[a] 6 m ideation (Israeli natives) = 8.7%[a]
Cross-national studies (3)			
Weissman et al. (1999)	Nine countries, varying designs and surveys	Approximately 40,000+ adults	LT ideation (range) = 2.1%–18.5% LT attempts (range) = 0.7%–5.9%
Bertolote et al. (2005)	10 countries, same community-based survey in 10 hospital catchment areas	69,797 children, adolescents, and adults (5+ years)	LT ideation (range) = 2.6%–25.4% LT plans (range) = 1.1%–15.6% LT attempts (range) = 0.4%–4.2%
Nock et al. (2008a)	17 countries, same household survey, most samples are nationally representative	84,850 adults	LT ideation (range) = 3.0%–15.9% LT plans (range) = 0.7%–5.6% LT attempts (range) = 0.5%–5.0% LT ideation (pooled) = 9.2% LT plans (pooled) = 3.1% LT attempts (pooled) = 2.7%

LT = lifetime; 1 m = 1-month; 6 m = 6-month; 12 m = 12-month.
[a] Not included in prevalence estimates in text due to differences in measurement.

examined shows an increase, and the overall rate increases from 113.4 to 132.0/100,000 (16.5%). Data from our systematic review suggest that the estimated 12-month prevalence of suicidal behaviors among adults in the U.S. has remained stable in recent years. One recent study revealed that although service utilization increased dramatically among suicidal adults in the decade between 1990–1992, and 2001–2003, the 12-month prevalence did not change significantly for suicide ideation (2.8%→3.3%), suicide plans

(0.7%→1.0%), or suicide attempts (0.4%→0.6%) (Kessler et al., 2005a). Data on the 12-month prevalence of suicidal behaviors among adolescents from the CDC YRBS are more encouraging and indicate that from 1991 to 2005 there was a decrease in the rate of suicide ideation (29.0%→16.9%) and plans (18.6%→13.0%), although there was no such decrease for attempts (7.3%→8.4%) (CDC, 2007b).

Onset and course

The earliest onset ever reported for suicidal behaviors is in children as young as 4–5 years (Bridge et al., 2006; Conwell & Duberstein, 2001; Kessler et al., 1999; Nock & Kazdin, 2002; Pfeffer, 2001; Tishler et al., 2007); however, many authors suggest that children younger than 10 years old are rarely capable of understanding the finality of death and therefore cannot make a suicide attempt (Cuddy-Casey & Orvaschel, 1997; Pfeffer, 1997). The most consistently reported pattern is that the risk of first onset for suicidal behavior increases significantly at the start of adolescence (12 years), peaks at age 16, and remains elevated into the early 20s. This means that adolescence and early adulthood are the times of greatest risk for first onset of suicidal behaviors (Bolger et al., 1989; Kessler et al., 1999). Early stressors such as parental absence and family history of suicidal behaviors have been associated with an earlier AOO (Bolger et al., 1989; Roy, 2004).

Relatively few studies have examined the course of suicidal behaviors. Data using retrospective recall of AOO suggest that 34% of lifetime suicide ideators go on to make a suicide plan, that 72% of those with a suicide plan go on to make a suicide attempt, and that 26% of ideators without a plan make an unplanned attempt (Kessler et al., 1999). The majority of these transitions occur within the first year after onset of suicide ideation (60% for planned first attempts and 90% for unplanned first attempts) (Kessler et al., 1999). These findings indicate that the presence of suicide ideation and plan significantly increase the risk for suicide attempt and that risk of suicide attempt among those without a plan is limited primarily to the first year after onset of ideation. Prior suicidal behaviors are among the strongest predictors of subsequent suicidal behaviors (Borges et al., 2006; Goldsmith et al., 2002; Goldstein et al., 1991; Joiner et al., 2005b); however, suicide ideation in the continued absence of a plan or attempt is associated with

decreasing risk of suicide plans and attempts over time (Borges et al., 2007).

Suicidal behaviors cross-nationally

Current

As with suicide death, there is considerable cross-national variability in the prevalence of suicidal behaviors. Across all studies identified that assessed lifetime prevalence among adults in individual countries, estimates varied widely for suicide ideation from 3.1% to 56.0% (IQR=8.0%–24.9%), suicide plans (0.9%–19.5%, IQR=1.5%–9.4%), and suicide attempts (0.4%–5.1%, IQR=1.3%–3.5%). Estimates of the 12-month prevalence of suicidal behaviors among adults also showed wide variability for suicide ideation (1.8%–21.3%, IQR=2.4%–8.8%), plans (0.5%–12.2%, IQR=0.9%–6.2%), and attempts (0.1%–3.8%, IQR=0.4%–1.5%). As in the U.S., prevalence estimates were consistently higher for adolescents for the lifetime prevalence of suicide ideation (21.7%–37.9%, IQR=21.7%–37.9%), plans (3.0%; one study), and attempts (1.5%–12.1%, IQR=2.2%–8.8%), as well as for the 12-month prevalence of suicide ideation (11.7%–26.0%, IQR=14.8%–22.9%), plans (5.0%–15.0%, IQR=5.0%–15.0%), and attempts (1.8%–8.4%, IQR=2.7%–4.7%) (see Table 2.1).

One important limitation in comparing results from across studies of suicidal behaviors is that different studies use different questions to assess these behaviors and so it is not clear how much of the variability observed across studies is due to differences in measurement methods. Three recent, cross-national studies have attempted to remedy this problem by using consistent measurement strategies across countries. These are: (1) the WHO/EURO Multicentre Study on Parasuicide (n=22,665) (De Leo et al., 2001; Michel et al., 2000; Platt et al., 1992), which included individuals engaging in "parasuicide" (i.e., combining suicidal and non-suicidal self-injury) who presented to medical centers in 15 European countries; (2) the WHO Multi-site Intervention Study on Suicidal Behaviors (SUPRE-MISS; n=69,797) (Bertolote & Fleischmann, 2005; Bertolote et al., 2005; Fleischmann et al., 2005), which included community samples in eight countries; and (3) the WHO World Mental Health (WMH) Survey Initiative, which provides data on the epidemiology of suicidal behaviors in 28 countries in the Americas, Europe, Asia, Africa, the Middle East, and the Pacific. Interestingly, all three studies revealed wide cross-national variation in suicidal behaviors. For instance, analyses for the first 17 WMH countries (n=84,850) yielded prevalence estimates for suicide ideation (3.0%–15.9%, IQR=4.4%–11.7%), plans (0.7%–5.6%, IQR=1.6%–4.0%), and attempts (0.5%–5.0%, IQR=1.5%–3.2%) that were consistent with those reviewed above. The pooled cross-national prevalence estimates (standard errors) in this study were reported for suicide ideation: 9.2% (0.1), plans: 3.1% (0.1), and attempts: 2.7% (0.1) (Nock et al., 2008a) (see Table 2.1). Interestingly, rates of suicidal behaviors do not mirror the geographic pattern reported for suicide death (e.g., high rates in Eastern Europe, low rates in South America), nor do they differ systematically between developed and developing countries (Nock et al., 2008a).

Trends

Our search did not yield any cross-national studies of trends in suicidal behaviors. However, it is notable that the prevalence estimates found in the studies that we reviewed are quite consistent with those obtained in an earlier cross-national review of nine studies of adult suicidal behavior conducted in the 1980s (Weissman et al., 1999), suggesting, but by no means confirming, that there has been no major change in trends over time. Trends in suicidal behaviors within individual countries also appear fairly steady over time (Borges et al., 2007; Gibb & Beautrais, 2004; Kessler et al., 2005a; Statham et al., 1998). The fact that within-country trends show internal consistency (i.e., greater agreement on prevalence estimates and evidence of stable patterns over time) means that there must be some stable between-country differences in the determinants of the prevalence and trends in suicidal behaviors that remain to be discovered.

Onset and course

Data on the onset and course of suicidal behaviors appear to be quite consistent cross-nationally and look similar to the previously mentioned data from studies in the U.S. Data from the WMH Surveys indicate that for all countries examined, the risk of first onset of suicide ideation increases sharply during adolescence and young adulthood and then stabilizes in early mid-life (Nock et al., 2008a). There is consistency in the timing and probability of transitioning from suicide ideation to suicide plans and attempts, with 33.6% of ideators going on to make a suicide plan (IQR=29.8%–35.6%) and 29.0% of ideators making

an attempt (IQR=21.2%–33.1%) (Nock et al., 2008b). In addition, the high risk of transitioning from ideation to plan and attempt during the first year after onset of ideation that was found in the U.S. (Kessler et al., 1999) was replicated across all countries examined, with the transition from ideation to attempt occurring during the first year more than 60% of the time across all countries (Nock et al., 2008a). These findings indicate that the onset and course of suicidal behaviors are quite consistent cross-nationally.

Risk factors

We review evidence on risk factors for both suicide and suicidal behaviors below, given the substantial overlap in the risk factors reported to predict these behaviors (Beautrais, 2003; Nock & Kessler, 2006), although it is noted that several studies have reported differences in some risk factors for suicide and suicidal behaviors (Brent et al., 1988; Brent et al., 1993a). Most of the studies reviewed on prevalence above also contained information about risk factors for suicidal behaviors. We do not distinguish between studies conducted in different countries given that the risk factors reported have been consistent across virtually all countries examined. As there is a large and ever-expanding literature on risk factors for suicidal behaviors, we provide a summary of only the strongest and most consistently reported factors.

Demographic factors

Demographic risk factors for suicide include male gender, being non-Hispanic white and Native American (in the U.S.), and being an adolescent or older adult. Demographic risk factors for suicidal behaviors (in the U.S. and cross-nationally) include being female, of younger age, unmarried, of lower educational attainment, and unemployed (Bertolote & Fleischmann, 2002; Bertolote et al., 2005; Nock et al., 2008a; Platt et al., 1992; Vijayakumar et al., 2005a; Weissman et al., 1999). The male-to-female ratio differences often are attributed to the use of more lethal suicide attempt methods, greater aggressiveness, and higher intent to die among men (Beautrais, 2002; Nock & Kessler, 2006). As mentioned earlier in connection with India and China, gender-specific lethality of methods may vary cross-nationally. The other demographic factors mentioned (younger age, lack of education, and unemployment) may represent increased risk for suicidal behavior associated with social disadvantage, although the mechanisms through which these factors may lead to suicidal behaviors are not yet understood.

Psychiatric factors

The presence of a psychiatric disorder is among the most consistently reported risk factors for suicidal behaviors (Gould et al., 1998; Kessler et al., 1999; Mann et al., 1999; Nock et al., 2008b; Petronis et al., 1990; Shaffer et al., 1996; Vijayakumar & Rajkumar, 1999). Psychological autopsy studies reveal that 90%–95% of the people who die by suicide had a diagnosable psychiatric disorder at the time of the suicide (Cavanagh et al., 2003), although this percentage is lower in non-Western countries such as China (Phillips et al., 2002; Vijayakumar, 2005). Mood, impulse-control, alcohol/substance use, psychotic, and personality disorders convey the highest risk for suicide and suicidal behaviors (Hawton et al., 2003; Kessler et al., 1999; Linehan et al., 2000; Mann et al., 1999; Nock et al., 2008b; Nock & Kessler, 2006; Shaffer et al., 1996; Shafii et al., 1985; Yen et al., 2003b), and the presence of multiple disorders is associated with especially elevated risk (Hawton et al., 2003; Kessler et al., 1999; Nock et al., 2008b; Shafii et al., 1988).

Psychological factors

Researchers have begun to examine more specific constructs that may explain exactly *why* psychiatric disorders are associated with suicidal behaviors. Several such risk factors include the presence of hopelessness (Beck et al., 1985; Brezo et al., 2006; Brown et al., 2000), anhedonia (Fawcett et al., 1990; Nock & Kazdin, 2002), impulsiveness (Fawcett, 2001; Fawcett et al., 1997; Mann et al., 1999; Zouk et al., 2006), and high emotional reactivity (Fawcett, 2001; Fawcett et al., 1990; Nock et al., 2008c), each of which may increase psychological distress to a point that is unbearable and leads a person to seek escape via suicide (Baumeister, 1990; Fawcett et al., 1997; Hawton et al., 1982; Williams & Pollock, 2000).

Biological factors

Family, twin, and adoption studies provide evidence for a heritable risk for suicide and suicidal behaviors (Baldessarini & Hennen, 2004; Fu et al., 2002; Glowinski et al., 2001; Joiner et al., 2005a; Roy & Segal, 2001; Roy et al., 1991). Much of the family history of suicidal behaviors may be explained by the risk associated with mental disorders (Kendler & Prescott, 2007); however, some studies provide evidence for

family transmission of suicidal behaviors even after controlling for mood and psychotic disorders (Mann, 2003). Researchers have not identified genetic loci for suicide in molecular genetics studies in light of the complex nature of the phenotype (Kendler, 2005a, 2005b), but instead have searched for biological correlates of suicidal behavior that may arise through gene–environment interactions (Baca-Garcia et al., 2002; Caspi et al., 2003; Courtet et al., 2001; De Luca et al., 2006; Mann et al., 1997; Yen et al., 2003a). The biological factors most consistently correlated with suicidal behaviors involve disruptions in the functioning of the inhibitory neurotransmitter serotonin. Those dying by suicide have lower levels of serotonin metabolites in their cerebrospinal fluid (Asberg et al., 1976; Mann & Malone, 1997; Roggenbach et al., 2002; Samuelsson et al., 2006), higher serotonin receptor binding in platelets (Mann et al., 1992; Pandey, 1997), and fewer presynaptic serotonin transporter sites and greater postsynaptic serotonin receptors in specific brain areas such as the prefrontal cortex (Mann, 2003; Oquendo et al., 2003), suggesting deficits in the ability to inhibit impulsive behavior (Mann, 2003; Traskman-Bendz & Mann, 2000). Notably, however, similar deficits in serotonergic functioning are found in other impulsive/aggressive behaviors such as violence and fire-setting (Virkkunen et al., 1994) and appear nonspecific to suicide.

Stressful life events

Most theoretical models of suicidal behaviors propose a diathesis–stress model in which the psychiatric, psychological, and biological factors above predispose a person to suicidal behaviors, while stressful life events interact with such factors to increase risk. Consistent with such a model, suicidal behaviors often are preceded by stressful events including family and romantic conflicts and the presence of legal/disciplinary problems (Brent et al., 1993b; Phillips et al., 2002; Vijayakumar & Rajkumar, 1999; Yen et al., 2005). The experience of persistent stress also may explain why some occupations may be associated with a higher rate of suicidal behaviors, such as physicians (Center et al., 2003), military personnel (Boxer et al., 1995; Helmkamp, 1996; Mahon et al., 2005; Marzuk et al., 2002), and police officers (Violanti et al., 1996); however, this increased risk may be explained by the demographic and personality characteristics of people who select such occupations (Agerbo et al., 2007; Marzuk et al., 2002). More distal stressors, such as perinatal conditions and child maltreatment, also have been linked to subsequent suicidal behaviors (Glassman et al., 2007; Joiner et al., 2007; Riordan et al., 2006; Salk et al., 1985; Wedig & Nock, 2007). One goal for future research is to begin to specify the mechanisms through which such factors may increase risk.

Other factors

The list of risk factors outlined above is not exhaustive, and there is emerging evidence for a range of others, such as: access to lethal means such as firearms and high doses of medication (Agerbo et al., 2007; Beautrais et al., 2007; Brent et al., 1988; Mann et al., 2005; Marzuk et al., 1992), chronic or terminal illness (Conwell et al., 2002; Stenager & Stenager, 2000), homosexuality (de Graaf et al., 2006; Fergusson et al., 1999; Herrell et al., 1999), the presence of suicidal behaviors among one's peers (Gould, 1990, 2001; Gould et al., 1990; Joiner, 2003), and time of year (with higher rates consistently reported in May and June) (Dixon et al., 2007; Nakaji et al., 2004; Petridou et al., 2002; Preti et al., 2000). Improvement in the ability to predict suicidal behaviors through the continued identification of specific risk factors represents one of the most important directions for future studies in this area.

Protective factors

Protective factors are those that decrease the probability of an outcome in the presence of elevated risk. Although formal tests of protective factors are rare in the suicide research literature, several studies of factors associated with lower risk of suicidal behaviors have yielded interesting results. Religious beliefs, religious practice, and spirituality have been associated with a decreased probability of suicide attempts (Blum et al., 2003; Clarke et al., 2003; Dervic et al., 2004; Garroutte et al., 2003). Potential mediators of this relation, such as moral objections to suicide (Oquendo et al., 2005) and social support (Meadows et al., 2005), also seem to protect against suicide attempts among those at risk. In addition, perceptions of social and family support and connectedness have been studied outside the context of religious affiliation and shown to be significantly associated with lower rates of suicidal behaviors (Anteghini et al., 2001; Borowsky et al., 2001; Marion & Range, 2003; O'Donnell et al., 2004;

Resnick et al., 1997). Being pregnant and having young children in the home also are protective against suicide (Marzuk et al., 1997; Qin & Mortensen, 2003); however, the presence of young children is associated with a significantly *increased* risk of first onset of suicide ideation. These findings highlight the importance of attending carefully to the dependent variable in question when examining risk and protective factors for suicidal behaviors.

Prevention/intervention programs

The relatively stable rates of suicide and suicidal behaviors over time highlight the need for greater attention to prevention and intervention efforts. A recent systematic review of suicide prevention programs revealed that restricting access to lethal means and training physicians to recognize and treat depression and suicidal behavior have shown impressive effects in reducing suicide rates (Mann et al., 2005). Means restriction programs can decrease suicide rates by 1.5%–23% (Bridges, 2004; Carrington, 1999; Kreitman, 1976; Lester, 1990; Oliver & Hetzel, 1972) while primary care physician education and training programs show reductions of 22%–73% (Rihmer et al., 2001; Rutz et al., 1989; Szanto et al., 2007; Takahashi et al., 1998). Although effective prevention programs exist, the fact that many people experiencing suicidal behaviors do not receive treatment of any kind (Kessler et al., 2005a; Vijayakumar, 2004; Vijayakumar et al., 2005b; WMH Consortium, 2004) underscores the need for greater dissemination and further development of prevention efforts (Jenkins, 2002; Jenkins & Singh, 2000; United Nations, 1996).

Discussion

Summary of findings

The past decade of research on the epidemiology of suicide has yielded several key findings. First, global estimates suggest suicide continues to be a leading cause of death and disease burden and that the number of suicide deaths will increase substantially over the next several decades. Second, the significant cross-national variability reported in rates of suicide and suicidal behaviors appears to reflect the true nature of this behavior and is not due to variation in research methods. Third, there is cross-national consistency in the early AOO of suicide ideation, rapid transition from suicidal thoughts to suicidal behaviors, and importance of several key risk factors. Fourth, despite significant developments in treatment research and increased service utilization among suicidal individuals in the U.S., there appears to have been little change in the rates of suicide or suicidal behaviors over the past decade. The 11.1% decrease in the U.S. suicide rate since 1990 is encouraging. Enthusiasm is tempered, however, by knowledge of the fact that the current suicide rate is at approximately the same level it was in 1950 and even 1900, with periodic fluctuation between 10.0 and 19.0/100,000 over the past 100 years (Goldsmith et al., 2002; Monk, 1987; Weed, 1985). Similar stable patterns have been observed in other countries (Ajdacic-Gross et al., 2006). Moreover, data on nonfatal self-injury show a 16.5% increase in such behaviors in only the past six years, especially for youth. It is possible that the decrease in youth suicide over this period coupled with the increase in nonfatal self-injury treated in emergency departments is the result of decreased lethality of youth suicidal behavior (perhaps due to safer medication and less access to firearms). An alternative possibility is that the increase in nonfatal self-injury is explained largely by increases in the occurrence of non-suicidal self-injury. More careful assessment of the intent of self-injury is needed to address this question. Regardless of the ultimate answers to these questions, it is clear that major advances are needed to enhance understanding of the causes of suicidal behaviors and to further decrease the loss of life due to suicide.

Research directions

The next generation of epidemiological studies in this area must move beyond reporting of prevalence estimates and known risk factors. Below, we review several developing lines of research that could be used to improve research on the epidemiology of suicidal behaviors. In doing so we propose an agenda for future studies in this area that address many existing gaps in our understanding of suicidal behaviors.

Testing theoretical models

There is no debate among epidemiologists and clinical investigators that suicidal behaviors are complex, multi-determined phenomena. Yet, most studies continue to test bivariate associations between atheoretical demographic or psychiatric factors and suicidal behaviors with little regard for existing theoretical models. Several notable exceptions exist, such as the testing of diathesis–stress models (Mann et al., 1999) and gene–environment interactions (Caspi et al., 2003). True advances in understanding of suicidal behaviors are likely to come only through increased testing of these and other models.

A related issue is that while most studies examining suicide ideation, plans, and attempts have shown that similar risk factors predict these outcomes, virtually no studies have more specifically tested which factors predict transitions from ideation to plans and attempts. Such an approach has been useful in other areas, such as the study of drug and alcohol problems where, for instance, factors that predict ever drinking differ from those that predict developing a drinking problem among drinkers, which are different from predictors of alcohol dependence among problem drinkers (Power et al., 2005; Ridenour et al., 2006; Sartor et al., 2007). In the suicide literature, interventions that reduce rates of suicide attempts often do not show similar reductions in ideation (Brown et al., 2005; Linehan et al., 2006), suggesting their effect may be in decreasing the probability of transitioning from ideation to attempt rather than in reducing ideation altogether. Understanding this kind of specificity can help us strengthen theories about causal processes and develop more effective interventions.

Incorporating methodological advances

Key methodological obstacles in the study of suicidal behaviors include the low base-rate of suicidal behaviors and the motivation to conceal suicidal thoughts and intentions. These problems have hindered suicide research for decades; however, recent methodological advances now offer novel solutions to each problem.

Low base-rate problem

New developments in survey methodology make it easier than ever before to conduct a large survey using inexpensive methods such as interactive voice response telephone surveys (Heisler et al., 2007; Academic ED SBIRT Research Collaborative, 2007; Kim et al., 2007) and web-based surveys (Rademacher & Lippke, 2007; Smith et al., 2007; Tomic & Janata, 2007). These methods are most effective when respondents have a known relationship to the researchers, as in the case of clinical samples. Although clinical epidemiology is an underdeveloped research area, advances in the use of electronic medical records and electronic clinical decision support tools will almost certainly lead to an expansion of this field. Prospective research on risk and protective factors for suicide and suicidal behaviors could be dramatically improved by such developments.

One important direction is using such methods to study high-risk samples prospectively. For instance, given that nearly 20% of high-school students report 12-month suicide ideation and that suicide is the second leading cause of death among college students in the U.S., researchers could screen large samples of college students before their first semester, identify those with recent suicide ideation, and follow that group over time in order to identify risk factors for suicide attempts among this high-risk group. The structure of the college setting (e.g., availability of internet, e-mail, four-year timeline) greatly increases the feasibility of such studies. On a larger scale, given that approximately 3% of U.S. adults report 12-month suicide ideation, resources like the CDC Behavioral Risk Factor Surveillance System (CDC, 2007a), which interviews over 350,000 people per year, could identify 10,500 suicide ideators who could be followed prospectively to examine risk factors for suicide attempt. Psychological autopsy studies could be done with a matched control group of non-attempting ideators, which would yield valuable information about more specific risk factors for suicide. These are only a few of the many directions now possible given these exciting technological advances.

Detection of suicidal behaviors

Researchers studying sensitive and potentially shameful topics such as illicit drug use, sexual practices, and suicidal behaviors have long realized that people often under-report such behaviors in order to avoid embarrassment or intervention (Tourangeau & Yan, 2007). Methods for limiting the influence of social desirability include using computer-based interviews (Turner et al., 1998), presenting survey items in written form rather than reading aloud (Kessler & Üstün, 2004), or using anonymous surveys, which have been shown to yield rates of suicidal behaviors as much as two to three times higher than non-anonymous surveys (Evans et al., 2005; Safer, 1997). Another important advance is the development of behavioral methods for assessing implicit thoughts about self-injurious behaviors. Methods have been developed recently that use a person's response times to self-injury-related stimuli presented in a brief computer-based test to measure implicit associations with self-injury. Such tests

circumvent the use of self-report and have been shown to accurately detect and predict suicidal behaviors (Nock & Banaji, 2007a, 2007b). Such methods could be used to supplement self-reports and to test the percentage of cases identified via behavioral methods that also are detected by standard self-report methods to gain a better understanding of the current extent of under-reporting of suicidal behaviors.

Conducting epidemiological experiments

Perhaps the most important directions for research on the epidemiology of suicidal behaviors is increased use of epidemiological experiments of prevention and intervention procedures. Such studies will serve multiple purposes. First, they allow for tests of causation not possible with the correlational designs that dominate this area of research. Second, they address the biggest shortcoming in suicide research to date: the inability to dramatically decrease the rate of suicidal behaviors and mortality despite decades of research and associated resources.

As a preliminary step, descriptive data are needed on rates of treatment utilization among those with suicidal behaviors, including data on treatment adequacy and the presence of potentially modifiable barriers to treatment (e.g., Wang et al., 2005a; Wang et al., 2005b). Following this, efforts are required to build on findings from recent natural experiments, quasi-experiments, and true experiments of suicide prevention methods (Mann et al., 2005).

Natural experiments

Changes in social policy or historical events provide valuable opportunities to study factors that may influence suicidal behaviors. For instance, one of the biggest controversies in the study and treatment of suicidal behaviors is whether the recent development of selective serotonin reuptake inhibitors (SSRIs) has led to a decrease, or a paradoxical increase, in suicidal behaviors among children and adolescents. Epidemiologists are perfectly poised to test this question, especially given advances in the development and maintenance of electronic health records. Several studies have documented a decrease in suicide following the development of, and associated with the prescription of, SSRIs (Gibbons et al., 2007b; Gibbons et al., 2005, 2006; Isacsson, 2000). However, there has been a decrease in prescriptions of SSRIs to children and adolescents following the implementation of the FDA's "black box" warning and an increase in adolescent suicide (Gibbons et al., 2007a;

Nemeroff et al., 2007). Epidemiological studies are underway to test differences in suicide trends before and after the black box warning as mediated by disaggregated changes in sales levels of SSRIs among youth.

Quasi-experiments

Quasi-experimental designs strengthen the case for causality and are a useful alternative when true experiments are not feasible, as is often the case in epidemiological research. One recent example from the suicide literature is the test of the U.S. Air Force Suicide Prevention Program, which was shown to reduce the rate of suicide death by 33% within this population (Knox et al., 2003). Many services currently provided to the public for the purposes of suicide prevention (e.g., suicide hotlines, inpatient hospitalization) have not been adequately tested. Epidemiological quasi-experimental studies could begin to address services provided in such settings.

True experiments

Some of the most effective suicide prevention programs to date are simple, efficient, and cost effective but have not been widely tested or disseminated. For instance, one intervention involved simply sending supportive letters four times per year to randomly selected patients following hospital discharge, which significantly decreased the rate of suicide death among such patients (Motto & Bostrom, 2001). Moving forward, many such conceptual and methodological changes are needed in order to decrease the significant levels of death and disability caused by these dangerous behaviors.

Acknowledgements

Reproduced from Nock, M. K., Borges, G., Bromet, E. J., et al. (2008b) Suicide and suicidal behavior. *Epidemiologic Reviews*, 30, 133–154, by permission of Oxford University Press.

References

Academic ED SBIRT Research Collaborative. (2007). The impact of screening, brief intervention, and referral for treatment on emergency department patients' alcohol use. *Annals of Emergency Medicine*, 50(6), 699–710.

Agerbo, E., Gunnell, D., Bonde, J. P., Bo Mortensen, P., & Nordentoft, M. (2007). Suicide and occupation: the impact of socio-economic, demographic and psychiatric differences. *Psychological Medicine*, 37(8), 1131–1140.

Agoub, M., Moussaoui, D., & Kadri, N. (2006). Assessment of suicidality in a Moroccan metropolitan area. *Journal of Affective Disorders*, 90(2–3), 223–226.

Ajdacic-Gross, V., Bopp, M., Gostynski, M., et al. (2006). Age-period-cohort analysis of Swiss suicide data, 1881–2000. *European Archives of Psychiatry and Clinical Neuroscience*, 256(4), 207–214.

Akyuz, G., Sar, V., Kugu, N., & Dogan, O. (2005). Reported childhood trauma, attempted suicide and self-mutilative behavior among women in the general population. *European Psychiatry*, 20(3), 268–273.

Alaimo, K., Olson, C. M., & Frongillo, E. A. (2002). Family food insufficiency, but not low family income, is positively associated with dysthymia and suicide symptoms in adolescents. *Journal of Nutrition*, 132(4), 719–725.

Anteghini, M., Fonseca, H., Ireland, M., & Blum, R. W. (2001). Health risk behaviors and associated risk and protective factors among Brazilian adolescents in Santos, Brazil. *Journal of Adolescent Health*, 28(4), 295–302.

Asberg, M., Traskman, L., & Thoren, P. (1976). 5-HIAA in the cerebrospinal fluid. A biochemical suicide predictor? *Archives of General Psychiatry*, 33(10), 1193–1197.

Baca-Garcia, E., Vaquero, C., Diaz-Sastre, C., et al. (2002). A gender-specific association between the serotonin transporter gene and suicide attempts. *Neuropsychopharmacology*, 26(5), 692–695.

Baldessarini, R. J., & Hennen, J. (2004). Genetics of suicide: an overview. *Harvard Review of Psychiatry*, 12(1), 1–13.

Baumeister, R. F. (1990). Suicide as escape from self. *Psychological Review*, 97(1), 90–113.

Beautrais, A., Fergusson, D., Coggan, C., et al. (2007). Effective strategies for suicide prevention in New Zealand: a review of the evidence. *New Zealand Medical Journal*, 120(1251), U2459.

Beautrais, A. L. (2002). Gender issues in youth suicidal behaviour. *Emergency Medicine (Fremantle)*, 14(1), 35–42.

Beautrais, A. L. (2003). Suicide and serious suicide attempts in youth: a multiple-group comparison study. *American Journal of Psychiatry*, 160(6), 1093–1099.

Beautrais, A. L., Wells, J. E., McGee, M. A., & Oakley Browne, M. A. (2006). Suicidal behaviour in Te Rau Hinengaro: the New Zealand Mental Health Survey. *Australian and New Zealand Journal of Psychiatry*, 40(10), 896–904.

Beck, A. T., Steer, R. A., Kovacs, M., & Garrison, B. (1985). Hopelessness and eventual suicide: a 10-year prospective study of patients hospitalized with suicidal ideation. *American Journal of Psychiatry*, 142(5), 559–563.

Bernal, M., Haro, J. M., Bernert, S., et al. (2007). Risk factors for suicidality in Europe: results from the ESEMED study. *Journal of Affective Disorders*, 101(1–3), 27–34.

Bertolote, J. M., & Fleischmann, A. (2002). A global perspective in the epidemiology of suicide. *Suicidologi*, 7(2), 6–8.

Bertolote, J. M., & Fleischmann, A. (2005). Suicidal behavior prevention: WHO perspectives on research. *American Journal of Medical Genetics Part C: Seminars in Medical Genetics*, 133(1), 8–12.

Bertolote, J. M., Fleischmann, A., De Leo, D., et al. (2005). Suicide attempts, plans, and ideation in culturally diverse sites: the WHO SUPRE-MISS community survey. *Psychological Medicine*, 35(10), 1457–1465.

Blum, R. W., Halcon, L., Beuhring, T., et al. (2003). Adolescent health in the Caribbean: risk and protective factors. *American Journal of Public Health*, 93(3), 456–460.

Bolger, N., Downey, G., Walker, E., & Steininger, P. (1989). The onset of suicidal ideation in childhood and adolescence. *Journal of Youth and Adolescence*, 18(2), 175–190.

Borges, G., Angst, J., Nock, M. K., et al. (2006). A risk index for 12-month suicide attempts in the National Comorbidity Survey Replication (NCS-R). *Psychological Medicine*, 36(12), 1747–1757.

Borges, G., Angst, J., Nock, M. K., Ruscio, A. M., & Kessler, R. C. (2007). Risk factors for the incidence and persistence of suicide-related outcomes: A 10-year follow-up study using the National Comorbidity Surveys. *Journal of Affective Disorders*, 105(1–3), 25–33.

Borges, G., Anthony, J. C., & Garrison, C. Z. (1995). Methodological issues relevant to epidemiologic investigations of suicidal behaviors of adolescents. *Epidemiologic Reviews*, 17(1), 228–239.

Borges, G., Nock, M. K., Medina-Mora, M. E., et al. (2008). The epidemiology of suicide-related outcomes in Mexico. *Suicide and Life-Threatening Behavior*, 37(6), 627–640.

Borowsky, I. W., Ireland, M., & Resnick, M. D. (2001). Adolescent suicide attempts: risks and protectors. *Pediatrics*, 107(3), 485–493.

Boxer, P. A., Burnett, C., & Swanson, N. (1995). Suicide and occupation: a review of the literature. *Journal of Occupational and Environmental Medicine*, 37(4), 442–452.

Brener, N. D., Hassan, S. S., & Barrios, L. C. (1999). Suicidal ideation among college students in the United States. *Journal of Consulting and Clinical Psychology*, 67(6), 1004–1008.

Brent, D. A., Perper, J. A., Goldstein, C. E., et al. (1988). Risk factors for adolescent suicide. A comparison of adolescent suicide victims with suicidal inpatients. *Archives of General Psychiatry*, 45(6), 581–588.

Brent, D. A., Perper, J. A., Moritz, G., et al. (1993a). Psychiatric risk factors for adolescent suicide: a case-control study. *Journal of the American Academy of Child and Adolescent Psychiatry*, 32(3), 521–529.

Brent, D. A., Perper, J. A., Moritz, G., et al. (1993b). Stressful life events, psychopathology, and adolescent suicide: a case control study. *Suicide and Life-Threatening Behavior*, 23(3), 179–187.

Brezo, J., Paris, J., & Turecki, G. (2006). Personality traits as correlates of suicidal ideation, suicide attempts, and suicide completions: a systematic review. *Acta Psychiatrica Scandinavica*, 113(3), 180–206.

Bridge, J. A., Goldstein, T. R., & Brent, D. A. (2006). Adolescent suicide and suicidal behavior. *Journal of Child Psychology and Psychiatry*, 47(3–4), 372–394.

Bridges, F. S. (2004). Gun control law (Bill C-17), suicide, and homicide in Canada. *Psychological Report*, 94(3 Pt 1), 819–826.

Bromet, E. J., Havenaar, J. M., Tintle, N., et al. (2007). Suicide ideation, plans and attempts in Ukraine: findings from the Ukraine World Mental Health Survey. *Psychological Medicine*, 37(6), 807–819.

Brown, G. K., Beck, A. T., Steer, R. A., & Grisham, J. R. (2000). Risk factors for suicide in psychiatric outpatients: a 20-year prospective study. *Journal of Consulting and Clinical Psychology*, 68(3), 371–377.

Brown, G. K., Ten Have, T., Henriques, G. R., et al. (2005). Cognitive therapy for the prevention of suicide attempts: a randomized controlled trial. *Journal of the American Medical Association*, 294(5), 563–570.

Cantor, C. H. (2000). Suicide in the Western World. In K. Hawton & K. van Heeringen (eds.), *International handbook of suicide and attempted suicide*, pp. 9–28. Chichester, England: John Wiley & Sons.

Cantor, C. H., Leenaars, A. A., Lester, D., et al. (1996). Suicide trends in eight predominantly English-speaking countries 1960–1989. *Social Psychiatry and Psychiatric Epidemiology*, 31(6), 364–373.

Carrington, P. J. (1999). Gender, gun control, suicide and homicide in Canada. *Archives of Suicide Research*, 5, 71–75.

Caspi, A., Sugden, K., Moffitt, T. E., et al. (2003). Influence of life stress on depression: Moderation by a polymorphism in the 5-HTT gene. *Science*, 301(5631), 386–389.

Cavanagh, J. T., Carson, A. J., Sharpe, M., & Lawrie, S. M. (2003). Psychological autopsy studies of suicide: a systematic review. *Psychological Medicine*, 33(3), 395–405.

CDC. (2007a). Behavioral Risk Factor Surveillance System. URL: http://www.cdc.gov/brfss/. Retrieved November 29, 2007.

CDC. (2007b). *National Youth Risk Behavior Survey: 1991–2005: Trends in the prevalence of suicide ideation and attempts*, (http://www.cdc.gov/HealthyYouth/yrbs/trends.htm). Retrieved November 12, 2007, from http://www.cdc.gov/HealthyYouth/yrbs/trends.htm.

CDC. (2008a). *Web-based Injury Statistics Query and Reporting System (WISQARS) Fatal Injuries: Mortality Reports.* Retrieved March 7, 2008, from http://www.cdc.gov/nipc/wisqars.

CDC. (2008b). *Web-based Injury Statistics Query and Reporting System (WISQARS) Nonfatal Injuries: Nonfatal Injury Reports.* Retrieved March 7, 2008, from http://www.cdc.gov/nipc/wisqars.

Center, C., Davis, M., Detre, T., et al. (2003). Confronting depression and suicide in physicians: a consensus statement. *Journal of the American Medical Association,* **289**(23), 3161–3166.

Cheng, A. T., & Lee, C. (2000). Suicide in Asia and the Far East. In K. Hawton & K. van Heeringen (eds.), *International handbook of suicide and attempted suicide,* pp. 29–48. Chichester, England: John Wiley & Sons.

Clarke, C. S., Bannon, F. J., & Denihan, A. (2003). Suicide and religiosity – Masaryk's theory revisited. *Social Psychiatry and Psychiatric Epidemiology,* **38**(9), 502–506.

Conwell, Y., & Duberstein, P. R. (2001). Suicide in elders. *Annals of the New York Academy of Sciences,* **932**, 132–147; discussion 147–150.

Conwell, Y., Duberstein, P. R., & Caine, E. D. (2002). Risk factors for suicide in later life. *Biolical Psychiatry,* **52**(3), 193–204.

Courtet, P., Baud, P., Abbar, M., et al. (2001). Association between violent suicidal behavior and the low activity allele of the serotonin transporter gene. *Molecular Psychiatry,* **6**(3), 338–341.

Crawford, M. J., Nur, U., McKenzie, K., & Tyrer, P. (2005). Suicidal ideation and suicide attempts among ethnic minority groups in England: results of a national household survey. *Psychological Medicine,* **35**(9), 1369–1377.

Cuddy-Casey, M., & Orvaschel, H. (1997). Children's understanding of death in relation to child suicidality and homicidality. *Clinical Psychology Review,* **17**(1), 33–45.

de Graaf, R., Sandfort, T. G., & ten Have, M. (2006). Suicidality and sexual orientation: differences between men and women in a general population-based sample from the Netherlands. *Archives of Sexual Behavior,* **35**(3), 253–262.

De Leo, D., Cerin, E., Spathonis, K., & Burgis, S. (2005). Lifetime risk of suicide ideation and attempts in an Australian community: prevalence, suicidal process, and help-seeking behaviour. *Journal of Affective Disorders,* **86**(2–3), 215–224.

De Leo, D., Padoani, W., Scocco, P., et al. (2001). Attempted and completed suicide in older subjects: results from the WHO/EURO Multicentre Study of Suicidal Behaviour. *International Journal of Geriatric Psychiatry,* **16**(3), 300–310.

De Luca, V., Hlousek, D., Likhodi, O., et al. (2006). The interaction between TPH2 promoter haplotypes and clinical-demographic risk factors in suicide victims with major psychoses. *Genes, Brain, and Behavior,* **5**(1), 107–110.

Department of Health and Human Services. Healthy People 2010. (2000). *Washington, DC: U.S. Department of Health and Human Services.*

Dervic, K., Akkaya-Kalayci, T., Kapusta, N. D., et al. (2007). Suicidal ideation among Viennese high school students. *Wiener Klinische Wochenschrift,* **119**(5–6), 174–180.

Dervic, K., Oquendo, M. A., Grunebaum, M. F., et al. (2004). Religious affiliation and suicide attempt. *American Journal of Psychiatry,* **161**(12), 2303–2308.

Dixon, P. G., McDonald, A. N., Scheitlin, K. N., et al. (2007). Effects of temperature variation on suicide in five U.S. counties, 1991–2001. *International Journal of Biometeorology,* **51**(5), 395–403.

Dube, S. R., Anda, R. F., Felitti, V. J., et al. (2001). Childhood abuse, household dysfunction, and the risk of attempted suicide throughout the life span: findings from the Adverse Childhood Experiences Study. *Journal of the American Medical Association,* **286**(24), 3089–3096.

Eisenberg, M. E., Neumark-Sztainer, D., & Story, M. (2003). Associations of weight-based teasing and emotional well-being among adolescents. *Archives of Pediatrics and Adolescent Medicine,* **157**(8), 733–738.

Elklit, A. (2002). Victimization and PTSD in a Danish national youth probability sample. *Journal of the American Academy of Child and Adolescent Psychiatry,* **41**(2), 174–181.

Evans, E., Hawton, K., Rodham, K., & Deeks, J. (2005). The prevalence of suicidal phenomena in adolescents: a systematic review of population-based studies. *Suicide and Life-Threatening Behavior,* **35**(3), 239–250.

Fairweather, A. K., Anstey, K. J., Rodgers, B., Jorm, A. F., & Christensen, H. (2007). Age and gender differences among Australian suicide ideators: prevalence and correlates. *Journal of Nervous and Mental Disease,* **195**(2), 130–136.

Fawcett, J. (2001). Treating impulsivity and anxiety in the suicidal patient. *Annals of the New York Academy of Sciences,* **932**, 94–102.

Fawcett, J., Busch, K. A., Jacobs, D., Kravitz, H. M., & Fogg, L. (1997). Suicide: a four-pathway clinical-biochemical model. *Annals of the New York Academy of Sciences,* **836**, 288–301.

Fawcett, J., Scheftner, W. A., Fogg, L., et al. (1990). Time-related predictors of suicide in major affective disorder. *American Journal of Psychiatry,* **147**(9), 1189–1194.

Fergusson, D. M., Horwood, L. J., & Beautrais, A. L. (1999). Is sexual orientation related to mental health problems and suicidality in young people? *Archives of General Psychiatry,* **56**(10), 876–880.

Fleischmann, A., Bertolote, J. M., De Leo, D., et al. (2005). Characteristics of attempted suicides seen in emergency-care settings of general hospitals in eight low- and middle-income countries. *Psychological Medicine*, **35**(10), 1467–1474.

Fortuna, L. R., Perez, D. J., Canino, G., Sribney, W., & Alegria, M. (2007). Prevalence and correlates of lifetime suicidal ideation and suicide attempts among Latino subgroups in the United States. *Journal of Clinical Psychiatry*, **68**(4), 572–581.

Fu, Q., Heath, A. C., Bucholz, K. K., et al. (2002). A twin study of genetic and environmental influences on suicidality in men. *Psychological Medicine*, **32**(1), 11–24.

Garroutte, E. M., Goldberg, J., Beals, J., Herrell, R., & Manson, S. M. (2003). Spirituality and attempted suicide among American Indians. *Social Science and Medicine*, **56**(7), 1571–1579.

Gibb, S., & Beautrais, A. (2004). Epidemiology of attempted suicide in Canterbury Province, New Zealand (1993–2002). *New Zealand Medical Journal*, **117**(1205), U1141.

Gibbons, R. D., Brown, C. H., Hur, K., et al. (2007a). Early evidence on the effects of regulators' suicidality warnings on SSRI prescriptions and suicide in children and adolescents. *American Journal of Psychiatry*, **164**(9), 1356–1363.

Gibbons, R. D., Brown, C. H., Hur, K., et al. (2007b). Relationship between antidepressants and suicide attempts: an analysis of the Veterans Health Administration data sets. *American Journal of Psychiatry*, **164**(7), 1044–1049.

Gibbons, R. D., Hur, K., Bhaumik, D. K., & Mann, J. J. (2005). The relationship between antidepressant medication use and rate of suicide. *Archives of General Psychiatry*, **62**(2), 165–172.

Gibbons, R. D., Hur, K., Bhaumik, D. K., & Mann, J. J. (2006). The relationship between antidepressant prescription rates and rate of early adolescent suicide. *American Journal of Psychiatry*, **163**(11), 1898–1904.

Glassman, L. H., Weierich, M. R., Hooley, J. M., Deliberto, T. L., & Nock, M. K. (2007). Child maltreatment, non-suicidal self-injury, and the mediating role of self-criticism. *Behaviour Research and Therapy*, **45**(10), 2483–2490.

Glowinski, A. L., Bucholz, K. K., Nelson, E. C., et al. (2001). Suicide attempts in an adolescent female twin sample. *Journal of the American Academy of Child and Adolescent Psychiatry*, **40**(11), 1300–1307.

Gmitrowicz, A., Szymczak, W., Kropiwnicki, P., & Rabe-Jablonska, J. (2003). Gender influence in suicidal behaviour of Polish adolescents. *European Child and Adolescent Psychiatry*, **12**(5), 205–213.

Goldney, R. D., Smith, S., Winefield, A. H., Tiggeman, M., & Winefield, H. R. (1991). Suicidal ideation: its enduring nature and associated morbidity. *Acta Psychiatrica Scandinavica*, **83**(2), 115–120.

Goldsmith, S. K., Pellmar, T. C., Kleinman, A. M., & Bunney, W. E. (eds.). (2002). *Reducing suicide: A national imperative*. Washington, DC: The National Academies Press.

Goldstein, R. B., Black, D. W., Nasrallah, A., & Winokur, G. (1991). The prediction of suicide. Sensitivity, specificity, and predictive value of a multivariate model applied to suicide among 1906 patients with affective disorders. *Archives of General Psychiatry*, **48**(5), 418–422.

Gould, M. S. (1990). Teenage suicide clusters. *Journal of the American Medical Association*, **263**(15), 2051–2052.

Gould, M. S. (2001). Suicide and the media. *Annals of the New York Academy of Sciences*, **932**, 200–221; discussion 221–204.

Gould, M. S., King, R., Greenwald, S., et al. (1998). Psychopathology associated with suicidal ideation and attempts among children and adolescents. *Journal of the American Academy of Child and Adolescent Psychiatry*, **37**(9), 915–923.

Gould, M. S., Wallenstein, S., & Kleinman, M. (1990). Time-space clustering of teenage suicide. *American Journal of Epidemiology*, **131**(1), 71–78.

Gunnell, D., Harbord, R., Singleton, N., Jenkins, R., & Lewis, G. (2004). Factors influencing the development and amelioration of suicidal thoughts in the general population. Cohort study. *British Journal of Psychiatry*, **185**, 385–393.

Gureje, O., Kola, L., Uwakwe, R., et al. (2007). The profile and risks of suicidal behaviours in the Nigerian Survey of Mental Health and Well-Being. *Psychological Medicine*, **37**(6), 821–830.

Hawton, K., Cole, D., O'Grady, J., & Osborn, M. (1982). Motivational aspects of deliberate self-poisoning in adolescents. *British Journal of Psychiatry*, **141**, 286–291.

Hawton, K., Houston, K., Haw, C., Townsend, E., & Harriss, L. (2003). Comorbidity of Axis I and Axis II disorders in patients who attempted suicide. *American Journal of Psychiatry*, **160**(8), 1494–1500.

Heisler, M., Halasyamani, L., Resnicow, K., et al. (2007). "I am not alone": the feasibility and acceptability of interactive voice response-facilitated telephone peer support among older adults with heart failure. *Congestive Heart Failure*, **13**(3), 149–157.

Helmkamp, J. C. (1996). Occupation and suicide among males in the US Armed Forces. *Annals of Epidemiology*, **6**(1), 83–88.

Herrell, R., Goldberg, J., True, W. R., et al. (1999). Sexual orientation and suicidality: a co-twin control study in adult men. *Archives of General Psychiatry*, **56**(10), 867–874.

Hintikka, J., Viinamaki, H., Tanskanen, A., Kontula, O., & Koskela, K. (1998). Suicidal ideation and parasuicide in the Finnish general population. *Acta Psychiatrica Scandinavica*, **98**(1), 23–27.

Horan, J. M., & Mallonee, S. (2003). Injury surveillance. *Epidemiologic Reviews*, 25, 24–42.

Ialongo, N., McCreary, B. K., Pearson, J. L., et al. (2002). Suicidal behavior among urban, African American young adults. *Suicide and Life-Threatening Behavior*, **32**(3), 256–271.

Isacsson, G. (2000). Suicide prevention – a medical breakthrough? *Acta Psychiatrica Scandinavica*, **102**(2), 113–117.

Jenkins, R. (2002). Addressing suicide as a public health problem. *Lancet*, **359**(9309), 813–814.

Jenkins, R., & Singh, B. (2000). General population strategies of suicide prevention. In K. Hawton & K. van Heeringen (eds.), *International handbook of suicide and attempted suicide*, pp. 631–644. Chichester, England: John Wiley & Sons.

Joe, S., Baser, R. E., Breeden, G., Neighbors, H. W., & Jackson, J. S. (2006). Prevalence of and risk factors for lifetime suicide attempts among blacks in the United States. *Journal of the American Medical Association*, **296**(17), 2112–2123.

Joiner, T. (2003). Contagion of suicidal symptoms as a function of assortative relating and shared relationship stress in college roommates. *Journal of Adolescence*, **26**(4), 495–504.

Joiner, T. E., Jr., Brown, J. S., & Wingate, L. R. (2005a). The psychology and neurobiology of suicidal behavior. *Annual Review of Psychology*, **56**, 287–314.

Joiner, T. E., Conwell, Y., Fitzpatrick, K. K., et al. (2005b). Four studies on how past and current suicidality relate even when "everything but the kitchen sink" is covaried. *Journal of Abnormal Psychology*, **114**(2), 291–303.

Joiner, T. E., Jr., Sachs-Ericsson, N. J., Wingate, L. R., et al. (2007). Childhood physical and sexual abuse and lifetime number of suicide attempts: a persistent and theoretically important relationship. *Behavior Research and Therapy*, **45**(3), 539–547.

Kaltiala-Heino, R., Rimpela, M., Marttunen, M., Rimpela, A., & Rantanen, P. (1999). Bullying, depression, and suicidal ideation in Finnish adolescents: school survey. *British Medical Journal*, **319**(7206), 348–351.

Kebede, D., & Alem, A. (1999). Suicide attempts and ideation among adults in Addis Ababa, Ethiopia. *Acta Psychiatrica Scandinavica Supplement*, **397**, 35–39.

Kendler, K. S. (2005a). "A gene for . . .": The nature of gene action in psychiatric disorders. *American Journal of Psychiatry*, **162**(7), 1243–1252.

Kendler, K. S. (2005b). Toward a philosophical structure for psychiatry. *American Journal of Psychiatry*, **162**(3), 433–440.

Kendler, K. S., & Prescott, C. A. (2007). *Genes, environment, and psychopathology: Understanding the causes of psychiatric and substance use disorders*. New York, NY: Guilford Press.

Kerkhof, A. J. F. M. (2000). Attempted suicide: Patterns and trends. In K. Hawton & K. van Heeringen (eds.), *International handbook of suicide and attempted suicide*, pp. 49–64. Chichester, England: John Wiley & Sons.

Kessler, R. C., Berglund, P., Borges, G., Nock, M. K., & Wang, P. S. (2005a). Trends in suicide ideation, plans, gestures, and attempts in the United States, 1990–1992 to 2001–2003. *Journal of the American Medical Association*, **293**(20), 2487–2495.

Kessler, R. C., Borges, G., & Walters, E. E. (1999). Prevalence of and risk factors for lifetime suicide attempts in the National Comorbidity Survey. *Archives of General Psychiatry*, **56**(7), 617–626.

Kessler, R. C., Demler, O., Frank, R. G., et al. (2005b). Prevalence and treatment of mental disorders, 1990 to 2003. *New England Journal of Medicine*, **352**(24), 2515–2523.

Kessler, R. C., & McRae, J. A., Jr. (1983). Trends in the relationship between sex and attempted suicide. *Journal of Health and Social Behavior*, **24**(2), 98–110.

Kessler, R. C., & Üstün, T. B. (2004). The World Mental Health (WMH) Survey Initiative Version of the World Health Organization (WHO) Composite International Diagnostic Interview (CIDI). *International Journal of Methods in Psychiatric Research*, **13**(2), 93–121.

Khokher, S., & Khan, M. M. (2005). Suicidal ideation in Pakistani college students. *Crisis*, **26**(3), 125–127.

Kim, H., Bracha, Y., & Tipnis, A. (2007). Automated depression screening in disadvantaged pregnant women in an urban obstetric clinic. *Archives of Women's Mental Health*, **10**(4), 163–169.

King, R. A., Schwab-Stone, M., Flisher, A. J., et al. (2001). Psychosocial and risk behavior correlates of youth suicide attempts and suicidal ideation. *Journal of the American Academy of Child and Adolescent Psychiatry*, **40**(7), 837–846.

Kjoller, M., & Helweg-Larsen, M. (2000). Suicidal ideation and suicide attempts among adult Danes. *Scandinavian Journal of Public Health*, **28**(1), 54–61.

Knox, K. L., Litts, D. A., Talcott, G. W., Feig, J. C., & Caine, E. D. (2003). Risk of suicide and related adverse outcomes after exposure to a suicide prevention programme in the US Air Force: cohort study. *British Medical Journal*, **327**(7428), 1376.

Kreitman, N. (1976). The coal gas story. United Kingdom suicide rates, 1960–71. *British Journal of Preventive and Social Medicine*, **30**(2), 86–93.

Kumar, V. (2003). Burnt wives–a study of suicides. *Burns*, **29**(1), 31–35.

Kuo, W. H., Gallo, J. J., & Tien, A. Y. (2001). Incidence of suicide ideation and attempts in adults: the 13-year follow-up of a community sample in Baltimore, Maryland. *Psychological Medicine*, **31**(7), 1181–1191.

Lee, S., Fung, S. C., Tsang, A., et al. (2007). Lifetime prevalence of suicide ideation, plan, and attempt in metropolitan China. *Acta Psychiatrica Scandinavica*, **116**(6), 429–437.

Lee, S., & Kleinman, A. (2003). Suicide as resistance in Chinese society. In E. J. Perry & M. Selden (eds.), *Chinese Society: Change, Conflict and Resistance, second edition*, pp. 289–311. London, England: Routledge.

Lester, D. (1990). The effect of the detoxification of domestic gas in Switzerland on the suicide rate. *Acta Psychiatrica Scandinavica*, **82**(5), 383–384.

Levi, F., La Vecchia, C., Lucchini, F., et al. (2003). Trends in mortality from suicide, 1965–99. *Acta Psychiatrica Scandinavica*, **108**(5), 341–349.

Linehan, M. M., Comtois, K. A., Murray, A. M., et al. (2006). Two-year randomized controlled trial and follow-up of dialectical behavior therapy vs therapy by experts for suicidal behaviors and borderline personality disorder. *Archives of General Psychiatry*, **63**(7), 757–766.

Linehan, M. M., Rizvi, S. L., Welch, S. S., & Page, B. (2000). Psychiatric aspects of suicidal behaviour: Personality disorders. In K. Hawton & K. van Heeringen (eds.), *International handbook of suicide and attempted suicide*, pp. 147–178. Chichester, England: John Wiley & Sons.

Liu, K. Y., Chen, E. Y., Chan, C. L., et al. (2006). Socio-economic and psychological correlates of suicidality among Hong Kong working-age adults: results from a population-based survey. *Psychological Medicine*, **36**(12), 1759–1767.

Liu, X., Tein, J. Y., Zhao, Z., & Sandler, I. N. (2005). Suicidality and correlates among rural adolescents of China. *Journal of Adolescent Health*, **37**(6), 443–451.

Mahon, M. J., Tobin, J. P., Cusack, D. A., Kelleher, C., & Malone, K. M. (2005). Suicide among regular-duty military personnel: A retrospective case-control study of occupation-specific risk factors for workplace suicide. *American Journal of Psychiatry*, **162**(9), 1688–1696.

Mann, J. J. (2003). Neurobiology of suicidal behaviour. *Nature Reviews Neuroscience*, **4**(10), 819–828.

Mann, J. J., Apter, A., Bertolote, J., et al. (2005). Suicide prevention strategies: a systematic review. *Journal of the American Medical Association*, **294**(16), 2064–2074.

Mann, J. J., & Malone, K. M. (1997). Cerebrospinal fluid amines and higher-lethality suicide attempts in depressed inpatients. *Biological Psychiatry*, **41**(2), 162–171.

Mann, J. J., Malone, K. M., Nielsen, D. A., et al. (1997). Possible association of a polymorphism of the tryptophan hydroxylase gene with suicidal behavior in depressed patients. *American Journal of Psychiatry*, **154**(10), 1451–1453.

Mann, J. J., McBride, P. A., Brown, R. P., et al. (1992). Relationship between central and peripheral serotonin indexes in depressed and suicidal psychiatric inpatients. *Archives of General Psychiatry*, **49**(6), 442–446.

Mann, J. J., Waternaux, C., Haas, G. L., & Malone, K. M. (1999). Toward a clinical model of suicidal behavior in psychiatric patients. *American Journal of Psychiatry*, **156**(2), 181–189.

Marion, M. S., & Range, L. M. (2003). African American college women's suicide buffers. *Suicide and Life-Threatening Behavior*, **33**(1), 33–43.

Marzuk, P. M., Leon, A. C., Tardiff, K., et al. (1992). The effect of access to lethal methods of injury on suicide rates. *Archives of General Psychiatry*, **49**(6), 451–458.

Marzuk, P. M., Nock, M. K., Leon, A. C., Portera, L., & Tardiff, K. (2002). Suicide among New York City police officers, 1977–1996. *American Journal of Psychiatry*, **159**(12), 2069–2071.

Marzuk, P. M., Tardiff, K., Leon, A. C., et al. (1997). Lower risk of suicide during pregnancy. *American Journal of Psychiatry*, **154**(1), 122–123.

Mathers, C. D., Bernard, C., Iburg, K. M., et al. (2003). *Global burden of disease in 2002: Data sources, method and results. Global Programme on Evidence for Health Policy Discussion Paper No. 54.* Geneva, Switzerland: World Health Organization.

Mathers, C. D., & Loncar, D. (2006). Projections of global mortality and burden of disease from 2002 to 2030. *PLoS Medicine*, **3**(11), e442.

Meadows, L. A., Kaslow, N. J., Thompson, M. P., & Jurkovic, G. J. (2005). Protective factors against suicide attempt risk among African American women experiencing intimate partner violence. *American Journal of Community Psychology*, **36**(1–2), 109–121.

Miauton, L., Narring, F., & Michaud, P. A. (2003). Chronic illness, life style and emotional health in adolescence: results of a cross-sectional survey on the health of 15–20-year-olds in Switzerland. *European Journal of Pediatrics*, **162**(10), 682–689.

Michel, K., Ballinari, P., Bille-Brahe, U., et al. (2000). Methods used for parasuicide: results of the WHO/EURO Multicentre Study on Parasuicide. *Social Psychiatry and Psychiatric Epidemiology*, **35**(4), 156–163.

Mohammadi, M. R., Ghanizadeh, A., Rahgozart, M., et al. (2005). Suicidal attempt and psychiatric disorders in Iran. *Suicide and Life-Threatening Behavior*, **35**(3), 309–316.

Monk, M. (1987). Epidemiology of suicide. *Epidemiologic Reviews*, **9**, 51–69.

Moscicki, E. K. (1999). Epidemiology of suicide. In D. G. Jacobs (ed.), *The Harvard Medical School guide to suicide assessment and intervention*, pp. 40–51. San Francisco, CA: Jossey-Bass.

Motto, J. A., & Bostrom, A. G. (2001). A randomized controlled trial of postcrisis suicide prevention. *Psychiatric Services*, **52**(6), 828–833.

Murray, C. L., & Lopez, A. D. (eds.). (1996). *The global burden of disease: A comprehensive assessment of mortality and disability from diseases, injuries, and risk factors in 1990 and projected to 2020*. Cambridge, MA: Harvard University Press.

Nakaji, S., Parodi, S., Fontana, V., et al. (2004). Seasonal changes in mortality rates from main causes of death in Japan (1970–1999). *European Journal of Epidemiology*, **19**(10), 905–913.

Nemeroff, C. B., Kalali, A., Keller, M. B., et al. (2007). Impact of publicity concerning pediatric suicidality data on physician practice patterns in the United States. *Archives of General Psychiatry*, **64**(4), 466–472.

Nock, M. K., & Banaji, M. R. (2007a). Assessment of self-injurious thoughts using a behavioral test. *American Journal of Psychiatry*, **164**(5), 820–823.

Nock, M. K., & Banaji, M. R. (2007b). Prediction of suicide ideation and attempts among adolescents using a brief performance-based test. *Journal of Consulting and Clinical Psychology*, **75**(5), 707–715.

Nock, M. K., Borges, G., Bromet, E. J., et al. (2008a). Cross-national prevalence and risk factors for suicidal ideation, plans, and attempts in the WHO World Mental Health Surveys. *British Journal of Psychiatry*, **192**(2), 98–105.

Nock, M. K., Borges, G., Bromet, E. J., et al. (2008b). Suicide and suicidal behavior. *Epidemiologic Reviews*, **30**, 133–154.

Nock, M. K., Joiner, T. E. Jr., Gordon, K. H., Lloyd-Richardson, E., & Prinstein, M. J. (2006). Non-suicidal self-injury among adolescents: Diagnostic correlates and relation to suicide attempts. *Psychiatry Research*, **144**(1), 65–72.

Nock, M. K., & Kazdin, A. E. (2002). Examination of affective, cognitive, and behavioral factors and suicide-related outcomes in children and young adolescents. *Journal of Clinical Child and Adolescent Psychology*, **31**(1), 48–58.

Nock, M. K., & Kessler, R. C. (2006). Prevalence of and risk factors for suicide attempts versus suicide gestures: Analysis of the National Comorbidity Survey. *Journal of Abnormal Psychology*, **115**(3), 616–623.

Nock, M. K., & Prinstein, M. J. (2005). Contextual features and behavioral functions of self-mutilation among adolescents. *Journal of Abnormal Psychology*, **114**(1), 140–146.

Nock, M. K., Wedig, M. M., Holmberg, E. B., & Hooley, J. M. (2008c). The emotion reactivity scale: development, evaluation, and relation to self-injurious thoughts and behaviors. *Behavior Therapy*, **39**(2), 107–116.

Nojomi, M., Malakouti, S. K., Bolhari, J., & Poshtmashhadi, M. (2007). A predictor model for suicide attempt: evidence from a population-based study. *Archives of Iranian Medicine*, **10**(4), 452–458.

O'Carroll, P. W., Berman, A. L., Maris, R. W., et al. (1996). Beyond the Tower of Babel: a nomenclature for suicidology. *Suicide and Life-Threatening Behavior*, **26**(3), 237–252.

O'Donnell, L., O'Donnell, C., Wardlaw, D. M., & Stueve, A. (2004). Risk and resiliency factors influencing suicidality among urban African American and Latino youth. *American Journal of Community Psychology*, **33**(1–2), 37–49.

Oliver, R. G., & Hetzel, B. S. (1972). Rise and fall of suicide rates in Australia: relation to sedative availability. *Medical Journal of Australia*, **2**(17), 919–923.

Olsson, G. I., & von Knorring, A. L. (1999). Adolescent depression: prevalence in Swedish high-school students. *Acta Psychiatrica Scandinavica*, **99**(5), 324–331.

Oquendo, M. A., Dragatsi, D., Harkavy-Friedman, J., et al. (2005). Protective factors against suicidal behavior in Latinos. *Journal of Nervous and Mental Disease*, **193**(7), 438–443.

Oquendo, M. A., Placidi, G. P., Malone, K. M., et al. (2003). Positron emission tomography of regional brain metabolic responses to a serotonergic challenge and lethality of suicide attempts in major depression. *Archives of General Psychiatry*, **60**(1), 14–22.

Ovuga, E., Boardman, J., & Wasserman, D. (2006). Undergraduate student mental health at Makerere University, Uganda. *World Psychiatry*, **5**(1), 51–52.

Pandey, G. N. (1997). Altered serotonin function in suicide: Evidence from platelet and neuroendocrine studies. *Annals of the New York Academy of Sciences*, **836**, 182–201.

Pescosolido, B. A., & Mendelsohn, R. (1986). Social causation or social construction of suicide? An investigation into the social organization of official rates. *American Sociological Review*, **51**, 80–101.

Petridou, E., Papadopoulos, F. C., Frangakis, C. E., Skalkidou, A., & Trichopoulos, D. (2002). A role of sunshine in the triggering of suicide. *Epidemiology*, **13**(1), 106–109.

Petronis, K. R., Samuels, J. F., Moscicki, E. K., & Anthony, J. C. (1990). An epidemiologic investigation of potential risk factors for suicide attempts. *Social Psychiatry and Psychiatric Epidemiology*, **25**(4), 193–199.

Pfeffer, C. R. (1997). Childhood suicidal behavior. A developmental perspective. *Psychiatric Clinics of North America*, **20**(3), 551–562.

Pfeffer, C. R. (2001). Diagnosis of childhood and adolescent suicidal behavior: unmet needs for suicide prevention. *Biological Psychiatry*, **49**(12), 1055–1061.

Phillips, M. R., Yang, G., Zhang, Y., et al. (2002). Risk factors for suicide in China: A national case-control psychological autopsy study. *Lancet*, **360**(9347), 1728–1736.

Platt, S., Bille-Brahe, U., Kerkhof, A., et al. (1992). Parasuicide in Europe: the WHO/EURO multicentre study on parasuicide. I. Introduction and preliminary analysis for 1989. *Acta Psychiatrica Scandinavica*, **85**(2), 97–104.

Ponizovsky, A. M., Ritsner, M. S., & Modai, I. (1999). Suicidal ideation and suicide attempts among immigrant adolescents from the former Soviet Union to Israel. *Journal of the American Academy of Child and Adolescent Psychiatry*, **38**(11), 1433–1441.

Posner, K., Oquendo, M. A., Gould, M., Stanley, B., & Davies, M. (2007). Columbia Classification Algorithm of Suicide Assessment (C-CASA): Classification of suicidal events in the FDA's pediatric suicidal risk analysis of antidepressants. *American Journal of Psychiatry*, **164**(7), 1035–1043.

Power, T. G., Stewart, C. D., Hughes, S. O., & Arbona, C. (2005). Predicting patterns of adolescent alcohol use: a longitudinal study. *Journal of Studies on Alcohol*, **66**(1), 74–81.

Preti, A., Miotto, P., & De Coppi, M. (2000). Season and suicide: recent findings from Italy. *Crisis*, **21**(2), 59–70.

Qin, P., & Mortensen, P. B. (2003). The impact of parental status on the risk of completed suicide. *Archives of General Psychiatry*, **60**(8), 797–802.

Rademacher, J. D., & Lippke, S. (2007). Dynamic online surveys and experiments with the free open-source software dynQuest. *Behavior Research Methods*, **39**(3), 415–426.

Ramberg, I. L., & Wasserman, D. (2000). Prevalence of reported suicidal behaviour in the general population and mental health-care staff. *Psychological Medicine*, **30**(5), 1189–1196.

Rancans, E., Lapins, J., Salander Renberg, E., & Jacobsson, L. (2003). Self-reported suicidal and help seeking behaviours in the general population in Latvia. *Social Psychiatry and Psychiatric Epidemiology*, **38**(1), 18–26.

Renberg, E. S. (2001). Self-reported life-weariness, death-wishes, suicidal ideation, suicidal plans and suicide attempts in general population surveys in the north of Sweden 1986 and 1996. *Social Psychiatry and Psychiatric Epidemiology*, **36**(9), 429–436.

Resnick, M. D., Bearman, P. S., Blum, R. W., et al. (1997). Protecting adolescents from harm. Findings from the National Longitudinal Study on Adolescent Health. *Journal of the American Medical Association*, **278**(10), 823–832.

Rey Gex, C., Narring, F., Ferron, C., & Michaud, P. A. (1998). Suicide attempts among adolescents in Switzerland: prevalence, associated factors and comorbidity. *Acta Psychiatrica Scandinavica*, **98**(1), 28–33.

Ridenour, T. A., Lanza, S. T., Donny, E. C., & Clark, D. B. (2006). Different lengths of times for progressions in adolescent substance involvement. *Addictive Behaviors*, **31**(6), 962–983.

Rihmer, Z., Belso, N., & Kalmar, S. (2001). Antidepressants and suicide prevention in Hungary. *Acta Psychiatrica Scandinavica*, **103**(3), 238–239.

Riordan, D. V., Selvaraj, S., Stark, C., & Gilbert, J. S. (2006). Perinatal circumstances and risk of offspring suicide. Birth cohort study. *British Journal of Psychiatry*, **189**, 502–507.

Rodriguez, A. H., Caldera, T., Kullgren, G., & Renberg, E. S. (2006). Suicidal expressions among young people in Nicaragua: a community-based study. *Social Psychiatry and Psychiatric Epidemiology*, **41**(9), 692–697.

Roggenbach, J., Muller-Oerlinghausen, B., & Franke, L. (2002). Suicidality, impulsivity and aggression – is there a link to 5HIAA concentration in the cerebrospinal fluid? *Psychiatry Research*, **113**(1–2), 193–206.

Roy, A. (2004). Family history of suicidal behavior and earlier onset of suicidal behavior. *Psychiatry Research*, **129**(2), 217–219.

Roy, A., & Segal, N. L. (2001). Suicidal behavior in twins: a replication. *Journal of Affective Disorders*, **66**(1), 71–74.

Roy, A., Segal, N. L., Centerwall, B. S., & Robinette, C. D. (1991). Suicide in twins. *Archives of General Psychiatry*, **48**(1), 29–32.

Rudatsikira, E., Muula, A. S., & Siziya, S. (2007). Prevalence and associated factors of suicidal ideation among school-going adolescents in Guyana: results from a cross sectional study. *Clinical Practice and Epidemiology in Mental Health*, **3**, 13.

Rutz, W., von Knorring, L., & Walinder, J. (1989). Frequency of suicide on Gotland after systematic postgraduate education of general practitioners. *Acta Psychiatrica Scandinavica*, **80**(2), 151–154.

Safer, D. J. (1997). Self-reported suicide attempts by adolescents. *Annals of Clinical Psychiatry*, **9**(4), 263–269.

Salk, L., Lipsitt, L. P., Sturner, W. Q., Reilly, B. M., & Levat, R. H. (1985). Relationship of maternal and perinatal conditions to eventual adolescent suicide. *Lancet*, **1**(8429), 624–627.

Samuelsson, M., Jokinen, J., Nordstrom, A. L., & Nordstrom, P. (2006). CSF 5-HIAA, suicide intent and hopelessness in the prediction of early suicide in male high-risk suicide attempters. *Acta Psychiatrica Scandinavica*, **113**(1), 44–47.

Sartor, C. E., Lynskey, M. T., Bucholz, K. K., et al. (2007). Childhood sexual abuse and the course of alcohol dependence development: findings from a female twin sample. *Drug and Alcohol Dependence*, **89**(2–3), 139–144.

Scocco, P., & De Leo, D. (2002). One-year prevalence of death thoughts, suicide ideation and behaviours in an elderly population. *International Journal of Geriatric Psychiatry*, **17**(9), 842–846.

Shaffer, D., Gould, M. S., Fisher, P., et al. (1996). Psychiatric diagnosis in child and adolescent suicide. *Archives of General Psychiatry*, **53**(4), 339–348.

Shafii, M., Carrigan, S., Whittinghill, J. R., & Derrick, A. (1985). Psychological autopsy of completed suicide in children and adolescents. *American Journal of Psychiatry*, **142**(9), 1061–1064.

Shafii, M., Steltz-Lenarsky, J., Derrick, A. M., Beckner, C., & Whittinghill, J. R. (1988). Comorbidity of mental disorders in the post-mortem diagnosis of completed suicide in children and adolescents. *Journal of Affective Disorders*, **15**(3), 227–233.

Sidhartha, T., & Jena, S. (2006). Suicidal behaviors in adolescents. *Indian Journal of Pediatrics*, **73**(9), 783–788.

Silverman, M. M., Berman, A. L., Sanddal, N. D., O'Carroll P, W., & Joiner, T. E. (2007a). Rebuilding the tower of Babel: A revised nomenclature for the study of suicide and suicidal behaviors. Part 1: Background, rationale, and methodology. *Suicide and Life-Threatening Behavior*, **37**(3), 248–263.

Silverman, M. M., Berman, A. L., Sanddal, N. D., O'Carroll P, W., & Joiner, T. E. (2007b). Rebuilding the tower of Babel: A revised nomenclature for the study of suicide and suicidal behaviors. Part 2: Suicide-related ideations, communications, and behaviors. *Suicide and Life-Threatening Behavior*, **37**(3), 264–277.

Silviken, A., & Kvernmo, S. (2007). Suicide attempts among indigenous Sami adolescents and majority peers in Arctic Norway: prevalence and associated risk factors. *Journal of Adolescence*, **30**(4), 613–626.

Smith, B., Smith, T. C., Gray, G. C., & Ryan, M. A. (2007). When epidemiology meets the Internet: web-based surveys in the Millennium Cohort Study. *American Journal of Epidemiology*, **166**(11), 1345–1354.

Spirito, A., & Esposito-Smythers, C. (2006). Attempted and completed suicide in adolescence. *Annual Review of Clinical Psychology*, **2**, 237–266.

Statham, D. J., Heath, A. C., Madden, P. A., et al. (1998). Suicidal behaviour: an epidemiological and genetic study. *Psychological Medicine*, **28**(4), 839–855.

Stenager, E. N., & Stenager, E. (2000). Physical illness and suicidal behaviour. In K. Hawton & K. van Heeringen (eds.), *International handbook of suicide and attempted suicide*, pp. 405–420. Chichester, England: John Wiley & Sons.

Szanto, K., Kalmar, S., Hendin, H., Rihmer, Z., & Mann, J. J. (2007). A suicide prevention program in a region with a very high suicide rate. *Archives of General Psychiatry*, **64**(8), 914–920.

Takahashi, K., Naito, H., Morita, M., et al. (1998). [Suicide prevention for the elderly in Matsunoyama Town, Higashikubiki County, Niigata Prefecture: psychiatric care for elderly depression in the community]. *Seishin Shinkeigaku Zasshi*, **100**(7), 469–485.

Tishler, C. L., Reiss, N. S., & Rhodes, A. R. (2007). Suicidal behavior in children younger than twelve: a diagnostic challenge for emergency department personnel. *Academic Emergency Medicine*, **14**(9), 810–818.

Tomic, S. T., & Janata, P. (2007). Ensemble: a web-based system for psychology survey and experiment management. *Behavior Research Methods*, **39**(3), 635–650.

Toros, F., Bilgin, N. G., Sasmaz, T., Bugdayci, R., & Camdeviren, H. (2004). Suicide attempts and risk factors among children and adolescents. *Yonsei Medical Journal*, **45**(3), 367–374.

Tourangeau, R., & Yan, T. (2007). Sensitive questions in surveys. *Psychological Bulletin*, **133**(5), 859–883.

Tousignant, M., Habimana, E., Biron, C., et al. (1999). The Quebec Adolescent Refugee Project: psychopathology and family variables in a sample from 35 nations. *Journal of the American Academy of Child and Adolescent Psychiatry*, **38**(11), 1426–1432.

Tran Thi Thanh, H., Tran, T. N., Jiang, G. X., Leenaars, A., & Wasserman, D. (2006). Life time suicidal thoughts in an urban community in Hanoi, Vietnam. *BMC Public Health*, **6**, 76.

Traskman-Bendz, L., & Mann, J. J. (2000). Biological aspects of suicidal behaviour. In K. Hawton & K. van Heeringen (eds.), *The international handbook of suicide and attempted suicide*, pp. 65–77. Chichester, England: John Wiley & Sons.

Turner, C. F., Ku, L., Rogers, S. M., et al. (1998). Adolescent sexual behavior, drug use, and violence: increased reporting with computer survey technology. *Science*, **280**(5365), 867–873.

U.S. Public Health Service. (1999). *The Surgeon General's call to action to prevent suicide*. Washington, DC.

United Nations. *Prevention of suicide guidelines for the formulation and implementation of national strategies.* (1996). New York, NY: United Nations.

Vijayakumar, L. (2004). Suicide prevention: the urgent need in developing countries. *World Psychiatry*, **3**(3), 158–159.

Vijayakumar, L. (2005). Suicide and mental disorders in Asia. *International Review of Psychiatry*, **17**(2), 109–114.

Vijayakumar, L., John, S., Pirkis, J., & Whiteford, H. (2005a). Suicide in developing countries (2): risk factors. *Crisis*, **26**(3), 112–119.

Vijayakumar, L., Pirkis, J., & Whiteford, H. (2005b). Suicide in developing countries (3): prevention efforts. *Crisis*, **26**(3), 120–124.

Vijayakumar, L., & Rajkumar, S. (1999). Are risk factors for suicide universal? A case-control study in India. *Acta Psychiatrica Scandinavica*, **99**(6), 407–411.

Violanti, J. M., Vena, J. E., & Marshall, J. R. (1996). Suicides, homicides, and accidental death: a comparative risk assessment of police officers and municipal workers. *American Journal of Industrial Medicine*, **30**(1), 99–104.

Virkkunen, M., Rawlings, R., Tokola, R., et al. (1994). CSF biochemistries, glucose metabolism, and diurnal activity rhythms in alcoholic, violent offenders, fire setters, and healthy volunteers. *Archives of General Psychiatry*, **51**(1), 20–27.

Waldrop, A. E., Hanson, R. F., Resnick, H. S., et al. (2007). Risk factors for suicidal behavior among a national sample of adolescents: Implications for prevention. *Journal of Traumatic Stress*, **20**(5), 869–879.

Wang, P. S., Berglund, P., Olfson, M., et al. (2005a). Failure and delay in initial treatment contact after first onset of mental disorders in the National Comorbidity Survey Replication. *Archives of General Psychiatry*, **62**(6), 603–613.

Wang, P. S., Lane, M., Olfson, M., et al. (2005b). Twelve-month use of mental health services in the United States: results from the National Comorbidity Survey Replication. *Archives of General Psychiatry*, **62**(6), 629–640.

Wedig, M. M., & Nock, M. K. (2007). Parental expressed emotion and adolescent self-injury. *Journal of the American Academy of Child and Adolescent Psychiatry*, **46**(9), 1171–1178.

Weed, J. A. (1985). Suicide in the United States: 1958–1982. In C. A. Taube & S. A. Barrett (eds.), *Mental Health, United States: 1985*. Rockville, MD: DHHS publication no (ADM), pp. 85–1378.

Weissman, M. M. (1974). The epidemiology of suicide attempts, 1960 to 1971. *Archives of General Psychiatry*, **30**(6), 737–746.

Weissman, M. M., Bland, R. C., Canino, G. J., et al. (1999). Prevalence of suicide ideation and suicide attempts in nine countries. *Psychological Medicine*, **29**(1), 9–17.

Wexler, L., Weissman, M. M., & Kasl, S. V. (1978). Suicide attempts 1970–75: updating a United States study and comparisons with international trends. *British Journal of Psychiatry*, **132**, 180–185.

WHO. (1996). *Prevention of suicide: guidelines for the formulation and implementation of national strategies.* Geneva: World Health Organization.

WHO. (2007). *World Health Organization: Suicide Prevention (SUPRE)*. Retrieved November 15, 2007, from http://www.who.int/mental_health/prevention/suicide/suicideprevent/en/.

Williams, J. M. G., & Pollock, L. R. (2000). The psychology of suicidal behaviour. In K. Hawton & K. van Heeringen (eds.), *The international handbook of suicide and attempted suicide*, pp. 79–94. Chichester, England: John Wiley & Sons.

WMH Consortium. (2004). WHO World Mental Health Consortium. Prevalence, severity, and unmet need for treatment of mental disorders in the World Health Organization World Mental Health Surveys. *Journal of the American Medical Association*, **291**(21), 2581–2590.

Yen, F. C., Hong, C. J., Hou, S. J., Wang, J. K., & Tsai, S. J. (2003a). Association study of serotonin transporter gene VNTR polymorphism and mood disorders, onset age and suicide attempts in a Chinese sample. *Neuropsychobiology*, **48**(1), 5–9.

Yen, S., Pagano, M. E., Shea, M. T., et al. (2005). Recent life events preceding suicide attempts in a personality disorder sample: findings from the collaborative longitudinal personality disorders study. *Journal of Consulting and Clinical Psychology*, **73**(1), 99–105.

Yen, S., Shea, M. T., Pagano, M., et al. (2003b). Axis I and axis II disorders as predictors of prospective suicide attempts: findings from the collaborative longitudinal personality disorders study. *Journal of Abnormal Psychology*, **112**(3), 375–381.

Yip, P. S., Liu, K. Y., Lam, T. H., et al. (2004). Suicidality among high school students in Hong Kong, SAR. *Suicide and Life-Threatening Behavior*, **34**(3), 284–297.

Young, R., Sweeting, H., & West, P. (2006). Prevalence of deliberate self harm and attempted suicide within contemporary Goth youth subculture: Longitudinal cohort study. *British Medical Journal*, **332**(7549), 1058–1061.

Zemaitiene, N., & Zaborskis, A. (2005). Suicidal tendencies and attitude towards freedom to choose suicide among Lithuanian schoolchildren: results from three cross-sectional studies in 1994, 1998, and 2002. *BMC Public Health*, **5**, 83.

Zouk, H., Tousignant, M., Seguin, M., Lesage, A., & Turecki, G. (2006). Characterization of impulsivity in suicide completers: clinical, behavioral and psychosocial dimensions. *Journal of Affective Disorders*, **92**(2–3), 195–204.

Chapter

3

Methods of the World Mental Health Surveys

Ronald C. Kessler, Janet Harkness, Steven G. Heeringa, Beth-Ellen Pennell, Alan M. Zaslavsky, Guilherme Borges, Yutaka Ono, and Matthew K. Nock

The World Mental Health (WMH) Survey Initiative is a World Health Organization (WHO) initiative designed to help countries carry out and analyze epidemiological surveys of the burden of mental disorders in their populations (www.hcp.med.harvard.edu/wmh). Twenty-eight countries have so far completed WMH Surveys and others are in progress. The vast majority of these surveys are nationally representative, although a few are representative of only a single region (e.g., the São Paulo metropolitan area in Brazil) or regions (e.g., six metropolitan areas in Japan). Results from 22 surveys carried out in 21 of those countries are reported in this volume. These are all the surveys that have so far been completed and processed.

All WMH Surveys use the same standardized procedures for sampling, interviewing, and data analysis. They also all use the same diagnostic interview, the WHO Composite International Diagnostic Interview (CIDI) Version 3.0 (Haro et al., 2008). The CIDI is a fully-structured research diagnostic interview designed for use by trained lay interviewers who do not have clinical experience. It generates diagnoses of mental disorders according to the definitions and criteria of both the International Classification of Diseases (ICD) and Diagnostic and Statistical Manual of Mental Disorders (DSM) systems, although only DSM-IV criteria are used here. Consistent WHO translation, back-translation, and harmonization procedures were used to modify the CIDI for use in each WMH country (Harkness et al., 2008). The same interviewer training materials, training programs, and quality control monitoring procedures were also used across WMH Surveys to guarantee cross-survey comparability of data (Pennell et al., 2008).

The use of these standardized procedures is key to WMH success, as the main mission of WMH is to allow countries that might not otherwise be able to implement mental health needs assessment surveys to do so by building on the existing WMH infrastructure. The use of standardized materials reduces costs for each country and makes it easier to implement high-quality surveys by building on tried and true procedures. This applies not only to instrument development and data collection but also to analysis, as WMH uses a centralized data processing and cross-national peer consultation model that allows less experienced collaborators to work with world-class statisticians and psychiatric epidemiologists to analyze, interpret, and write scientific reports about their data.

The current chapter presents information about these standardized materials and procedures. We begin by reviewing the WMH sample design. We then present an overview of the measures of suicidal behaviors and risk factors for suicidal behaviors that are used in this volume. The next section discusses interviewer training and quality control monitoring procedures. The final section discusses the statistical methods used in this volume to study patterns and predictors of suicidal behaviors.

The WMH samples

The sampling procedures used in the WMH Surveys are closely related to those originally developed for the World Fertility Survey (WFS) program, one of the first and largest efforts to coordinate a global gathering of survey data (Verma et al., 1980). The decisions made in developing sample designs for the WMH Surveys drew heavily on the lessons of the WFS experience. Like the WFS and more recent successful international programs of community survey research, the WMH Surveys required collaborating countries to employ probability sample designs to select nationally or

Suicide, eds. Matthew K. Nock, Guilherme Borges, and Yutaka Ono. Published by Cambridge University Press.
© World Health Organization 2012.

regionally representative samples of adults for the survey interview. The aim of sampling in the WMH Surveys was to obtain a representative sample of the household population in the country or region under study. This usually involved drawing a multistage clustered area probability sample of households in the population and then selecting one, or in some cases two, respondents from each sampled household using probability methods without replacement. These sample designs were standardized across countries based on the principles of probability sampling, but with less emphasis placed on the specific probability sample design features employed across countries in recognition of the fact that countries varied widely in the information available to develop a sample frame from which the WMH sample could be selected.

In order to achieve the level of coordination in sampling required across countries, we established a WMH Data Collection Coordination Centre at the Institute for Social Research (ISR) at the University of Michigan in the U.S. The Survey Research Center (SRC) at ISR is one of the leading academic survey research organizations in the world, with a long history of leadership in the development and implementation of large community surveys (www.src.isr.umich.edu). The Survey Sampling group at SRC, under the direction of Steve Heeringa, supervised WMH sampling, while the Survey Implementation group, under the supervision of Beth-Ellen Pennell, supervised WMH interviewer training and field implementation.

Focusing first on sampling, the SRC group began by developing a list containing a common set of requirements and performance standards that the probability sample design in each WMH Survey was required to meet. Unique opportunities available in individual countries were then used to develop a sampling plan that achieved these requirements and to meet the WMH standards. The staff of the WMH Data Collection Coordination Centre worked closely with local collaborators to develop these sample design plans. The plans were reviewed by a panel of technical experts and revised based on feedback from this panel. Once the design was finalized, day-to-day oversight of implementation was the responsibility of the local research team.

Most WMH countries developed a similar sampling plan that featured multistage area probability sampling. Several countries, though, adopted an alternative probability sampling procedure, such as the use of a national registry or combined uses of area probability methods and registry sampling to achieve the required probability sampling of the designated target population. All these samples, however, were probability samples. No WMH Survey used a convenience sample, an interviewer-managed quota sample, or any other nonprobability method of sample selection.

The target populations

Probability sample surveys are designed to describe a *target population* of elements that spans a specific geographic space during a specific window of time. Although it might seem obvious how to do this, a number of important considerations arise as soon as one begins to consider the possibilities. Should persons who were temporary residents, guest workers, or those who had legal claim to medical treatment or services be included in the sample? What about people who were incapable of participating in the survey because they were institutionalized, or cognitively or physically impaired, and people living in remote places that would require disproportionate amounts of survey resources to sample and interview? In the end, a decision was made to allow the answers to these questions to vary across countries within a range of options described as follows.

The *survey population* is defined as the subset of the target population that is truly eligible for sampling under the survey design (Groves et al., 2004). A decision was needed to decide what restrictions would apply in each participating WMH country to establish a survey population definition that would conform to the survey's scientific objectives, available sample frames, and budget limitations. Multiple dimensions were included here. One of these involved the age range of the sample. WMH was designed to focus on adults. However, the age that defines adulthood (commonly referred to as the "age of majority") varies across countries (most typically either 18 or 21 years old). In addition, some countries decided to impose an upper age limit on the sample (usually 65 years). Other dimensions that defined the survey population involved geographic scope limitations (most typically excluding otherwise eligible people who lived in remote areas of the country), language restrictions, citizenship requirements, and whether to include special populations such as persons living in military barracks and group quarters or persons who were institutionalized at the time of the survey (e.g., hospital patients, prison inmates). These varied somewhat across countries.

Table 3.1 provides a summary of the survey populations for the 22 WMH Surveys included in this volume. Starting with the different age limits, the

Table 3.1. WMH sample characteristics by World Bank income categories[a]

Country by income category	Survey[b]	Sample characteristics[c]	Field dates	Age range (years)	Sample size			Response rate[e]
					Part 1	Part 2	Part 2 and age ≤ 44[d]	
I. Low- and lower-middle-income countries								
Colombia	NSMH	All urban areas of the country (approximately 73% of the total national population)	2003	18–65	4426	2381	1731	87.7
India	WMHI	Pondicherry region	2003–2005	18–97	2992	1373	642	98.8
Nigeria	NSMHW	21 of the 36 states in the country, representing 57% of the national population. The surveys were conducted in Yoruba, Igbo, Hausa, and Efik languages	2002–2003	18–100	6752	2143	1203	79.3
China	B-WMH S-WMH	Beijing and Shanghai metropolitan areas	2002–2003	18–70	5201	1628	570	74.7
China	Shenzhen	Shenzhen metropolitan area. Included temporary residents as well as household residents	2006–2007	18–88	7132	2476	1993	80.0
Ukraine	CMDPSD	Nationally representative	2002	18–91	4724	1720	541	78.3
Total					31,227	11,721	6680	
II. Upper-middle-income countries								
Brazil	São Paulo Megacity	Stratified multistage clustered area probability sample of household residents in the São Paulo metropolitan area	2005–2007	18–93	5037	2942	–	81.3
Bulgaria	NSHS	Nationally representative	2003–2007	18–98	5318	2233	741	72.0
Lebanon	LEBANON	Nationally representative	2002–2003	18–94	2857	1031	595	70.0
Mexico	M-NCS	Stratified multistage clustered area probability sample of household residents in all urban areas of the country (approximately 75% of the total national population)	2001–2002	18–65	5782	2362	1736	76.6

Table 3.1. (cont.)

Country by income category	Survey[b]	Sample characteristics[c]	Field dates	Age range (years)	Sample size			Response rate[e]
					Part 1	Part 2	Part 2 and age ≤ 44[d]	
Romania	RMHS	Nationally representative	2005–2006	18–96	2357	2357	–	70.9
South Africa[f]	SASH	Nationally representative	2003–2004	18–92	4315	4315	–	87.1
Total					25,666	15,240	3072	
III. High-income countries								
Belgium	ESEMeD	Nationally representative. The sample was selected from a national register of Belgium residents	2001–2002	18–95	2419	1043	486	50.6
France	ESEMeD	Nationally representative. The sample was selected from a national list of households with listed telephone numbers	2001–2002	18–97	2894	1436	727	45.9
Germany	ESEMeD	Nationally representative	2002–2003	18–95	3555	1323	621	57.8
Israel	NHS	Nationally representative	2002–2004	21–98	4859	4859	–	72.6
Italy	ESEMeD	Nationally representative. The sample was selected from municipality resident registries	2001–2002	18–100	4712	1779	853	71.3
Japan	WMHJ2002–2006	Eleven metropolitan areas. Although samples from a clustered household sample, there was no within-household clustering due to setting the sampling fraction so that some households were skipped after enumeration because residents fall below the specified sampling fraction	2002–2006	20–98	4129	1682	547	55.1
Netherlands	ESEMeD	Nationally representative. The sample was selected from municipal postal registries	2002–2003	18–95	2372	1094	516	56.4
New Zealand[f]	NZMHS	Nationally representative	2003–2004	18–98	12,790	7312	4119	73.3

Spain	ESEMeD	Nationally representative	2001–2002	18–98	5473	2121	960	78.6
United States	NCS-R	Nationally representative	2002–2003	18–99	9281	5692	3197	70.9
Total					52,484	28,341	12,026	
IV. Total					**109,377**	**55,302**	**21,778**	**72.1**

[a] The World Bank. (2008).

[b] NSMH (The Colombian National Study of Mental Health); WMHI (World Mental Health); WMHI (World Mental Mental Health India); NSMHW (The Nigerian Survey of Mental Health and Wellbeing); B-WMH (The Beijing World Mental Health Survey); S-WMH (The Shanghai World Mental Health Survey); CMDPSD (Comorbid Mental Disorders during Periods of Social Disruption); NSHS (Bulgaria National Survey of Health and Stress); LEBANON (Lebanese Evaluation of the Burden of Ailments and Needs of the Nation); M-NCS (The Mexico National Comorbidity Survey); RMHS (Romania Mental Health Survey); SASH (South Africa Health Survey); ESEMeD (The European Study of the Epidemiology of Mental Disorders); NHS (Israel National Health Survey); WMHJ2002–2006 (World Mental Health Japan Survey); NZMHS (New Zealand Mental Health Survey); NCS-R (The US National Comorbidity Survey Replication).

[c] Most WMH Surveys are based on stratified multistage clustered area probability household samples in which samples of areas equivalent to counties or municipalities in the U.S. were selected in the first stage followed by one or more subsequent stages of geographic sampling (e.g., towns within counties, blocks within towns, households within blocks) to arrive at a sample of households, in each of which a listing of household members was created and one or two people were selected from this listing to be interviewed. No substitution was allowed when the originally sampled household resident could not be interviewed. These household samples were selected from Census area data in all countries other than France (where telephone directories were used to select households) and the Netherlands (where postal registries were used to select households). Several WMH Surveys (Belgium, Germany, Italy) used municipal resident registries to select respondents without listing households. The Japanese sample is the only totally unclustered sample, with households randomly selected in each of the four sample areas and one random respondent selected in each sample household. 18 of the 22 surveys are based on nationally representative household samples.

[d] Brazil, Israel, Romania, and South Africa did not have an age restricted Part 2 sample. All other countries, with the exception of India, Nigeria, People's Republic of China, and Ukraine (which were age restricted to ≤ 39 years) were age restricted to ≤ 44 years.

[e] The response rate is calculated as the ratio of the number of households in which an interview was completed to the number of households originally sampled, excluding from the denominator households known not to be eligible either because of being vacant at the time of initial contact or because the residents were unable to speak the designated languages of the survey. The weighted average response rate is 72.1%.

[f] South Africa and New Zealand interviewed respondents of 16+ years but for the purposes of cross-national comparisons, we limit the sample to those of 18+ years.

vast majority of the surveys had a minimum age of 18 years. The lowest minimum age was 16 (New Zealand) and the oldest was 21 years (Israel). For maximum age requirements, Colombia, Mexico, and the regional surveys carried out in Beijing and Shanghai mandated that respondents be no older than 65 or 70 years. Turning to the geographic scope of the survey population, 14 of the 22 surveys defined the geographic scope of their survey population as the entire country; Brazil, India, Japan, Nigeria, and China restricted their survey populations to specific regions, states/provinces, or cities. Colombia and Mexico conducted national surveys but limited their survey populations to urban places above a specified population size (e.g., more than 2500 persons in Mexico).

Sampling frames

Probability sampling requires a sampling frame that provides a high level of coverage for the defined survey population. The sampling frame is defined as the list or equivalent enumeration procedure that identifies all population elements and enables the sampler to assign non-zero selection probabilities to each element (Kish, 1965). We carefully reviewed the available choices of sample frames with the collaborators in each WMH country before deciding on a final frame. Options could have included population registries, new or existing area probability sampling frames, postal address lists, voter registration lists, and telephone subscriber lists. The final choice of the frame for each country was determined by a number of factors, including the extent of coverage and statistical efficiency of available frame alternatives, the cost of developing and using the frame for sample selection, and the experience of the data collection organization in the use of the sample frame.

The final sampling frames for the WMH Surveys were generally of three types: (1) a database of individual contact information provided in the form of national population registries, voter registration lists, postal address lists, or household telephone directories; (2) a multistage area probability sample frame (Kish, 1965); or (3) a hybrid multistage frame that combined area probability methods in the initial stages and a registry or population list in the penultimate and/or final stages of sample selection. Table 3.1 identifies the sample frame type chosen in each of the participating surveys.

Complex sample designs for the WMH Surveys

The goal of all survey sample designs is either to minimize sampling variance and bias for a fixed total cost or to minimize total cost while meeting predetermined analysis objectives. The analysis objectives are typically formulated as fixed targets for the variance and bias components of the total survey error for key survey estimates or the parameter estimates for important population models. In the WMH Survey program, there was no single path to this goal. The surveys shared a set of common analysis objectives, primarily centered on the estimation of the population prevalence and correlates of mental disorders. Survey cost structures were highly variable from one country to another, depending on factors such as availability and accessibility of survey infrastructure (government or commercial survey organizations), availability and costs for databases and map materials required to develop sample frames, labor rates for field interviewers and team leaders, and transportation costs for getting trained interviewers to distributed samples of households. Total funding for the surveys also varied widely across countries. In many cases, funding restrictions limited not only the total size of the interviewed sample but also the scope of the survey populations or the use of costly sample design options.

The individual WMH sample designs employed the full range of probability sampling techniques that survey statisticians can use to improve sample precision and reduce costs. Stratification of the samples by geographic regions and demographic characteristics was used to increase sample precision and control sample allocation. Multistage designs with modest clustering in the initial stages of sampling were used to control travel time and expenses. A version of the "double sampling" technique (Cochran, 1977) was used in the vast majority of surveys to determine the subsample of initial Part 1 CIDI screening interview respondents who would complete the more intensive Part 2 CIDI diagnostic questionnaire.

The variety of designs used in different WMH Surveys is a reflection of the differences in the essential survey conditions faced by the collaborators. With the exception of a small number of studies that sampled adults directly from high-quality population registries, the great majority of WMH Surveys used a multistage area probability sampling method. The population registry approach is very attractive when this option is available because it avoids within-household selection and weighting. A few other countries chose a first-stage probability sample of households directly from national postal lists (e.g., the Netherlands) or telephone directories (e.g., France) and then chose random respondents within the selected households. Germany used a two-stage design that involved a first-stage sampling of municipalities and a second-stage sampling of adults from population registries available within each of the selected municipalities. A number of other countries used a similar design but added an intermediate second-stage sampling of electoral or postal districts before selecting eligible adults from a district registry (e.g., Italy) or an enumerated list of residents within selected districts (e.g., Ukraine).

The vast majority of WMH Surveys, though, used three-stage or four-stage area probability designs. The three-stage designs began with a primary stage sample of a probability sample of census enumeration districts or neighborhood units selected with probabilities proportional to size followed by a second-stage sampling of households within the first-stage units and a third-stage random selection of an eligible adult within the sampled household. Countries that used four-stage designs expanded this same basic approach by beginning with the selection of large county or municipal units and then progressing to selection of area segment blocks, then to households, and then to respondents within households. All WMH Surveys that used within-household selection of respondents did so with an objective household selection table method developed by Kish (1949). In a probability subsample of households in some countries, the spouses of selected respondents who were married were also selected to take part in the survey.

It is important to note that considerable effort was required to construct the frames for the WMH samples in countries where preexisting survey frames did not exist. In Lebanon, for example, area probability methods were used to build the frame and select a multistage sample due to the fact that only limited population data existed in Lebanon. The primary stage of sampling consequently selected area segments (sectors) from a comprehensive list developed by the WMH collaborators, stratified by region and urbanicity. From this list, 342 area segments were selected with probabilities proportional to size. Prior to the second stage of sampling, the Lebanese team sent trained field staff to each selected area segment to create a comprehensive list of all housing units in the segment. Once this enumerative list was completed for each area segment, a second-stage sample was selected of housing units and then of respondents within households.

The WMH guidelines specified a target response rate target of 65% based on a precise method required to calculate the response rate (American Association for Public Opinion Research, 2000). This target response rate was achieved by 18 of the surveys, with eight having response rates in the range 70%–75%, five in the range 75%–80%, and four over 80%. The five surveys that failed to meet the target had response rates in the range 45.9%–57.8%. It is noteworthy that these five were all high-income countries (Belgium, France, Germany, Japan, and the Netherlands). This is consistent with other evidence that difficulties contacting respondents because they are away from the household are greatest in high-income countries, where people have a higher probability than elsewhere of being away from home in the evening and on weekends, and also that marketing surveys have become so common in high-income countries that the willingness of people to participate in surveys has declined substantially over time (Couper & de Leeuw, 2003). Surveys remain sufficiently novel in lower-income countries, though, that response rates are generally higher than in high-income countries. Survey response rates are, of course, also influenced by many other factors, including government privacy rules, population resistance to survey participation, the experience and norms of the chosen data collection organization, and availability of financial resources to invest in incentives or other refusal aversion efforts.

Nonresponse surveys

Collaborators in all countries were encouraged to carry out systematic nonresponse surveys in an effort to evaluate and, to the extent possible, correct for the effects of systematic survey nonresponse. The basic design of the nonresponse survey was to select a stratified probability subsample of initial survey nonrespondents who were approached one last time and asked to participate in a *brief* (typically 10–20 minutes of interview time) interview that would provide the investigators with basic information about people who were not able to participate in the full survey.

Respondents were typically offered a financial incentive to participate in this brief survey. The survey was usually carried out either by telephone or face-to-face. The questions in the survey included a small number of basic sociodemographics (e.g., age, gender, education, marital status) and diagnostic stem questions for diagnoses of core mental and substance disorders. Importantly, identical questions were asked in the main survey. Comparison of responses to these questions in the main sample and the nonrespondent sample was used to make inferences about nonresponse bias, while weighting adjustments described as follows were used to adjust the main sample for these biases.

Weighting

Person–level analysis weights that incorporated sample selection, nonresponse, and poststratification factors were constructed for each WMH Survey dataset. In a number of cases these weights were developed by survey statisticians on the individual country research teams, while weights were constructed in other cases by the staff of the WMH Data Analysis Coordination Centre at Harvard Medical School (HMS) using sample design and population control data supplied by the local project teams. The case-specific analysis weights were used in computing estimates of descriptive statistics for the survey population and for estimating the descriptive statistics reported in this volume.

Construction of analysis weights

In general, the final analysis weight for each WMH Survey respondent was computed as the product of the three weight components:

$$W_{final,i} = W_{sel,i} \cdot W_{nr,i} \cdot W_{psc,i}$$

where:

$W_{sel,i}$ = the selection weight factor for respondent $i = 1, \ldots, n$;

$W_{nr,i}$ = the nonresponse weight adjustment factor for respondent $i = 1, \ldots, n$;

$W_{psc,i}$ = the poststratification factor for respondent $i = 1, \ldots, n$.

The exact sequence of weight calculation steps differed slightly across surveys. In some countries, a separate nonresponse adjustment step was skipped and the final weight was derived as the product of the sample selection factor and a final, all-encompassing, poststratification to external population controls.

The sample selection weight was designed to compensate for the differing sampling probabilities for selecting individuals as WMH respondents. The selection weight factor, W_{sel}, is generally the product of the reciprocals of three probabilities: $W_{sel,hh}$, the reciprocal of the multistage probability of selecting the respondent's housing unit selection from the sample frame; $W_{sel,resp}$, the reciprocal of the conditional probability of selecting the WMH respondent at random within the eligible household (Kish, 1965); and $W_{sel,Part\,2}$, the reciprocal of the probability that an eligible WMH Survey respondent was subsampled to complete the in-depth Part 2 diagnostic section of the WMH interview. It is noteworthy in this regard that all WMH respondents completed Part 1 of the WMH interview. Based on the results of Part 1, the majority of the country surveys selected a stratified subsample of respondents to complete Part 2 of the interview, over-sampling Part 1 respondents who met criteria for any of the mental disorders assessed in that first half of the interview.

The nonresponse adjustment weight, W_{nr}, could be computed to account for differential patterns of response across categories of eligible respondents for a country-specific survey. When this weight was applied, nonresponse adjustments to survey weights were based on endogenous data; that is, on data from the sample frame that was known for both sample respondents and nonrespondents. In baseline or cross-sectional surveys such as the WMH studies described here, the data available to develop nonresponse adjustments is often limited to geographic and possibly demographic information available for respondents and nonrespondents in the sample frame, such as population census data collected by the government.

In cases where nonresponse adjustment was implemented, a nonrespondent survey of the sort described previously was used to generate this weight. The nonresponse sample was first weighted to be representative of all nonrespondents using within-household probability of selections weights (see later) and then this weighted subsample was compared to the similarly weighted main sample in an effort to determine if the two samples differed meaningfully on the variables assessed in both samples. When differences of this sort were found, either a weighting class method or a propensity modeling approach (Little & Rubin, 2002) was used to develop the adjustment factors.

The weight calculations for most of the WMH Survey datasets, however, did not include a separate nonresponse adjustment. Instead, an adjustment for differential nonresponse and sample noncoverage of the survey population was integrated into one consolidated adjustment in the poststratification weighting step, which is described later. In such cases, the factor W_{nr} can be viewed as taking a value of 1.0 in the final composite weight calculation. Readers who are interested in detailed case studies of nonresponse adjustment weighting for selected WMH datasets are referred to Alonso et al. (2004) and Kessler & Üstün (2004).

The final component in the WMH individual analysis weight is a poststratification factor, W_{ps}. The poststratification weighting adjustment differs from the nonresponse adjustment factors in that poststratification weighting uses data that are exogenous to the survey design to calibrate the weights for survey estimation. The WMH poststratification used estimates of population values from external sources such as a recent national census or demographic population estimation program to standardize the sampling weights to known population distribution values, such as the distribution of the population of the cross-classification of age (in categories), gender, and education. The logic of the general procedure used in each country involved forming a matrix of adjustment cells by cross-classifying age, gender, and major geographic regions (data permitting) of the survey population. Within each cell of this matrix, the poststratification weight factors were computed as the ratio of the external population count for each cell to the sum of computed sample selection weights for the WMH Survey cases assigned to that cell:

$$W_{pstrat,c,i} = \frac{\hat{N}_c}{\sum_{i \in c}^{n_c} W_{sel,i} \cdot W_{nr,i}}$$

where:

$W_{pstrat,c,i}$ = the poststratification factor for all cases in cell c;

$\hat{N}_c$ = the WMH country population estimate for cell c;

n_c = WMH country sample size in cell c;

$W_{sel,i}$ = the composite sample selection weight for case i = 1,..., n_c;

$W_{nr,i}$ = the nonresponse adjustment for case i = 1, ..., n_c.

In some countries, it was possible to include much more information than a few sociodemographic and geographic variables due to the availability of much more detailed population data on a wide range of social and demographic variables that were also assessed in the WMH Survey. In cases of this sort, logistic regression analyses were carried out to compare the WMH Survey data, with other weights imposed on the data, to the population data in an effort to pinpoint any variables that were meaningfully discrepant between the two. When the number of such variables was small, a modified poststratification weighting of the sort described in the last paragraph could have been implemented using poststratification tables constructed from only those variables. When a large number of poststratification variables were available, though, we used as many of them as feasible in the poststratification weighting step, based on the logistic regression equation that assigned a predicted probability of participation to each respondent based on a comparison of population data with survey data (Deville & Särndal, 1992). This regression-based weighting approach tends to make the weighted sample more representative of the population and, in particular, to avoid the risk when fewer variables are controlled of creating discrepancies between the weighted sample and the population on other variables that were originally nondiscrepant. A cross-tabulation of many variables, in comparison, would create an excessive number of cells with a small or zero sample size. Instead, in the regression-based approach, logistic regression analysis was able to produce a more stable estimate based on a dichotomous outcome that discriminated between the WMH sample and the population in an analysis that included both the sample data and individual-level population data. This prediction equation allowed for interactions among the poststratification variables and sequentially evaluated a wide range of predictors, arriving at a final model that included core variables (i.e., age, gender, education, geography) and significant discriminating variables. Appropriately weighted predicted probabilities generated from this final equation were used to adjust the final WMH sample to approximate the multivariate distribution of the population on these variables.

Although poststratification can potentially reduce sampling variances for survey estimates, the primary purpose of weighting is to eliminate potential sources of bias that would be present in an unweighted analysis. Those biases could arise due to differences in the original selection probabilities for respondents, differential nonresponse (probabilities of observation), and differential sample noncoverage for elements of the target population. However, the pursuit of "unbiasedness" can have a price in the form of increased variance of survey estimates compared to an unweighted estimate based on the same sample size. Weighting effects on standard errors arise due to several factors, including the association between the distributions of the weights and the variables of interest and variance of the weight values assigned to the individual cases. In the process of developing the final analysis weights for the WMH datasets, sensitivity analyses were conducted to determine the effect of extreme weight values on the estimated sampling errors and potential bias of key survey estimates. If sampling variances proved highly sensitive to the most extreme weight values, the computed weights in the extreme lower and upper ranges were trimmed using methods that retained the sum of weights but distributed those weights across cases at each tail of the distribution. This trimming was typically carried out for respondents with the highest and lowest 1%–2% of weights and in extreme cases for those in the highest and lowest 5% of weights. For a detailed example of how this was done in one WMH Survey, see Kessler et al. (2004).

Sampling error and inference from the WMH Survey data

The WMH Surveys are based on a variety of probability sample designs – each design adapted to the resources, experiences, and cost structures that are unique to the collaborating countries. Despite the variations in probability sample design, each survey is designed to support robust, design-based estimation of population statistics, such as prevalence of mental health in a chosen survey population.

The survey literature refers to designs like the ones used in the WMH Surveys as *complex designs*, a loosely used term meant to denote the fact that the sample incorporates special design features such as stratification, clustering, and differential selection probabilities (i.e., weighting) that analysts must consider in computing sampling errors and confidence intervals for sample estimates of descriptive statistics and model parameters. Standard programs in statistical analysis software packages assume simple random sampling (SRS) or independence of observations in computing standard errors for sample estimates. In general, the

SRS assumption results in underestimation of variances of estimates of descriptive statistics and model parameters from surveys with clustered or multistage designs. This means that the confidence intervals based on computed variances that assume independence of observations will be biased (generally too narrow) and design-based inferences will be affected accordingly. This section focuses on sampling error estimation and construction of confidence intervals for WMH Survey estimates of descriptive statistics such as means, proportions, ratios, and coefficients for linear and logistic regression models.

Over the past 50 years, advances in survey sampling theory have guided the development of a number of methods for estimating variances from complex sample datasets correctly. Several sampling error programs that implement these complex sample variance estimation methods are available to WMH data analysts. The two most common approaches are the Taylor Series Linearization method (and corresponding approximation to its variance) and resampling variance estimation methods such as the Balanced Repeated Replication method and the Jackknife Repeated Replication (JRR) method (Rust, 1985). The sampling error estimates presented in the substantive chapters of this volume were, for the most part, estimated in SUDAAN Version 9 (Research Triangle Institute, 2002) using the Taylor Series Linearization method, although some of the more complex estimates required the use of the JRR method, which we implemented in special SAS macros (SAS Institute Inc., 2008) written by staff of the WMH Data Collection Coordination Centre.

As noted earlier in this chapter in the discussion of the WMH sample designs, the WMH Surveys, like most other sample designs in health-related surveys, use stratification and clustering. Stratification is introduced to increase the statistical and administrative efficiency of the sample. Sample elements are selected as clusters in multistage designs to reduce travel costs and improve interviewing efficiency. Disproportionate sampling of population elements may be used to increase the sample sizes for subpopulations of special interest, resulting in the need to employ weighting in the estimation of population prevalence or other descriptive statistics. Relative to simple random sampling, each of these complex sample design features influences the size of standard errors for survey estimates. Figure 3.1 illustrates the effects of these design features on standard errors of estimates. The curve

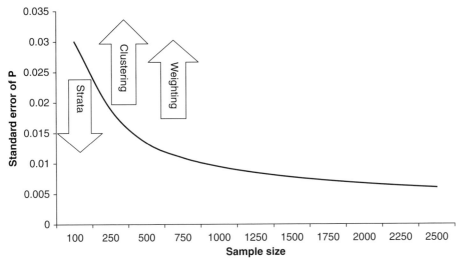

Figure 3.1. Complex sample design effects on standard errors of prevalence estimates. (Illustration for p = 0.10). Originally appeared in Heeringa et al. (2008). © 2008. World Health Organization. Used with permission.

plotted in this figure represents the SRS standard error of an estimate as a function of sample size. At any chosen sample size, the effect of sample stratification is generally a reduction in standard errors relative to SRS. Clustering of sample elements and designs that require weighting for unbiased estimation generally have larger standard errors than an SRS sample of equal size (Kish, 1965).

The combined effects of stratification, clustering, and weighting on the standard errors of estimates are termed the *design effect* (D^2) and are measured by the ratio:

$$D^2 = \frac{SE(p)^2_{complex}}{SE(p)^2_{srs}} = \frac{Var(p)_{complex}}{Var(p)_{srs}}$$

where:

D^2 = the design effect;

$Var(p)_{complex}$ = the complex sample design variance of the sample statistic p;

$Var(p)_{srs}$ = the simple random variance of p.

Table 3.2 provides the design effects for estimates of the lifetime prevalence of the suicidal behaviors that are the focus of analysis in this volume. With only a small number of exceptions, design effects are greater than 1.0 but relatively modest in elevation, with the mean across countries being 1.7 for suicide ideation, 1.5 for suicide plans, 1.3 for suicide attempts, 1.4 for suicide plans among ideators, 1.3 for suicide attempts among ideators, 1.3 for attempts among planners, and

1.4 for attempts among ideators without a plan. The same general patterns hold for 12-month prevalence of suicidal behaviors (see Appendix Table 3.1).

Design effects are for the most part somewhat larger when results are pooled across countries compared to when they are estimated within countries. For example, the range of mean design effects across outcomes in the total sample is 1.4–2.1 compared to 1.1–1.6 for within-country mean design effects. It needs to be remembered, though, that the sample size increases dramatically when data are combined across countries, resulting in substantial decreases in standard errors of estimates despite these relatively small increases in design effects.

Measures

Suicidal behavior

We have had a preview of the main suicidal behaviors in Table 3.2. These behaviors were assessed in the WMH Surveys in a special module that included an assessment of the lifetime occurrence, age-of-onset (AOO), and recency of suicide ideation, plans, and attempts. Based on evidence that reports of such potentially embarrassing behaviors are higher in self-administered than interviewer-administered surveys (Turner et al., 1998), these questions were printed in a self-administered booklet and referred to by letter. For example, the question about suicide ideation was

Table 3.2. Design effects of lifetime prevalence estimates of suicide ideation, plans, and attempts in the WMH Surveys[a]

Country specific	In the total sample			Among 12-month ideators			
	Ideation	Plan	Attempt	Plan	Attempt	Attempt among planners	Attempt among non-planners
I. Low- and lower-middle-income countries							
Colombia	2.1	1.9	1.7	1.7	1.5	1.5	2.4
India-Pondicherry	1.0	0.9	1.3	0.7	1.3	1.2	1.4
Nigeria	1.2	1.0	0.9	1.4	1.3	1.1	0.8
China-Beijing, China-Shanghai	1.1	1.6	1.5	1.6	1.4	1.3	1.4
China-Shenzhen	2.1	1.8	2.3	1.8	2.2	1.0	3.0
China (total)	1.8	1.8	1.9	1.8	1.8	1.1	2.3
Ukraine	1.5	1.2	1.3	1.1	1.3	1.1	1.4
II. Upper-middle-income countries							
Brazil	1.4	1.1	1.0	1.4	1.2	1.0	2.7
Bulgaria	1.3	1.0	0.5	1.1	0.7	0.7	0.8
Lebanon	2.8	2.3	1.7	1.2	1.3	1.3	1.3
Mexico	2.0	1.6	1.9	1.5	1.8	2.0	1.4
Romania	1.5	1.0	1.1	0.7	1.3	2.2	1.0
South Africa	2.5	1.6	1.4	0.9	1.2	1.4	1.0
III. High-income countries							
Belgium	2.6	1.6	0.9	1.1	0.8	0.7	0.3
France	1.4	1.1	1.3	1.6	1.3	1.1	1.4
Germany	1.9	1.5	1.5	1.3	1.2	1.3	1.3
Israel	1.0	1.2	1.2	1.2	1.2	1.1	1.0
Italy	1.1	1.4	1.8	1.2	1.8	1.2	1.4
Japan	1.0	1.3	0.9	1.3	1.0	0.9	0.7
Netherlands	1.1	2.0	1.2	2.2	1.1	0.9	1.4
New Zealand	2.5	2.2	1.8	1.9	1.7	1.8	1.7
Spain	1.6	1.8	1.0	1.8	1.0	1.2	1.5
United States	1.9	1.8	1.6	1.6	2.0	2.2	1.4
IV. Cross-national combination of countries							
Low-income countries	1.6	1.4	1.4	1.4	1.5	1.2	2.1
Middle-income countries	1.9	1.4	1.4	1.3	1.4	1.4	1.8
High-income countries	2.2	1.9	1.5	1.7	1.5	1.7	1.4
Total	2.1	1.7	1.4	1.5	1.5	1.5	1.6

[a] As described in more detail in the text, the design effect (DE) is the square of the ratio of the standard error of the prevalence estimate using design-based methods divided by the standard error of the prevalence estimate assuming a simple random sample. DE represents the extent to which the design-based sample would have to increase in size to obtain the same standard error as that obtained in a simple random sample of the observed size. For example, the DE of 2.1 in Colombia means that the Part 2 sample of 2381 respondents would have to be 5238 (i.e., 2.1 × 2381) to achieve a design-based standard error equal in size to the standard error in a simple random sample of 2381 respondents.

asked by referring the respondent to a particular page in the Respondent Booklet (RB; see Subsection: Question comprehension) and asked "Did experience A ever happen to you?" In the RB, the entry under A was "You seriously thought about committing suicide". In cases in which the respondent was unable to read, the interviewer read the questions aloud.

Respondents who reported the lifetime occurrence of suicide ideation were asked about AOO ("How old were you the first time this happened?") and about 12-month prevalence ("Did experience A happen at any time in the past 12 months?"). Among respondents who no longer had ideation in the 12 months before the interview, we then asked about recency of ideation ("How old were you the last time this experience happened to you?"). This series was followed by a parallel series of questions about lifetime occurrence, AOO, 12-month occurrence, and recency of suicide plans ("Experience B: You made a plan for committing suicide") and suicide attempts ("Experience C: You attempted suicide"). In the case of suicide attempts, we also asked about number of lifetime attempts and about the methods used in the first and most recent attempts.

Mental disorders

As noted earlier in this chapter, mental disorders were assessed with the WHO Composite International Diagnostic Interview (CIDI; Kessler & Üstün, 2004), a fully structured lay-administered research diagnostic interview. DSM-IV criteria were used in making diagnoses. The disorders assessed include anxiety disorders (panic disorder, generalized anxiety disorder, specific phobia, social phobia, agoraphobia with or without a history of panic disorder, posttraumatic stress disorder (PTSD), obsessive-compulsive disorder, separation anxiety disorder), mood disorders (major depressive disorder, dysthymic disorder, bipolar disorder), disruptive behavior disorders (oppositional-defiant disorder, conduct disorder, intermittent explosive disorder, eating disorders, pathological gambling disorder), substance disorders (alcohol and drug abuse and dependence among abusers, nicotine dependence), and a screen for non-affective psychosis. In each case, the CIDI assessed lifetime prevalence of the disorder and then obtained retrospective data about AOO, 12-month prevalence, and recency.

A clinical reappraisal study using the DSM-IV Axis I Disorders, Research Version, Non-patient Edition of the Structured Clinical Interview for DSM-IV (SCID;

First et al., 2002) was carried out in several high-income WMH countries, and generally good concordance was found between diagnoses based on the CIDI and clinical diagnoses based on blinded clinical re-interviews (Haro et al., 2006; Haro et al., 2008).

Concordance of lifetime diagnosis based on the CIDI with diagnoses based on blinded SCID clinical reappraisal interviews was good for the majority of diagnoses considered, with the area under the receiver operator characteristic curve (AUC; Hanley & McNeil, 1982), a measure of concordance that is relatively insensitive to disorder prevalence (Kraemer et al., 2003), in the range 0.7–0.8. Concordance was higher, in comparison, for bipolar disorder, agoraphobia, and alcohol abuse (AUC in the range 0.8 to >0.9) and in the range 0.6–0.7 for specific phobia, social phobia, PTSD, and drug dependence. The majority of SCID cases were detected by the CIDI (SN) for anxiety disorders (54.4%; 38.3%–62.6%), major depression (55.3%), bipolar disorder (86.8%), substance dependence (73.6%), and any disorder (62.8%). Concordance was also assessed for 12-month disorders. Because of the narrower time frame, though, the number of respondents with individual CIDI disorders was much smaller than for lifetime prevalence. As a result, CIDI-SCID 12-month diagnostic consistency was assessed by focusing on summary measures of any anxiety disorder, any mood disorder, and any overall disorder. Concordance for 12-month prevalence was substantial (AUC in the range 0.8–0.9) for any mood disorder, any anxiety disorder, and any overall disorder. The majority of 12-month SCID cases were detected by the CIDI for any anxiety (83.7%), any mood (69.1%), and any overall disorder (77.9%).

Other measures

The CIDI measures a great many other variables that were used in the analyses reported in this volume. In addition to basic sociodemographics, these include measures of a variety of variables that are thought to be causal risk factors for the onset and/or persistence of suicidal behaviors, including parental psychopathology when respondents were young, other childhood adversities (e.g., physical and sexual abuse, neglect, family violence), other lifetime traumatic stresses, mental disorders, and physical disorders. The Chapters in Section 3 of this volume are organized by these presumed risk factors. Rather than describe them here, all of these measures other than respondent mental disorders are introduced in the chapters where they are the central focus.

CIDI version 3.0 modifications

Retrospective reporting of lifetime suicidal behaviors, mental disorders, childhood adversities, and other traumatic stressors plays a central part in the analyses presented in this volume. We use those retrospective reports as the bases for survival analyses, which are discussed later in this chapter, and we use reports about differences in ages of first occurrence of risk factors and suicidal behaviors to generate estimates of the associations of temporally prior predictors with the subsequent first onset and persistence of suicidal behaviors. It is important, in light of this central role of retrospective reports, that considerable evidence suggests that these reports can be inaccurate (Giuffra & Risch, 1994; Moffitt et al., 2010; Patten, 2003; Simon & Von Korff, 1995). Two main types of evidence exist. The first comes from analyses of AOO reports in cross-sectional surveys, which show implausible distributions (Patten, 2003; Simon et al., 1995). The typical pattern is for AOO reports to be too recent. For example, Simon and colleagues (Simon et al., 1995) found that close to half of all reported lifetime cases of major depression in one survey reported first lifetime onsets within five years before the interview no matter how old the respondent. Simulations show that this kind of implausible data pattern can be reproduced by assuming a relatively plausible rate of recall failure that accumulates over time (Giuffra & Risch, 1994; Patten, 2003).

The second kind of evidence comes from longitudinal surveys in which respondents are followed over time and interviewed repeatedly. Surveys of this type often find that respondents report lifetime disorders in follow-up interviews that they did not report in their first interviews but that are subsequently reported to have started prior to their first interviews. These differences are sometimes very substantial. In the Epidemiologic Catchment Area (ECA) study, for example, when respondents were interviewed a second time either six or twelve months after their original interview, consolidated lifetime prevalence estimates increased by as much as 50% (Eaton et al., 1989). It is, of course, implausible to think that the number of lifetime mental disorders actually increased this dramatically in such a short period of time and, in fact, retrospective AOO reports in the follow-up survey

showed that the vast majority of newly reported lifetime disorders in the follow-up interview were said to have started many years earlier than the baseline interview. In addition, longitudinal studies that assess recent prevalence of mental disorders in each interview show that cumulative lifetime prevalence estimates far exceed the lifetime prevalence estimates obtained in cross-section surveys using retrospective reports (Moffitt et al., 2010; Patten, 2009).

These problems with lifetime reporting are not unique to interviews about mental disorders. The same sorts of problems have been recognized by survey methodologists for years and a considerable amount of methodological research has been carried out by survey methodologists to address these problems (e.g., Sudman et al., 1996; Tanur, 1992; Turner & Martin, 1985). This research has advanced considerably over the past two decades as cognitive psychologists have become interested in the survey interview as a natural laboratory for studying cognitive processes (Schwarz & Sudman, 1994; Schwarz & Sudman, 1996; Sirken et al., 1999). A number of important insights have emerged from these studies about practical ways to improve the accuracy of retrospective reports. However, psychiatric epidemiologists have been largely unaware of these developments and consequently have not used them to improve their assessments of lifetime mental disorders.

These insights and methods were used, though, to develop CIDI 3.0, the instrument used in the WMH Surveys (Kessler & Üstün, 2004; Kessler & Üstün, 2008). We review the aspects of these improvements most relevant to the study of suicidal behavior in this subsection. Before doing so, though, we note that methodological analyses of the WMH data provide compelling evidence for the success of these improvements. This is true in two ways. First, the problem found in previous psychiatric epidemiological surveys of AOO reports being substantially over-represented in the five years before interview do not occur in the WMH Surveys (Kessler et al., 2007b; Kessler et al., 2008). The distributions of AOO reports are much more substantively plausible and, in fact, are very consistent with those obtained in long-term longitudinal studies that follow cohorts of respondents from childhood through adulthood (Kessler et al., 2007a). Second, a ten-year follow-up survey of the respondents in the WMH Survey carried out in the U.S. did not find the problem seen in previous longitudinal psychiatric epidemiological surveys of a large number of respondents in the follow-up who reported pre-baseline lifetime disorders that were not noted in the baseline interview (Borges et al., 2008).

These improvements were achieved by beginning with evaluations of problems in earlier versions of the CIDI made by survey methodologists in preparation for an earlier U.S. survey that was the foundation for the WMH Surveys (Kessler et al., 1998; Kessler et al., 1999; Kessler et al., 2000). Four main methodological challenges highlighted in those evaluations that became the focus of CIDI 3.0 revision efforts are: (1) that respondents might not understand some of the CIDI questions about lifetime prevalence, a number of which include multiple clauses and vaguely defined terms; (2) that some respondents might not understand the task implied by the lifetime prevalence questions, which requires careful memory search that is unlikely to be carried out unless respondents are clearly instructed to do so; (3) that respondents might not be motivated to put in the hard work required to think back over their entire lives and answer lifetime recall questions accurately, especially in light of the fact that many CIDI questions deal with potentially embarrassing and stigmatizing experiences; and (4) that respondents might not be able to answer some CIDI questions accurately, especially those that ask about characteristics of mental disorders that are difficult to remember. Age-of-onset comes in as especially important as part of this fourth challenge, as previous research has shown that age-of-onset is often difficult to recall accurately even when respondents are motivated to do so (Belli, 1998; Prohaska et al., 1998). The strategies used in CIDI 3.0 to address these four challenges are discussed in detail elsewhere (Kessler & Üstün, 2004; Kessler & Üstün, 2008) and will only be briefly reviewed here.

Question comprehension

It is obvious that ambiguous questions are likely to be misconstrued, but it is perhaps less obvious just how ambiguous most structured survey is questions are and how often respondents must "read between the lines" to make sense of questions. Debriefing studies of earlier versions of the CIDI found that a great many respondents misunderstood important aspects of key diagnostic questions. The reason for this lies partly in the fact that many terms in surveys are vaguely defined. But beyond this is the more fundamental fact that the survey interview situation is a special kind of interaction in which the standard rules of conversation – rules that help fill in the gaps in

meaning that exist in most speech – do not apply. Unlike the situation in normal conversational practice, the respondent in the survey interview often has only a vague notion of the person to whom he is talking or the purpose of the conversation (Cannell et al., 1968). The person who asks the questions (the interviewer) is not the person who formulated the questions (the researcher), and the questioner is often unable to clarify the respondent's uncertainties about the intent of the questions. Furthermore, the flow of questions in the survey interview is established prior to the beginning of the conversation, which means that normal conversational rules of give and take in question and answer sequences do not apply. This leads to more misreading than in normal conversations even when questions are seemingly straightforward (Clark & Schober, 1992), a problem that is compounded when the topic of the interview is one that involves emotional experiences that are, in many cases, difficult to describe with clarity.

In an effort to investigate this problem, debriefing interviews were carried out with community respondents who were administered sections of the CIDI and were asked to explain what they thought the questions meant and why they answered the way they did (Kessler et al., 1998; Kessler, 1999). Four discriminating features were found among questions that had high versus low levels of misunderstanding. First, some questions were too complex. Second, some questions involved vaguely defined terms. Third, some questions asked about odd experiences that could plausibly be interpreted in more than one way, such as questions about seeing and hearing things that others do not. Many respondents were found to have a tendency to normalize these questions and to respond positively when the correct answer was actually negative. Fourth, some questions were misunderstood because of *contextual* misunderstanding; that is, a misunderstanding that derived more from the position of the question in the flow of the interview than from lack of clarity in the question.

Based on these results, we carried out detailed CIDI debriefing interviews with volunteer respondents in methodological studies to support the development of CIDI 3.0 by pinpointing questions with each of the above four types of comprehension problems. Misunderstandings based on complex questions were addressed by breaking down the original CIDI questions into less complex subquestions. Especially complex questions were presented in a Respondent

Booklet that provided a visual aid to respondents as the questions were being read by the interviewer. Misunderstandings based on the vagueness of terms were addressed by introducing clarifications and examples. Misunderstandings based on normalization of questions about odd experiences were addressed by prefacing the questions with clarification that we were actually asking about odd experiences and informing respondents that it was important for us to learn how often these experiences occur. Contextual misunderstandings were resolved by reordering questions to remove the contextual effects and by adding clarifying clauses in questions where residual confusion might exist. The number of modifications of this sort was large, see Kessler, R. C., & Üstün, T. B. (2008) pp. 85–90 for one example of each of the main types of modifications.

Task comprehension

Respondents also sometimes misunderstand the fundamental task they are being asked to carry out. Debriefing studies showed this was especially common with the diagnostic stem questions in the CIDI (Kessler et al., 2000). These stem questions are the first questions asked in each diagnostic section. They are used to determine whether a lifetime syndrome of a particular sort might have ever occurred. These questions provide what are, in effect, brief vignettes and ask the respondent whether they ever had an experience of this sort. If a diagnostic stem question is endorsed, additional questions are asked to assess the specifics of the syndrome. If all diagnostic stem questions for a particular disorder are denied, the remaining questions about this syndrome are skipped.

Our methodological studies found that substantial confusion arises from respondent failure to understand the purpose of diagnostic stem questions. In particular, only about half of pilot respondents in our studies of the earlier version of CIDI interpreted these questions as they were intended; namely, as a request to engage in active memory search and to report the lifetime occurrence of episodes of the sort in the question. The other respondents interpreted the question as a request to report whether a memory of such an episode was readily accessible. These latter respondents did not believe that they were being asked to engage in active memory search and did not do so. Not surprisingly, the latter respondents were much less likely than those who understood the intent of the question to remember lifetime episodes.

Why did so many respondents misinterpret the intent of these lifetime recall questions? As Marquis and Cannell (1969) discovered in their early research on standard interview practice, respondents are generally ill informed about the purposes of the research and poorly motivated to participate actively. Furthermore, cues from interviewers often reinforce the inclination of respondents to participate in a halfhearted way. For example, when an interviewer asks a question that requires considerable thought, the respondent is likely to assume, in the absence of instructions to the contrary, that the interviewer is operating under normal conversational rules and, as such, is really asking for an immediate and appropriate answer. Cannell and colleagues (1981) showed that this conversational artifact can be minimized by explicitly instructing respondents to answer completely and accurately and that the use of such instruction can substantially improve the quality of data obtained in surveys. Based on this result, we built in clarifying statements throughout CIDI 3.0 aimed at informing respondents that accuracy was important. The number of modifications of this sort was large, see Kessler, R. C., & Üstün, T. B. (2008) pp. 85–90 for one example of each of the main types of modifications.

Motivation

One problem with emphasizing to respondents the need to work hard at a series of demanding and potentially embarrassing recall tasks is that more respondents than otherwise may refuse to engage in the task. Recognition of this problem among survey methodologists has led to the development of motivational techniques intended to increase the chances that respondents will accept the job of answering completely and accurately. Two techniques that have proven to be particularly useful in this regard were used in CIDI 3.0. The first is the use of motivational components in instructions; that is, introductory remarks at the beginning of a survey that clarify the research aims in order to motivate respondents to provide a more complete and accurate report than they would otherwise. Respondents are known to be willing to undertake laborious and possibly painful memory searches if they recognize some altruistic benefit of doing so (Cannell et al., 1981). Based on this evidence, we developed and presented a statement containing a clear rationale for administering the interview and emphasized the importance of the survey for social policy purposes.

The second technique is contingent reinforcement embedded in the interviewer feedback probes. Consistent with research on behavioral modification of verbal productions through reinforcement (e.g., Centers, 1963), several survey researchers have demonstrated that verbal reinforcers such as "thanks" and "that's useful" can significantly affect the behavior of survey respondents (Marquis & Cannell, 1969). Based on this observation, Cannell and his associates developed a method for training interviewers to use systematic feedback – both positive and negative – to reinforce respondent effort in reporting (Oksenberg et al., 1979). The central feature of this method is the use of structured feedback statements coordinated with the content and timing of instructions aimed at reinforcing respondent performance. It is important to recognize that it is performance that is being reinforced rather than the content of particular answers. For example, a difficult recall question may be prefaced with the instruction "This next question may be difficult, so please take your time before answering". In contingent feedback instruction, interviewers issue some expression of gratitude whenever the respondent seems to consider his or her answer carefully, whether they remember anything or not. Alternatively, the interviewer might instruct the precipitous respondent: "You answered that awfully quickly. Was there anything (else), even something small?" Such invitations to reconsider would occur whenever the respondent gives an immediate answer, whether or not anything was reported. Experiments document clearly that the combined use of these contingent reinforcement probes with instructions explaining the importance of careful and accurate reporting leads to substantial improvement in recall of health-related events in general population surveys, including validated dates of medical events (Miller & Cannell, 1977; Vinokur et al., 1979). Importantly, their results also showed that self-enhancing response biases are reduced when these strategies are used, as indicated by both a decreased tendency to under-report potentially embarrassing conditions and behaviors (e.g., gynecological problems, seeing an X-rated movie) and a decreased tendency to over-report self-enhancing behaviors (e.g., number of books read in the last three months, having read the editorial page of the newspaper the previous day). Based on these results, the contingent feedback approach was included as a fundamental part of the interviewer training materials developed for CIDI 3.0.

The ability to answer accurately

Research on basic cognitive processes has shown that memories are organized and stored in structured sets of information packages commonly called schemas (Markus & Zajonc, 1985). When the respondent has a history of many instances of the same experience that cannot be discriminated, the separate instances tend to blend together in memory to form a special kind of memory schema called a "semantic memory," a general memory for a prototypical experience (Jobe et al., 1990; Means & Loftus, 1991). For example, the person may have a semantic memory of what panic attacks are like but, due to the fact that he has had many such attacks in his lifetime, cannot specify details of any particular panic attack. In comparison, when a respondent has had only a small number of lifetime experiences of a certain sort or when one instance stands out in memory as much different from the others, a memory can likely be recovered for that particular episode. This is called an "episodic memory."

In the case of memories of illness experiences, memory schemas tend to include not only semantic memories of prototypic symptoms but also personal theories about causes, course, and cure (Leventhal et al., 1984; Skelton & Croyle, 1991). Some of these theories will conceptualize the experience in illness terms, while other theories will conceptualize the experience as a moral failing, a punishment from God, or a normal reaction to stress (Gilman, 1988). These interpretations can influence the extent to which different memory cues are capable of triggering the schemas. The effects of memory schemas and the difference between semantic and episodic memories are central themes in research on autobiographical memory. In the survey context, a critical issue related to this research is whether the respondent is able to recover episodic memories in answering a particular survey question or if the respondent is answering the question by drawing inferences of what the past must have been like on the basis of more general semantic memories.

Research shows that people are more likely to recover episodic memories for experiences that are recent, distinctive, and unique, while people are more likely to rely on semantic memories for experiences that are frequent, typical, and regular (Belli, 1988; Brewer, 1986; Menon, 1994). When a survey question is designed to ask about a particular instance of an experience, it must be posed in such a way that the respondent knows he is being asked to recover an episodic memory. Furthermore, the researcher must have some basis for assuming that an episodic memory can be recovered for this experience. If it cannot, a question that asks for such a memory implicitly invites the respondent to guess rather than to remember and this can have adverse effects on quality of reporting later in the interview (Pearson et al., 1992). In comparison, when a question is designed to recover a semantic memory or to use semantic memories to arrive at an answer by estimation, that should be made clear.

One difficulty with these injunctions in the case of retrospective recall questions about lifetime mental disorders is uncertainty about what level of recall accuracy to expect. Therefore, as part of the CIDI pilot work in preparation for the WMH Surveys, we debriefed pilot respondents with an explicit eye toward pinpointing questions that were difficult to answer on the basis of episodic memory. When questions of this sort were discovered, an attempt was made to revise the questions to reduce the memory problem either by allowing explicitly for estimation (e.g., explicitly asking respondents to provide a rough estimate), by providing categorical responses that reduce the complexity of the task, or by decomposing the question into subquestions that mimic effective memory search processes.

Age-of-onset questions are of special importance in this regard, as our pilot data showed that some people had quite a vivid memory of their first (and often only) episode of some mental disorders, especially when these disorders had rapid onsets, as in the case of panic attacks, whereas other people had only a vague memory of their first onset. The latter cases tended to involve accretion disorders (i.e., disorders that come on slowly) that occurred to people who subsequently had a great many other episodes. Based on a good deal of exploratory pilot work, we finally developed an approach to this problem that proved to be simple and very effective: to ask people at the beginning of the AOO sequence if they had a *clear* memory of their first episode. As it turned out, the vast majority of people are able to answer this meta-question with no difficulty. We then varied subsequent questions depending on the answer to that first question. Respondents who reported having a clear memory were asked a follow-up question that simply asked them for their age when that first episode occurred. Respondents who reported not having a clear memory,

in comparison, were asked a more complex set of questions about the earliest age they could clearly remember a particular episode and their best estimate of *about* how old they were when they had their first episode. We carried out an experimental study to evaluate the effects of these questions by randomly assigning a group of community respondents to receive either a standard AOO question or our more complex series of AOO probes. The results were dramatic in showing that our new AOO probes resulted in much more substantially plausible AOO reports than those obtained in response to standard AOO questions (Knäuper et al., 1999). In particular, the implausible pattern found in earlier studies of AOO reported clustered in the five years before interview was not found in responses to our AOO questions.

Combining strategies

We also used some additional strategies to deal with two or more of these problems at once. The most important of these is a life review section that we developed for use in CIDI 3.0 near the beginning of the interview in an effort both to motivate and to facilitate active memory search in answering diagnostic stem questions. This section starts out with an introduction that explains to respondents that the next questions might be difficult to answer because they require respondents to review their entire lives. The introduction then goes on to say that despite this difficulty it is very important for the research that these questions are answered accurately. The introduction ends with the injunction to "please take your time and think carefully before answering".

The diagnostic stem questions for all core CIDI diagnoses are administered directly following this commitment question. The questions are all included in the RB with a written instruction to "take your time and think carefully before answering". Interviewers are instructed to read the diagnostic stem questions slowly in an effort to emphasize their importance and to use motivational probes to encourage active memory search. Our intent in developing this section was both to explain the serious and difficult nature of the task and to motivate respondents to engage in the active memory search we hoped to stimulate by combining all the stem questions after a fairly detailed motivational introduction. We also recognized, based on our debriefing studies, that CIDI respondents quickly learn the logic of the stem–branch structure after a few sections and recognize that they can shorten the interview considerably by saying no to the stem questions. This problem is removed by asking all the stem questions near the beginning of the interview before the logic of the stem–branch structure becomes clear. Another important reason for including the section near the beginning of the interview is that pilot study respondents told us in debriefing interviews that their energy flagged as the interview progressed, making it much more difficult to carry out a serious memory search later in the interview than at the beginning.

We carried out an experiment to evaluate the effects of using this lifetime review section in conjunction with motivational probes. A random sample of 200 community respondents was randomized either to an earlier version of CIDI or to a version that was identical except that it included the life review section at the beginning of the interview. As reported in more detail elsewhere (Kessler et al., 1998), this experiment documented that the life review section led to a significant increase in the proportion of respondents who endorsed diagnostic stem questions. For example, while 26.7% of respondents in the standard CIDI condition endorsed a diagnostic stem question for major depression, a significantly higher 40.6% did so in the life review condition. Importantly, a clinical validity study documented that this increased prevalence of stem endorsement was not accompanied by a reduction in sensitivity with regard to clinical diagnoses, documenting that additional true cases were discovered by the use of the life review section and the accompanying commitment and motivation probes. These results were the basis of adopting the lifetime review section in CIDI 3.0.

Translation

The innovations in CIDI 3.0 measurement were all developed initially in English. One of the fundamental challenges in an undertaking such as the WMH Survey Initiative is to achieve both equivalence in meaning and consistency in measurement across surveys and have multiple languages. This is a special challenge in studying mental disorders, as the symptoms of mental disorders are described and interpreted differently in different cultures (Cheng, 2001; Prince & Tcheng-Laroche, 1987), making it necessary in some cases to use substantially different terms or even questions in different countries to assess the presence versus absence of these symptoms. Another complexity is that the CIDI

source language, English, has a larger lexicon (stock of vocabulary) than any other known language. This can mean that distinctions made in English cannot be matched in one or more target languages. The opposite can also be true with respect to certain areas of lexical or grammatical distinctions, in which the source language may not specify enough detail necessary for translation into a given target language.

WMH collaborators were given guidelines for translation and adaptation of the CIDI aimed at achieving both equivalence in meaning and consistency in measurement across surveys. A detailed discussion of these guidelines is presented elsewhere (Harkness et al., 2008) and will not be repeated here. We merely note that these guidelines were modifications of longstanding WHO guidelines for translation and back-translations that were updated by the staff of the WHO Data Collection Coordination Centre under the direction of B. E. Pennell in collaboration with the WMH Co-Principal Investigators.

Countries were instructed that the central aim of the translation process was to achieve target language versions of the English questionnaire that were *conceptually equivalent* in each of the countries/cultures rather than literal equivalence in terms of word-for-word translation. It was emphasized that the translation should sound natural in each language (in as far as that is possible in standardized instruments) and to perform in comparable fashion across the populations and languages. Independent assessors who were experts on cross-national translation reviewed the CIDI translations and found that these aims were generally achieved, but that some of the translations were, at times, too close to the English questionnaire language formulation and structure to sound "natural".

Countries were required to follow a six-step process in achieving these aims. These steps included: (1) forward translation; (2) expert panel review; (3) independent back-translation; (4) harmonization of vocabulary and formulation across different country versions of a shared language (if appropriate); (5) pretesting and cognitive interviewing; and (6) final revision, creation, and documentation of a final version of the translated questionnaire. A detailed description of each of these steps is presented elsewhere (Harkness et al., 2008).

Pretesting

Consistent with best-practices recommendations (Converse & Presser, 1986; Groves et al., 2004;

Harkness et al., 2004; Sheatsley, 1983; Smith, 2004), pretests of the instrument and procedures were carried out in each WMH Survey prior to main study implementation. The pretests were designed to mirror the main study in most aspects, except in some cases using experienced interviewers for pretest data collection. Pretest interviews were evaluated by debriefing interviewers to identify potential problem areas with the instrument and survey procedures, checking the distributions of items for high rates of missing data and out-of-range values, and using behavior coding of audio-taped pretest interviews to pinpoint questions that were often misread or often elicited respondent requests for clarification.

Pretesting is especially important in cross-national studies (Smith 2004) because of the challenges associated with working in many different languages and social contexts (Smith 2004). A separate series of pretests was consequently required in each WMH country. Initial pretests focused on evaluating the translations. Later pretests evaluated the interview schedule and field procedures. The number of the latter pretest rounds varied from one to three, with approximately two-thirds of the countries conducting just one round of pretests and most others two rounds. The pretest debriefing sessions identified country-specific difficulties with questionnaire wording and response categories that were modified prior to the beginning of production interviewing. These sessions, along with quantitative analyses of responses, also detected skip pattern errors in the PAPI version and programming errors in the CAPI version that were corrected prior to the beginning of production interviewing. The pretests also allowed the investigators to evaluate the adequacy of survey procedures and sample management systems.

Interviewer training and quality control monitoring

Although large-scale cross-national surveys have been undertaken for decades (Heath et al., 2005 provide a concise history), there is surprisingly little written research on the practical aspects of training and supervising interviewers to achieve high-quality survey data. The necessity of cultural adaptation of survey methods is widely recognized in order to achieve equivalence in measurement across countries (Bulmer, 1998; Jowell, 1998; Kuechler, 1998; Lynn, 2001). However, few details are provided in the literature as to how to

achieve this equivalence across the many phases of a project's development. In the absence of such standards of practice, many cross-national projects have been left to accept the research traditions of individual countries, which vary widely in methodological rigor. An approach at the other extreme is to implement a "one-size-fits-all" methodology that naively imposes the same procedure and protocols across all countries and cultures based on the assumption that good practice in one culture will be good practice in other cultures (Harkness et al., 2002).

The WMH Survey Initiative sought to implement an approach between these two extremes by establishing guidelines that set minimum standards for each phase of project implementation but allowed for country-specific adaptations. We saw this earlier in the chapter in the discussion of probability sampling methods that allowed for country-specific variations. The difficulty for the staff of the WMH Data Collection Coordination Centre was determining when variations in approach were necessary and appropriate rather than simply expedient. Staying with the above sampling example, survey organizations in some parts of the world have a tradition of quota sampling and respondent substitution that violates the WMH requirement of probability sampling. This kind of potential conflict between local practice and best practices was found in every phase of the WMH Survey implementation.

A detailed description of the WMH data quality control standards established by the WMH Data Collection Coordination Centre and the ways in which these standards were implemented in the individual WMH countries is presented elsewhere (Pennell et al., 2008). These standards were subsequently used by the senior members of the WMH Data Collection Coordination Centre to take the lead in developing internationally recognized guidelines for best practices in cross-national comparative survey research more generally (www.ccsg.isr.umich.edu). Issues of interviewer recruitment and training, research ethics, field structure, data collection procedures and quality control, and data preparation are all included in these guidelines. We will not discuss here the main practical decisions made in establishing WMH field procedures, such as the decision to have interviews carried out face-to-face rather than by telephone and the decision to use both paper and pencil and computer-assisted versions of the survey and to allow individual countries to choose which of the two modes they were able to use, but refer the reader to a detailed discussion of these decisions elsewhere (Pennell et al., 2008).

Interviewer hiring and training

The previous section made it clear that CIDI 3.0 is a complex instrument. Successful implementation of such an instrument requires interviewers to be highly trained. We consequently placed high importance on careful interviewer training and quality assurance monitoring. In some countries, the research team was responsible for interviewer recruitment and management, while in other countries the interviewing component was subcontracted to an external survey organization. Before starting the interviewer recruitment and training process, each country sent at least two interviewer supervisors to a "train-the-trainer" session presented by the WMH Data Collection Coordination Centre at the University of Michigan in the U.S. These sessions lasted an average of six days and were designed to prepare the interviewer supervisors to train and monitor interviewer performance, as well as to manage data collection and data processing in their country. Through these sessions, research teams obtained all of the information and materials necessary to train their own interviewing staff using consistent procedures. These trainers, who in almost all countries came from a pool of experienced interviewers, then trained a team of supervisors to help in interviewer recruitment, training, and field quality control monitoring. Many countries were required to recruit and hire new interviewers for the WMH Survey, while others were able to use existing field staff from ongoing survey organizations. In most countries where new interviewers were recruited, recruitment was carried out in the general population. In a few countries, though, interviewers were recruited exclusively from among college students. Careful centralized screening procedures were used in this hiring process.

Interviewer training was divided into two parts: general interviewing techniques and CIDI-specific training. General interviewing training (GIT) was designed to introduce interviewers to the basic components of standardized questionnaire administration (e.g., question reading, appropriate techniques for probing and seeking clarification, providing feedback, and accurate data recording). General interviewing training sessions ranged from two to three days in most countries. In addition, countries that used computer-assisted interviewing had a GIT component focused on computer hardware and software use. Some countries added other country-specific topics in their GIT session, such as New Zealand's inclusion of cultural empathy to Maori and Pacific Islander households and Colombia's special training on interacting with governmental authorities and armed guerrilla and paramilitary groups. All interviewers were required to demonstrate competence with GIT concepts and procedures through a variety of tests before moving on to study-specific training.

Study-specific training averaged 30 hours across countries. The content was presented as a mix of lecture and round-robin practice sessions focused on general project background and importance, rules for obtaining informed consent, definitions of eligibility and respondent selection procedures, specifics of the precise interview procedures, and discussion of production requirements. Hands-on practice was stressed throughout. Trainers assessed the skill level of each interviewer in small group exercises and often held tailored "after-hours" special sessions to address areas where interviewers needed additional assistance and practice. Most countries included in the training team a clinical consultant, typically a psychiatric social worker or clinical psychologist, who provided interviewers with background information about the kinds of symptoms of emotional problems they would encounter during production interviewing. This clinical contact person (CCP) was also a resource person for both interviewers and respondents during data collection to address the needs of respondents who might require a referral for follow-up and interviewers who might need to debrief after a particularly difficult interview. In most cases, the CCP was available to interviewers 24 hours a day, seven days a week. Many countries developed protocols that allowed interviewers to contact their CCP privately, without first going through a supervisor to provide interviewers a unique opportunity to speak freely about their own and their respondents' experiences.

Quality control monitoring

Importantly, all countries required interviewers to pass a certification test before being approved for production work. Interviewers who did not pass the certification process were either terminated from the project or received additional retraining and another opportunity to obtain certification. Interviewer training often continued during the production phase of the project through such means as periodic in-person seminars, telephone conference calls, and bulletins or newsletters.

Special procedures were also developed to monitor interviewer performance during production. Systematic monitoring is critical to survey data quality assurance (Billiet & Loosveldt, 1988; Fowler & Mangione, 1990). Consistent with best-practices guidelines for survey implementation (Biemer & Lyberg, 2003), four areas of performance were the main targets of quality assurance monitoring: detection and prevention of falsified information, compliance with the interviewing rules and guidelines set forth in the training manual, performance of non-interview tasks, and identification of interviewer–questionnaire interface problems.

These areas were evaluated by a number of methods including supervisor reinterview of selected cases, supervisor verification of key survey elements through spot recontact of respondents, direct observation of interviews, audio-recording, questionnaire review, analysis of performance and production measures, keystroke/trace file analysis (files that record keystrokes and movement of the interviewer through the computerized instrument), and mock interviews/tests of knowledge and practice. Interviewers were terminated from production interviewing if they were found through these methods not to be able to perform up to required standards. The recommended supervisor-to-interviewer ratio of one supervisor for every 8–10 interviewers was used in the majority of countries that used paper and pencil data collection, while lower ratios were used in countries with computer administration based on the greater control over the data collection process afforded by computerized interviewing (Lavrakas, 1993; Williams, 1986).

Statistical analysis methods

The outcome variables

The main focus of this volume is on the predictors of first lifetime onset of suicidal behaviors, predictors of the transitions among different suicidal behaviors, and predictors of the persistence of these behaviors over the life course. As noted in the subsection on measures, the CIDI assessed three lifetime suicidal behaviors: ideation, plans, and attempts, but plans and

attempts occur in the context of ideation, so it is also of interest to note examples of the *conditional* outcomes of suicide plans among people with preexisting lifetime ideation, suicide attempts among lifetime ideators with a preexisting plan, and suicide attempts among lifetime ideators without a preexisting plan. The third of these three represents people who made impulsive (i.e., unplanned) suicide attempts. As we will see in the next chapter, quite a high proportion of attempts are impulsive/unplanned and the risk factor profile of these attempts is rather different from the profile of planned attempts.

In the substance analyses of lifetime and 12-month prevalence reported in this volume, we focus primarily on five outcomes: the two unconditional outcomes of ideation and attempts in the total sample; and the three conditional outcomes of suicide plans among people with preexisting lifetime ideation, suicide attempts among lifetime ideators with a preexisting plan, and suicide attempts among lifetime ideators without a preexisting plan. In cases where sample sizes are too small for separate analyses of the last two conditional outcomes, we sometimes combine the two into a single measure of suicide among ideators with a statistical control for the existence of a plan.

Cumulative lifetime prevalence curves

For each of the previously given five outcomes (two unconditional and three conditional), we use simple cross-tabulations to calculate lifetime and 12-month prevalence in the total sample as well as in important subsamples. In addition, given that we asked about AOO of each suicidal behavior, we are able to calculate *cumulative lifetime probability* curves for each of these outcomes. The actuarial method (Halli et al., 1992) is used to make these calculations. The actuarial method is somewhat different from and preferable to the more conventional Kaplan-Meier method (Lee & Go, 1997) in the way it handles ties. A cumulative lifetime prevalence curve (also referred to as a survival curve), as the name implies, plots the probability of the outcome ever occurring as of a given age for every year of life. The values in the cumulative probability curve can never decrease with increasing age.

In the case of the three unconditional outcomes, the cumulative lifetime probability curves tell us about the age ranges at which suicidal behaviors are most likely to begin. The curves also give us information about the speed with which transitions typically occur between first onset of ideation and development of a suicide plan, between first development of a plan and first suicide attempt, and between first onset of ideation among ideators without a plan and first impulsive/unplanned suicide attempt. Subgroup analyses can then be used to investigate the extent to which these various transition rates differ depending on AOO of the earlier stage in the progression (e.g., whether unplanned/impulsive attempts are more likely to occur after early onset compared to later-onset ideation).

Predicting onset of suicidal behaviors

Discrete-time survival analysis with person–year used as the unit of analysis (Willett & Singer, 1993) was used to study the predictors of first onset of the five outcomes. The discrete-time approach was chosen over the more traditional Cox proportional hazards analysis approach for two reasons: because our information about timing of onsets was available only for discrete intervals of time (i.e., years of age); and because the discrete-time approach handles the use of multiple time-varying predictor variables, which is a central feature of our models, much more easily than does the Cox modeling approach (Clayton & Hills, 1993). The discrete-time models were operationalized as logistic regression models with person–year as the unit of analysis and first onset of the suicidal behaviors as outcomes. The predictors included the variables alluded to previously in the section on measures: socio-demographics, parental psychopathology and other childhood family adversities, other lifetime traumatic stresses, mental disorders, and physical disorders.

While some of these predictors are true of the respondent throughout his or her life (e.g., the respondent is either male or female and was born in a given country in a specific year), an important feature of the analysis is that many of these predictors are *time-varying*; that is, they occurred at a discrete time in the life course (e.g., the respondent's parents divorced when he/she was 14 years old; the respondent was sexually assaulted and developed posttraumatic stress disorder at age 16, finished junior college at age 20, and entered the labor force at age 21 years) and, in some cases, were reversed over time (e.g., the respondent married at age 22, divorced at age 29, and remarried at age 34 years). First onset of the suicidal behaviors of interest to us could have occurred either before or after the occurrence of any of these predictors. As a result,

in order to maintain the temporal sequence between predictors and outcomes, it is necessary to take timing into consideration in estimating risk factor models. We can do this using discrete-time survival analysis by coding each year of each respondent's life separately for each predictor and allowing values to change over time for a single individual depending on the timing of predictors. For example, the first 19 years of a given respondent's life might be coded as *never married*, the 20th through 29th years as *married*, the 30th through 34th years as *divorced*, and the 35th and subsequent years as *remarried*.

This kind of within-person variation in coding is easily achieved in the discrete-time survival approach because each year of each person's life is treated as a separate observational record. To be specific and using suicide ideation as an illustrative outcome: the total WMH sample we are working with consists of 109,377 respondents across 21 countries, 10,018 of whom reported ever having suicide ideation. The earliest retrospectively reported AOO of ideation was 4 years and the latest was 94 years. As all 109,377 respondents were older than 4 years at the time of interview, we could estimate a logistic regression equation in which we predicted onset of suicide ideation at age 4 in the total sample of 109,377 from characteristics of these respondents as of age 3 years. Given that only 38 respondents reported first onset of suicide ideation at age 4, there were 109,339 other respondents who never had suicide ideation as of age 4 years. However, as another 23 reported first onset of ideation at age 5, we could estimate a second logistic regression equation in this sample of 109,339 (i.e., 109,377–38) that predicted first onset of ideation as of age 5 from characteristics of these respondents as of age 4, and so on for first onsets at ages 6, 7, etc., up through age 94 years, yielding 91 separate equations (i.e., one for each age of life in the age range 4–94 years), each time reducing the sample under investigation to remove those respondents who had first onsets prior to the index year and also excluding respondents who were younger at the time of interview than the age under investigation.

Given that the number of first onsets will be low in each of these 91 years considered one at a time, there will be little statistical power to detect significant effects in any of the 91 equations. This problem can be resolved, though, by pooling across years; that is, by stacking the 109,377 person–year observations in the equation for age 4 years with the 109,339 observations in the equation for age 5, etc., into a single data file, including a separate dummy variable for each person–year to distinguish among the 91 component data files, and estimating a single pooled equation that combines information across all person–years and implicitly assumes that regression coefficients are constant in value over all these years. The full pooled data file of this sort has a total of 8,680,239 person–years, 10,018 representing first onsets of suicide ideation and the other 8,670,221 representing years in the lives of respondents prior to ever having suicide ideation. Note that the years of life prior to the onset of ideation among respondents who subsequently developed ideation are included in the data file. Note, too, that some unknown number of respondents that never experienced ideation as of the time of our survey might do so in the future.

As noted in the last paragraph, this pooled model assumes that the associations of predictors with outcomes are constant across age. However, this assumption can be evaluated and revised by including interaction terms in the equation between person–year (i.e., the dummy variables used to distinguish among the 91 component data files or a continuous variable that provides a linear summary of the ages represented in those dummy variables) and the substantive predictors. Those kinds of interactions are included in the analyses described in this volume. We consistently evaluate the significance of differences in regression coefficients predicting onsets in childhood (ages 4–12), adolescence (ages 13–19), young adulthood (ages 20–29), and subsequently (ages 30+ years). These age ranges were selected not only because they represent meaningful divisions in the life course, but also because inspection of AOO curves show that they divide up the actual distributions of first onsets of suicidal behaviors into rough quartiles. We also examined interactions of predictors with country income level, distinguishing countries classified by the World Bank as low-/lower-middle-income countries from those classified as higher-middle, and high-income countries.

A practical problem with the pooled model is that it is computationally intensive because of including 8,680,239 records. This problem was solved by using *case-control sampling* to reduce the number of observations. In this approach, the 10,018 onsets of suicide ideation were compared to a probability sample of 100,180 control person–years (i.e., ten times the 10,018 onsets of ideation) selected with stratification

from the full set of 8,670,221 such person–years and weighted to have a sum of weights equal to the sum of weights in the full set. As the logistic link function is used in these models, the coefficients are not biased by selecting a subsample of controls. Furthermore, the ratio of ten controls for every one case is large enough that any increase in statistical power achieved by adding more controls would be trivial (Schlesselman, 1982).

The six chapters in Section III that focus on individual classes of predictors (Chapters 6–11) use a consistent method of beginning with bivariate analyses of each predictor (net of controls for the predictors considered in earlier chapters) with each of the five outcomes and then considering the multivariate associations of the individually significant predictors based on an additive model. In most of these chapters, we consider lists of predictors that might be considered roughly equivalent predictors – a variety of parental mental disorders (Chapter 6), of other childhood adversities (Chapter 7), of other lifetime traumatic experiences (Chapter 8), of mental disorders (Chapter 9), and of chronic physical disorders (Chapter 10). In each of these cases, a question could be asked whether the *number* of these experiences that occurred to the respondent might not be as important as, or even more important than, the *types* of experiences in predicting the subsequent onset of suicidal behaviors. There is also the possibility that number and type have distinct associations with the outcomes. In order to investigate this possibility, we estimated a model that included counts of the number of experiences (e.g., number of lifetime traumatic events experienced by the respondent) as predictors of subsequent suicidal behaviors. We also estimated a model that included information about both types and number of these experiences as predictors.

It is noteworthy that the models including both type and number as predictors included a separate dummy predictor variable for each experience along with a series of dummy predictor variables for number of experiences that began with *two*. A detailed discussion of the logic of this approach is described elsewhere (Kessler et al., 2010) and will only be summarized here. To begin, a logistic regression model that includes only a series of dummy predictor variables for type of experiences (in the case of traumatic life events, for example, exposure to a natural disaster, a life-threatening automobile accident, physical assault, the unexpected death of a loved one, etc.)

implicitly assumes that the joint effects of exposure to multiple experiences in predicting suicidal behaviors is the product of the odds ratios (ORs) for the component experienced.

A model that includes only a series of dummy variables for number of predictor experiences, in comparison, implicitly allows for interactions in the sense that the odds ratios (ORs) associated with having exactly two or exactly three or n of the n predictor experiences can be significantly different from the square or cube or nth power of the OR associated with having exactly one experience. However, by excluding information about the content of the experiences, the main effect coefficients for the various component experiences are assumed to be the same.

The model that includes terms for both type and number, though, allows both for differences in effects of the different experiences and also allows for interactions. Specifically, the ORs associated with types of experiences can be interpreted as the ORs of the outcome among individuals who had one and only one specific component experience compared to respondents with none of the experiences, while the ORs associated with number of experiences are multipliers of the products of the ORs associated with the component experienced. For example, if the ORs associated with exposure to a natural disaster, life-threatening automobile accident, physical assault, and unexpected death of a loved one are 1.8, 2.0, 2.2, and 2.4, respectively, while the ORs associated with having exactly two, three, and four experiences are 1.3, 1.4, and 1.5, respectively, then the predicted OR for a respondent who was exposed to only the first three of these experiences would be 11.1 (i.e., $1.8 \times 2.0 \times 2.2 \times 1.4$) compared to a respondent with no exposures, while the predicted OR for a respondent who was exposed only to the first and last of these experiences would be 5.6 (i.e., $1.8 \times 2.4 \times 1.3$).

The simplifying assumption in the type–number model is that the interaction multiplier varies only with number of experiences. As described elsewhere (Kessler et al., 2010), other simplifying assumptions can be made, but our experience exploring several of them is that the assumption made in the type–number model is generally most consistent with the data. Simplifying assumptions of some sort are needed, of course, because it is impossible even in a dataset as large as the WMH series to work with unrestricted models that include a separate coefficient for each of the 2^t logically possibly multivariate profiles made up

by cross-classifying t types of conditions. If there are 20 types, for example, as there are in our analysis of traumatic life experiences, 2^n is greater than one million. It would be impossible to include this large a number of predictors in our models. Data mining methods exist that could be used to search through this enormous number of combinations to find a stable significantly predictive set (Kantardzic, 2003). However, we did not use this approach because we were more interested in developing models that could give us insights that are often obscured in data-mining about the importance of individual modifiable predictors.

Population attributable risk proportions

An informative way to summarize the strength of associations between a set of predictors and the subsequent onset of suicidal behaviors is by calculating the population attributable risk proportion (PARP) (Rockhill B et al., 1996). PARP can be interpreted in this context as the proportions of respondents with a lifetime history of suicidal behaviors who would not have had these behaviors in the absence of a particular set of predictors if the predictors were causal, and the regression equation accurately characterizes the functional form of the associations of the predictors with the outcome. We use PARP as a summary measure throughout the volume.

In the bivariate case with a dichotomous predictor, we can think of PARP as having two components. The first component is the individual-level association among respondents with the risk factor of interest. Let us say we have a dichotomous predictor associated with 20% higher risk of suicidal behavior than among respondents without the risk factor. The individual-level elevated risk would then be 1.2.

The second component is the population projection. If the risk factor occurs to 10% of the population, the 20% elevation in that subsample means that 10% of the population has a risk of $1.2r$, while the other 90% of the population has a risk of r. If the elevated risk were removed, total risk would be r rather than $1.02r$ (i.e., $1.2r \times 0.1 + 1r \times 0.9$). The proportion of total risk due to the elevation in the high-risk subsample is then roughly 2.0% $[1 - (1/1.02)]$. This would be our calculation of PARP in this particular case. If the risk factor occurred to 20% rather than 10% of the population, PARP would have been approximately 4.0%. If the elevation in risk is 50% rather than 20% and it occurs to 20% of the population, PARP will be approximately 9%.

Calculation of PARP is more complicated when multiple predictors are considered together, some of which might be continuous and involve non-additive associations among multiple variables. In a situation of this sort, simulation is used to calculate PARP. Specifically, we use the coefficients in the multiple regression equation to generate a predicted probability of the outcome for each respondent. The mean of these values represents the predicted risk of the outcome under the model (r_1). We then generate a second predicted probability for each respondent based on a modified version of the equation in which we change the coefficients for the predictors of interest to represent the absence of an association (e.g., logistic regression coefficients of 0.0). The mean of this second set of predicted probabilities represents the predicted risk of the outcome in the absence of the predictors of interest (r_2). PARP is then estimated as $1 - (r_2/r_1)$.

Recency curves

A common approach in studying course of illness retrospectively is to calculate the ratio of recent prevalence (e.g., presence in the year before interview) to lifetime (LT) prevalence (McLaughlin et al., 2010). Highly persistent disorders will have a high 12-month/LT prevalence ratio. Of course, this ratio is also a function of recency of onset, as 100% of the disorders that had first onsets in the past year will have been prevalent in the past 12 months. As a result, better information about course can be obtained by inspecting 12-month/LT prevalence ratios in subsamples defined by recency of onset. Even more insights into course of illness can be obtained if more detailed information is obtained in the survey than about lifetime and recent prevalence.

As noted above in the subsection on measures, we collected information on AOO and *age of recency* for each of the six suicidal behavior outcomes in the WMH Surveys. This is less detailed than the information we could have obtained by collecting a complete *event history* for suicidal behaviors; that is, by asking respondents to take us forward through time from their AOO to whether or not the behavior continued, remitted, or recurred in each subsequent year of their life or, in the case of suicide attempts, the number of additional attempts they made at each subsequent year of their life. From what cognitive science tells about memory processes, though, we felt that respondents would not have been able to provide accurate

information at this level of detail for history of either ideation or plans, although they probably could have reported their age at each of their lifetime suicide attempts (Williams et al., 2008). As a result, we settled for asking only about recency of ideation and plans and about number of lifetime suicide attempts along with age of recency of last attempt.

This information was used to make inferences about the course of suicidal behaviors, recognizing that this information was necessarily less complete than if we had complete event histories. The basic analysis approach was to examine recency curves; that is, curves that plotted the cumulative probability of each of the three unconditional suicidal behaviors we studied occurring most recently as of each age of life beginning with the AOO, where the cumulative probability reached 1.0 by definition as of the respondent's age at interview. However, unrestricted recency curves are not very informative, as 100% of the respondents whose suicidal behaviors started only a few years before the interview would, by definition, have a recency within that short period of time, whereas respondents whose suicidal behaviors started many years before interview might have many cumulative probabilities of recency in the first few years after onset. As a result, it was important to stratify recency curves by time since onset. Furthermore, as time since onset is a joint function of AOO and age at interview, we generated a separate series of curves for each of a large number of subsamples defined by the cross-classification of AOO and age at interview. As shown in Chapter 5, inspection of these curves yielded valuable information about the typical course of suicidal behaviors.

Predicting course of suicidal behaviors

As noted in the last subsection, a common approach to study course of illness is to calculate the 12-month/LT prevalence ratio. The predictors of course of illness are studied in that framework by using multiple regression analysis to estimate predictors of 12-month prevalence among lifetime cases, controlling for AOO and time-since-onset (McLaughlin et al., 2010). In order to maintain the temporal order between predictors and outcomes, predictors are often defined as characteristics of the respondent as of AOO. Given that predictors might vary as a function of AOO or time since onset or both, it might also be useful to examine interactions between predictors and these temporal variables in models of this sort, although we are unaware of previous research studies that have done this.

When the only data available about course of illness in a cross-section survey is AOO and recent prevalence, models of the sort described in the last paragraph are the only ones available to obtain even indirect information about predictors of course of illness. However, when data are also available about recency, as in the WMH Surveys, the analysis of course can be refined. On an intuitive level, one would expect that respondents with the most recent episodes would generally, although not always, have the most persistent course of illness; leading investigation of the baseline (i.e., as of AOO) predictors of recency will give us some insights into the predictors of course of illness.

Social demographers have developed models to analyze such recency data to make inferences about the predictors of time-to-next-event for such repeatable events as having a child (Scheike & Keiding, 2006) and making a residential move (Yamaguchi, 2003). These models are based on the fact that when the distribution of time between interview and last occurrence of a previously occurring repeatable event is a stationary renewal process governed by an accelerated failure–time (AFT) model, the same model will apply to the distribution of time-since-last-occurrence (Keiding et al., 2011).

As we were unwilling to make such strong assumptions about recurrence distributions, we did not estimate AFT models to study the predictors of time-since-last-occurrence. However, we did estimate discrete-time survival models to obtain basic information about significant predictors of time-since-last-occurrence. These predictors were defined as of AOO and were examined in models that controlled for AOO and time-since-onset. Importantly, we did not interpret the coefficients in these models in substantive terms (i.e., as suggesting that a 2.0 odds ratio implied a two-fold increased odds of recurrence), but rather used the results only in a qualitative sense as indicators of the predictors of persistent course of suicidal behaviors.

In addition to these general models, we also used logistic regression to study the associations of the same predictors with a series of five more specific aspects of course based on preliminary analyses of recency curves. As detailed in Chapter 5, those preliminary analyses found that 40%–50% of respondents with a lifetime history of suicide ideation never had a recurrence of their ideation beyond the year of onset no matter how many subsequent years had elapsed at the time of interview. Similar patterns with even higher proportions of nonrecurrence were found in recency curves for suicide plans and suicide attempts.

We also found that respondents whose suicidal behaviors continued beyond their AOO varied in persistence. For example, we found that among respondents who were 40 years or older at the time of interview and whose suicide ideation began before they entered their teenage years, 36.6% never had suicide ideation again after AOO. We might think of the remaining 63.4% of lifetime ideators as the more persistent cases. As it happens, 26.8% of these more persistent cases reported having ideation in the year of interview. If this percentage were a simple random sample of a homogeneous group of persistent cases, 26.8% of whom have ideation in any given year, we would expect that $[1-(1-0.268)^5] = 79.0\%$ of persistent cases would have ideation at some time within the five years before interview. The actual percent, though, is much smaller: 38.1%. This implies that some persistent cases are much more persistent than others, with the 38.1% of persistent cases who had ideation within five years of interview having it for an average of 3.5 of those five years if the 26.8% 12-month prevalence is stable over years.

This observation of variation in persistence among persistent cases means that a simple *mover–stayer model* of persistence (Goodman, 1961) – that is, a model in which the population is assumed to consist of two latent classes, one of which has a zero probability of persistence beyond a given start time and the other of which has a single fixed probability of persistence in each year that is independent of the value in the previous or earlier years – does not fit the observed data. But another possibility is that a mover–stayer Markov model fits the data. Under this scenario, each respondent's probability of ideation in a given year is a function of whether or not he had ideation in the previous year. Patterns in earlier years are irrelevant in the Markov model. If we consider the above example, where 26.8% of persistent cases reported ideation in the year of interview, we can calculate the Markov transition probabilities by noting that an additional 3.6% of persistent cases reported ideation in the year before interview. If we assume that the transition probabilities of ideation at time t are p_1 of time $t-1$ cases and p_2 of time $t-1$ non-cases, and if we further assume that the observed period prevalence of 26.8% is constant over years, then $p_1(0.268) = (0.268-0.036)$, which means that $p_1 = 0.86$. Furthermore, $3.6\% = p_2(1-0.268)$, which means that $p_2 = 0.05$. The proportion of all persistent cases who will have ideation in at least one year over the five years before interview will then be $0.268\,(1{-}0.86)\ (1{-}0.05)^4 + (1{-}0.268)\ (1{-}0.05)^5 = 60\%$, which is much higher than the observed 38.1%. This result shows clearly that a mover–stayer Markov model does not fit the data.

It was based on results such as these, which show consistently that simple models do not fit the observed data on persistence of suicidal behaviors, that we decided to estimate a series of simple logistic regression models rather than make strong assumptions about more complex underlying recurrence process distributions (Yamaguchi, 2003) to study predictors of the course of suicidal behaviors. The first of these five logistic regression models predicted whether each suicidal behavior occurred more than two years after AOO. This model was estimated among respondents whose AOO was at least five years before the time of interview and included controls for AOO and time-since-onset in addition to a number of substantive predictors. The remaining four models focused on respondents whose suicidal behaviors occurred more than two years after AOO. The first three of these four models predicted whether recency was within ten, five, and one years of interview among respondents whose AOO was 10 or 15 or more years before interview. The final model focused on respondents whose suicidal behavior occurred within five years of interview and predicted whether recency was within one year of interview. The intent here was to distinguish predictors of very high persistence from those of less high persistence. We could have selected other times than these five, but we believe this set of five models provides a good general sense of the predictors of the course of suicidal behavior patterns. Consequently we examine the associations of all the predictors considered here with each of these aspects of the persistence of suicide ideation, plans, and attempts.

Acknowledgements

Portions of this chapter appeared previously in: Harkness, J., Pennell, B. E., Villar, A., et al. (2008). Translation procedures and translation assessment in the World Mental Health Survey initiative. In R. C. Kessler, & T. B. Üstün (eds.). The WHO World Mental Health Surveys: Global Perspectives on the Epidemiology of Mental Disorders, pp. 91–113. New York, NY: Cambridge University Press; Haro, J. M., Arbabzadeh-Bouchez, S., Brugha, T. S., et al. (2008). Concordance of the Composite International Diagnostic Interview Version 3.0 (CIDI 3.0) with standardized clinical assessments in the WHO World Mental Health surveys. In R. C. Kessler, & T. B. Üstün (eds). The WHO World Mental Health Surveys: Global Perspectives on the Epidemiology of Mental Disorders, pp. 114–130. New York, NY: Cambridge University Press.; Heeringa, S. G., Wells, J. E., Hubbard, F. M., et al. (2008). Sample designs and sampling procedures. In R. C. Kessler, & T. B. Üstün (eds.). The WHO World Mental Health Surveys: Global perspectives on the epidemiology of mental disorders, pp. 14–32. New York, NY: Cambridge University Press.; Kessler, R. C., & Üstün, T. B. (2008). The World Health Organization Composite International Diagnostic Interview. In R. C. Kessler, & T. B. Üstün (eds.). The WHO World Mental Health Surveys: Global Perspectives on the Epidemiology of Mental Disorders, pp. 58–90. New York, NY: Cambridge University Press.; Pennell, B.-E., Mneimneh, Z., Bowers, A., et al. (2008). Implementation of the world mental health surveys. In R. C. Kessler, & T. B. Üstün (eds.). The WHO World Mental Health Surveys: Global Perspectives on the Epidemiology of Mental Disorders, pp. 33–57. New York, NY: Cambridge University Press. All © 2008. World Health Organization. Used with permission.

References

Alonso, J., Angermeyer, M. C., Bernert, S., et al. (2004). Sampling and methods of the European Study of the Epidemiology of Mental Disorders (ESEMeD) project. *Acta Psychiatrica Scandinavica Supplement*, 8–20.

American Association for Public Opinion Research. (2000). Standard definitions: Final dispositions of case codes and outcome rates for surveys. Retrieved April 17, 2011 from http://www.aapor.org.

Belli, R. F. (1988). Color blend retrievals: Compromise memories or deliberate compromise responses? *Memory and Cognition*, **16**(4), 314–326.

Belli, R. F. (1998). The structure of autobiographical memory and the event history calendar: potential improvements in the quality of retrospective reports in surveys. *Memory*, **6**(4), 383–406.

Biemer, P., & Lyberg, L. (2003). *Introduction to Survey Quality*. New York, NY: John Wiley & Sons.

Billiet, J., & Loosveldt, G. (1988). Interviewer training and quality of responses. *Public Opinion Quarterly*, **52**(2), 190–211.

Borges, G., Angst, J., Nock, M. K., Ruscio, A. M. & Kessler, R. C. (2008). Risk factors for the incidence and persistence of suicide-related outcomes: a 10-year follow-up study using the National Comorbidity Surveys. *Journal of Affective Disorders*, **105**(1–3), 25–33.

Brewer, W. F. (1986). What is autobiographical memory? In D. C. Rubin (ed.), *Autobiographical Memory*, pp. 25–49. New York, NY: Cambridge University Press.

Bulmer, M. (1998). The problem of exporting social survey research. *American Behavioral Scientist*, **42**(2), 153–167.

Cannell, C. F., Fowler, F. J., Jr. & Marquis, K. H. (1968). The influence of interviewer and respondent psychological and behavioral variables on the reporting in household interviews. *Vital and Health Statistics* **26**, 1–65.

Cannell, C. F., Miller, P. V. & Oksenberg, L. (1981). Research on interviewing techniques. In S. Leinhardt (ed.), *Sociological Methodology*, pp. 389–487. San Francisco, CA: Jossey-Bass Publishers.

Centers, R. (1963). A laboratory adaptation of the conversational procedure for the conditioning of verbal operants. *Journal of Abnormal Psychology*, **67**, 334–339.

Cheng, A. T. (2001). Case definition and culture: are people all the same? *British Journal of Psychiatry*, **179**, 1–3.

Clark, H. H., & Schober, M. F. (1992). Asking questions and influencing answers. In J. M. Tanur (ed.), *Questions about Questions: Inquiries Into the Cognitive Bases of Surveys*, pp. 15–48. New York, NY: Russell Sage Foundation.

Clayton, D., & Hills, M. (1993). *Statistical Models in Epidemiology*. New York, NY: Oxford University Press.

Cochran, W. G. (1977). *Sampling Techniques*. New York, NY: John Wiley & Sons.

Converse, J., & Presser, S. (1986). *Survey Questions: Handcrafting the Standardized Questionnaire, Sage Series No. 63*. Thousand Oaks, CA: Sage Publications.

Couper, M. P., & de Leeuw, E. D. (2003). Nonresponse in cross-cultural and cross-national surveys. In J. A. Harkness, F. J. R. Van de Vijver, & P. P. Mohler (eds.), *Cross-Cultural Survey Methods*, pp. 155–177. Hoboken, NJ: John Wiley & Sons.

Deville, J.-C., & Särndal, C.-E. (1992). Calibration estimators in survey sampling. *Journal of the American Statistical Association*, **87**, 376–382.

Eaton, W. W., Kramer, M., Anthony, J. C., et al. (1989). The incidence of specific DIS/DSM-III mental disorders: data from the NIMH Epidemiologic Catchment Area Program. *Acta Psychiatrica Scandinavica*, **79**(2), 163–178.

First, M. B., Spitzer, R. L., Gibbon, M. & Williams, J. B. W. (2002). *Structured Clinical Interview for DSM-IV Axis I Disorders, Research Version, Non-Patient Edition (SCID-I/NP)*. New York, NY: Biometrics Research, New York State Psychiatric Institute.

Fowler, F., & Mangione, T. (1990). *Standardized Survey Interviewing: Minimizing Interviewer-Related Error*. Newbury Park, CA: Sage Publications, Inc.

Gilman, S. (1988). *Disease and Depresentation: Images of Illness from Madness to AIDS*. Ithaca, NY: Cornell University Press.

Giuffra, L. A., & Risch, N. (1994). Diminished recall and the cohort effect of major depression: A simulation study. *Psychological Medicine*, **24**(2), 375–383.

Goodman, L. A. (1961). Statistical methods for the Mover-Stayer model. *Journal of the American Statistical Association*, **56**, 841–868.

Groves, R. M., Fowler, F. J., Jr., Couper, M. P., et al. (2004). *Survey Methodology*. New York, NY: John Wiley & Sons.

Halli, S. S., Rao, K. V. & Halli, S. S. (1992). *Advanced Techniques of Population Analysis*. New York, NY: Plenum.

Hanley, J. A., & McNeil, B. J. (1982). The meaning and use of the area under a receiver operating characteristic (ROC) curve. *Radiology*, **143**(1), 29–36.

Harkness, J., Pennell, B. E., Villar, A., et al. (2008). Translation procedures and translation assessment in the World Mental Health Survey initiative. In R. C. Kessler, & T. B. Üstün (eds.). *The WHO World Mental Health Surveys: Global Perspectives on the Epidemiology of Mental Disorders*, pp. 91–113. New York, NY: Cambridge University Press.

Harkness, J. A., Pennell, B. E. & Schoua-Glusberg, A. (2004). Survey questionnaire translation and assessment. In S. Presser, J. Rothgeb, M. P. Couper, et al. (eds.). *Methods for Testing and Evaluating Survey Questionnaires*, pp. 453–474. Hoboken, NJ: John Wiley & Sons.

Harkness, J. A., Van de Vijver, J. R. & Mohler, P. P. (2002). *Cross-Cultural Survey Methods*. New York, NY: John Wiley & Sons.

Haro, J. M., Arbabzadeh-Bouchez, S., Brugha, T. S., et al. (2006). Concordance of the Composite International Diagnostic Interview Version 3.0 (CIDI 3.0) with standardized clinical assessments in the WHO World Mental Health surveys. *International Journal of Methods in Psychiatric Research*, **15**(4), 167–180.

Haro, J. M., Arbabzadeh-Bouchez, S., Brugha, T. S., et al. (2008). Concordance of the Composite International Diagnostic Interview Version 3.0 (CIDI 3.0) with standardized clinical assessments in the WHO World Mental Health surveys. In R. C. Kessler, & T. B. Üstün (eds). *The WHO World Mental Health Surveys: Global Perspectives on the Epidemiology of Mental Disorders*, pp. 114–130. New York, NY: Cambridge University Press.

Heath, A., Fisher, S., & Smith, S. (2005). The globalization of public opinion research. *Annual Review of Political Science*, **8**, 297–333.

Heeringa, S. G., Wells, J. E., Hubbard, F. M., et al. (2008). Sample designs and sampling procedures. In R. C. Kessler, & T. B. Üstün (eds.). *The WHO World Mental Health Surveys: Global perspectives on the epidemiology of mental disorders*, pp. 14–32. New York, NY: Cambridge University Press.

Jobe, J. B., White, A. A., Kelley, C. L., et al. (1990). Recall strategies and memory for health-care visits. *Milbank Quarterly*, **68**(2), 171–189.

Jowell, R. (1998). How comparative is comparative research? *American Behavioral Scientist*, **42**, 168–177.

Kantardzic, M. (2003). *Data Mining: Concepts, Models, Methods, and Algorithms*. New York, NY: John Wiley & Sons.

Keiding, N., Fine, J. P., Hansen, H. O., & Slama, R. (2011). Accelerated failure time regression for backward recurrence times and current durations. *Statistics and Probability Letters*, **81**, 724–729.

Kessler, R. C. (1999). The World Health Organization International Consortium in Psychiatric Epidemiology (ICPE): Initial work and future directions – the NAPE Lecture 1998. Nordic Association for Psychiatric Epidemiology. *Acta Psychiatrica Scandinavica*, **99**(1), 2–9.

Kessler, R. C., Aguilar-Gaxiola, S., Alonso, J., et al. (2008). Lifetime prevalence and age of onset distributions of mental disorders in the World Mental Health Survey Initiative. In R. C. Kessler, & T. B. Üstün (eds.). *The WHO World Mental Health Surveys: Global Perspectives on the Epidemiology of Mental Disorders*, pp. 511–521. New York, NY: Cambridge University Press.

Kessler, R. C., Amminger, G. P., Aguilar-Gaxiola, S., et al. (2007a). Age of onset of mental disorders: a review of recent literature. *Current Opinion in Psychiatry*, **20**(4), 359–364.

Kessler, R. C., Angermeyer, M., Anthony, J. C., et al. (2007b). Lifetime prevalence and age-of-onset distributions of mental disorders in the World Health Organization's World Mental Health Survey Initiative. *World Psychiatry*, **6**(3), 168–176.

Kessler, R. C., Berglund, P., Chiu, W. T., et al. (2004). The US National Comorbidity Survey Replication (NCS-R): design and field procedures. *International Journal of Methods in Psychiatric Research*, **13**(2), 69–92.

Kessler, R. C., McLaughlin, K. A., Green, J. G., et al. (2010). Childhood adversities and adult psychopathology in the WHO World Mental Health Surveys. *British Journal of Psychiatry*, **197**(5), 378–385.

Kessler, R. C., Mroczek, D. K. & Belli, R. F. (1999). Retrospective adult assessment of childhood psychopathology. In D. Shaffer, C. P. Lucas, & J. E. Richters (eds.). *Diagnostic Assessment in Child and Adolescent Psychopathology*, pp. 256–284. New York, NY: Guilford Press.

Kessler, R. C., & Üstün, T. B. (2004). The World Mental Health (WMH) Survey Initiative Version of the World Health Organization (WHO) Composite International Diagnostic Interview (CIDI). *International Journal of Methods in Psychiatric Research*, **13**(2), 93–121.

Kessler, R. C., & Üstün, T. B. (2008). The World Health Organization Composite International Diagnostic Interview. In R. C. Kessler, & T. B. Üstün (eds.). *The WHO World Mental Health Surveys: Global Perspectives on the Epidemiology of Mental Disorders*, pp. 58–90. New York, NY: Cambridge University Press.

Kessler, R. C., Wittchen, H.-U., Abelson, J. M., et al. (1998). Methodological studies of the Composite International Diagnostic Interview (CIDI) in the US National Comorbidity Survey. *International Journal of Methods in Psychiatric Research*, **7**, 33–55.

Kessler, R. C., Wittchen, H. U., Abelson, J. M. & Zhao, S. (2000). Methodological issues in assessing psychiatric disorder with self-reports. In A. A. Stone, J. S. Turrkan, C. A. Bachrach, et al. (eds.). *The Science of Self-Report: Implications for Research and Practice*, pp. 229–255. Mahwah, NJ: Lawrence Erlbaum Associates.

Kish, L. (1949). A procedure for objective respondent selection within the household. *Journal of the American Statistical Association*, **44**, 380–7.

Kish, L. (1965). *Survey sampling*. New York, NY: John Wiley & Sons.

Knäuper, B., Cannell, C. F., Schwarz, N., Bruce, M. L. & Kessler, R. C. (1999). Improving accuracy of major depression age-of-onset reports in the US National Comorbidity Survey. *International Journal of Methods in Psychiatric Research*, **8**, 39–48.

Kraemer, H. C., Morgan, G. A., Leech, N. L., et al. (2003). Measures of clinical significance. *Journal of the American Academy of Child and Adolescent Psychiatry*, **42**(2), 1524–9.

Kuechler, M. (1998). The Survey Method: An indispensable tool for social science research everywhere? *American Behavioral Scientist*, **42**, 178–200.

Lavrakas, P. J. (1993). *Telephone Survey Methods: Sampling, Selection, and Supervision*. Thousand Oaks, CA: Sage Publications.

Lee, E. T., & Go, O. T. (1997). Survival analysis in public health research. *Annual Review of Public Health*, **18**, 105–34.

Leventhal, H., Nerenz, D., & Steele, D. J. (1984). Illness representations and coping with health threats. In A. Baum, S. E. Taylor, & J. E. Singer (eds.). *Handbook of Psychology and Health*, pp. 219–252. Hillsdale, NJ: Erlbaum Associates.

Little, R. J. A., & Rubin, D. B. (2002). *Statistical analysis with missing data, second edition.* New York, NY: John Wiley & Sons.

Lynn, P. (2001). Developing Quality Standards for Cross-National Survey Research: Five Approaches. Institute for Social and Economic Research Working Papers, Number 2001–2021.

Markus, H., & Zajonc, R. B. (1985). The cognitive perspective in social psychology. In G. Lindzey, & E. Aronson (eds.). *The Handbook of Social Psychology,* pp. 137–230. New York, NY: Random House.

Marquis, K. H., & Cannell, C. F. (1969). *A Study of Interviewer-Respondent Interaction in the Urban Employment.* Ann Arbor, MI: Survey Research Center, University of Michigan.

McLaughlin, K. A., Green, J. G., Gruber, M. J., et al. (2010). Childhood adversities and adult psychiatric disorders in the national comorbidity survey replication II: associations with persistence of DSM-IV disorders. *Archives of General Psychiatry,* **67**(2), 124–32.

Means, B., & Loftus, E. F. (1991). When personal history repeats itself: decomposing memories for recurring events. *Applied Cognitive Psychology,* **5**, 297–318.

Menon, A. (1994). Judgements of behavioral frequencies: Memory search and retrieval strategies. In N. Schwartz, & S. Sudman (eds.). *Autobiographical Memory and the Validity of Retrospective Reports,* pp. 161–172. New York, NY: Springer-Verlag.

Miller, P. V., & Cannell, C. F. (1977). Communicating measurement objectives in the survey interview. In D. M. Hirsch, P. V. Miller, & F. G. Kline (eds.). *Strategies for Communication Research,* pp. 127–151. Beverly Hills, CA: Sage Publications.

Moffitt, T. E., Caspi, A., Taylor, A., et al. (2010). How common are common mental disorders? Evidence that lifetime prevalence rates are doubled by prospective versus retrospective ascertainment. *Psychological Medicine,* **40**(6), 899–909.

Oksenberg, L., Vinokur, A., & Cannell, C. F. (1979). The effects of instructions, commitment and feedback on reporting in personal interviews. In C. F. Cannell, L. Oksenberg, & J. M. Converse (eds.). *Experiments in Interviewing Techniques. DHEW Publication No. (HRA) 78-3204,* pp. 133–199. Washington, DC: Department of Health, Education, and Welfare.

Patten, S. B. (2003). Recall bias and major depression lifetime prevalence. *Social Psychiatry and Psychiatric Epidemiology,* **38**(6), 290–6.

Patten, S. B. (2009). Accumulation of major depressive episodes over time in a prospective study indicates that retrospectively assessed lifetime prevalence estimates are too low. *BMC Psychiatry,* **9**, 19.

Pearson, R. W., Ross, M., & Dawes, R. M. (1992). Personal recall and the limits of retrospective questions in surveys. In J. M. Tanur (ed.). *Questions about Questions: Inquiries Into the Cognitive Bases of Surveys,* pp. 65–94. New York, NY: Russell Sage Foundation.

Pennell, B.-E., Mneimneh, Z., Bowers, A., et al. (2008). Implementation of the world mental health surveys. In R. C. Kessler, & T. B. Üstün (eds.). *The WHO World Mental Health Surveys: Global Perspectives on the Epidemiology of Mental Disorders,* pp. 33–57. New York, NY: Cambridge University Press.

Prince, R., & Tcheng-Laroche, F. (1987). Culture-bound syndromes and international disease classifications. *Cultural Medical Psychiatry,* **11**(1), 3–52.

Prohaska, V., Brown, N. R., & Belli, R. F. (1998). Forward telescoping: the question matters. *Memory,* **6**(4), 455–65.

Research Triangle Institute (2002). *SUDAAN: Professional Software for Survey Data Analysis.* Research Triangle Park, Durham, NC: Research Triangle Institute.

Rockhill, B., Newman, B., & Weinberg, C. (1996). Use and misuse of population attributable fractions. *American Journal of Public Health,* **88**(1), 15–19.

Rust, K. (1985). Variance estimation for complex estimators in sample surveys. *Journal of Official Statistics,* **1**, 381–397.

SAS Institute Inc. (2008). *SAS/STAT® Software, Version 9.2 for Windows.* Cary, NC: SAS Institute Inc.

Scheike, T. H., & Keiding, N. (2006). Design and analysis of time-to-pregnancy. *Statistical Methods in Medical Research,* **15**(2), 127–140.

Schlesselman, J. J. (1982). *Case-Control Studies: Design, Conduct, Analysis.* New York, NY: Oxford University Press.

Schwarz, N., & Sudman, S. (eds.). (1994). *Autobiographical Memory and the Validity of Retrospective Reports.* New York, NY: Springer-Verlag.

Schwarz, N., & Sudman, S. (eds.). (1996). *Answering Questions: Methodology for Determining Cognitive and Communicative Processes in Survey Research.* San Francisco, CA: Jossey-Bass Publishers.

Sheatsley, P. B. (1983). Questionnaire construction and item writing. In P. H. Rossi, J. D. Wright, & A. B. Anderson (eds.). *Handbook of Survey Research: Quantitative Studies in Social Relations,* pp. 195–230. New York, NY: Academy Press.

Simon, G. E., & Von Korff, M. (1995). Recall of psychiatric history in cross-sectional surveys: implications for epidemiologic research. *Epidemiologic Reviews,* **17**(1), 221–227.

Simon, G. E., Von Korff, M., Üstün, T. B., et al. (1995). Is the lifetime risk of depression actually increasing? *Journal of Clinical Epidemiology,* **48**(9), 1109–1118.

Sirken, M. G., Herrmann, D. J., Schechter, S., et al. (eds.). (1999). *Cognition and Survey Research*. New York, NY: John Wiley & Sons.

Skelton, J. A., & Croyle, R. T. (1991). *Mental Representation in Health and Illness*. New York, NY: Springer-Verlag.

Smith, T. W. (2004). Developing and evaluating cross-national survey instruments. In S. Presser, J. M. Rothgeb, M. P. Couper, et al. (eds.). *Methods for Testing and Evaluating Survey Questionnaires*, pp. 431–452. New York, NY: John Wiley & Sons.

Sudman, S., Bradburn, N., & Schwarz, N. (1996). *Thinking About Answers: The Application of Cognitive Processes to Survey Methodology*. San Francisco, CA: Jossey-Bass Publishers.

Tanur, J. M. (1992). *Questions about Questions: Inquiries Into the Cognitive Bases of Surveys*. New York, NY: Russell Sage Foundation.

Turner, C., & Martin, E. (1985). *Surveying Subjective Phenomena*. New York, NY: Russell Sage Foundation.

Turner, C. F., Ku, L., Rogers, S. M., et al. (1998). Adolescent sexual behavior, drug use, and violence: increased reporting with computer survey technology. *Science*, **280**(5365), 867–873.

Verma, V., Scott, C., & O'Muircheartaigh, C. (1980). Sample designs and sampling errors for the World Fertility Survey. *Journal of the Royal Statistical Society*, **143**, 431–473.

Vinokur, A., Oksenberg, L., & Cannell, C. F. (1979). Effects of feedback and reinforcement on the report of health information. In C. F. Cannell, L. Oksenberg, & J. M. Converse (eds.). *Experiments in Interviewing Techniques*, Ann Arbor, MI: Survey Research Center, University of Michigan.

Willett, J. B., & Singer, J. D. (1993). Investigating onset, cessation, relapse, and recovery: Why you should, and how you can, use discrete-time survival analysis to examine event occurrence. *Journal of Consulting and Clinical Psychology*, **61**(6), 952–965.

Williams, B. J. (1986). Suggestions for the application of advanced technology in Canadian collection operations. *Journal of Official Statistics*, **2**(4), 555–560.

Williams, H. L., Conway, M. A. & Cohen, G. (2008). Autobiographical memory. In G. Cohen, & M. A. Conway (eds.). *Memory in the Real World, third Edition*, pp. 21–90. Hove, England: Psychology Press.

The World Bank. (2008). Data and Statistics. Accessed May 12, 2009 at: http://go.worldbank.org/D7SN0B8YU0

Yamaguchi, K. (2003). Accelerated failure-time mover-stayer regression models for the analysis of last-episode data. *Sociological Methodology*, **33**, 81–110.

Chapter

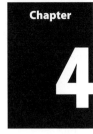

4

Prevalence, onset, and transitions among suicidal behaviors

Guilherme Borges, Wai Tat Chiu, Irving Hwang, Bharat N. Panchal,
Yutaka Ono, Nancy A. Sampson, Ronald C. Kessler, and Matthew K. Nock

Introduction

The prevalence of suicide around the world has been a topic of great interest and discussion since the early work of Durkheim (1951). Epidemiological studies have examined the problem in many different countries around the world. Unfortunately, very little research is available to document the possible cross-national differences (if any) in the rates of suicidal behavior (i.e., suicide ideation, plans, and attempts), and less still on the possible sources of those observed differences. Two exceptions are the work of Bertolote et al. (2005) and Weissman et al. (1999). Weissman et al. (1999) found that in nine countries, the lifetime rates of suicide ideation ranged from 2.09%–18.51% and rates of suicide attempts ranged from 0.72%–5.93%. Bertolote et al. (2005) reported lifetime prevalence rates in eight countries for suicide attempts (range 0.4%–4.2%), plans (range 1.1%–15.6%), and ideation (range 2.6%–25.4%). More recently, Nock et al. (2008b) reviewed all available studies on epidemiology of suicidal behavior published from 1997 to 2007 and found that lifetime prevalence of these suicidal behaviors varied widely across countries for suicide ideation (3.1%–56.0%; IQR=8.0–24.9), suicide plans (0.9%–19.5%; IQR=1.5–9.4), and suicide attempts (0.4%–5.1%; IQR=1.3–3.5). These prior studies document the large differences in prevalence rates of suicidal behaviors; however, they are based on comparisons among surveys that used different methods and assessment strategies to measure the presence of these behaviors (Nock et al., 2008b; Weissman et al., 1999), or on small surveys in catchment areas for health services that varied in scope across sites (Bertolote et al., 2005).

Most recently, Nock et al. (2008a) for the first time used consistent assessment methods to study suicidal behavior across 17 nationally representative and large samples of the general population, which permitted the largest and most representative examination of suicidal behavior ever conducted. In this chapter, we build on this prior work in several ways. First, the current study adds the results from five additional surveys, bringing the total to 22 different surveys around the world. Second, we examine the results on a country-specific level in much finer detail than in our earlier paper. Third, we extend our discussion on the transitions from suicide ideation to suicide plan and attempt. Our goal is to present new data on the prevalence, age-of-onset (AOO), probability and timing of transitions among suicidal behaviors, and associations between AOO and the probability and speed of transitions among these behaviors. Other chapters in this book discuss possible explanations based on the risk and protective factors identified across these surveys.

Method

A detailed description of the respondent samples, study procedures, interview measures, and statistical analyses is provided in Chapter 3 of this volume.

Results

Prevalence and transitions across suicidal behaviors

There is large variability in prevalence of suicidal behaviors across individual countries (see Table 4.1). The prevalence of suicide ideation varies from 2.6% (Romania) to 15.9% (New Zealand); the prevalence of plan varies between 0.7% (Bulgaria, Italy, Romania) and 6.2% (India); and the prevalence of suicide attempt varies from 0.5% (Bulgaria, Italy) to 5.0% (United States). There is no distinct

Suicide, eds. Matthew K. Nock, Guilherme Borges, and Yutaka Ono. Published by Cambridge University Press.

Table 4.1. Lifetime prevalence of suicide outcomes across World Mental Health countries in the Part 1 sample

Countries	Ideation			Plan			Attempt		
	%	SE	n	%	SE	n	%	SE	n
The Americas									
Brazil	12.2	0.6	650	4.6	0.3	257	4.0	0.3	224
Colombia	12.4	0.7	587	4.1	0.4	204	4.7	0.4	224
Mexico	8.1	0.5	488	3.2	0.3	192	2.7	0.3	166
United States	15.6	0.5	1462	5.4	0.3	507	5.0	0.2	469
Europe									
Belgium	8.4	0.9	209	2.7	0.4	77	2.5	0.4	66
Bulgaria	3.2	0.3	170	0.7	0.1	48	0.5	0.1	36
France	12.4	0.7	391	4.4	0.4	143	3.4	0.4	115
Germany	9.7	0.7	347	2.2	0.3	78	1.7	0.3	64
Italy	3.0	0.3	144	0.7	0.1	33	0.5	0.1	26
Netherlands	8.2	0.6	223	2.7	0.5	78	2.3	0.3	64
Romania	2.6	0.4	67	0.7	0.2	19	0.8	0.2	20
Spain	4.4	0.3	272	1.4	0.2	84	1.5	0.2	80
Ukraine	8.2	0.5	389	2.7	0.3	126	1.8	0.2	80
Africa and the Middle East									
Israel	5.5	0.3	268	1.9	0.2	93	1.4	0.2	66
Lebanon	4.3	0.6	117	1.7	0.4	39	2.0	0.3	54
Nigeria	3.2	0.2	238	1.0	0.1	70	0.7	0.1	46
South Africa	9.1	0.7	394	3.8	0.4	171	2.9	0.3	140
Asia and the Pacific									
China (Beijing and Shanghai)	3.1	0.2	160	0.9	0.2	42	1.0	0.2	49
India	14.2	0.6	455	6.2	0.4	203	4.1	0.4	131
Japan	10.0	0.5	400	1.8	0.2	74	1.5	0.2	67
China (Shenzhen)	5.0	0.4	375	1.1	0.2	72	0.7	0.1	53
New Zealand	15.9	0.5	2212	5.6	0.3	814	4.6	0.3	688

geographical pattern in these data. Although, in general, the prevalence of suicide ideation, plan, and attempt is higher as a group in the Americas, high prevalence of ideation also is seen in individual countries in Asia and the Pacific, and high prevalence of plans and attempts are seen in countries in Europe and Asia. In addition, we rearranged the data from Table 4.1, grouping the countries according to their income (high-income, middle-income, and low-income), but again no consistent trend is found (see Table 4.2). As an example, the prevalence of suicide attempt ranges from 0.5% (Israel) to 5.0% (United States) in high-income countries, from 0.5% (Bulgaria) to 4.0% (Brazil) in middle-income countries, and from 0.7% (Nigeria and Shenzhen) to 4.7% (Colombia) in low-income countries.

We show the conditional prevalence of plan among ideators, attempt among ideators with a plan, and attempt among ideators without a plan in Table 4.3. Between 18.4% (Japan) and 43.5% (India) of those with suicide ideation ever made a plan. Among those with ideation and plan, between 26.8% (Shenzhen) and 73.3% (Spain) ever made a suicide attempt. In all the surveys, unplanned suicide attempts occurred much less often (1.9%–30.1% of those with ideation but no plan make an attempt) than attempts among those who have a suicide plan (26.8%–73.3%). There was no geographical pattern of distribution of unplanned (or "impulsive") attempts across these regions as high levels of impulsive attempts are found in the Americas (Colombia 22.7%), Europe (Romania 16.7%), Africa and the Middle East (Lebanon 30.1%), as well as Asia

Table 4.2. Lifetime prevalence of suicide outcomes across World Mental Health countries by income

Countries by income category	Ideation			Plan			Attempt		
	%	SE	n	%	SE	n	%	SE	n
High-income countries									
Belgium	8.4	0.9	209	2.7	0.4	77	2.5	0.4	66
France	12.4	0.7	391	4.4	0.4	143	3.4	0.4	115
Germany	9.7	0.7	347	2.2	0.3	78	1.7	0.3	64
Israel	5.5	0.3	268	1.9	0.2	93	1.4	0.2	66
Italy	3.0	0.3	144	0.7	0.1	33	0.5	0.1	26
Japan	10.0	0.5	400	1.8	0.2	74	1.5	0.2	67
Netherlands	8.2	0.6	223	2.7	0.5	78	2.3	0.3	64
New Zealand	15.9	0.5	2212	5.6	0.3	814	4.6	0.3	688
Spain	4.4	0.3	272	1.4	0.2	84	1.5	0.2	80
United States	15.6	0.5	1462	5.4	0.3	507	5.0	0.2	469
Middle-income countries									
Brazil	12.2	0.6	650	4.6	0.3	257	4.0	0.3	224
Bulgaria	3.2	0.3	170	0.7	0.1	48	0.5	0.1	36
Lebanon	4.3	0.6	117	1.7	0.4	39	2.0	0.3	54
Mexico	8.1	0.5	488	3.2	0.3	192	2.7	0.3	166
Romania	2.6	0.4	67	0.7	0.2	19	0.8	0.2	20
South Africa	9.1	0.7	394	3.8	0.4	171	2.9	0.3	140
Low-income countries									
China (Beijing and Shanghai)	3.1	0.2	160	0.9	0.2	42	1.0	0.2	49
Colombia	12.4	0.7	587	4.1	0.4	204	4.7	0.4	224
India	14.2	0.6	455	6.2	0.4	203	4.1	0.4	131
Nigeria	3.2	0.2	238	1.0	0.1	70	0.7	0.1	46
China (Shenzhen)	5.0	0.4	375	1.1	0.2	72	0.7	0.1	53
Ukraine	8.2	0.5	389	2.7	0.3	126	1.8	0.2	80

and the Pacific region (China [Beijing and Shanghai] 26.1%).

Ages of onset for suicidal behaviors

The distribution of ages of onset for suicide ideation in the 22 surveys is presented in Figure 4.1. In most countries, suicide ideation is very rarely reported before adolescence. In general, these curves are strikingly similar in showing low increases before the teens and then sharp increases up to young adulthood. In all surveys, the risk of first onset of suicide ideation increases rapidly from adolescence to young adulthood, with India, Bulgaria, and Romania starting a little later (late teens–early 20s). Another group of countries, the United States, Japan, and New Zealand, showed higher slopes between the middle and latter teens.

Suicidal behaviors as risk factors for transitioning from suicide ideation to plan

Figure 4.2 shows that in all samples, in general, there is a rapid transition from ideation to plan with most of the transitions occurring within the first year of onset of ideation. In some countries, such as Bulgaria and Italy, there was little transition in any other year after the first year of ideation. Other countries, such as India and Mexico, showed more transitions after the first year.

Table 4.4 presents results from a discrete-time survival model for the transition from suicide ideation to the development of a suicide plan, considering AOO of ideation and time since ideation – both continuous variables in years. The square term of AOO of ideation was also included to account for nonlinearity in the data. Consistent with Figure 4.1, the main

Table 4.3. Conditional lifetime prevalence of suicide outcomes across World Mental Health countries in the Part 1 sample

Countries	Plan among ideators			Attempt among ideators with a lifetime plan			Attempt among ideators without a lifetime plan		
	%	SE	n	%	SE	n	%	SE	n
The Americas									
Brazil	37.1	2.3	257	58.6	3.8	152	17.9	3.1	72
Colombia	33.2	2.6	204	68.3	3.5	147	22.7	3.2	77
Mexico	39.0	2.7	192	61.3	4.8	118	16.3	2.6	48
United States	34.5	1.6	507	54.4	3.1	284	19.9	1.4	185
Europe									
Belgium	32.2	3.4	77	65.7	7.0	50	12.2	3.4	16
Bulgaria	21.7	3.3	48	49.9	6.0	24	7.1	1.8	12
France	35.9	3.1	143	50.4	4.6	75	14.2	3.1	40
Germany	22.1	2.5	78	64.7	5.8	50	4.0	1.3	14
Italy	24.6	4.0	33	48.8	11.2	16	8.2	3.0	10
Netherlands	33.4	4.6	78	58.6	7.4	46	12.0	3.2	18
Romania	26.5	4.7	19	64.9	16.7	14	16.7	6.9	6
Spain	33.1	3.8	84	73.3	5.8	57	14.4	3.4	23
Ukraine	32.9	2.5	126	38.2	5.0	48	13.4	2.3	32
Africa and the Middle East									
Israel	35.3	3.2	93	55.5	5.5	51	8.3	2.1	15
Lebanon	38.4	5.0	39	72.4	6.9	29	30.1	6.3	25
Nigeria	29.7	3.6	70	64.8	7.2	43	1.9	0.9	3
South Africa	41.7	2.3	171	60.5	4.5	107	11.2	2.3	33
Asia and the Pacific									
China (Beijing and Shanghai)	29.5	4.6	42	47.1	10.0	21	26.1	4.7	28
India	43.5	1.9	203	53.6	3.9	109	10.1	2.3	22
Japan	18.4	2.2	74	50.6	5.4	38	7.5	1.5	29
China (Shenzhen)	22.3	2.9	72	26.8	5.4	23	9.4	1.8	30
New Zealand	35.1	1.4	814	51.2	2.2	447	16.6	1.4	241

finding of this analysis is that as more time passes after the first onset of ideation, respondents are less likely to make a suicide plan. In all countries, the risk of transition from ideation to plan diminishes with increasing time from the first onset of ideation (see Table 4.4, third column). The odds ratios (ORs) for this association range from a low OR of 0.1 (Bulgaria and Italy) to a high OR of 0.8 (Spain and Colombia).

Suicidal behaviors as risk factors for the transition from suicide ideation to attempt

Figure 4.3 shows that there is a rapid transition from ideation to a suicide attempt in all samples, with most of the transitions again occurring within the first year after onset of ideation. Some variations of this general rule also are apparent in the graph, as in China (Beijing and Shanghai). For example, there are some transitions that emerge after 35 years since the onset of ideation, such as in Colombia where transitions are reported as late as 40 years after the first onset of ideation.

Table 4.5 presents the discrete-time survival model for suicidal characteristics as risk factors for the transition from ideation to attempt. This model is a little more complex than the one described in Table 4.4, as we also included the presence of a plan, and interaction terms for AOO of ideation and time since ideation, AOO of ideation and plan, and time since ideation and

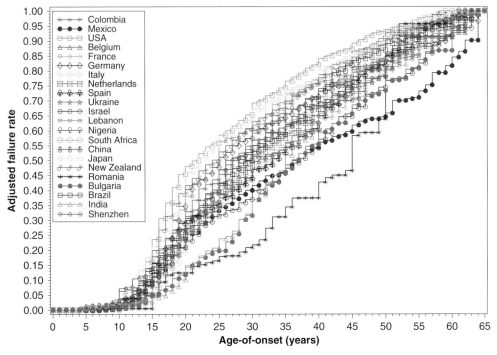

Figure 4.1. Cumulative age-of-onset distribution for suicide ideation in each country. (See color plate section.)

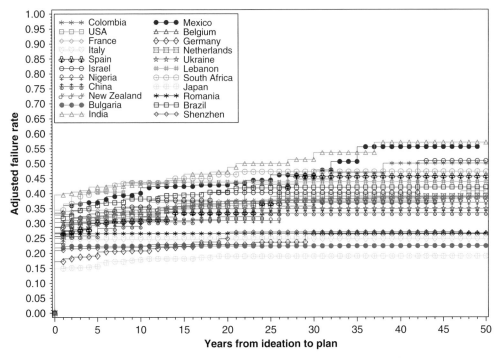

Figure 4.2. Cumulative speed of transition from ideation to plan in each country. (See color plate section.)

Table 4.4. Association between age-of-onset of ideation and transitioning to a plan from ideation among ideators across World Mental Health countries

Countries	Age-of-onset of ideation[a] OR (95% CI)	Age-of-onset^2 of ideation[b] OR (95% CI)	Time since ideation OR (95% CI)
The Americas			
Brazil	0.8 (0.5–1.4)	1.0 (0.9–1.1)	0.5* (0.4–0.7)
Colombia	1.6 (0.7–3.6)	0.9 (0.8–1.1)	0.8* (0.7–0.9)
Mexico	0.8 (0.4–1.7)	1.0 (0.9–1.2)	0.7* (0.6–0.8)
United States	0.6* (0.4–0.8)	1.1 (1.0–1.1)	0.7* (0.6–0.7)
Europe			
Belgium	2.4* (1.0–5.5)	0.9* (0.8–1.0)	0.6* (0.4–0.8)
Bulgaria	0.3* (0.1–0.8)	1.2* (1.0–1.3)	0.1* (0.1–0.1)
France	0.8 (0.4–1.7)	1.0 (0.9–1.1)	0.5* (0.3–0.7)
Germany	1.1 (0.5–2.8)	1.0 (0.9–1.1)	0.7* (0.6–0.9)
Italy	1.0 (0.2–3.9)	1.0 (0.8–1.2)	0.1* (0.0–0.1)
Netherlands	1.3 (0.5–3.1)	1.0 (0.8–1.1)	0.7* (0.5–0.9)
Romania	1.4 (0.1–3.6)	1.1 (0.9–1.4)	0.0* (0.0–0.0)
Spain	0.5* (0.3–0.8)	1.1* (1.0–1.2)	0.8* (0.6–0.9)
Ukraine	0.7 (0.4–1.3)	1.0 (1.0–1.1)	0.3* (0.2–0.5)
Africa and the Middle East			
Israel	1.4 (0.6–3.0)	1.0 (0.9–1.1)	0.7* (0.5–0.8)
Lebanon	0.7 (0.1–3.5)	1.0 (0.8–1.3)	0.5* (0.2–0.9)
Nigeria	1.8 (0.6–5.4)	0.9 (0.8–1.1)	0.5* (0.3–1.0)
South Africa	1.6 (0.6–4.5)	0.9 (0.8–1.1)	0.5* (0.4–0.7)
Asia and the Pacific			
China (Beijing and Shanghai)	0.9 (0.3–2.7)	1.0 (0.9–1.2)	0.6* (0.4–0.9)
India	1.5 (0.9–2.5)	0.9 (0.9–1.0)	0.7* (0.5–0.8)
Japan	1.0 (0.4–2.2)	1.0 (0.9–1.1)	0.7* (0.6–1.0)
China (Shenzhen)	1.3 (0.5–3.6)	1.0 (0.8–1.1)	0.5* (0.3–0.7)
New Zealand	0.8 (0.6–1.1)	1.0 (1.0–1.1)	0.6* (0.5–0.7)

* Significant at the 0.05 level, two-sided test.
0.0* (0.0–0.0) OR is ≤ 0.05 indicating very low risk.
[a] AOO (age-of-onset) of ideation is divided by 10.
[b] AOO^2 of ideation is divided by 100.

plan. Three main findings are apparent in these results. Generally, having a suicide plan increases the odds of making a suicide attempt. Positive ORs ranged from 1.1 (Nigeria) to 109.1 (Germany), with eight ORs reaching statistical significance. The exceptions to this pattern are France, China (Beijing and Shanghai), and Shenzhen, in which lower (but non-significant) odds are found among those with a plan. Null results are seen in two countries (Netherlands and Spain). As was the case for suicide plan, longer time since ideation is associated with lower ORs for transition to attempt, meaning the longer one goes with suicide ideation without making an attempt, the less likely one is to make an attempt. Another point worth mentioning is the interaction term in the last column of this table. The interaction term tells us that among those with a plan, the longer the period of ideation, the greater the risk of attempt. Increased ORs are found for all countries except Brazil, Bulgaria, Ukraine, and Israel. Null results are seen for South Africa. This is

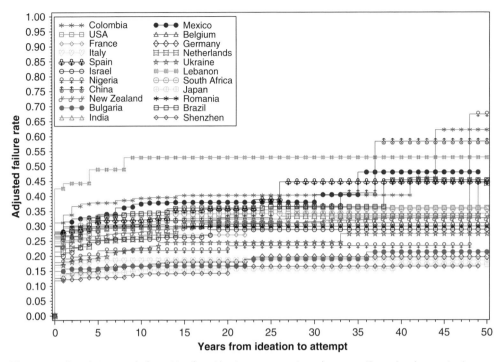

Figure 4.3. Cumulative speed of transition from ideation to attempt in each country. (See color plate section.)

interesting because we see that the main variable – time since ideation – is negatively associated with attempt so that the longer the time since one had ideation the less likely one is to make an attempt, but among planners that was not the case.

Discussion

The results of this study are limited in four important ways. First, our analysis was based on retrospective self-reports, which may contain inaccuracies due to bias or forgetting (Angold et al., 1996). Second, although the overall response rate was at an acceptable level, response rates varied across countries and in some cases were below commonly accepted standards. We controlled for differential response using poststratification adjustments, but it is possible that response rates were related to the presence of suicidal behaviors or mental disorders, which could have biased cross-national comparisons. Third, there may have been cross-national differences in the willingness to report on suicidal behavior. Significant efforts were dedicated to carefully translating and back-translating the WHO-CIDI used in this study in order to minimize such concerns (Kessler & Üstün, 2004). However, differences in factors such as the stigma about suicide are likely to

persist cross-nationally despite these efforts. Fourth, we only examined a limited set of potential risk factors for transitions across suicide ideation to plan and attempt (the characteristics of suicidal behavior) and did not include factors known to be associated with suicidal behavior (e.g., demographic variables and psychiatric disorders). These topics will all be the subject of further inquiries in the following chapters of this book.

With these limitations in mind, this study documented three noteworthy results. First, we expanded the number of participating sites compared to the prior work of Nock et al. (2008a) to document large cross-national variability in the prevalence of suicidal behavior. Suicide ideation varied from 2.6% to 15.9%, the prevalence of plan varied between 0.7% and 6.2%, and suicide attempt varied between 0.5% and 5.0%. The reasons for these differences are currently unknown, and no apparent pattern of variation was found for countries from a similar geographical region or income status. As this is the first study to document and provide data on these prevalence rates using a unified set of definitions and a similar protocol for data collection, we can only speculate on the reasons for the variability. The first obvious question is whether the rates of suicidal behavior observed here map onto the rates of suicide

Table 4.5. Association between age-of-onset of ideation and transitioning to an attempt among ideators

Countries	Age-of-onset of ideation[a] OR (95% CI)	Age-of-onset^2 of ideation[b] OR (95% CI)	Time since ideation OR (95% CI)	Plan OR (95% CI)	Age-of-onset of ideation x time since ideation OR (95% CI)	Age-of-onset of ideation x plan OR (95% CI)	Time since ideation x plan OR (95% CI)
The Americas							
Brazil	1.5 (0.5–4.7)	0.9 (0.8–1.1)	1.1 (0.8–1.4)	10.1* (2.2–46.3)	1.0* (1.0–1.0)	1.0 (1.0–1.0)	0.8 (0.5–1.1)
Colombia	1.7 (0.5–6.4)	0.8 (0.7–1.0)	1.2 (0.9–1.5)	1.5 (0.3–7.0)	1.0* (0.9–1.0)	1.1* (1.0–1.1)	1.1 (0.9–1.3)
Mexico	1.6 (0.5–5.4)	0.9 (0.7–1.1)	1.0 (0.5–2.1)	3.3 (0.7–16.0)	1.0* (0.9–1.0)	1.0 (1.0–1.1)	1.5 (0.8–2.6)
United States	1.1 (0.6–2.0)	1.0 (0.9–1.1)	0.9 (0.6–1.2)	5.5* (2.3–13.1)	1.0* (1.0–1.0)	1.0 (0.9–1.0)	1.2 (0.9–1.6)
Europe							
Belgium	4.0* (1.0–16.3)	0.9 (0.7–1.1)	0.9 (0.3–2.6)	10.2 (0.3–353.8)	1.0 (0.9–1.0)	1.0 (0.9–1.1)	1.3 (0.5–3.5)
Bulgaria	2.4 (0.5–11.1)	0.9 (0.8–1.1)	0.8 (0.4–1.7)	41.1* (1.2–1381.4)	1.0 (1.0–1.0)	1.0 (0.9–1.1)	0.9 (0.4–2.1)
France	1.0 (0.2–4.6)	1.0 (0.8–1.2)	0.3* (0.2–0.4)	0.6 (0.1–2.6)	1.0 (1.0–1.0)	1.0* (1.0–1.1)	4.2* (3.4–5.2)
Germany	2.2 (0.5–10.6)	0.9 (0.7–1.1)	0.3* (0.2–0.4)	109.1* (9.9–1199.1)	1.0 (1.0–1.0)	0.9 (0.8–1.0)	2.2* (1.5–3.1)
Italy	2.0 (0.2–25.7)	0.9 (0.7–1.3)	0.6 (0.3–1.2)	38.5* (2.2–687.9)	0.9* (0.9–1.0)	0.9 (0.9–1.0)	1.8 (0.8–3.8)
Netherlands	8.6 (0.7–112.3)	0.6* (0.4–1.0)	0.8 (0.5–1.3)	1.0 (0.1–13.7)	1.0 (0.9–1.0)	1.1 (1.0–1.2)	1.4 (0.9–2.1)
Romania	10.3* (1.9–55.6)	0.8* (0.6–0.9)	0.3 (0.1–1.3)	3.1 (0.1–77.3)	1.0 (0.9–1.0)	1.0 (1.0–1.0)	1.3 (0.2–6.8)
Spain	1.2 (0.4–3.2)	0.9 (0.8–1.1)	0.8 (0.5–1.4)	1.0 (0.1–8.4)	1.0* (0.9–1.0)	1.1* (1.0–1.2)	1.8* (1.0–3.1)
Ukraine	2.0 (0.6–6.2)	0.9 (0.8–1.1)	1.1 (0.8–1.6)	3.9 (0.9–17.7)	1.0 (0.9–1.0)	1.0 (1.0–1.1)	0.9 (0.7–1.3)
Africa and the Middle East							
Israel	1.6 (0.6–4.4)	0.9 (0.8–1.0)	0.7 (0.3–1.6)	4.5 (0.8–25.8)	1.0 (1.0–1.0)	1.0 (1.0–1.0)	0.8 (0.5–1.4)
Lebanon	6.2* (1.6–24.6)	0.7* (0.6–0.9)	0.0* (0.0–0.1)	1.5 (0.1–20.1)	1.0 (0.9–1.0)	1.0 (0.9–1.1)	22.6* (11.8–43.3)
Nigeria	0.4 (0.1–2.4)	1.0 (0.7–1.5)	0.3* (0.2–0.5)	1.1 (0.0–36.9)	0.9* (0.9–1.0)	1.2 (1.0–1.3)	5.5* (3.7–8.3)
South Africa	0.8 (0.2–2.6)	1.0 (0.9–1.2)	0.3* (0.2–0.5)	7.8 (2.2–27.5)	1.0 (1.0–1.0)	1.0 (1.0–1.1)	1.0 (0.6–1.5)
Asia and the Pacific							
China (Beijing and Shanghai)	4.8 (0.7–34.6)	0.8 (0.5–1.1)	0.7 (0.3–1.8)	0.0 (0.0–1.3)	1.0 (1.0–1.0)	1.1* (1.0–1.2)	1.6 (0.8–3.3)
India	0.4* (0.2–0.8)	1.1* (1.0–1.2)	0.3* (0.1–0.6)	4.5* (1.1–18.9)	0.9* (0.9–1.0)	1.0 (1.0–1.1)	3.9* (2.2–7.1)
Japan	0.6 (0.3–1.4)	1.1 (0.9–1.2)	0.2* (0.2–0.3)	3.5 (0.8–6.2)	1.0 (1.0–1.0)	1.0 (1.0–1.0)	4.0* (3.0–5.4)
China (Shenzhen)	6.0* (1.2–31.1)	0.7 (0.5–1.0)	1.1 (0.5–2.3)	0.2 (0.0–.9)	0.9* (0.9–1.0)	1.2* (1.0–1.3)	1.4 (0.7–2.9)
New Zealand	1.2 (0.7–2.1)	1.0 (0.9–1.0)	1.0 (0.8–1.2)	4.3* (2.2–8.5)	1.0* (1.0–1.0)	1.0 (1.0–1.0)	1.1 (0.9–1.4)

* Significant at the 0.05 level, two-sided test.
[a] AOO (age-of-onset) of ideation is divided by 10.
[b] AOO^2 of ideation is divided by 100.

death across the same countries. Using data retrieved from the WHO suicide database (http://www.who.int/mental_health/prevention/suicide_rates/en/index.html, accessed June 30, 2010), we observed that the rate of suicide death and suicide attempt have a small, negative correlation ($r = -0.20$), further highlighting the difference between suicide completers and suicide attempters (Paris, 2006). Differences in rates of alcohol use, psychiatric disorders, and other known socioeconomic variables are possible reasons for this global variability of rates of suicidal behavior, following prior work on completed suicide. Other chapters of this book delve into these and other possible explanatory factors.

A second finding was that even though there is variability in lifetime prevalence, there are important commonalities in our results. Suicide ideation rarely is reported before the early teens, increases rapidly in mid- to late-teens and early adulthood, and although suicide ideation can have its onset throughout the life course, the likelihood of new-onset ideation diminishes in later life. In all countries, suicide attempt is reported more often among those with a plan than among those without a plan. In all countries, the highest risk period for transitioning from ideation to plan or to attempt occurs during the first year after the onset of ideation. The similarity of results regarding the rapid transition from ideation to plan and attempt is perhaps one of the most striking findings of this report. Indeed, the fact that the majority of those with suicide ideation who subsequently make a plan and attempt do so within the first year of onset of ideation suggests that the window of opportunity for preventive interventions after the onset of ideation is quite narrow. In essence, intervention efforts need to focus on prevention of ideation rather than prevention of the transition from ideation to more serious outcomes. This finding is consistent with, and provides further support for, earlier work from our group using data from the U.S. (Kessler et al., 1999) and suggests cross-national consistency in this very important pattern of rapid transition from onset of ideation to onset of plan and attempt. Understanding who among those with suicide ideation will transition to make a suicide plan and attempt suicide has become a priority in current suicide research due to its possible impact on clinical practice (Borges et al., 2006).

Third, and perhaps most importantly, we showed that in all countries, prior history of suicide ideation is a key risk factor for a future suicide plan, and that a history of ideation, the presence of a plan, and the history of ideation among planners are all key factors to understanding the transition to attempt among suicide ideators. These findings on the importance of retrospectively assessed AOO of suicide ideation, time since ideation, and the presence of a suicide plan are similar to prior longitudinal reports in the National Comorbidity Survey (NCS) that used baseline suicidal behavior as predictors of later reported suicidal behavior in the NCS-2 (Borges et al., 2008).

Future directions

This study provides data on the lifetime prevalence of suicide ideation, plans, and attempts among the largest ever available nationally representative sample, with a common set of definitions and data gathering protocol. As new countries continue to join the WMH Surveys project, the representativeness of this dataset will continue to expand. As our study was based on retrospective self-report of suicidal behavior, longitudinal work on large and representative samples of the general population is needed. Given the cost and great length of time required to conduct such surveys, it is likely that results from cross-sectional surveys such as ours will be needed for preventive purposes, at least as a first approximation. In this regard, it is very reassuring that our results are consistent with the extant longitudinal work on the topic (Borges et al., 2008; Brezo et al., 2007).

Acknowledgements

Portions of this chapter are based on Nock, M. K., Borges, G., Bromet, E. J., et al. (2008a). Cross-national prevalence and risk factors for suicidal ideation, plans and attempts. *British Journal of Psychiatry*, 192(2), 98–105. Copyright © 2008. The Royal College of Psychiatrists. Reproduced with permission.

References

Angold, A., Erkanli, A., Costello, E. J., & Rutter, M. (1996). Precision, reliability and accuracy in the dating of symptom onsets in child and adolescent psychopathology. *Journal of Child Psychology and Psychiatry*, **37**(6), 657–664.

Bertolote, J. M., Fleischmann, A., De Leo, D., et al. (2005). Suicide attempts, plans, and ideation in culturally diverse sites: the WHO SUPRE-MISS community survey. *Psychological Medicine*, **35**(10), 1457–1465.

Borges, G., Angst, J., Nock, M. K., Ruscio, A. M., & Kessler, R. C. (2008). Risk factors for the incidence and persistence of suicide-related outcomes: a 10-year follow-up study using the National Comorbidity Surveys. *Journal of Affective Disorders*, **105**(1–3), 25–33.

Borges, G., Angst, J., Nock, M. K., et al. (2006). A risk index for 12-month suicide attempts in the National Comorbidity Survey Replication (NCS-R). *Psychological Medicine*, **36**(12), 1747–1757.

Brezo, J., Paris, J., Tremblay, R., et al. (2007). Identifying correlates of suicide attempts in suicidal ideators: a population-based study. *Psychological Medicine*, **37**(11), 1551–1562.

Durkheim, É. (1951). *Suicide*. New York, NY: Free Press.

Kessler, R. C., Borges, G., & Walters, E. E. (1999). Prevalence of and risk factors for lifetime suicide attempts in the National Comorbidity Survey. *Archives of General Psychiatry*, **56**(7), 617–626.

Kessler, R. C., & Üstün, T. B. (2004). The World Mental Health (WMH) Survey Initiative Version of the World Health Organization (WHO) Composite International Diagnostic Interview (CIDI). *International Journal of Methods in Psychiatric Research*, **13**(2), 93–121.

Nock, M. K., Borges, G., Bromet, E. J., et al. (2008a). Cross-national prevalence and risk factors for suicidal ideation, plans and attempts. *British Journal of Psychiatry*, **192**(2), 98–105.

Nock, M. K., Borges, G., Bromet, E. J., et al. (2008b). Suicide and suicidal behaviors. *Epidemiologic Reviews*, **30**, 133–154.

Paris, J. (2006). Predicting and preventing suicide: do we know enough to do either? *Harvard Review of Psychiatry*, **14**(5), 233–240.

Weissman, M. M., Bland, R. C., Canino, G. J., et al. (1999). Prevalence of suicide ideation and suicide attempts in nine countries. *Psychological Medicine*, **29**(1), 9–17.

Chapter

5

Persistence of suicidal behaviors over time

Ronald C. Kessler, Sergio Aguilar-Gaxiola, Guilherme Borges,
Wai Tat Chiu, John Fayyad, Mark Oakley Browne, Yutaka Ono,
Nancy A. Sampson, Alan M. Zaslavsky, and Matthew K. Nock

The vast majority of research on suicidal behavior (i.e., suicide ideation, plans, and attempts) has focused on the identification of correlates or risk factors for the occurrence or first onset of such behavior (Hawton & van Heeringen, 2000; Nock et al., 2008). In contrast, few studies have documented the course of suicidal behavior; as a result, surprisingly little is known about the extent to which suicidal behavior, once present, persists over time. Prior data consistently document that suicidal behavior is reported at much higher rates among adolescents than among adults (Centers for Disease Control, 2008; Nock et al., 2008). The rates of suicidal behavior are so high among adolescents that some have suggested that the experience of such thoughts and behaviors are a normative part of adolescence (Lieberman, 1993). On the other hand, we know from decades of research that the best predictor of future suicidal behavior is a history of past suicidal behavior. Therefore, an important task for suicide research is to determine: (a) In what proportion of cases is suicidal behavior a one-time, transient event vs. an ongoing, more persistent problem in need of clinical attention? (b) When suicidal behavior does persist, what does its course look like over time? and (c) What factors predict an extended pattern of persistence? This chapter addresses each of these questions by providing a comprehensive examination of the persistence of suicide ideation, plans, and attempts among respondents in the WMH Surveys.

The few studies that have examined the persistence of suicidal behavior over time provide useful preliminary results about the pattern of persistence, and also highlight several ways in which research in this area can be improved. Several studies have documented that among people experiencing suicide ideation at baseline, approximately one-third continue to report ideation at 12 months (36.7%; Raue et al., 2007), two years (31.3%; ten Have et al., 2009), and 10 years (35.0%; Borges et al., 2008). A smaller percentage report the persistence of suicide attempt – with 7.4% reporting the persistence of such behavior at two years (ten Have et al., 2009), and 15.4% at 10 years (Borges et al., 2008). Several other studies report on persistence but provide only crude measures, such as whether suicide ideation was reported in two or more of: "adolescence", "adulthood", and "current" (Brezo et al., 2007) or whether lifetime suicide ideation also was endorsed in the subsequent 12 months (Zhang et al., 2011); report only on differences between people who have made single vs. multiple suicide attempts (Rudd et al., 1996); or examine only a narrow developmental period (e.g., age 15–30 years; Reinherz et al., 2006) and/or a small clinical sample. In summary, several earlier studies suggest suicide ideation and attempts persist over 1–10 years for a substantial minority of people; however, there are many as yet unanswered questions about the patterns and predictors of the persistence of suicidal behavior over time.

In the WMH Surveys, as described in Chapter 3, we used the information obtained about age-of-onset (AOO) and recency to study persistence of suicidal behaviors over time. The main problem with this kind of information is that it is *right-censored* (Lagakos, 1979); that is, we do not know anything about the transition probabilities for persistence or recurrence of the behaviors going forward, but only current prevalence and, among people who did not have any suicidal behavior in the year of interview, time since last occurrence. Although some information about course of suicidal behaviors can be gleaned from such right-censored data, this information is limited.

Suicide, eds. Matthew K. Nock, Guilherme Borges, and Yutaka Ono. Published by Cambridge University Press.
© World Health Organization 2012.

Methods

Suicidal behaviors

We consider persistence of three suicidal behaviors in this chapter: ideation among lifetime ideators, plans among lifetime planners, and repeat attempts among people with a lifetime history of making one or more prior attempts. We know AOO of each of these behaviors. We know each respondent's age at interview and we know age of recency of each behavior. AOO can be subtracted from age at interview to obtain a measure of time between AOO and interview. We can also subtract AOO from age of recency to obtain a measure of duration of the suicidal behavior, but with the caveat that the right-censoring of the data makes it impossible to know the proportion of respondents defined as having low duration who might in the future have a recurrence.

Statistical analysis

As described in Chapter 3, we begin by examining recency curves that plot the cumulative probability of a given outcome occurring most recently as a function of age at interview, AOO, and age at recency. As unrestricted recency curves are uninformative, these curves are stratified by how many years ago the behaviors started (i.e., time between AOO and interview). We noted in Chapter 3 that the patterns of persistence among respondents with a history of suicidal behaviors do not fit a simple mover–stayer model. We nonetheless estimated a general backward recency model to predict number of years since most recent suicidal behavior controlling for AOO and time since onset and using predictors that were true of the respondent as of AOO. In addition, we estimated the five logistic regression models described in Chapter 3 for each outcome in order to break down significant associations seen in the general backward recency model and see the parts of the process in which they are important. These five include: whether or not the behavior persisted beyond two years after AOO; if so, whether recency was in the ten, five, or one year(s) of interview; and whether recency among cases with a most recent episode in the five years before interview was in the one year before interview.

Recency distributions

Recency of ideation was plotted for the 10,018 WMH respondents who reported ever having suicide ideation

and having AOO at least three years before interview. These curves were plotted separately in subgroups defined by number of years between AOO and time of interview in five-year intervals (+/− two years from the mid-point of the interval) of 5, 10, 15, 20, 25, and 30+ years since onset. The X-axis in the figure represents the number of years between AOO and recency. A score of 0 consequently means that the suicidal behavior never occurred beyond the age of onset, whereas scores of 5, 10, or 15 mean that the behavior most recently occurred either 5, 10, or 15 years after onset. A very striking result can be seen in this figure: that 47%–55% of lifetime ideators (exclusive of those whose ideation started within the three years of interview) never have suicidal thoughts beyond the year the thoughts first started no matter how many years pass between AOO and age at interview (Figure 5.1). The remainder of cases have recencies that are relatively evenly distributed across years. A similar pattern can be seen for recency of suicide plans, where 54%–64% of lifetime cases report never again having a plan beyond the year of onset, while recency for the remainder of cases is well distributed across the subsequent years (Figure 5.2). The same basic pattern is found for recency of suicide attempts, where 63%–77% of lifetime cases never make an attempt beyond the year of their first attempt, while recency for the remainder of cases is well distributed across the subsequent years (Figure 5.3). With regard to attempts, 62.1% of lifetime attempters report only one attempt, 18.4% two, 9.2% three, 3.2% four, 1.7% five, and 5.4% more than five (see Table 5.1).

Another perspective on recency comes from examining the number of years before interview (rather than since AOO) when the suicidal behavior most recently occurred in the same samples as the earlier figures, again plotting curves separately in subgroups defined by number of years between AOO and time of interview. When this is done, we see that between 13% and 23% of lifetime ideators continue to have thoughts of suicide in the year of interview no matter how many years passed between AOO and age at interview (Figure 5.4). Given that the results reported previously in Figure 5.1 showed that 47%–55% of lifetime ideation does not persist beyond AOO, the results in Figure 5.4 imply that 25%–45% of all lifetime ideators with any persistence beyond AOO continue to have ideation in the year of interview. As seen in Figures 5.5 and 5.6, the unconditional proportions are a good deal lower for suicide plans (7%–19%) and attempts

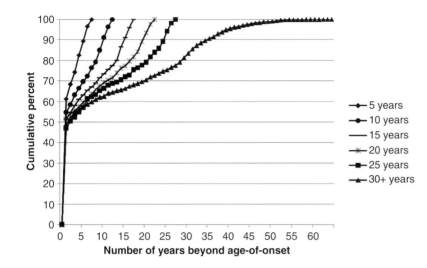

Figure 5.1. Recency of suicide ideation by number of years beyond age-of-onset in subgroups defined by time between age-of-onset and interview (+/− 2).

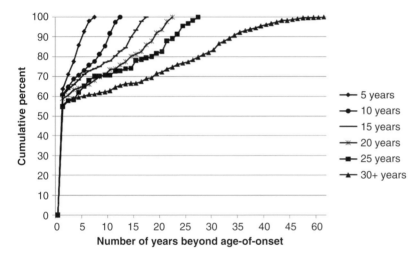

Figure 5.2. Recency of suicide plan by number of years beyond age-of-onset in subgroups defined by time between age-of-onset and interview (+/− 2).

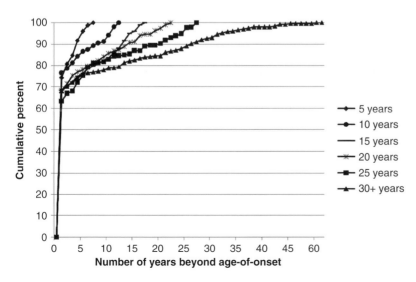

Figure 5.3. Recency of suicide attempt by number of years beyond age-of-onset in subgroups defined by time between age-of-onset and interview (+/− 2).

Table 5.1. Number of lifetime suicide attempts among WMH respondents who made attempts (n = 2928)

	Among WMH respondents who made attempts	
Number of lifetime suicide attempts	**%**	**(SE)**
1	62.1	(1.1)
2	18.4	(1.0)
3	9.2	(0.7)
4	3.2	(0.5)
5	1.7	(0.3)
6–7	1.0	(0.2)
8–10	1.2	(0.2)
11–15	0.7	(0.1)
16–20	1.4	(0.3)
21+	1.1	(0.2)
Total	100.0	

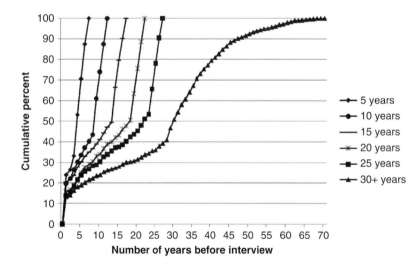

Figure 5.4. Recency of suicide ideation by number of years before interview in subgroups defined by time between age-of-onset and interview (+/− 2).

(4%–14%), but these represent 15%–51% of respondents with plans that persisted beyond AOO and 14%–61% of respondents who make repeated suicide attempts.

Associations of persistence with age of onset and time between age-of-onset and interview

We went through an illustrative series of calculations in **Chapter 3** to demonstrate that the patterns of persistence seen in the previous figures cannot be reproduced by assuming the existence of underlying processes with simple characteristics. However, there is also more structure in the data than shown in the figures. This can be seen by breaking down the patterns in the figures more finely by cross-classifying AOO with time between AOO and interview. We examine this cross-classification here for illustrative values of AOO and time between AOO and interview. Appendix Tables 5.1–5.3 show the cross-classification for a more complete set of values.

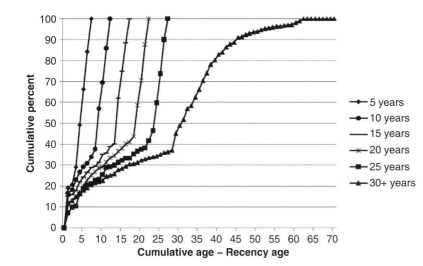

Figure 5.5. Recency of suicide plan by number of years before interview in subgroups defined by time between age-of-onset and interview (+/− 2).

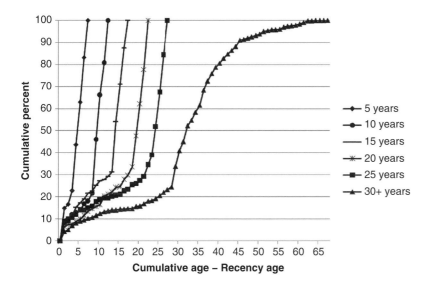

Figure 5.6. Recency of suicide attempt by number of years before interview in subgroups defined by time between age-of-onset and interview (+/− 2).

Focusing first on persistence of ideation, we see that early onset is consistently associated with high persistence. This can be seen in the finding that the proportions of lifetime cases with either no persistence (i.e., age at recency is the same as AOO) or low persistence (i.e., recency is no more than five years after AOO) are substantially lower among respondents with early rather than later AOO after controlling for time between AOO and interview (see Table 5.2, Parts I–II). The positive association of early AOO with persistence can also be seen in the finding that the proportions of cases with high persistence (i.e., within either five or one year [s] of interview) are higher for early than later-onset cases (see Table 5.2, Parts III–IV). The

pattern becomes increasingly pronounced as time between AOO and interview increases.

Persistence is also negatively associated with time between AOO and interview after controlling for AOO, although this association is more pronounced for measures of high persistence (i.e., recency within five years of interview) than no-low persistence (i.e., recency no more than five years after AOO). It is important to realize that the outcomes in Parts I–II of Table 5.2 can only decrease within cohorts as time between AOO and interview increases. They can never increase, as any future recurrence of ideation among respondents who, up to a given time, had no recurrence beyond the first five years after AOO would

Table 5.2. Recency of suicide ideation among respondents with a lifetime history of ideation as a joint function of age-of-onset and time between age-of-onset and interview[a]

	Number of years (+/− 2) between Age-of-onset and interview					
	10		20		30+	
Age-of-onset	% (SE)	(n)	% (SE)	(n)	% (SE)	(n)
I. Ideation did *not* continue beyond AOO						
≤12	43.8 (5.3)	(128)	37.3 (5.9)	(100)	36.6 (4.0)	(222)
20–24	56.6 (3.8)	(258)	57.8 (4.8)	(164)	60.1 (3.7)	(267)
35+	67.4 (2.9)	(410)	67.2 (3.8)	(195)	65.5 (4.4)	(158)
II. Ideation did *not* continue beyond five years after AOO						
≤12	62.0 (5.2)	(128)	46.8 (6.1)	(100)	41.8 (4.1)	(222)
20–24	68.0 (3.6)	(258)	62.4 (4.4)	(164)	65.3 (3.6)	(267)
35+	76.0 (2.7)	(410)	73.6 (3.5)	(195)	73.4 (4.0)	(158)
III. Ideation continued to within five years of interview						
≤12	45.7 (5.5)	(128)	30.1 (5.7)	(100)	27.9 (3.6)	(222)
20–24	34.9 (3.7)	(258)	22.3 (4.0)	(164)	16.4 (2.7)	(267)
35+	26.6 (2.7)	(410)	16.1 (3.1)	(195)	12.2 (2.8)	(158)
IV. Ideation continued to the year of interview						
≤12	23.6 (5.0)	(128)	16.9 (4.5)	(100)	17.0 (2.8)	(222)
20–24	24.2 (3.4)	(258)	12.0 (2.9)	(164)	12.1 (2.5)	(267)
35+	18.3 (2.4)	(410)	10.1 (2.4)	(195)	11.0 (2.7)	(158)

AOO, age-of-onset.
[a] Reported only for illustrative values of AOO and time between AOO and interview. Results for a complete set of these values are reported in Appendix Table 5.1.

move such individuals out of this no-low persistence category. We would consequently expect, all else equal, that these proportions would decrease in Table 5.2 within subsamples defined by AOO as time between AOO and interview increases. The fact that very little evidence of such a time trend exists in the data other than for respondents with early AOO is striking. This finding implies that risk of subsequent recurrence among cases initially classified in the no-low recurrence category is very small if it does not occur by approximately one decade after AOO.

The entries in Parts III–IV of Table 5.2, in comparison, could either increase, decrease, or remain unchanged within cohorts as time between AOO and interview increases, as the proportion of cases with recent episodes will increase if recurrence rates increase over time, decrease if recurrence rates fall over time, and remain the same if recurrence rates are constant over time. As it happens, we see consistent

evidence of decreases with increasing time from AOO within subsamples defined by AOO. This evidence of decreases associated with time between AOO and interview in Parts III–IV is consistent with the absence of increases in Parts I–II.

The results in Table 5.3 show that AOO is less consistently associated with persistence of suicide plans than Table 5.2 showed it to be with suicide ideation. Specifically, the proportions of cases with both no-low persistence and high persistence are higher among respondents with early than later-onset of plans after controlling for time between AOO and interview. Time between AOO and interview, in comparison, has a consistently negative association with persistence of suicide plans. This can be seen in the fact that high proportions of lifetime cases have no-low persistence that shows no strong pattern of decreasing as time between AOO and interview increases other than for respondents with early AOO

Table 5.3. Recency of suicide plans among respondents with a lifetime history of a plan as a joint function of age-of-onset and time between age-of-onset and interview[a]

| Age-of-onset | Number of years (+/– 2) between Age-of-onset and interview | | | | | |
| | 10 | | 20 | | 30+ | |
	% (SE)	(n)	% (SE)	(n)	% (SE)	(n)
I. Ideation did *not* continue beyond AOO						
≤12	53.1 (11.0)	(42)	35.9 (11.8)	(32)	33.0 (7.4)	(56)
20–24	67.1 (6.5)	(91)	70.4 (7.5)	(52)	64.4 (5.5)	(95)
35+	65.2 (5.2)	(154)	77.7 (7.8)	(52)	75.3 (7.4)	(45)
II. Ideation did *not* continue beyond five years after AOO						
≤12	63.6 (11.2)	(42)	45.9 (11.7)	(32)	39.7 (8.1)	(56)
20–24	72.8 (6.2)	(91)	73.8 (7.5)	(52)	67.3 (5.5)	(95)
35+	73.7 (4.5)	(154)	85.0 (6.4)	(52)	75.3 (7.4)	(45)
III. Ideation continued to within five years of interview						
≤12	36.4 (11.2)	(42)	34.9 (10.6)	(32)	15.0 (5.5)	(56)
20–24	27.2 (6.2)	(91)	20.4 (7.2)	(52)	22.0 (5.1)	(95)
35+	28.8 (4.6)	(154)	13.5 (6.2)	(52)	14.5 (6.3)	(45)
IV. Ideation continued to the year of interview						
≤12	27.8 (11.3)	(42)	13.1 (5.7)	(32)	10.0 (4.7)	(56)
20–24	18.4 (6.0)	(91)	6.5 (3.4)	(52)	13.1 (4.4)	(95)
35+	18.4 (3.6)	(154)	4.1 (2.3)	(52)	12.4 (6.0)	(45)

AOO, age-of-onset.
[a] Reported only for illustrative values of AOO and time between AOO and interview. Results for a complete set of these values are reported in Appendix Table 5.2.

(see Table 5.3, Parts I–II). The negative association of persistence with time between AOO and interview can also be seen in the finding that the proportion of lifetime cases with recent episodes decreases within subsamples defined by AOO with increasing time between AOO and interview.

The results in Table 5.4 show similar patterns for recurrence of suicide attempts. As with ideation and plans, the proportion of lifetime attempters who never make another attempt beyond five years of AOO increases with increasing AOO and shows no evidence of decreasing with increasing time between AOO and interview within subsamples defined by AOO other than among those who made their first suicide attempt before entering their teens (Parts I–II). In a similar fashion, the proportion of lifetime attempters who made recent repeat attempts decreases with AOO as well as with increasing time between AOO and interview (Parts III–IV).

The persistence models

The basic persistence models

The basic associations of AOO and time between AOO and interview can be seen in the models described in Chapter 3 to study the predictors of persistence of suicidal behavior. As noted in Chapter 3, these models include a general backward recency model that summarizes information on the associations of predictors (measured as of AOO) with overall persistence as well as five more specific logistic regression models that break down these overall associations into finer components that include predictors of: whether or not the suicidal behavior persisted beyond two years after AOO; if so, whether recency was within the ten, five, or one year(s) of interview; and whether recency among cases with a most recent episode in the five years before interview was also in the past one year.

Table 5.4. Recency of suicide attempts among respondents with a lifetime history of attempts as a joint function of age-of-onset and time between age-of-onset and interview[a]

	Number of years (+/− 2) between Age-of-onset and interview					
	10		20		30+	
Age-of-onset	% (SE)	(n)	% (SE)	(n)	% (SE)	(n)
I. Ideation did *not* continue beyond AOO						
≤12	79.1 (6.5)	(36)	56.6 (11.3)	(27)	57.9 (7.6)	(56)
20–24	80.5 (6.7)	(81)	81.4 (5.8)	(57)	78.9 (5.3)	(98)
35+	85.6 (3.6)	(98)	78.3 (7.9)	(50)	89.9 (5.2)	(29)
II. Ideation did *not* continue beyond five years after AOO						
≤12	89.9 (4.2)	(36)	60.7 (11.2)	(27)	59.4 (7.5)	(56)
20–24	86.5 (6.0)	(81)	85.9 (4.9)	(57)	85.5 (4.2)	(98)
35+	90.4 (3.4)	(98)	87.1 (5.0)	(50)	92.3 (4.5)	(29)
III. Ideation continued to within five years of interview						
≤12	10.1 (4.2)	(36)	20.0 (8.7)	(27)	17.3 (6.1)	(56)
20–24	13.8 (6.0)	(81)	6.7 (3.9)	(57)	4.9 (2.5)	(98)
35+	11.6 (3.7)	(98)	3.2 (2.5)	(50)	5.4 (3.9)	(29)
IV. Ideation continued to the year of interview						
≤12	10.1 (4.2)	(36)	9.6 (7.0)	(27)	9.3 (4.8)	(56)
20–24	11.8 (5.9)	(81)	2.1 (2.1)	(57)	0.0 (0.0)	(98)
35+	5.4 (2.2)	(98)	0.0 (0.0)	(50)	2.4 (2.5)	(29)

AOO, age-of-onset.
[a] Reported only for illustrative values of AOO and time between AOO and interview. Results for a complete set of these values are reported ion Appendix Table 5.3.

Information about the predictors of persistence associated with these components has the potential to be important in targeting interventions aimed at intervening to affect the course of suicidal behaviors. Whereas we consider five outcomes in studying the *onset* of suicidal behaviors (i.e., ideation and attempts in the total sample; plans among ideators; and attempts separately among ideators with and without a plan), we consider only three outcomes (ideation, plans, attempts) in studying *persistence*.

As shown in Table 5.5, AOO and time between AOO and interview are both significant predictors of persistence of all three suicidal behaviors in the overall backward recency model. These odds ratios (ORs) are all less than 1.0, which means that odds of recurrence are positively associated with early AOO. The negative OR of time between AOO and interview means that persistence decreases as time since AOO increases within subsamples defined by AOO. These results are consistent with the patterns seen in Tables 5.2–5.4.

These overall patterns are decomposed in the five logistic regression models in Table 5.6. Focusing first on AOO, we see that the only consistently significant association in the logistic regression models related to the negative association in the overall backward recency models is that AOO predicts low persistence (i.e., recency no more than two years after AOO). This association is significant for all three outcomes (i.e., ideation, plans, and attempts) with ORs in the range 0.94–0.96. Given that the standard deviation of AOO of ideation in roughly a decade in most countries (see Figure 4.1) and the transitions to first onset of plan and attempt are typically rapid (see Figures 4.2–4.3), these ORs suggest that the odds that suicidal behaviors will persist beyond AOO among people whose AOO is one standard deviation above the mean are only between half (0.94^{10}) and two-thirds (0.96^{10}) of the odds of people whose AOO is at the mean. People whose AOO is one standard deviation below the mean, in comparison, are assumed by this model to have odds

Table 5.5. Joint associations of age-of-onset and time between age-of-onset and interview with persistence of suicidal behaviors in the overall backward recency model[a]

	Ideation	Plan	Attempt
	OR (95% CI)	OR (95% CI)	OR (95% CI)
AOO	0.97[*] (1.0–1.0)	0.97[*] (1.0–1.0)	0.95[*] (0.9–1.0)
Time between AOO and interview	0.97[*] (1.0–1.0)	0.97[*] (1.0–1.0)	0.96[*] (1.0–1.0)

AOO, age-of-onset.
[*] Significant at the 0.05 level, two-sided test.
[a] A discrete-time survival model estimated among respondents with a lifetime history of the suicidal behavior and an AOO more than one year before interview. Person–year is the unit of analysis. The outcome is number of years since most recent occurrence of the suicidal behavior. See the text for a more detailed description of the model.

Table 5.6. Joint associations of age-of-onset and time between age-of-onset and interview with persistence of suicidal behaviors in the logistic regression models for components of recency

	Model 1[a]	Model 2[b]	Model 3[c]	Model 4[d]	Model 5[e]
	OR (95% CI)	OR (95% CI)	OR (95% CI)	OR (95% CI)	OR (95% CI)
I. Suicide ideation					
AOO	0.96[*] (1.0–1.0)	0.98[*] (1.0–1.0)	0.99 (1.0–1.0)	1.01 (1.0–1.0)	1.02[*] (1.0–1.0)
Time between AOO and interview	1.01[*] (1.0–1.0)	0.94[*] (0.9–1.0)	0.95[*] (0.9–1.0)	0.98[*] (1.0–1.0)	1.02 (1.0–1.0)
II. Suicide plans					
AOO	0.96[*] (1.0–1.0)	1.03 (1.0–1.1)	1.02 (1.0–1.0)	1.03[*] (1.0–1.0)	1.02 (1.0–1.1)
Time between AOO and interview	1.01[*] (1.0–1.0)	0.95[*] (0.9–1.0)	0.95[*] (0.9–1.0)	0.99 (1.0–1.0)	1.03 (1.0–1.1)
III. Suicide attempts					
AOO	0.94[*] (0.9–1.0)	1.00 (1.0–1.0)	0.99 (1.0–1.0)	0.99 (1.0–1.0)	1.01 (0.9–1.1)
Time between AOO and interview	1.02[*] (1.0–1.0)	0.96[*] (0.9–1.0)	0.95[*] (0.9–1.0)	0.98 (0.9–1.0)	1.03 (1.0–1.1)

AOO, age-of-onset.
[*] Significant at the 0.05 level, two-sided test.
[a] A logistic regression model estimated among respondents with a lifetime history of the suicidal behavior and an AOO five or more years before interview. The outcome is a dichotomy for recency more than two years (coded 1) vs. 0–2 years (coded 0) after AOO.
[b] A logistic regression model estimated among respondents with a lifetime history of the suicidal behavior, an AOO fifteen or more years before interview, and recency more than two years after AOO. The outcome is a dichotomy for recency within ten years of interview (coded 1) vs. 11 + years earlier than interview (coded 0).
[c] A logistic regression model estimated among respondents with a lifetime history of the suicidal behavior, an AOO ten or more years before interview, and recency more than two years after AOO. The outcome is a dichotomy for recency within five years of interview (coded 1) vs. 6+ years earlier than interview (coded 0).
[d] A logistic regression model estimated among respondents with a lifetime history of the suicidal behavior, an AOO ten or more years before interview, and recency more than two years after AOO. The outcome is a dichotomy for recency within the year of interview (coded 1) vs. 1+ years earlier than interview (coded 0).
[e] A logistic regression model estimated among respondents with a lifetime history of the suicidal behavior, an AOO ten or more years before interview, and recency within five years of interview. The outcome is a dichotomy for recency within the year of interview (coded 1) vs. 1+ years earlier than interview (coded 0).

of persistence beyond AOO that are 1.5–2.0 times those of people whose AOO is at the mean.

The associations of AOO with the other four dichotomous outcomes in Table 5.6 are inconsistent in sign and largely insignificant. There are three significant coefficients in this set. First, AOO has a significant negative association with persistence in the ten years before interview (among people with recency more than two years after AOO) of suicide ideation. Second, AOO has a significant positive association with persistence of ideation in the year of interview (among people with recency within five years of interview). Third, AOO has a positive association with persistence of plans in the year of interview (among people with recency more than two years after AOO). Taken together, these results suggest that while late AOO is a consistent predictor of suicidal behaviors never persisting beyond their AOO, some aspects of persistence among those who do persist beyond AOO are stronger for later- than earlier-onset cases.

We also see inconsistent signs in the associations of time between AOO and interview with persistence. As noted above, these associations are consistently negative in the general backward recency model, but they are consistently positive in predicting recency more than two years after AOO although the effect is modest. Specifically, the odds of reporting suicidal behaviors persisting beyond two years after AOO increase by only 10%–20% for a 10-year increase in time from AOO to interview. Time between AOO and interview has significant negative associations, in comparison, with persistence in the ten (ideation plans, and attempts), five (ideation and plans), and one (ideation and plans) years before interview among people with recency more than two years after AOO. The strongest effects are for recency within either five years of interview or within ten years of interview, suggesting that the odds of persistence into recent years among respondents with time between AOO and interview a decade above the mean are between half and two-thirds the odds of people at the mean, while people interviewed a decade earlier than the mean interval after AOO are predicted to have odds of persistence in this time range 1.5–2.0 times those of people at the mean.

More complex persistence models

These associations of AOO, and especially of time between AOO and interview, with persistence were included in our prediction equations largely as methodological controls to adjust for the fact that we assessed persistence only indirectly (i.e., by asking about recency rather than asking the more detailed set of questions needed to reconstruct a complete event history) and retrospectively. We consequently want to use controls for these variables to adjust as best as possible for methodological confounds associated with time at risk and length of recall. The linear specification in Tables 5.5–5.6 might not be optimal for this purpose even though it provides an easy-to-grasp overview assessment of the significant patterns in the data. We consequently elaborated this model after using it to get a general overview of the basic shape of the associations.

The elaboration took into consideration the fact that respondent age is the sum of AOO and time between AOO and interview and that only two of these three variables can be included as predictors in any single equation because the third variable in the set is perfectly defined by the other two. However, once we consider nonlinear associations, it is possible to include all three variables because the identity for the linear components does not extend to nonlinear components. For example, although a respondent with AOO of 15 years who is age 25 years at interview has a time between AOO and interview (10 years) that equals 25 – 15, the square of this difference (i.e., 10^2 = 100) is not the difference between the square of age at interview and AOO ($25^2 – 15^2 = 625 – 225 = 400$). It is consequently possible to include in a single prediction equation any two of the three linear terms plus all three quadratics to investigate the significance of nonlinear joint associations with persistence of AOO, time between AOO and interview, and age at interview.

We estimated quadratic models of this sort to predict persistence in the general backward recency model separately in low/lower-middle, upper-middle, and high-income countries and then plotted nonlinear associations in cases where the quadratic terms were significant. Based on the shape of the nonlinearities, we fitted regression splines to capture these nonlinear associations (de Boor, 2001). Splines were used instead of less complex polynomial models because they captured the structure in the data better. Splines were used instead of more complex recursive partitioning or adaptive splines (Zhang & Singer, 2010) because we wanted to avoid over-fitting the relatively sparse data. Detailed results of the spline regression models are presented in Appendix Tables 5.4–5.6. The

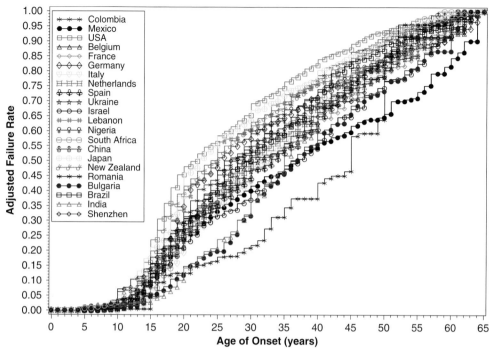

Figure 4.1. Cumulative age of onset distribution for suicide ideation in each country.

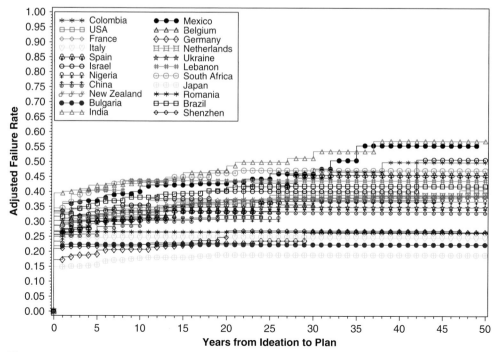

Figure 4.2. Cumulative speed of transition from ideation to plan in each country (not go to 1.0).

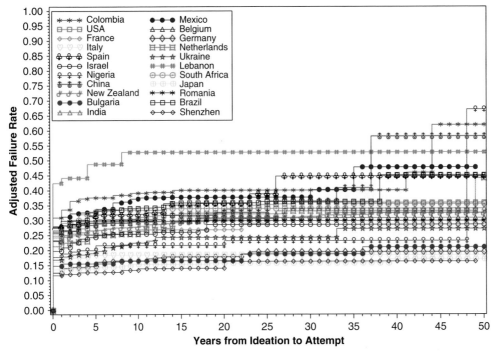

Figure 4.3. Cumulative speed of transition from ideation to attempt in each country (not go to 1.0).

associations in these models are similar to those in the general backward recency models in that AOO and time between AOO and recency are both negatively associated with recency, but unlike that general model they include piecewise components that capture important nonlinearities in these associations. These components are included as controls in all the substantive models presented in Part III.

Discussion

The results in this chapter have shown that persistence of suicidal behaviors is complex. A substantial proportion of suicidal behavior is short-lived, resolving within the year of onset and never recurring. But the remainder is often highly persistent. Persistence is higher among early onset than later-onset cases. Time between AOO and interview is also significantly associated with persistence of suicidal behaviors in the WMH data, although this might be due, at least in part, to the fact that we assessed persistence only indirectly. The associations of persistence with both AOO and time between AOO and interview are significantly nonlinear, leading us to develop regression spline models to control for the effects of AOO and time between AOO and interview in the more complex models examined in Section III. The models in those chapters will examine the predictors that distinguish between the substantial proportion of suicidal behaviors that remit within a year of onset and those that persist and, among those that persist, the predictors of degree of persistence.

References

Borges, G., Angst, J., Nock, M. K., Ruscio, A. M., & Kessler, R. C. (2008). Risk factors for the incidence and persistence of suicide-related outcomes: a 10-year follow-up study using the National Comorbidity Surveys. *Journal of Affective Disorders*, **105**(1–3), 25–33.

Brezo, J., Paris, J., Tremblay, R., et al. (2007). Identifying correlates of suicide attempts in suicidal ideators: a population-based study. *Psychological Medicine*, **37**(11), 1551–1562.

Centers for Disease Control. (2008). Web-based Injury Statistics Query and Reporting System (WISQARS) Nonfatal Injuries: Nonfatal Injury Reports. Retrieved March 7, 2008, from (http://www.cdc.gov/nipc/wisqars).

de Boor, C. (2001). *A Practical Guide to Splines*, revised edition. New York, NY: Springer-Verlag.

Hawton, K., & van Heeringen, K., Eds. (2000). *The International Handbook of Suicide and Attempted Suicide*. West Sussex, England: John Wiley & Sons.

Lagakos, S. W. (1979). General right censoring and its impact on the analysis of survival data. *Biometrics*, **35**(1), 139–156.

Lieberman, E. J. (1993). Suicidal ideation and young adults. *American Journal of Psychiatry*, **150**, 171.

Nock, M. K., Borges, G., Bromet, E. J., et al. (2008). Suicide and suicidal behavior. *Epidemiologic Reviews*, **30**, 133–154.

Raue, P. J., Meyers, B. S., Rowe, J. L., Heo, M., & Bruce, M. L. (2007). Suicidal ideation among elderly homecare patients. *International Journal of Geriatric Psychiatry*, **22**(1), 32–37.

Reinherz, H. Z., Tanner, J. L., Berger, S. R., Beardslee, W. R., & Fitzmaurice, G. M. (2006). Adolescent suicidal ideation as predictive of psychopathology, suicidal behavior, and compromised functioning at age 30. *American Journal of Psychiatry*, **163**(7), 1226–1232.

Rudd, M. D., Joiner, T., & Rajab, M. H. (1996). Relationships among suicide ideators, attempters, and multiple attempters in a young-adult sample. *Journal of Abnormal Psychology*, **105**(4), 541–550.

ten Have, M., de Graaf, R., van Dorsselaer, S., et al. (2009). Incidence and course of suicidal ideation and suicide attempts in the general population. *Canadian Journal of Psychiatry*, **54**(12), 824–833.

Zhang, H., & Singer, B. H. (2010). *Recursive Partitioning and Applications*, second edition. New York, NY: Springer.

Zhang, Y., Law, C. K., & Yip, P. S. (2011). Psychological factors associated with the incidence and persistence of suicidal ideation. *Journal of Affective Disorders*, **133**(3), 584–590.

Sociodemographic risk factors for suicidal behavior: results from the WHO World Mental Health Surveys

Matthew K. Nock, Charlene A. Deming, Christine B. Cha, Wai Tat Chiu, Irving Hwang, Nancy A. Sampson, Hristo Hinkov, Jean-Pierre Lépine, Yutaka Ono, and Annette Beautrais

Introduction

Sociodemographic factors are among the strongest and most consistently reported risk factors for suicidal behavior. Foremost among these, factors such as female gender,[1] younger age, fewer years of education, and being previously married (i.e., being divorced, separated, or widowed) all have been consistently shown to predict suicide ideation, plans, and attempts (Nock et al., 2008b; Nock et al., 2008c; Schmidtke et al., 1996; Weissman et al., 1999). These associations have been known for several decades (e.g., Paykel et al., 1974; Weissman, 1974; Wexler et al., 1978); however, most studies have either simply documented such associations, or have controlled for them in order to examine the effects of what are considered to be more important risk factors, such as the presence of mental disorders or certain personality traits. As a result, important questions remain about the nature of the associations between sociodemograhic factors and suicidal behavior.

First, surprisingly little is known about the extent to which these sociodemographic factors predict suicide attempts beyond their association with suicide ideation. Recent studies have shown that some of the strongest risk factors for suicide attempts (e.g., mental disorders) are actually most useful in predicting the onset of suicide ideation, but are much less useful in predicting which people with suicide ideation go on to make suicide plans and attempts (Nock et al., 2009; Nock et al., 2010). Obtaining a better understanding of how sociodemographic factors relate to different aspects of the pathway to suicide attempts will advance our understanding of the development of suicidal behavior and also will be valuable for guiding prevention efforts.

Second, little is known about the extent to which the associations between sociodemographic factors and suicidal behavior vary over the lifespan. For instance, although lower educational attainment is associated with the lifetime occurrence of suicidal behavior (Kessler et al., 1999; Nock et al., 2008b), it may be that having less education is not important during adolescence and young adulthood, but has a stronger effect on the development of suicidal behavior as people grow older due to the cumulative loss of occupational or financial opportunities.

Third, little is known about whether these sociodemographic factors also predict the *persistence* of suicidal behavior over time. Virtually all prior studies have tested risk factors for the onset or presence of suicide ideation, plans, and attempts, but have not examined what factors predict the length of time for which people will continue to experience each of these behaviors. This is an important but as yet unexplored aspect of the experience of suicidal behavior given that greater persistence of suicidal behavior may increase the likelihood that a person ultimately dies by suicide (Forman et al., 2004; Miranda et al., 2008; Rudd et al., 1996).

Fourth, there is debate regarding the extent to which these sociodemographic factors consistently

---

[1] Female gender is associated with a higher risk of non-fatal suicidal behavior; however, male gender is associated with a higher risk of suicide death. Because WMH data are based on surveys of living respondents, we focus only on non-fatal suicidal behavior in this volume.

Suicide, eds. Matthew K. Nock, Guilherme Borges, and Yutaka Ono. Published by Cambridge University Press.
© World Health Organization 2012.

predict suicidal behavior across high-, middle-, and low-income countries. Some studies have reported consistency in the importance of these risk factors (Nock et al., 2008b; Weissman et al., 1999), whereas other studies have suggested that there are differences cross-nationally (Girard, 1993; Vijayakumar et al., 2005). A limitation of prior work is that often it is difficult to know whether differences observed across studies are due to variation in the measurement methods used or whether they reflect true cross-national differences.

The purpose of the current study was to advance the understanding of the associations between sociodemographic factors and suicidal behavior by conducting a comprehensive analysis of these relations using data from the WHO-World Mental Health (WMH) Surveys. Given their strong associations with suicidal behavior in prior studies, we were especially interested in examining gender, age, educational attainment, and marital status as predictors of suicidal behavior. The specific objectives of this study were to test: (1) the associations between sociodemographic factors and multiple forms of suicidal behavior (i.e., suicide ideation, plans, and attempts); (2) the extent to which the observed associations differ over the course of the lifespan; (3) the associations between sociodemographic factors and the persistence of suicidal behavior over time; and (4) the extent to which these associations are observed consistently across high-, middle-, and low-income countries. The WMH Surveys provided a unique opportunity to test each of these previously unanswered questions.

Method

A detailed description of the respondent samples, study procedures, statistical analyses, and assessment of suicidal behavior is provided in Chapter 3 of this volume.

Assessment of sociodemographic factors

Sociodemographic factors were assessed using the WMH-Composite International Diagnostic Interview (CIDI) Screening, Demographics, and Marriage modules (Kessler & Üstün, 2004). The CIDI Screening Section assessed respondents: (1) gender as reported by the interviewer, and (2) current age as reported by the respondent. The Demographics module assessed current employment status (e.g., student) and number

of years of education. The following education categories were created based on number of years of education and were standardized across participating countries: currently a student, low, low-average, high-average, and high. The Marriage module assessed current marital status and history of first marriage (e.g., start and end date, if applicable due to divorce or death of a spouse), upon which the following marital status categories were calculated: never married, previously married, and currently in first marriage. Respondents also were asked how old they were when they got married for the first time, and if separated or divorced from their first spouse, the age they separated for the last time, and if their first spouse died, the age when that happened. In several countries (i.e., European countries and New Zealand), spousal separation/divorce/death was not recorded and so a separate variable was created for these countries called "history of marriage, current status unknown" that started (i.e., was endorsed or "turned on" in the person–year files) during their first year of marriage and remained endorsed for the remainder of their person–years.

Results

Sociodemographic risk factors for the onset of suicidal behavior

Multivariate survival analyses were used to test the associations between gender, age cohort, education level, and marital status and each type of suicidal behavior. Results for the total WMH sample are reported in Table 6.1, with odd ratios (ORs) representing the unique association between each demographic factor and each form of suicidal behavior. Results of similar analyses for high-, middle-, and low-income countries are presented in Appendix Tables 6.1, 6.2, and 6.3, respectively, at the end of this chapter.

Gender

As shown in Table 6.1, women are at a significantly increased risk for suicide ideation and attempts. Among those with suicide ideation, being a woman is associated with significantly increased odds of making both planned and unplanned suicide attempts. The increased risk associated with being a woman is generally consistent across high-, middle-, and low-income countries (see Appendix Tables 6.1–6.3).

Table 6.1. Sociodemographic risk factors for lifetime suicidal behavior[a] (all countries combined)

Demographics	Among total sample		Among ideators		
	Ideation	Attempt	Plan	Planned attempt	Unplanned attempt
	OR (95% CI)	OR (95% CI)	OR (95% CI)	OR (95% CI)	OR (95% CI)
Gender					
Female	1.4* (1.3–1.5)	1.8* (1.6–2.0)	1.1 (1.0–1.2)	1.3* (1.0–1.6)	1.5* (1.2–1.9)
Male					
χ^2 (p-value)	100.6 (<0.001)*	113.0 (<0.001)*	1.6 (0.20)	4.0 (0.05)*	12.5 (<0.001)*
Age group (years)					
18–34	9.4* (8.1–10.8)	11.4* (8.9–14.7)	1.2 (0.8–1.6)	1.1 (0.6–2.1)	1.7 (0.9–2.9)
35–49	4.5* (3.9–5.2)	5.4* (4.2–6.9)	1.1 (0.8–1.5)	1.3 (0.7–2.3)	1.6 (0.9–2.9)
50–64	2.6* (2.2–2.9)	3.1* (2.3–4.0)	1.0 (0.8–1.4)	1.4 (0.8–2.5)	1.6 (0.9–2.8)
65+					
χ^2 (p-value)	1173.6 (<0.001)*	502.6 (<0.001)*	1.6 (0.65)	1.9 (0.60)	3.2 (0.36)
5-Category education					
Currently a student	1.1 (0.9–1.2)	1.2 (0.9–1.5)	1.3 (1.0–1.7)	1.5 (0.9–2.3)	0.9 (0.6–1.5)
Low	1.5* (1.3–1.7)	2.1* (1.7–2.6)	1.4* (1.1–1.7)	2.0* (1.4–3.0)	1.9* (1.3–2.9)
Low-average	1.2* (1.0–1.3)	1.6* (1.3–2.0)	1.3* (1.1–1.7)	1.7* (1.2–2.4)	1.6* (1.0–2.5)
High-average	1.2* (1.0–1.3)	1.4* (1.1–1.8)	1.1 (0.9–1.4)	1.2 (0.9–1.8)	1.2 (0.7–1.8)
High					
χ^2 (p-value)	61.9 (<0.001)*	76.8 (<0.001)*	11.0 (0.03)*	18.9 (<0.001)*	24.8 (<0.001)*
Marital status					
Never married	1.2* (1.1–1.3)	1.5* (1.2–1.7)	0.9 (0.8–1.1)	1.6* (1.2–2.2)	1.2 (0.9–1.6)
Previously married	1.9* (1.7–2.2)	2.6* (2.1–3.2)	1.1 (0.9–1.4)	1.5* (1.1–2.2)	1.6* (1.1–2.4)
History of marriage, current marital status unknown	1.8* (1.6–2.1)	2.2* (1.7–2.7)	1.7* (1.4–2.3)	2.1* (1.4–3.2)	1.6* (1.0–2.5)
Currently in first marriage					
χ^2 (p-value)	137.3 (<0.001)*	100.9 (<0.001)*	26.7 (<0.001)*	18.5 (<0.001)*	8.1 (0.04)*

* Significant at the 0.05 level, two-sided test.
[a] Each column is a separate multivariate model in survival framework, with all rows as predictors controlling for person–years and countries. Outcome variable indicated in each column header.

Age cohort

In the total sample, there also are significant associations between age cohort and suicidal behavior, with younger cohorts having greater risk of suicide ideation and attempts (see Table 6.1). The association between age cohort and suicide attempts appears to be explained by the prediction of suicide ideation, as age cohort is not predictive of which suicide ideators go on to make a suicide plan or attempt. In other words, respondents from younger age cohorts have higher levels of suicide ideation, but are not more likely to make a suicide

plan or attempt after accounting for the presence of suicide ideation. When assessed across income levels, the same pattern is present in high-income countries. However, in middle- and low-income countries, respondents from younger age cohorts are more likely to make suicide plans and planned attempts among those with ideation (see Appendix Tables 6.1–6.3).

Education

Fewer years of education is associated with a significantly greater risk of suicide ideation and attempts, as well as with greater risk of making suicide plans and attempts among ideators in the total sample (see Table 6.1). Notably, respondents who are currently still a student are not at increased risk for suicidal behavior. Examination of these effects across high-, middle-, and low-income countries reveals that lower educational level is associated with increased risk of suicidal behavior in high-income countries, but such associations are largely absent in middle- and low-income countries. Moreover, the cross-national effects of currently being a student are mixed. In high-income countries, currently being a student is associated with higher risk of suicide attempt in the total sample, and with suicide plan and planned attempts among ideators, whereas in low-income countries, currently being a student is associated with significantly *lower* risk of suicide ideation and attempt. Similar to the results of looking at all countries combined, in middle-income countries, current student status is not associated with increased or decreased risk for suicidal behavior (see Appendix Tables 6.1–6.3).

Marital status

Relative to respondents who are currently in their first marriage, those who have never been married are at significantly increased risk for suicide ideation and attempts, as well as planned suicide attempts among ideators (see Table 6.1). People who have been previously married – whether they are still divorced, have remarried, or their current marital status is unknown – are at even greater risk for suicide ideation and attempts, and show an increased risk of planned and unplanned suicide attempts among those with suicide ideation. Examination of these effects cross-nationally reveals that having never married is associated with increased risk of suicide ideation and attempts, as well as with planned attempts among ideators in high-income countries only. In contrast, being previously married is associated with higher odds of suicide ideation and attempts across all countries (high-, middle-, and low-income categories), and with making planned and unplanned attempts among ideators in high-income countries (see Appendix Tables 6.1–6.3).

Interactions between respondent age and sociodemographic factors in predicting suicidal behavior

In order to test whether the associations between these sociodemographic risk factors and suicidal behavior

vary over the lifespan, we also tested multivariate models that included the interaction of each risk factor and respondent age. As shown in Table 6.2, in the total sample the odds of suicide ideation are increased among those who are older (i.e., 13+ years) and of high-average education and have a history of marriage, whereas the odds of ideation are decreased among those who are older and either never married or previously married. The odds of suicide attempt in the total sample are increased after age 13 years among young cohorts (i.e., those <65 years of age at the time of interview). That is, the odds of first suicide attempt seem to occur later among younger cohorts. History of marriage also is associated with greater odds of suicide attempt among those age 13–19 years (relative to those age 4–12 years). There is not a clear pattern of findings in the prediction of plans and attempts among ideators, with most significant effects showing decreased odds of suicide plan and attempt among those with lower educational attainment and previously married status. These effects are reported separately for high-, middle-, and low-income countries in Appendix Tables 6.4, 6.5, and 6.6, respectively.

Sociodemographic risk factors for childhood-, adolescent-, young adulthood- and later adulthood-onset suicidal behavior

Next, we tested the extent to which each sociodemographic factor predicts the onset of suicidal behavior during childhood (4–12 years), adolescence (13–19 years), young adulthood (20–29 years), and later adulthood (30+ years). Results for childhood-, adolescent-, young adulthood-, and late adulthood-onset are presented separately in Tables 6.3, 6.4, 6.5, and 6.6, respectively. Results are reported separately for high-, middle-, and low-income countries (see Appendix Tables 6.7–6.10, 6.11–6.14, and 6.15–6.18, respectively).

Gender

Among the total sample, women are at a greater risk of adolescent- and young adulthood-onset of suicidal behavior (see Tables 6.3–6.6), with ORs equal to or exceeding those in Table 6.1. These ORs begin to decrease after adolescence and once in late adulthood, only remain statistically significant for the prediction of suicide ideation and attempts. A similar pattern

Table 6.2. Interactions between sociodemographic factors and respondent age (4–12, 13–19, 20–29, 30+ years) in the prediction of suicidal behavior[a] (all countries combined)

		Among total sample			Among ideators	
		Ideation	Attempt	Plan	Planned attempt	Unplanned attempt
Interactions		OR (95% CI)	OR (95% CI)	OR (95% CI)	OR (95% CI)	OR (95% CI)
Gender						
Female	13–19	1.3 (1.0–1.7)	1.3 (0.8–2.0)	1.0 (0.5–2.0)	2.5 (0.6–10.4)	1.7 (0.6–4.9)
	20–29	1.1 (0.9–1.5)	1.1 (0.7–1.7)	1.0 (0.5–2.0)	3.6 (0.9–14.9)	1.5 (0.6–4.0)
	30+	1.1 (0.8–1.4)	0.9 (0.6–1.3)	0.8 (0.4–1.6)	2.5 (0.6–10.3)	1.2 (0.4–3.3)
Male	13–19					
	20–29					
	30+					
χ^2 (p-value)		6.9 (0.07)	8.8 (0.03)*	2.6 (0.45)	5.8 (0.12)	2.4 (0.48)
Age group (years)						
18–34	13–19	1.3 (0.8–2.1)	3.0* (1.7–5.4)	0.3 (0.0–3.0)	2.2 (0.3–18.8)	–
	20–29	1.1 (0.7–1.8)	2.5* (1.3–4.9)	0.8 (0.1–6.2)	1.2 (0.2–9.2)	–
	30+	0.9 (0.6–1.5)	2.2* (1.2–4.1)	2.0 (0.2–16.4)	4.0 (0.5–31.9)	–
35–49	13–19	1.2 (0.7–1.9)	2.2* (1.1–4.3)	0.6 (0.1–6.4)	4.9 (0.5–46.7)	–
	20–29	1.1 (0.7–1.9)	1.8 (0.8–3.8)	1.3 (0.1–11.4)	2.3 (0.3–20.7)	–
	30+	1.2 (0.8–1.8)	2.1* (1.2–3.9)	3.3 (0.4–28.1)	6.4 (0.8–54.3)	–
50–64	13–19	1.0 (0.6–1.7)	1.9 (0.9–3.8)	1.3 (0.1–14.1)	–	1.5 (0.3–7.8)
	20–29	1.2 (0.7–1.9)	3.1* (1.4–6.8)	3.1 (0.3–28.4)	–	4.4 (0.9–21.0)
	30+	1.2 (0.8–1.8)	1.9* (1.1–3.6)	3.2 (0.4–28.8)	–	2.3 (0.5–10.8)
65+	13–19					
	20–29					
	30+					
χ^2 (p-value)		11.7 (0.23)	35.4 (<0.001)*	53.2 (<0.001)*	23.7 (<0.001)*	11.9 (0.01)*
5-Category education						
Currently a student	13–19	0.5 (0.1–1.9)	1.7 (0.3–11.0)	0.3 (0.0–3.1)	0.0* (0.0–0.0)	–
	20–29	0.5 (0.1–2.1)	1.6 (0.2–10.8)	0.6 (0.1–6.9)	0.0* (0.0–0.0)	–
	30+	–	0.2 (0.0–1.3)	0.0* (0.0–0.0)	–	–
Low	13–19	0.4 (0.1–1.6)	1.3 (0.2–10.6)	0.7 (0.1–10.4)	0.0* (0.0–0.0)	–
	20–29	0.3 (0.1–1.5)	1.0 (0.1–8.3)	1.0 (0.1–18.4)	0.0* (0.0–0.0)	–
	30+	0.3 (0.1–1.5)	1.3 (0.2–10.5)	1.1 (0.1–18.8)	0.0* (0.0–0.0)	–
Low-average	13–19	0.5 (0.1–2.5)	0.7 (0.1–6.8)	0.0* (0.0–0.0)	0.0* (0.0–0.0)	2.4 (0.3–21.0)
	20–29	0.4 (0.1–2.1)	0.6 (0.1–5.8)	0.0* (0.0–0.0)	0.0* (0.0–0.0)	2.1 (0.2–19.0)
	30+	0.3 (0.1–1.7)	0.6 (0.1–5.6)	0.0* (0.0–0.0)	0.0* (0.0–0.0)	3.9 (0.4–35.2)
High-average	13–19	1.6* (1.0–2.5)	1.3 (0.6–3.0)	0.8 (0.3–2.0)	1.0 (0.3–3.0)	0.5 (0.2–1.1)
	20–29	1.4* (1.1–1.7)	1.2 (0.8–1.8)	1.4 (0.9–2.1)	1.9* (1.0–3.5)	0.7 (0.4–1.4)
	30+					
High	13–19					
	20–29					
	30+					
χ^2 (p-value)		21.6 (0.03)*	55.1 (<0.001)*	585.5 (<0.001)*	416.4 (<0.001)*	6.0 (0.30)

Table 6.2. (cont.)

Interactions		Among total sample			Among ideators	
		Ideation	Attempt	Plan	Planned attempt	Unplanned attempt
		OR (95% CI)	OR (95% CI)	OR (95% CI)	OR (95% CI)	OR (95% CI)
Marital status						
Never	13–19	0.5* (0.3–0.8)	1.2 (0.6–2.2)	1.3 (0.3–5.8)	–	–
married	20–29	0.5* (0.3–0.7)	0.9 (0.5–1.6)	1.0 (0.2–4.9)	–	–
	30+	0.4* (0.2–0.6)	0.8 (0.4–1.6)	0.8 (0.2–3.5)	–	–
Previously	13–19	–	–	0.0* (0.0–0.0)	4.3 (0.6–30.5)	–
married	20–29	0.0* (0.0–0.0)	4.4 (0.7–26.7)	0.0* (0.0–0.0)	1.7 (0.9–3.2)	1.0 (0.5–1.6)
	30+	0.0* (0.0–0.0)	2.5 (0.4–15.5)	0.0* (0.0–0.0)	–	–
History of	13–19	2.5* (1.3–4.8)	4.7* (2.1–10.5)	4.5 (0.9–23.0)	–	0.7 (0.1–6.8)
marriage,	20–29	1.3* (1.0–1.8)	1.2 (0.8–1.8)	1.4 (0.9–2.1)	–	0.8 (0.3–1.9)
current	30+					
marital						
status						
unknown						
Currently in	13–19					
first marriage	20–29					
	30+					
χ^2 (p-value)		28.1 (<0.001)*	24.6 (0.002)*	9.2 (0.24)	3.8 (0.15)	1810.0 (<0.001)*

* Significant at the 0.05 level, two-sided test.
– Not included due to small cell size.
0.0* (0.0–0.0) OR is ≤ 0.05 indicating very low risk.
[a] Each column is a separate multivariate model in survival framework; models control for all the demographic predictors in each row, life course intervals (4–12, 13–19, 20–29, 30+ years), and countries. Only the results of interaction terms for life course interval variables by each sociodemographic variable are shown. Outcome variable indicated in each column header.

is seen in high- and middle-income countries for adolescent- and young adulthood-onset, with women generally being more at risk for four of the five suicidal behaviors (see Appendix Tables 6.7–6.14). In low-income countries, female gender is not significantly associated with increased odds of any of the suicidal outcomes for children or adolescents, but is significant for young adulthood-onset (see Appendix Tables 6.15–6.18).

Age cohort

In the total sample, the younger age cohort is associated with greater odds of childhood-, adolescent-, young adulthood-, and later adulthood-onset of suicide ideation and attempts, with the strongest effects seen for childhood-onset suicidal behavior and progressively decreasing across onset periods (see

Tables 6.3–6.6). Notably, the younger age cohort also is significantly associated with increased risk for suicide plans, planned attempts, and unplanned attempts with later adulthood-onset.

Examination of age cohort effects across income levels reveals generally similar findings for high-, middle-, and low-income countries; the younger age group is associated with increased odds for suicide ideation and attempt at all onset periods (see Appendix Tables 6.7–6.18). Among high-income countries, the magnitude of this association reaches its peak during childhood and steadily decreases over the subsequent onset periods, whereas the effects are mixed in middle- and low-income countries (e.g., in middle-income countries, ORs decrease from childhood- to adolescent-onset, but then begin to increase from adolescent- to young adulthood- and later adulthood-onset).

Table 6.3. Sociodemographic risk factors for suicidal behavior during childhood (person–years: 4–12)[a] (all countries combined)

Demographics	Among total sample			Among ideators	
	Ideation	Attempt	Plan	Planned attempt	Unplanned attempt
	OR (95% CI)	OR (95% CI)	OR (95% CI)	OR (95% CI)	OR (95% CI)
Gender					
Female	1.2 (1.0–1.6)	1.9* (1.2–3.0)	1.3 (0.7–2.4)	0.2 (0.0–2.5)	1.8 (0.6–5.0)
Male					
X^2 (p-value)	2.6 (0.11)	7.3 (0.01)*	0.6 (0.43)	1.4 (0.23)	1.2 (0.26)
Age group (years)					
18–34	20.8* (9.5–45.7)	15.9* (4.1–62.0)	2.7 (0.3–22.9)	0.0* (0.0–0.0)	0.0* (0.0–0.0)
35–49	10.0* (4.5–22.4)	9.3* (2.3–37.1)	1.4 (0.1–13.1)	0.0* (0.0–0.0)	0.0* (0.0–0.0)
50–64	5.2* (2.3–11.8)	3.0 (0.7–13.1)	0.7 (0.1–6.4)	0.0* (0.0–0.0)	0.0* (0.0–0.0)
65+					
X^2 (p-value)	101.4 (<0.001)*	31.7 (<0.001)*	11.7 (0.01)*	125.1 (<0.001)*	63.5 (<0.001)*
5-Category education					
Currently a student	0.7 (0.2–2.0)	0.2* (0.1–0.8)	0.0* (0.0–0.0)	0.5 (0.0–33.9)	3.6 (0.0–314.8)
Low	1.5 (0.4–5.4)	0.6 (0.1–2.8)	0.0* (0.0–0.0)	–	1.3 (0.0–104.4)
Low-average					
High-average					
High					
X^2 (p-value)	7.3 (0.03)*	8.1 (0.02)*	230.4 (<0.001)*	221.4 (<0.001)*	1.4 (0.50)
Marital status					
Never married	–	–	0.0* (0.0–0.0)	–	–
Previously married	–	0.5 (0.1–3.3)	–	–	–
History of marriage, current marital status unknown					
Currently in first marriage					
X^2 (p-value)	–	276.9 (<0.001)*	45.4 (<0.001)*	–	–

* Significant at the 0.05 level, two-sided test.
– Not included due to small cell size.
0.0* (0.0–0.0) OR is ≤0.05 indicating very low risk.
[a] Each column is a separate multivariate model in survival framework, with all rows as predictors controlling for person–years and countries. Outcome variable indicated in each column header.

Table 6.4. Sociodemographic risk factors for suicidal behavior during adolescence (person–years: 13–19)[a] (all countries combined)

Demographics	Among total sample			Among ideators	
	Ideation	Attempt	Plan	Planned attempt	Unplanned attempt
	OR (95% CI)	OR (95% CI)	OR (95% CI)	OR (95% CI)	OR (95% CI)
Gender					
Female	1.5* (1.3–1.7)	2.1* (1.7–2.5)	1.1 (0.9–1.5)	1.2 (0.8–1.9)	1.9* (1.3–2.7)
Male					
X^2 (p-value)	50.2 (<0.001)*	59.5 (<0.001)*	1.0 (0.31)	0.9 (0.34)	11.1 (<0.001)*
Age group (years)					
18–34	11.7* (8.6–15.8)	12.5* (8.4–18.6)	0.5 (0.2–1.2)	2.1 (0.6–7.5)	1.6 (0.6–4.3)
35–49	4.9* (3.6–6.6)	5.3* (3.6–8.0)	0.4 (0.2–1.0)	2.0 (0.5–7.6)	1.6 (0.6–4.3)
50–64	2.5* (1.8–3.4)	2.4* (1.5–3.8)	0.5 (0.2–1.3)	2.4 (0.6–10.6)	0.7 (0.2–2.1)
65+					
X^2 (p-value)	554.6 (<0.001)*	238.8 (<0.001)*	4.7 (0.20)	1.4 (0.70)	9.2 (0.03)*
5-Category education					
Currently a student	0.5 (0.3–1.1)	0.2* (0.1–0.4)	0.5 (0.1–1.9)	0.7 (0.1–6.2)	0.1* (0.0–0.9)
Low	0.7 (0.4–1.6)	0.3* (0.2–0.7)	0.4 (0.1–1.7)	0.6 (0.1–6.0)	0.2 (0.0–1.5)
Low-average	0.6 (0.3–1.4)	0.3* (0.1–0.6)	0.3 (0.1–1.4)	0.6 (0.1–5.4)	0.2 (0.0–1.3)
High-average	0.7 (0.3–1.5)	0.3* (0.1–0.6)	0.4 (0.1–1.6)	0.3 (0.0–3.1)	0.1* (0.0–0.9)
High					
X^2 (p-value)	21.5 (<0.001)*	38.0 (<0.001)*	4.9 (0.30)	3.7 (0.44)	9.2 (0.06)
Marital status					
Never married	0.8 (0.6–1.2)	0.8 (0.6–1.2)	0.7 (0.4–1.2)	0.8 (0.3–1.9)	1.0 (0.5–2.0)
Previously married	2.6* (1.2–5.5)	–	1.0 (0.3–3.5)	2.7 (0.4–17.4)	–
History of marriage, current marital status unknown	1.9 (0.9–4.0)	3.1* (1.4–6.8)	3.5 (0.7–18.3)	1.0 (0.2–7.0)	0.8 (0.1–10.6)
Currently in first marriage					
X^2 (p-value)	15.5 (0.001)*	12.4 (0.01)*	5.9 (0.11)	2.1 (0.54)	329.3 (<0.001)*

* Significant at the 0.05 level, two-sided test.
– Not included due to small cell size.
[a] Each column is a separate multivariate model in survival framework, with all rows as predictors controlling for person–years and countries. Outcome variable indicated in each column header.

Table 6.5. Sociodemographic risk factors for suicidal behavior during young adulthood (person–years: 20–29)[a] (all countries combined)

Demographics	Among total sample			Among ideators	
	Ideation	Attempt	Plan	Planned attempt	Unplanned attempt
	OR (95% CI)	OR (95% CI)	OR (95% CI)	OR (95% CI)	OR (95% CI)
Gender					
Female	1.4* (1.2–1.5)	1.8* (1.5–2.2)	1.2 (1.0–1.5)	1.7* (1.2–2.3)	1.5* (1.0–2.2)
Male					
χ^2 (p-value)	25.4 (<0.001)*	33.5 (<0.001)*	3.1 (0.08)	8.1 (0.004)*	4.7 (0.03)*
Age group (years)					
18–34	8.6* (6.3–11.7)	11.5* (6.3–21.3)	1.1 (0.6–1.8)	1.4 (0.6–3.4)	3.1 (0.7–13.5)
35–49	4.3* (3.2–5.9)	5.3* (2.9–9.8)	0.9 (0.5–1.5)	1.4 (0.6–3.4)	2.6 (0.6–11.1)
50–64	2.6* (1.9–3.6)	4.7* (2.5–8.8)	1.3 (0.7–2.3)	2.8* (1.1–7.5)	3.7 (0.8–16.7)
65+					
χ^2 (p-value)	293.7 (<0.001)*	120.9 (<0.001)*	6.1 (0.11)	7.7 (0.05)	4.0 (0.26)
5-Category education					
Currently a student	1.2 (0.9–1.5)	1.2 (0.8–1.8)	1.5 (0.9–2.5)	2.0* (1.1–3.9)	0.6 (0.2–1.4)
Low	1.4* (1.1–1.8)	1.8* (1.3–2.6)	1.4 (1.0–2.0)	2.1* (1.2–3.9)	1.9* (1.1–3.4)
Low-average	1.2 (1.0–1.5)	1.7* (1.2–2.2)	1.8* (1.3–2.5)	2.2* (1.3–3.4)	1.2 (0.6–2.3)
High-average	1.3* (1.0–1.6)	1.6* (1.2–2.1)	1.3 (0.9–1.9)	1.8* (1.1–3.0)	1.2 (0.6–2.1)
High					
χ^2 (p-value)	10.5 (0.03)*	17.5 (0.002)*	12.6 (0.01)*	11.1 (0.03)*	12.1 (0.02)*
Marital status					
Never married	1.3* (1.1–1.5)	1.5* (1.2–1.8)	1.1 (0.9–1.5)	1.8* (1.2–2.7)	1.3 (0.8–2.0)
Previously married	2.8* (2.2–3.6)	3.6* (2.5–5.1)	1.4 (0.9–2.3)	2.1* (1.2–3.7)	1.5 (0.8–2.9)
History of marriage, current marital status unknown	2.2* (1.7–3.0)	2.4* (1.6–3.5)	2.0* (1.3–3.2)	3.6* (1.7–7.6)	1.6 (0.7–3.5)
Currently in first marriage					
χ^2 (p-value)	94.3 (<0.001)*	64.4 (<0.001)*	11.4 (0.01)*	16.1 (0.001)*	2.7 (0.44)

* Significant at the 0.05 level, two-sided test.
[a] Each column is a separate multivariate model in survival framework, with all rows as predictors controlling for person–years and countries. Outcome variable indicated in each column header.

Table 6.6. Sociodemographic risk factors for suicidal behavior during later adulthood (person–years: 30+)[a] (all countries combined)

Demographics	Among total sample			Among ideators	
	Ideation	Attempt	Plan	Planned attempt	Unplanned attempt
	OR (95% CI)	OR (95% CI)	OR (95% CI)	OR (95% CI)	OR (95% CI)
Gender					
Female	1.3* (1.1–1.4)	1.4* (1.2–1.7)	1.0 (0.8–1.2)	1.2 (0.9–1.6)	1.2 (0.8–1.7)
Male					
χ^2 (p-value)	17.8 (<0.001)*	13.1 (<0.001)*	0.1 (0.70)	1.2 (0.27)	0.9 (0.35)
Age group (years)					
18–34	6.9* (5.0–9.5)	10.2* (6.7–15.8)	2.8* (1.6–4.6)	2.6* (1.2–5.6)	2.2 (0.8–5.9)
35–49	4.4* (3.8–5.2)	6.4* (4.7–8.8)	2.2* (1.6–3.1)	2.3* (1.4–3.7)	2.9* (1.6–5.3)
50–64	2.6* (2.2–3.0)	2.9* (2.2–4.0)	1.3 (0.9–1.8)	1.4 (0.8–2.3)	1.9* (1.1–3.3)
65+					
χ^2 (p-value)	345.4 (<0.001)*	172.3 (<0.001)*	40.2 (<0.001)*	15.0 (0.002)*	11.9 (0.01)*
5-Category education					
Low	1.4* (1.2–1.7)	2.2* (1.6–3.0)	1.4* (1.0–1.8)	1.9* (1.2–3.0)	2.5* (1.3–4.8)
Low-average	1.0 (0.8–1.1)	1.5* (1.1–2.1)	1.3 (0.9–1.7)	1.5 (0.9–2.4)	2.7* (1.4–5.3)
High-average	1.0 (0.8–1.1)	1.2 (0.9–1.7)	1.0 (0.8–1.4)	0.9 (0.5–1.4)	1.6 (0.8–3.4)
High					
χ^2 (p-value)	36.1 (<0.001)*	34.0 (<0.001)*	6.1 (0.11)	14.3 (0.003)*	12.2 (0.01)*
Marital status					
Never married	1.3* (1.1–1.6)	2.0* (1.5–2.8)	0.9 (0.7–1.2)	2.6* (1.6–4.2)	1.1 (0.6–1.9)
Previously married	1.9* (1.6–2.2)	2.7* (2.0–3.6)	1.0 (0.7–1.3)	1.3 (0.8–2.1)	1.6 (0.9–2.7)
History of marriage, current marital status unknown	2.3* (1.9–2.8)	3.2* (2.2–4.5)	1.9* (1.4–2.7)	2.1* (1.2–3.6)	1.7 (0.9–3.3)
Currently in first marriage					
χ^2 (p-value)	120.1 (<0.001)*	78.9 (<0.001)*	17.1 (<0.001)*	16.7 (<0.001)*	5.7 (0.13)

* Significant at the 0.05 level, two-sided test.
[a] Each column is a separate multivariate model in survival framework, with all rows as predictors controlling for person–years and countries. Outcome variable indicated in each column header.

Education

Among the total sample, being in school or having lower educational attainment is associated with decreased odds of suicide attempt during the ages of 4–19 years. However, these effects flip for those >20 years, among whom we see that those with lower educational attainment have increased odds of suicidal behavior (see Tables 6.3–6.6).

Looking cross-nationally, the above effects appear to be driven primarily by middle- and low-income countries, which show the same general pattern as that described above. This pattern is absent in high-income countries, where there is no protective effect of being a student (see Appendix Tables 6.8–6.18).

Marital status

Compared to those who are married (and still in their first marriage), those who have never been married have increased odds of suicidal behavior, with the strength of this effect increasing with age. More specifically, there is no effect during adolescence (ORs = 0.7–1.0), some significant effects during early adulthood (ORs=1.1–1.8), and stronger effects during later adulthood (ORs=0.9–2.6). The effects are even stronger for those who were previously married or have a history of marriage; however, these effects are fairly stable across adolescence (ORs=0.8–3.5), early adulthood (ORs = 1.4–3.6), and later adulthood (ORs=1.0–3.2) (see Tables 6.3–6.6).

Looking cross-nationally, the effects for marital status in the total sample appear to be driven largely by high-income countries, which show the same general pattern as that reported above. This pattern is largely absent in middle- and low-income countries. Low- and middle-income countries show some increase in the odds of suicide ideation and attempt among those who were previously married. However, there are no ill effects of being never married in middle-income countries, and there is a slight protective effect of being never married during adolescence in low-income countries (see Appendix Tables 6.8–6.18).

Sociodemographic risk factors for persistence of suicidal behaviors over time

The results from the backwards recurrence models predicting the persistence of suicidal behavior are reported in Table 6.7. As shown, none of the

sociodemographic risk factors examined consistently predicts suicide ideation, plan, or attempt. More specifically, in the total sample only two of the 24 ORs tested are statistically significant: a positive association between lower education and persistence of suicide ideation and a positive association between currently being a student and persistence of suicide plans, but no consistent pattern emerged. Cross-nationally, there is no consistent pattern of findings supporting the prediction of persistence of suicidal behavior in high-, middle-, or low-income countries, with the exception of lower levels of education predicting more persistent suicide plans in low-income countries (see Appendix Tables 6.19–6.21). Results from the more fine-grained logistic regression models predicting persistence (results not reported in tables) similarly reveal some evidence of an association between lower education and greater persistence of suicide ideation, with the strongest associations for models predicting very high persistence (i.e., persistence into the year prior to interview), with ORs ranging from 1.8–3.2 for low through low-average education, all obtaining statistical significance. Low through low-average education also predicts very high persistence of suicide plan (ORs = 2.3–5.3), but such effects were absent in the case of suicide attempt. However, male gender is associated with persistence of suicide attempt beyond two years after AOO, with significant ORs of 0.4 in three out of the five models.

Discussion

These results should be interpreted in the context of several noteworthy limitations. First, although the WMH Surveys achieved an acceptable overall response rate, response rates varied across countries and it is possible that this variation could have influenced the results. Differential response was controlled statistically using poststratification adjustments; however, some potential for bias remains. Another shortcoming is that although data are mostly from large and nationally representative samples from 21 different countries around the world, it is important to bear in mind that some samples were not nationally representative and the WMH countries represent only a small sampling of all countries. These factors limit the generality of the results.

Second, these data are based on retrospective self-reports of the occurrence and timing of suicidal

Table 6.7. Association between sociodemographic factors and persistence of suicidal behavior[a] (all countries combined)

Demographics	Ideation OR (95% CI)	Plan OR (95% CI)	Attempt OR (95% CI)
Gender			
Female	1.1 (0.9–1.2)	0.9 (0.8–1.1)	1.0 (0.8–1.3)
Male			
χ^2 (p-value)	1.0 (0.31)	0.3 (0.58)	0.0 (0.92)
Education as of the age of each outcome			
Currently a student	1.2 (0.9–1.5)	1.5* (1.0–2.2)	0.9 (0.5–1.7)
Low	1.3* (1.0–1.6)	1.3 (0.9–1.9)	1.3 (0.7–2.3)
Low-average	1.2 (1.0–1.5)	1.2 (0.8–1.7)	1.2 (0.7–2.2)
High-average	1.1 (0.9–1.4)	1.3 (0.9–1.9)	1.4 (0.8–2.5)
High			
χ^2 (p-value)	5.6 (0.23)	5.1 (0.28)	6.9 (0.14)
Marital status as of the age of each outcome			
Never married	1.1 (0.9–1.3)	1.1 (0.9–1.5)	1.2 (0.9–1.7)
Previously married	0.9 (0.7–1.1)	1.2 (0.8–1.6)	1.0 (0.6–1.7)
History of marriage, current marital status unknown	0.9 (0.7–1.1)	1.1 (0.7–1.6)	0.8 (0.4–1.4)
Currently in first marriage			
χ^2 (p-value)	5.3 (0.15)	1.1 (0.77)	4.3 (0.23)

* Significant at the 0.05 level, two-sided test.
[a] Results are based on multivariate discrete time survival model with countries and age-related variables as a control.

behavior, which introduces potential problems with under-reporting and biased recall (Angold et al., 1996). On balance, the sociodemographic factors are either time-invariant (i.e., gender) or represent major life events that are likely to be reported with a high degree of accuracy (i.e., age, educational attainment, marital status), which limits such concerns. Moreover, systematic reviews have suggested that people can recall significant life events with sufficient accuracy to provide valuable information (Brewin et al., 1993; Hardt & Rutter, 2004) and that such data are especially useful when prospective data are not available (Schlesselman, 1982), as in the current case. These mitigating factors notwithstanding, the retrospective nature of the data on suicidal behavior remains an important limitation of this work. Another limitation related to the reporting of suicidal behavior is that cultural factors may have influenced respondents' willingness to report on suicidal behavior due to perceived stigma (Alonso et al., 2008) or to varying interpretations of questions about clinical constructs like suicidal thoughts or attempts (Lopez & Guarnaccia, 2000; Thakker & Ward, 1998).

A third limitation is that we examined the sociodemographic factors simultaneously in order to test the unique associations between each factor and each suicidal behavior; however, this strategy precluded us from examining interactions among sociodemographic factors. For instance, it has been suggested that factors such as being previously married are more predictive of suicidal behavior among men than women (Kposowa, 2000; Luoma & Pearson, 2002; Yeh et al., 2008). We were not able to examine such questions given the data analytical strategy used in this study, and so the investigation of these questions remains an important direction for future research.

Despite these limitations, this study advances the understanding of suicidal behavior in several important ways. Overall, the results of this study revealed that female gender, fewer years of education, being previously married, and being of younger age are most consistently and strongly associated with both suicide ideation and suicide attempts. Notably, the first three factors also predict the occurrence of planned and unplanned suicide attempts among ideators, whereas belonging to a younger age cohort does not. This demonstration of the usefulness of sociodemographic factors in predicting which people with suicide ideation go on to make plans and attempts replicates findings from a prior study conducted in the United States (Borges et al., 2006) and is particularly important given that other known risk factors for suicidal behavior have been shown to predict ideation, but to be much less useful in the prediction of suicide plans and attempts among ideators (Nock et al., 2009; Nock et al., 2010). Although sociodemographic factors proved useful in predicting the onset of suicidal behavior, they generally did not predict the persistence of suicidal behavior over time. Many of the associations observed between sociodemographic factors and suicidal behavior were consistent across income levels; however, some important differences emerged among respondents from high-, middle-, and low-income countries. Several noteworthy aspects of these findings warrant more detailed comment.

The finding that women are at higher risk for nonfatal suicidal behavior replicates the results of many prior studies (e.g., Kessler et al., 1999; Moscicki, 1994; Nock et al., 2008c; Wunderlich et al., 2001) and adds to earlier work by suggesting that this effect is consistent across high-, middle-, and low-income countries (Nock et al., 2008b; Weissman et al., 1999). This study also revealed that younger age cohorts report higher rates of suicide ideation and attempts than older cohorts. There are several possible interpretations of this finding. It may be that the prevalence of suicide ideation and attempts are increasing, that the onset of these outcomes occurs earlier now than it has in the past, or that this pattern of results is merely due to forgetting or denial among those in older age cohorts. Our analyses revealed that the risk of suicidal behavior among those in younger age cohorts is especially pronounced for childhood-onset suicidal behavior, which supports the idea that the overall age cohort effects are due to a change in the average age-of-onset of suicidal behavior over the past several decades. Such an interpretation is consistent with data on suicide mortality, which suggest that while the overall rate of suicide has not changed worldwide, suicide rates have been increasing among youth over the past several decades (Bertolote & Fleischmann, 2002). Our findings suggest that this increased risk among youth is present for non-fatal suicidal behavior as well.

The association between low educational attainment and suicidal behavior has been studied far less frequently than the other sociodemographic factors included in this study, perhaps because educational status is more difficult to measure and less commonly assessed in research studies. Among studies that have examined this link, findings have been mixed, with some studies reporting a negative association (Lorant et al., 2005; Petronis et al., 1990), and others reporting a positive association (Agerbo et al., 2007). The present study revealed that currently being a student or having lower education attainment is associated with decreased odds of suicidal behavior early in life, but with increased odds of such behavior later in life. There are several potential explanations for these effects. It is possible that low educational attainment and suicidal behavior are related because they are both consequences of some third variable, such as the presence of a mental disorder. However, the fact that educational attainment positively predicts middle- and late-onset suicidal behavior but not early onset suggests that suicidal behavior may result from some downstream negative effects of lower educational attainment (e.g., greater financial or occupational difficulties [Bureau of Labor Statistics, 2008, 2009]). The correlational nature of these data precludes any firm conclusions about the direction of the observed association or about potential mechanisms.

Similar to educational attainment, being previously married or never married has been shown to be positively associated with suicidal behavior and suicide risk in many prior studies (Kposowa, 2000; Luoma & Pearson, 2002; Nock et al., 2008a; Smith et al., 1988; Weissman et al., 1999; Yip & Thorburn, 2004), but negatively associated in other studies (Agerbo et al., 2007). We found that having never been married is a risk factor for suicidal behavior in all countries combined and in high-income countries, but that it does not predict suicidal behavior among middle- and low-income countries (and may be protective in low-income countries). Being previously married emerged as a risk factor for suicidal behavior across all countries combined, as well as divided by income level. One possible explanation for the association between marital status and suicidal behavior is that marriage provides interpersonal support that helps to buffer against negative outcomes (Durkheim, 1951; Hughes & Gove, 1981; Wyke & Ford, 1992). Never having this type of supportive relationship or losing this relationship via separation, divorce, or death not only removes that source of support, but also is associated with the experience of significant stress in itself (Hope et al., 1999). The current findings further support this view and suggest that the dissolution of the marital relationship may lead to suicidal behavior; however, here too the design of this study precludes firm conclusions about the true nature of this relationship. In order to better understand how and why marital status is related to suicidal behavior, future studies must take into account the presence of potential confounding variables (e.g., presence of a mental disorder) and should examine the potential effects of length of marriage, quality of marital relationship, specific reason for separation (e.g., divorced, widowed), and time-lag between change in marital status and onset of suicidal behavior.

Future directions

This chapter provided a comprehensive analysis of the associations between sociodemographic factors and suicidal behavior. Although it is vital that future research continues to advance the understanding of how sociodemographic factors may influence suicidal behavior, many additional factors are undoubtedly involved in the development of suicidal behavior and it is important that such factors are studied independent of the effects of sociodemographic factors. As such, the effects of sociodemographic factors must be consistently measured and accounted for in future studies of familial, environmental, and psychological/diagnostic influences on suicidal behavior. Consistent with this approach, the sociodemographic factors that emerged as significant predictors of each suicidal behavior in the current chapter are statistically controlled in the analyses conducted in subsequent chapters (see Appendix Tables 6.22–6.25 for a list of control variables). Although this approach is necessary in order to carefully study these other potential risk and protective factors, we strongly encourage future research directly focused on further delineating *how* and *why* sociodemographic factors may influence the onset and persistence of suicidal behavior.

References

Agerbo, E., Gunnell, D., Bonde, J. P., Bo Mortensen, P., & Nordentoft, M. (2007). Suicide and occupation: the impact of socio-economic, demographic and psychiatric differences. *Psychological Medicine*, 37(8), 1131–1140.

Alonso, J., Buron, A., Bruffaerts, R., et al. (2008). Association of perceived stigma and mood and anxiety disorders: results from the World Mental Health Surveys. *Acta Psychiatrica Scandinavica*, 118(4), 305–314.

Angold, A., Erkanli, A., Costello, E. J., & Rutter, M. (1996). Precision, reliability and accuracy in the dating of symptom onsets in child and adolescent psychopathology. *Journal of Child Psychology and Psychiatry*, 37(6), 657–664.

Bertolote, J. M., & Fleischmann, A. (2002). A global perspective in the epidemiology of suicide. *Suicidologi*, 7(2), 6–8.

Borges, G., Angst, J., Nock, M. K., et al. (2006). A risk index for 12-month suicide attempts in the National Comorbidity Survey Replication (NCS-R). *Psychological Medicine*, 36(12), 1747–1757.

Brewin, C. R., Andrews, B., & Gotlib, I. H. (1993). Psychopathology and early experience: a reappraisal of retrospective reports. *Psychological Bulletin*, 113(1), 82–98.

Bureau of Labor Statistics. (2008). *Education pays in higher earnings and lower unemployment rates.* Retrieved January 22, 2009, from http://www.bls.gov/emp/emptab7.htm.

Bureau of Labor Statistics. (2009). Usual weekly earnings of wage and salary workers: Fourth quarter 2008. *U.S. States Department of Labor.*

Durkheim, E. (1951). *Suicide.* New York, NY: The Free Press.

Forman, E. M., Berk, M. S., Henriques, G. R., Brown, G. K., & Beck, A. T. (2004). History of multiple suicide attempts as a behavioral marker of severe psychopathology. *American Journal of Psychiatry*, 161(3), 437–443.

Girard, C. (1993). Age, gender, and suicide: a cross-national analysis. *American Sociological Review*, 58(4), 553–574.

Hardt, J., & Rutter, M. (2004). Validity of adult retrospective reports of adverse childhood experiences: review of the evidence. *Journal of Child Psychology and Psychiatry*, 45(2), 260–273.

Hope, S., Rodgers, B., & Power, C. (1999). Marital status transitions and psychological distress: longitudinal evidence from a national population sample. *Psychological Medicine*, 29(2), 381–389.

Hughes, M., & Gove, W. R. (1981). Living alone, social integration, and mental health. *American Journal of Sociology*, 87(1), 48–74.

Kessler, R. C., Borges, G., & Walters, E. E. (1999). Prevalence of and risk factors for lifetime suicide attempts in the National Comorbidity Survey. *Archives of General Psychiatry*, 56(7), 617–626.

Kessler, R. C., & Üstün, T. B. (2004). The World Mental Health (WMH) Survey Initiative Version of the World Health Organization (WHO) Composite International Diagnostic Interview (CIDI). *International Journal of Methods in Psychiatric Research*, 13(2), 93–121.

Kposowa, A. J. (2000). Marital status and suicide in the National Longitudinal Mortality Study. *Journal of Epidemiology and Community Health*, **54**(4), 254–261.

Lopez, S. R., & Guarnaccia, P. J. (2000). Cultural psychopathology: uncovering the social world of mental illness. *Annual Review of Psychology*, **51**, 571–598.

Lorant, V., Kunst, A. E., Huisman, M., Bopp, M., & Mackenbach, J. (2005). A European comparative study of marital status and socio-economic inequalities in suicide. *Social Science and Medicine*, **60**(11), 2431–2441.

Luoma, J. B., & Pearson, J. L. (2002). Suicide and marital status in the United States, 1991–1996: is widowhood a risk factor? *American Journal of Public Health*, **92**(9), 1518–1522.

Miranda, R., Scott, M., Hicks, R., et al. (2008). Suicide attempt characteristics, diagnoses, and future attempts: comparing multiple attempters to single attempters and ideators. *Journal of the American Academy of Child and Adolescent Psychiatry*, **47**(1), 32–40.

Moscicki, E. K. (1994). Gender differences in completed and attempted suicides. *Annals of Epidemiology*, **4**(2), 152–158.

Nock, M. K., Borges, G., Bromet, E. J., et al. (2008a). Cross-national prevalence and risk factors for suicidal ideation, plans and attempts. *British Journal of Psychiatry*, **192**(2), 98–105.

Nock, M. K., Borges, G., Bromet, E. J., et al. (2008b). Cross-national prevalence and risk factors for suicidal ideation, plans, and attempts in the WHO World Mental Health Surveys. *British Journal of Psychiatry*, **192**, 98–105.

Nock, M. K., Borges, G., Bromet, E. J., et al. (2008c). Suicide and suicidal behaviors. *Epidemiologic Reviews*, **30**(1), 133–154.

Nock, M. K., Hwang, I., Sampson, N., et al. (2009). Cross-national analysis of the associations among mental disorders and suicidal behavior: findings from the WHO World Mental Health Surveys. *PLoS Medicine*, **6**(8), e1000123.

Nock, M. K., Hwang, I., Sampson, N., & Kessler, R. C. (2010). Mental disorders, comorbidity, and suicidal behaviors: Results from the National Comorbidity Survey Replication. *Molecular Psychiatry*, **15**(8), 868–876.

Paykel, E. S., Myers, J. K., Lindenthal, J. J., & Tanner, J. (1974). Suicidal feelings in the general population: a prevalence study. *British Journal of Psychiatry*, **124**(0), 460–469.

Petronis, K. R., Samuels, J. F., Moscicki, E. K., & Anthony, J. C. (1990). An epidemiologic investigation of potential risk factors for suicide attempts. *Social Psychiatry and Psychiatric Epidemiology*, **25**, 193–199.

Rudd, M. D., Joiner, T., & Rajab, M. H. (1996). Relationships among suicide ideators, attempters, and multiple attempters in a young-adult sample. *Journal of Abnormal Psychology*, **105**(4), 541–550.

Schlesselman, J. J. (1982). *Case-control studies: Design, conduct, and analysis.* New York, NY: Oxford University Press.

Schmidtke, A., Bille-Brahe, U., DeLeo, D., et al. (1996). Attempted suicide in Europe: rates, trends and sociodemographic characteristics of suicide attempters during the period 1989–1992. Results of the WHO/EURO Multicentre Study on Parasuicide. *Acta Psychiatrica Scandinavica*, **93**(5), 327–338.

Smith, J. C., Mercy, J. A., & Conn, J. M. (1988). Marital status and the risk of suicide. *American Journal of Public Health*, **78**(1), 78–80.

Thakker, J., & Ward, T. (1998). Culture and classification: the cross-cultural application of the DSM-IV. *Clinical Psychology Review*, **18**(5), 501–529.

Vijayakumar, L., John, S., Pirkis, J., & Whiteford, H. (2005). Suicide in developing countries (2): risk factors. *Crisis*, **26**(3), 112–119.

Weissman, M. M. (1974). The epidemiology of suicide attempts, 1960 to 1971. *Archives of General Psychiatry*, **30**(6), 737–746.

Weissman, M. M., Bland, R. C., Canino, G. J., et al. (1999). Prevalence of suicide ideation and suicide attempts in nine countries. *Psychological Medicine*, **29**(1), 9–17.

Wexler, L., Weissman, M. M., & Kasl, S. V. (1978). Suicide attempts 1970–75: updating a United States study and comparisons with international trends. *British Journal of Psychiatry*, **132**, 180–185.

Wunderlich, U., Bronisch, T., Wittchen, H. U., & Carter, R. (2001). Gender differences in adolescents and young adults with suicidal behaviour. *Acta Psychiatrica Scandinavica*, **104**(5), 332–339.

Wyke, S., & Ford, G. (1992). Competing explanations for associations between marital status and health. *Social Science and Medicine*, **34**(5), 523–532.

Yeh, J. Y., Xirasagar, S., Liu, T. C., Li, C. Y., & Lin, H. C. (2008). Does marital status predict the odds of suicidal death in taiwan? A seven-year population-based study. *Suicide and Life Threatening Behavior*, **38**(3), 302–310.

Yip, P. S., & Thorburn, J. (2004). Marital status and the risk of suicide: experience from England and Wales, 1982–1996. *Psychological Reports*, **94**(2), 401–407.

Parental psychopathology and the risk of suicidal behavior

Oye Gureje, Bibilola Oladeji, Charlene A. Deming, Wai Tat Chiu, Jordi Alonso, Guilherme Borges, Yanling He, Irving Hwang, Viviane Kovess-Masféty, José Posada-Villa, Nancy A. Sampson, Ronald C. Kessler, and Matthew K. Nock

Introduction

Worldwide, suicide is one of the leading causes of death and disease burden. Ranked as the 14th leading cause of death globally in 2002, it is projected to rise by 50% and become the 12th leading cause of death by 2030 (Mathers & Loncar, 2006; World Health Organization, 2007). Suicide rates among young people have been increasing in both developed and developing countries. In individuals aged 15–34 years, suicide is among the top three causes of death, representing a massive loss to societies of young persons, including their most productive years of life (World Health Organization, 2001; World Health Organization, UNAIDS, & UNICEF, 2007). Despite the public health impact of suicide, the prevention of suicide has not been adequately addressed in many nations of the world due to a lack of awareness of the burden associated with suicide and a lack of empirical data on which to base preventive strategies because our understanding of the factors that lead to suicide is still limited. Current evidence from family, adoption, and twin studies demonstrates that suicide and suicidal behavior run in families (Balderssarini & Hennen, 2004; Brent et al., 1996; Brent & Mann, 2005). However, the mechanism(s) through which this risk is transmitted from parent to offspring is still poorly understood (Brent et al., 1996; Melhem et al., 2007; Qin et al., 2002; Sorensen et al., 2009).

Although the increased rates of suicidal behavior demonstrated in biological relatives of persons with suicidal behavior in many studies suggests a genetic component to the transmission of risk for suicidal behavior (Balderssarini & Hennen, 2004; Brent & Mann, 2005; Brent & Melhem, 2008), other studies have shown that part of the risk can be attributed to the elevated rates of psychiatric disorders in affected families (Brent & Mann, 2005). To date, few studies have provided information about which familial or parental mental disorders increase the risk of suicide and suicidal behavior or how they might do so (Agerbo et al., 2002; Krakowski & Czobor, 2004; Mittendorfer-Rutz et al., 2008; Pfeffer et al., 1994, 1998; Stenager & Qin, 2008). For example, parental psychiatric disorders could exact their effect on increasing the risk of offspring suicidal behavior through their negative impact on family life and their association with reduced care for children (Brent & Melhem, 2008; Heider et al., 2007; Krakowski & Czobor, 2004).

Different parental factors may predict distinct aspects of the pathway to suicide. For example, the co-occurrence of suicide ideation in family members has been linked to increased familial rates of psychiatric disorders, especially depression, whereas suicide attempts have not been linked thus (Brent et al., 1996; Brent & Mann, 2005). Suicide attempts and completed suicides instead appear to be predicted by a family history of impulsive-aggressive behavior (Brent et al., 1996; Brent & Mann, 2005; Brent et al., 2002; Melhem et al., 2007) and "affective reaction" or impulsive-unstable (cluster B) personality disorders (Wender et al., 1986).

Prior studies have been unable to carefully examine the effects of comorbid parental mental disorders on offspring suicidal behavior and the effect of different parental psychopathology in predicting the transition from suicide ideation to attempts. In the meantime, recent epidemiological studies have shown more generally that different forms of psychopathology predict distinct stages of the pathway to suicide. For instance, although major depression predicts the onset of suicide ideation, it does not consistently predict which people with ideation go on to make a suicide attempt (Nock et al., 2009). The transition from suicidal thoughts to attempt has been better predicted by disorders characterized by impulsive-aggressive and anxious traits (Gureje et al., 2007; Nock et al., 2010; Nock et al., 2009). It will be important to discover whether similar relationships exist between parental psychopathology and offspring suicidal behavior, as this will provide a clue as to the factors related to the intergenerational transmission of suicidal behavior.

The World Mental Health (WMH) Surveys, a series of large-scale, community-based epidemiological surveys conducted in 21 countries around the world, provide a unique opportunity to expand the current knowledge on the intergenerational transmission of suicidal behavior. The large sample size permits the examination of which aspects of parental psychopathology are most strongly predictive of offspring suicidal behavior and allows insight into the extent to which the accumulation of parental disorder influences the associations. Specifically, the current report is designed to: (1) examine the associations between specific forms of parental psychopathology and distinct steps in the suicidal behavior pathway, (2) examine the associations between parental psychopathology and the persistence of suicidal behavior, and (3) test the extent to which such associations are consistent across high-, middle-, and low-income countries.

Method

A detailed description of the respondent samples, study procedures, statistical analyses, and assessment of suicidal behavior is provided in Chapter 3 of this volume. Assessment and analysis of sociodemographic factors included as covariates in the following analyses are described in Chapter 6.

Assessment of parental psychopathology

Five different forms of possible parental psychopathology experienced in the respondents' childhood, and as reported by them, are considered in the present report: major depression, panic disorder, generalized anxiety disorder (GAD), substance abuse, and antisocial personality disorder (ASPD), as well as parental suicide attempt or suicide death (hereafter referred to

as "parental suicidal behavior"). Such parental psychopathology was assessed with the expanded version of the Family History Research Diagnostic Criteria Interview (Andreasen et al., 1977; Kendler et al., 1997).

Results

Specificity of the relationship between parent with disorder and respondent disorder

There is no association between which parent (father or mother) or the number of parents (one versus both) who had the disorder and suicidal behavior in the respondent. However, there is a difference in the case of parental history of suicidal behavior. Here, there is an association between maternal and respondent suicidal behavior among female respondents and paternal and respondent suicidal behavior among male respondents. Therefore, subsequent analyses test the effects of the presence versus absence of psychopathology in either parent, but parental suicidal behavior is considered present only if it occurred in the parent of the same gender (i.e., fathers' suicidal behavior among male respondents and mothers' suicidal behavior among female respondents).

Prevalence of parental psychopathology among those with suicidal behavior

Data on the prevalence of each type of parental disorder assessed among those with suicidal behavior are presented in Table 7.1. Perhaps most interesting is the low prevalence of parental psychopathology present among those with each examined suicidal outcome. For example, among those making a suicide attempt, the most prevalent parental disorder is panic disorder (15.8%), followed by substance abuse (13.0%), and ASPD (9.3%); all other parental psychopathology occur at even lower rates. Overall, parental psychopathology is most common among offspring attempting suicide in the total sample and among those making unplanned attempts among ideators. The lowest rates of parental psychopathology are observed among offspring exhibiting suicide ideation.

A similar pattern of low parental psychopathology prevalence as related to suicidal outcomes is observed in high-, middle-, and low-income countries. Prevalence is generally higher among those making

Table 7.1. Prevalence of parental psychopathology among those with each type of suicidal behavior (all countries combined)

Parental disorder	In total sample						Among ideators			
	%[b] (SE) with parental disorder						%[b] (SE) with parental disorder			
	Ideation	No ideation	Attempt	No attempt	Plan	No plan	Planned attempt	No planned attempt	Unplanned attempt	No unplanned attempt
Type of parental disorder										
Depression	6.1 (0.4)	1.7 (0.1)	8.0 (0.7)	1.8 (0.1)	7.9 (0.7)	5.5 (0.6)	7.7 (0.9)	9.8 (1.2)	8.0 (1.4)	4.4 (0.5)
Panic disorder	11.4 (0.5)	4.4 (0.1)	15.8 (1.1)	4.6 (0.1)	14.2 (0.9)	10.6 (0.8)	15.2 (1.3)	11.7 (1.5)	15.2 (1.8)	8.9 (0.8)
Generalized anxiety disorder	6.8 (0.5)	1.7 (0.1)	8.9 (0.8)	1.8 (0.1)	8.9 (0.7)	5.4 (0.5)	8.3 (0.8)	12.7 (2.0)	9.6 (1.6)	4.4 (0.5)
Substance abuse	10.4 (0.5)	3.6 (0.1)	13.0 (1.0)	3.8 (0.1)	12.3 (1.0)	9.5 (0.8)	12.7 (1.2)	12.1 (1.7)	14.0 (1.7)	8.5 (0.9)
Antisocial personality disorder	6.2 (0.4)	1.6 (0.1)	9.3 (0.8)	1.7 (0.1)	7.7 (0.7)	5.0 (0.5)	8.9 (0.9)	6.7 (1.3)	11.1 (1.8)	3.9 (0.5)
Suicidal behavior	0.7 (0.1)	0.3 (0.0)	0.8 (0.3)	0.3 (0.0)	0.8 (0.2)	1.0 (0.4)	1.0 (0.4)	0.4 (0.2)	0.6 (0.3)	1.0 (0.5)
Number of parental disorders[c]										
1	14.7 (0.6)	6.5 (0.2)	17.3 (1.0)	6.7 (0.2)	15.9 (1.0)	14.4 (0.9)	16.2 (1.3)	15.8 (2.0)	18.9 (1.9)	13.8 (1.1)
2	5.7 (0.4)	1.8 (0.1)	7.6 (0.7)	1.9 (0.1)	7.6 (0.7)	5.1 (0.6)	7.5 (0.9)	7.5 (1.3)	7.5 (1.2)	4.3 (0.5)
3	2.8 (0.3)	0.7 (0.0)	3.0 (0.5)	0.7 (0.1)	3.5 (0.4)	2.4 (0.3)	2.9 (0.5)	4.3 (0.7)	6.3 (1.3)	2.7 (0.4)
4	0.9 (0.1)	0.2 (0.0)	3.2 (0.5)	0.3 (0.0)	2.4 (0.3)	1.2 (0.3)	3.2 (0.5)	2.3 (0.7)		
5+	0.7 (0.1)	0.1 (0.0)								
N[a]	(6088)	(164120)	(2077)	(169575)	(2417)	(5914)	(1297)	(1474)	(681)	(4509)

[a] Number of cases with the outcome variable; N represents the number of person–years.

[b] % represents the percentage of people with the parental disorder among the cases with the outcome variable indicated in the column header. Prevalence estimates are from person–year data. For example, the first cell is the % of those with parental depression among those with attempts.

[c] For number of parental disorders, the last OR represents the odds for that number of parental disorders or more. For example: for unplanned attempt, 3 represents $\geq$ 3 (that is, 3+).

suicide attempts in the total sample and among those ideators making unplanned attempts, whereas prevalence is generally lowest among those with suicide ideation (see Appendix Tables 7.1–7.3).

Associations between parental psychopathology and suicidal behavior

In bivariate survival models, each form of parental psychopathology examined is significantly associated with increased risk of the subsequent first onset of both suicide ideation and attempt among offspring (see Table 7.2). Parental suicidal behavior also is significantly associated with the onset of both lifetime suicide ideation and attempt. Looking more specifically at the associations between individual parental disorders and suicide plans and attempts among ideators, we see that only GAD predicts the development of a suicide plan among ideators; whereas only parental panic disorder predicts which people with suicide ideation are at increased risk for planned suicide attempt. Unplanned suicide attempt among ideators is related to parental panic disorder, GAD, and ASPD. Interestingly, parental GAD appears to protect against planned suicide attempt in people with suicidal thoughts. In multivariate models in which adjustments are made for the number of parental disorders, similar associations are found, though there is a slight attenuation of the results compared to those of bivariate analyses. In these models, parental GAD remains protective against planned attempts among ideators, parental panic remains the only positive predictor of planned attempts among ideators, and parental ASPD emerges as the only predictor of unplanned attempts among ideators.

Associations between number and type of parental disorders and suicidal behavior

The associations between the number of parental disorders present and the risk of suicidal behavior among offspring are presented in Table 7.3. The results show a dose–response relationship between number of parental disorders and suicide ideation as well as suicide attempt. A somewhat similar, albeit less consistent, pattern is seen for suicide plans and attempts among ideators.

In multivariate analysis, taking into account the number of parental disorders present, each form of parental psychopathology continues to predict suicide

ideation and attempt (see Table 7.4). Parental GAD remains protective against planned suicide attempt among those with ideation, and is now joined by parental substance abuse in this regard. Parental ASPD remains a significant predictor of unplanned attempts among ideators, and is now joined by parental panic disorder and GAD in this regard. Further, the multivariate model resulted in subadditive effects of increasing number of parental disorders such that, as the number of parental disorders increases, the relative odds of respondent suicidal behavior increases at a decreasing rate. For example, as the number of parental disorders increases from one to two, the odds of a suicide attempt in the respondent only increases by 60% of the product of the individual disorders and only by 20% when the number of parental disorders increase from two to three. We next examined the extent to which these associations were explained by respondents' mental disorders by repeating the analysis adjusting for respondents' lifetime mental disorders. We observed a similar pattern of associations with essentially no change in their strength.

Multivariate analyses examining the associations between the type and number of parental disorders and offspring suicidal behavior cross-nationally revealed that nearly every parental disorder measured continued to predict suicide ideation and attempt across high-, middle-, and low-income countries (see Appendix Tables 7.4–7.6). Exceptions to this are seen in middle-income countries where parental substance abuse fails to significantly predict suicide ideation and in low-income countries where parental depression and parental ASPD fail to significantly predict suicide ideation and attempt. Further, the associations between parental psychopathology and attempts among ideators lessen across income levels when compared to that in the total sample. Only in high-income countries does parental panic disorder continue to predict unplanned attempts among ideators. In middle-income countries, parental panic disorder predicts plan among ideators, whereas parental ASPD is protective against plan among ideators. Finally, in low-income countries, parental panic disorder is shown to be predictive of planned attempts, whereas parental GAD is protective against planned attempts. Interestingly, in this model among low-income countries, parental suicidal behavior was shown to be a stronger predictor of offspring suicide ideation and attempt than when examined in the total sample or any other income level. Finally, as observed in the total

Table 7.2. Bivariate and multivariate associations between parental psychopathology and lifetime suicidal behavior[a] (all countries combined)

Type of parental disorder	Among total sample				Among ideators					
	Ideation		Attempt		Plan		Planned attempt		Unplanned attempt	
	Bivariate OR (95% CI)	Multivariate additive OR (95% CI)	Bivariate OR (95% CI)	Multivariate additive OR (95% CI)	Bivariate OR (95% CI)	Multivariate additive OR (95% CI)	Bivariate OR (95% CI)	Multivariate additive OR (95% CI)	Bivariate OR (95% CI)	Multivariate additive OR (95% CI)
Depression	3.0* (2.6–3.6)	1.3* (1.1–1.6)	3.2* (2.6–4.0)	1.2 (0.9–1.6)	1.3 (1.0–1.7)	1.1 (0.8–1.5)	0.8 (0.6–1.2)	1.1 (0.6–1.8)	1.4 (0.9–2.2)	0.9 (0.5–1.6)
Panic disorder	2.3* (2.0–2.6)	1.7* (1.5–1.9)	3.0* (2.5–3.5)	2.2* (1.8–2.6)	1.2 (1.0–1.5)	1.2 (1.0–1.5)	1.5* (1.0–2.1)	1.6* (1.1–2.2)	1.5* (1.1–2.0)	1.3 (1.0–1.8)
Generalized anxiety disorder	3.2* (2.7–3.7)	1.5* (1.3–1.9)	3.3* (2.6–4.2)	1.5* (1.2–2.0)	1.3* (1.0–1.8)	1.2 (0.9–1.7)	0.6* (0.4–0.8)	0.5* (0.3–0.8)	1.8* (1.1–2.7)	1.5 (0.8–2.7)
Substance abuse	2.1* (1.8–2.4)	1.5* (1.3–1.7)	2.2* (1.9–2.7)	1.3* (1.1–1.6)	1.0 (0.8–1.3)	1.0 (0.8–1.2)	0.9 (0.6–1.3)	0.7 (0.5–1.1)	1.3 (0.9–1.9)	1.0 (0.7–1.4)
Antisocial personality disorder	2.8* (2.5–3.3)	1.6* (1.4–1.9)	3.5* (2.9–4.2)	2.1* (1.6–2.6)	1.1 (0.8–1.5)	1.0 (0.8–1.4)	1.1 (0.7–1.7)	1.4 (0.9–2.2)	2.0* (1.3–3.2)	1.8* (1.1–3.0)
Suicidal behavior	2.8* (1.7–4.4)	1.1 (0.7–1.8)	2.8* (1.4–5.3)	1.2 (0.6–2.3)	0.6 (0.2–1.4)	0.7 (0.3–1.6)	2.5 (0.2–26.6)	2.9 (0.4–19.2)	0.4 (0.1–2.0)	0.5 (0.1–2.1)

* Significant at the 0.05 level, two-sided test.

[a] Assessed in the Part 2 sample due to having Part 2 controls. Each row represents a bivariate model. Data from New Zealand and Israel were dropped from these models due to not having the variables for parental disorders. Models control for person–years, country, and significant variables from the chapter on sociodemographics.

Table 7.3. Multivariate associations between number of parental disorders and lifetime suicidal behavior[a] (all countries combined)

	Among total sample		Among ideators		
	Ideation	Attempt	Plan	Planned attempt	Unplanned attempt
Number of parental disorders[b]	OR (95% CI)	OR (95% CI)	OR (95% CI)	OR (95% CI)	OR (95% CI)
1	2.1* (1.9–2.3)	2.4* (2.1–2.7)	1.0 (0.8–1.2)	0.9 (0.7–1.3)	1.4* (1.1–1.8)
2	2.7* (2.4–3.1)	3.2* (2.7–3.8)	1.4* (1.1–1.8)	1.0 (0.7–1.5)	1.5* (1.0–2.1)
3	3.5* (2.8–4.4)	3.2* (2.3–4.6)	1.3 (0.9–1.9)	0.7 (0.4–1.1)	1.7* (1.1–2.8)
4	2.5* (1.7–3.6)	6.2* (4.5–8.7)	1.4 (0.8–2.5)	1.3 (0.6–2.6)	
5+	15.4* (10.3–23.0)				
χ² (p-value)	661.5 (<0.001)*	335.8 (<0.001)*	11.9 (0.02)*	2.6 (0.63)	12.8 (0.01)*

* Significant at the 0.05 level, two-sided test.
[a] Assessed in the Part 2 sample due to having Part 2 controls. Models control for person–years, country, and significant variables from the chapter on sociodemographics.
[b] For number of parental disorders, the last OR represents the odds for that number of parental disorders or more. For example, for unplanned attempt, 3 represents ≥3 (that is, 3+).

Table 7.4. Final multivariate models for associations between parental psychopathology and lifetime suicidal behavior[a] (all countries combined)

	Among total sample		Among ideators		
	Ideation	Attempt	Plan	Planned attempt	Unplanned attempt
Parental disorder	OR (95% CI)	OR (95% CI)	OR (95% CI)	OR (95% CI)	OR (95% CI)
Type of parental disorder					
Depression	2.4* (1.9–3.0)	2.2* (1.6–2.9)	1.0 (0.6–1.4)	0.9 (0.5–1.5)	1.4 (0.7–2.6)
Panic disorder	2.1* (1.9–2.4)	2.6* (2.2–3.2)	1.1 (0.8–1.4)	1.5 (0.9–2.3)	1.6* (1.1–2.4)
Generalized anxiety disorder	2.7* (2.2–3.3)	2.5* (1.9–3.3)	1.1 (0.7–1.6)	0.4* (0.2–0.8)	2.1* (1.1–4.0)
Substance abuse	2.0* (1.7–2.3)	1.7* (1.4–2.1)	0.9 (0.6–1.2)	0.7* (0.4–1.0)	1.3 (0.9–1.9)
Antisocial personality disorder	2.6* (2.1–3.1)	3.0* (2.3–3.9)	0.9 (0.6–1.4)	1.2 (0.7–2.0)	2.3* (1.3–4.1)
Suicidal behavior	1.9* (1.2–3.1)	1.6 (0.8–3.1)	0.6 (0.3–1.5)	2.0 (0.3–13.5)	0.6 (0.2–2.4)
6 df χ² test for 6 types	264.4 (<.001)*	152.3 (<.001)*	3.2 (0.78)	16.3 (0.01)*	15.6 (0.02)*
5 df χ² test for difference between types	16.3 (0.01)*	16.7 (0.01)*	3.5 (0.62)	16.0 (0.01)*	10.3 (0.07)
Number of parental disorders[b]					
2	0.6* (0.5–0.7)	0.6* (0.5–0.8)	1.5 (1.0–2.5)	1.2 (0.7–2.4)	0.6 (0.3–1.1)
3	0.3* (0.2–0.4)	0.2* (0.1–0.4)	1.3 (0.6–2.9)	1.2 (0.4–3.4)	0.3* (0.1–0.9)
4	0.1* (0.0–0.1)	0.2* (0.1–0.3)	1.7 (0.6–5.2)	2.9 (0.6–13.1)	
5+	0.3* (0.1–0.6)				
χ² (p-value)	101.5 (<0.001)*	37.7 (<0.001)*	3.9 (0.27)	2.9 (0.41)	4.8 (0.09)

* Significant at the 0.05 level, two-sided test.
[a] Assessed in the Part 2 sample due to having Part 2 controls. Models control for person–years, country, and significant variables from the chapter on sociodemographics.
[b] For number of parental disorders, the last OR represents the odds for that number of parental disorders or more. For example, for unplanned attempt, 3 represents ≥3 (that is, 3+).

sample, the final multivariate models revealed subadditive effects of increasing number of parental disorders such that, as the number of parental disorders increases, the relative odds of respondent suicidal behavior increases at a decreasing rate across high-, middle-, and low-income countries.

Interactions between parental disorders and respondent age in predicting suicidal behavior

In order to test whether the associations between the examined parental disorders and suicidal behavior vary over the lifespan, we tested multivariate survival models that included the interaction of each parental disorder and respondent age. As shown in Table 7.5, the effect of parental depression on suicide ideation and attempt are higher in those aged 13–19 years (relative to those aged 4–12 years), and are higher for suicide ideation among those aged 30+ years. The effect of parental panic disorder on suicide attempt is increased among those aged 13–29 years. Interestingly, the effects of parental suicidal behavior on the onset of suicide ideation are lower among adolescents (aged 13–19 years) and older adults (aged 30+ years) relative to children (aged 4–12 years). Similar to parental suicidal behavior, the presence of multiple parental disorders is associated with decreased odds of suicide attempt among those 13–29 years of age.

These effects are reported separately for high-, middle-, and low-income countries in Appendix Tables 7.7, 7.8, and 7.9, respectively. Among high-income countries, only parental suicidal behavior is shown to have a significant effect on offspring; such that parental suicidal behavior is again negatively associated with suicide ideation among adolescents (aged 13–19 years) and adults (aged 30+ years). In middle-income countries, the effects of parental depression and panic on offspring suicide ideation are increased among those aged 13–19 years, whereas the effect of parental suicidal behavior on suicide ideation is decreased among those 30+ years of age. Parental panic, GAD, and ASPD all are associated with a significant decrease in the odds of suicide plan among ideators among those 13+ years of age. Finally, in low-income countries, the effects of parental depression on suicide ideation are increased among those aged 13–19 and 30+ years, and parental ASPD increases the odds of suicide ideation among those 20–29 years of age.

Associations between parental psychopathology and the persistence of suicidal behavior

The results of the backwards recurrence models show that parental depression and panic disorder predict the persistence of suicide ideation, whereas only parental depression predicts the persistence of plan (see Table 7.6). Parental panic and suicidal behavior both predict the persistence of suicide attempt. The results of the more fine-grained, logistic-regression persistence models (results not reported in tables) are consistent with those described earlier. More specifically, parental depression (OR = 1.6) and panic (OR = 1.3) predict the persistence of suicide ideation beyond two years after age of onset; parental depression (OR=4.1) predicts the persistence of a suicide plan within the past 10 years; and parental panic predicts the persistence of suicide attempt beyond two years (OR=1.8) and into the year prior to interview (OR=6.9). Overall, these results suggest that parental depression is especially strongly associated with the persistence of suicide ideation and plans, whereas parental panic is strongly associated with the long-term persistence of suicide attempts.

When persistence of suicidal behavior was examined cross-nationally (see Appendix Tables 7.10, 7.11, and 7.12), findings were very similar to the pattern reported previously for middle-income countries (with the exception of parental depression no longer predicting the persistence of plan) and slightly different for high- and low-income countries. No form of parental psychopathology predicts the persistence of suicidal behavior in high-income countries, whereas in low-income countries, parental depression predicts the persistence of ideation and plan.

Discussion

The findings of this study corroborate and extend previous findings on parental psychopathology and suicidal behavior among offspring. Although previous reports have found parental psychiatric disorders to be related to offspring suicide (Agerbo et al., 2002; Stenager & Qin, 2008) and suicidal behavior (Brent et al., 1996; Mittendorfer-Rutz et al., 2008; Pfeffer et al., 1994), the large sample size available to us in this study has enabled us to examine which particular parental disorders predict distinct stages on the

Table 7.5. Interactions between parental psychopathology and respondent age in the prediction of suicidal behavior[a] (all countries combined)

Interactions		Among total sample			Among ideators	
		Ideation	Attempt	Plan	Planned attempt	Unplanned attempt
		OR (95% CI)	OR (95% CI)	OR (95% CI)	OR (95% CI)	OR (95% CI)
Type of parental disorder						
Depression	13–19	2.2* (1.1–4.3)	3.7* (1.4–10.0)	0.9 (0.1–8.6)	2.1 (0.1–34.3)	1.4 (0.2–11.4)
	20–29	1.6 (0.8–3.1)	2.7 (1.0–7.6)	1.1 (0.1–9.9)	1.9 (0.1–30.1)	1.0 (0.1–9.6)
	30+	2.1* (1.0–4.2)	2.2 (0.7–6.5)	0.9 (0.1–8.2)	1.3 (0.1–17.9)	0.5 (0.0–4.7)
χ^2 (p-value)		6.2 (0.10)	7.9 (0.05)*	0.2 (0.98)	0.8 (0.86)	3.5 (0.32)
Panic disorder	13–19	1.2 (0.7–2.1)	2.3* (1.1–4.6)	1.1 (0.3–4.2)	3.7 (0.2–54.7)	0.9 (0.1–4.9)
	20–29	1.0 (0.6–1.8)	2.1* (1.0–4.3)	1.5 (0.4–5.4)	4.3 (0.3–55.9)	0.5 (0.1–2.5)
	30+	1.0 (0.6–1.8)	1.9 (1.0–3.7)	2.6 (0.7–9.7)	4.9 (0.4–65.1)	0.6 (0.1–3.3)
χ^2 (p-value)		1.3 (0.72)	5.3 (0.15)	8.6 (0.04)*	1.7 (0.63)	2.6 (0.45)
Generalized anxiety disorder	13–19	1.3 (0.6–2.7)	1.6 (0.6–4.5)	1.1 (0.2–5.6)	1.2 (0.1–18.2)	–
	20–29	0.9 (0.4–1.9)	1.4 (0.5–4.1)	1.0 (0.2–5.9)	1.7 (0.1–27.6)	–
	30+	0.9 (0.4–2.0)	0.8 (0.3–2.4)	0.9 (0.2–4.1)	1.5 (0.1–21.8)	–
χ^2 (p-value)		3.5 (0.33)	4.4 (0.22)	0.3 (0.96)	0.3 (0.97)	–
Substance abuse	13–19	1.0 (0.6–1.5)	1.3 (0.6–2.6)	1.2 (0.3–4.4)	0.3 (0.0–3.0)	1.2 (0.3–5.8)
	20–29	0.9 (0.6–1.4)	1.3 (0.7–2.5)	1.0 (0.3–3.6)	0.4 (0.0–4.0)	1.1 (0.3–4.8)
	30+	0.7 (0.4–1.2)	0.9 (0.4–1.8)	0.9 (0.3–3.2)	0.3 (0.0–3.3)	0.6 (0.1–3.0)
χ^2 (p-value)		3.8 (0.28)	2.8 (0.43)	0.8 (0.86)	1.4 (0.70)	2.4 (0.50)
Antisocial personality disorder	13–19	1.5 (0.8–2.8)	2.1 (0.9–4.8)	2.6 (0.5–14.1)	4.1 (0.2–70.5)	1.1 (0.3–4.6)
	20–29	1.3 (0.7–2.5)	2.1 (0.9–4.6)	3.2 (0.6–16.2)	4.1 (0.2–77.9)	0.9 (0.2–4.0)
	30+	1.4 (0.7–2.7)	2.3 (0.9–5.9)	2.3 (0.4–13.0)	5.5 (0.3–109.3)	1.6 (0.3–7.9)
χ^2 (p-value)		1.7 (0.63)	3.9 (0.28)	2.5 (0.48)	1.4 (0.71)	1.0 (0.80)
Suicidal behavior	13–19	0.2* (0.1–0.7)	0.7 (0.1–3.8)	0.2 (0.0–4.6)	–	–
	20–29	0.5 (0.1–1.8)	1.2 (0.2–6.2)	0.5 (0.0–10.6)	–	–
	30+	0.1* (0.0–0.3)	0.4 (0.1–2.4)	0.6 (0.0–14.1)	–	–
χ^2 (p-value)		17.9 (<.001)*	2.0 (0.58)	1.9 (0.60)	–	–
18 df χ^2 test for all parental disorders		35.4 (0.01)*	23.7 (0.16)	18.2 (0.44)	5.3 (0.99)	9.8 (0.64)
30 df χ^2 test for all parental disorders and dummies for number of disorders		67.3 (<0.001)*	52.7 (0.002)*	28.2 (0.40)	14.4 (0.85)	22.5 (0.10)
Number of parental disorders[b]						
2	13–19	0.6 (0.3–1.4)	0.3* (0.1–0.9)	0.4 (0.1–3.3)	0.2 (0.0–8.4)	2.8 (0.3–26.4)
	20–29	0.6 (0.3–1.4)	0.2* (0.1–0.6)	0.3 (0.0–2.4)	0.1 (0.0–3.7)	2.3 (0.2–23.1)
	30+	0.8 (0.4–1.9)	0.5 (0.2–1.6)	0.4 (0.1–2.8)	0.1 (0.0–6.2)	6.5 (0.6–67.7)
3	13–19	0.4 (0.1–1.3)	0.1* (0.0–0.4)	0.9 (0.0–32.2)	0.0 (0.0–5.0)	
	20–29	0.5 (0.2–1.9)	0.1* (0.0–0.4)	0.5 (0.0–15.8)	0.0 (0.0–5.3)	
	30+	0.5 (0.1–1.7)	0.2 (0.0–1.3)	0.8 (0.0–24.1)	0.0 (0.0–5.5)	

Table 7.5. (cont.)

Interactions		Among total sample			Among ideators	
		Ideation	Attempt	Plan	Planned attempt	Unplanned attempt
		OR (95% CI)	OR (95% CI)	OR (95% CI)	OR (95% CI)	OR (95% CI)
4+	13–19	0.1* (0.0–0.9)	0.1* (0.0–0.8)	0.1 (0.0–20.8)		
	20–29	0.1* (0.0–1.0)	0.0* (0.0–0.6)	0.1 (0.0–14.7)		
	30+	0.2 (0.0–1.5)	0.1 (0.0–1.7)	0.3 (0.0–46.8)		
χ^2 (p-value)		8.9 (0.44)	17.5 (0.04)*	4.1 (0.90)	6.0 (0.43)	4.0 (0.26)

*Significant at the 0.05 level, two-sided test.
– Not included due to small cell size.
[a] Assessed in the Part 2 sample due to having Part 2 controls. Models control for life course intervals (4–12, 13–19, 20–29, 30+ years), country, significant interaction terms from the chapter on sociodemographics, and the interaction of the life course intervals and all controls. Only the interactions for parental psychopathology and life course intervals are shown.
[b] For number of parental disorders, the last OR represents the odds for that number of parental disorders or more. For example, for unplanned attempt, 2 represents ≥2 (that is, 2+).

Table 7.6. Parental psychopathology and risk of persistence of suicidal behavior in the respondent[a] (all countries combined)

Parental disorder	Ideation	Plan	Attempt
	OR (95% CI)	OR (95% CI)	OR (95% CI)
Type of parental disorder			
Depression	1.5* (1.2–2.0)	1.7* (1.0–2.7)	1.3 (0.7–2.4)
Panic disorder	1.2* (1.0–1.5)	1.3 (1.0–1.7)	1.7* (1.2–2.4)
Generalized anxiety disorder	1.1 (0.8–1.5)	1.0 (0.7–1.5)	1.0 (0.6–1.6)
Substance abuse	1.0 (0.8–1.3)	1.0 (0.7–1.4)	1.0 (0.7–1.4)
Antisocial personality disorder	1.2 (0.9–1.7)	1.0 (0.7–1.6)	0.9 (0.5–1.6)
Suicidal behavior	1.2 (0.6–2.3)	2.7 (1.0–7.3)	3.4* (1.0–11.1)
χ^2_6 (p-value)	13.1 (0.04)*	13.0 (0.04)*	13.4 (0.04)*
χ^2_5 (p-value)	6.5 (0.26)	11.6 (0.04)*	10.2 (0.07)
Number of parental disorders[b]			
2	1.0 (0.7–1.3)	0.8 (0.5–1.4)	1.1 (0.6–2.0)
3	0.8 (0.5–1.3)	0.5 (0.2–1.3)	0.7 (0.2–2.1)
4	0.8 (0.4–1.6)	0.7 (0.2–2.1)	0.8 (0.2–2.7)
5+	0.4 (0.2–1.1)	2.4 (0.49)	2.1 (0.55)
χ^2 (p-value)	5.8 (0.22)		

*Significant at the 0.05 level, two-sided test.
0.0* (0.0–0.0) OR is ≤0.05 indicating very low risk.
[a] Results are based on multivariate discrete time survival models. Models control for country, age-related variables, and significant variables from the chapter on sociodemographics.
[b] For number of parental disorders, the last OR represents the odds for that number of parental disorders or more. For example, for attempt, 4 represents ≥4 (that is, 4+).

pathway to suicide. Our bivariate analyses showed that although all forms of parental psychopathology that were measured predict offspring suicide ideation, only parental GAD increases the chances of offspring developing a suicide plan and only panic, ASPD, and GAD predict unplanned suicide attempt.

Most of these findings remained even after potential confounds (e.g., comorbidity, number of parental disorders) were controlled. Each parental disorder continued to predict suicide ideation and attempt, and parental panic, GAD, and ASPD continued to predict unplanned attempt.

One interesting and unexpected finding was that parental GAD was consistently associated with decreased odds of suicide attempt among ideators with a plan. One possible explanation for this result is that if people with a predisposition for GAD develop a suicide plan, their worry and rumination may preclude them from ever acting on the plan (e.g., due to concerns about the negative consequences of the attempt). The reason for the protective effect of GAD in this case is not clear, but this represents a very intriguing direction for future research.

The WMH Surveys also provide a unique opportunity to compare the association of parental psychiatric disorders and suicidal behavior among offspring across countries grouped by income level (i.e., among high-, middle-, and low-income countries). In the final multivariate model examined, across all the different country groups and after controlling for number of parental disorders, each disorder continues to predict offspring suicide ideation. However, only parental panic emerged as a predictor of plans and attempts among ideators. The replication of these associations cross-nationally suggests they are robust in nature. However, the reason for the observed associations remains unclear. Our analyses revealed that the effects of parental psychopathology on offspring suicidal behavior remain, although they are slightly attenuated, after controlling for offspring mental disorders. This may be because parental psychopathology is a marker (or are markers) for traits such as neuroticism/pessimism, rumination, impulsiveness, etc., that are not fully explained by documenting the presence of offspring mental disorders.

The strong and consistent relationship between parental panic and offspring suicide attempt gives empirical support for prior suggestions on the genetic

transmission of suicide and suicidal behavior. Findings from previous family studies suggest that suicide ideation is predicted by the presence of parental depressive disorders (Brent et al., 1996; Brent & Mann, 2005), as seen in the current study, whereas suicide attempt is more likely to be related to increased rates of impulsive aggression in relatives (Brent et al., 2003). Impulsive aggression has been found to predict the onset of suicide attempt and to mediate the familial transmission of suicidal behavior. The possible genetic transmission for suicidal behavior is supported by a prior report from the WMH Surveys indicating that the presence of mental disorders, especially mood disorders, was more likely to predict the onset of suicidal thoughts while anxiety and poor impulse-control disorders, such as panic disorder, intermittent explosive disorder, and substance use disorders, were the strongest predictors of suicide attempts (Nock et al., 2009).

The findings reported here need to be considered within the context of the limitations of the study. First, all of the information relating to parental disorders as well as suicidal behavior was obtained by retrospective self-report provided by the respondents, which could have been affected by recall bias. There is, however, some evidence suggesting that past events can be recalled with sufficient accuracy to support their validity (Hardt & Rutter, 2004). Second, our assessment of parental psychopathology was confined to a limited number of disorders and did not include some other conditions of potential relevance, such as personality disorders and non-affective psychosis. Third, we may have underestimated the association between parental disorders and respondents' suicidal behavior by not taking chronicity and severity of parental disorders into account. Fourth and finally, in view of the cross-sectional design of the surveys, we were unable to make a direct estimate of persistence from duration of incident episodes and subsequent time to recurrence of further episodes. Rather, we made an approximation of duration and risk of recurrence among those with a history of previous suicidal behavior.

The results presented here provide support for a number of findings and new directions for future research. Although prior research has suggested the trend for suicidal behavior to run in families, an understanding of the mode of transmission has been limited (Brent & Mann, 2005). Taken together, the probability exists that different aspects of the suicidal spectrum of behaviors might have different genetic origins, an area that will require further investigation. However, the role of family environmental factors also is worth considering in this association. Parental psychiatric disorders and poor impulse control predisposes a family to instability and to inadequate parental care which may increase the likelihood for abuse, psychopathology, and suicidal behavior in the offspring (Brent & Melhem, 2008; Stenager & Qin, 2008).

Acknowledgements

Adapted by permission from Macmillan Publishers Ltd: Molecular Psychiatry (Gureje et al., 2010, doi: 10.1038/mp. 2010. 111), copyright © 2010.

References

Agerbo, E., Nordentoft, M., & Mortensen, P. B. (2002). Familial, psychiatric, and socioeconomic risk factors for suicide in young people: nested case-control study. *British Medical Journal*, **325**(7355), 74.

Andreasen, N., Endicott, J., Spitzer, R., & Winokur, G. (1977). The family history method using diagnostic criteria: reliability and validity. *Archives of General Psychiatry*, **34**(10), 1229–1235.

Balderssarini, R. J., & Hennen, J. (2004). Genetics of suicide: an overview. *Harvard Review of Psychiatry*, **12**(1), 1–13.

Brent, D. A., Bridge, J., Johnson, B. A., & Connolly, J. (1996). Suicidal behavior runs in families. A controlled family study of adolescent suicide victims. *Archives of General Psychiatry*, **53**(12), 1145–1152.

Brent, D. A., & Mann, J. J. (2005). Family genetic studies, suicide, and suicidal behavior. *American Journal of Medical Genetics Part C: Seminars in Medical Genetics*, **133C**(1), 13–24.

Brent, D. A., & Melhem, N. (2008). Familial transmission of suicidal behavior. *Psychiatric Clinics of North America*, **31**(2), 157–177.

Brent, D. A., Oquendo, M., Birmaher, B., et al. (2002). Familial pathways to early-onset suicide attempt: risk for suicidal behavior in offspring of mood-disordered suicide attempters. *Archives of General Psychiatry*, **59**(9), 801–807.

Brent, D. A., Oquendo, M., Birmaher, B., et al. (2003). Peripubertal suicide attempts in offspring of suicide attempters with siblings concordant for suicidal behavior. *American Journal of Psychiatry*, **160**(8), 1486–1493.

Gureje, O., Kola, L., Uwakwe, R., et al. (2007). The profile and risks of suicidal behaviours in the Nigerian Survey of Mental Health and Well-Being. *Psychological Medicine*, **37**(6), 821–830.

Gureje, O., Oladeji, B., Hwang, I., et al. (2010). Parental psychopathology and the risk of suicidal behavior in their offspring: results from the World Mental Health surveys. *Molecular Psychiatry*. [E-pub ahead of print, November 16.]

Hardt, J., & Rutter, M. (2004). Validity of adult retrospective reports of adverse childhood experiences: review of the evidence. *Journal of Child Psychology and Psychiatry*, **45**(2), 260–273.

Heider, D., Bernert, S., Matschinger, H., et al. (2007). Parental bonding and suicidality in adulthood. *Australian and New Zealand Journal of Psychiatry*, **41**(1), 66–73.

Kendler, K., Davis, C., & Kessler, R. (1997). The familial aggregation of common psychiatric and substance use disorders in the National Comorbidity Survey: a family history study. *British Journal of Psychiatry*, **170**, 541–548.

Krakowski, M. I., & Czobor, P. (2004). Psychosocial risk factors associated with suicide attempts and violence among psychiatric inpatients. *Psychiatric Services*, **55**(12), 1414–1419.

Mathers, C. D., & Loncar, D. (2006). Projections of global mortality and burden of disease from 2002 to 2030. *PLoS Medicine*, **3**(11), e442.

Melhem, N. M., Brent, D. A., Ziegler, M., et al. (2007). Familial pathways to early-onset suicidal behavior: familial and individual antecedents of suicidal behavior. *American Journal of Psychiatry*, **164**(9), 1364–1370.

Mittendorfer-Rutz, E., Rasmussen, F., & Wasserman, D. (2008). Familial clustering of suicidal behaviour and psychopathology in young suicide attempters. A register-based nested case control study. *Social Psychiatry and Psychiatric Epidemiology*, **43**(1), 28–36.

Nock, M. K., Hwang, I., Sampson, N. A., & Kessler, R. C. (2010). Mental disorders, comorbidity and suicidal behavior: Results from the National Comorbidity Survey Replication. *Molecular Psychiatry*, **15**(8), 868–876.

Nock, M. K., Hwang, I., Sampson, N. A., et al. (2009). Cross-national analysis of the associations among mental disorders and suicidal behavior: findings from the WHO World Mental Health Surveys. *PLoS Medicine*, **6**(8), e1000123.

Pfeffer, C. R., Normandin, L., & Kakuma, T. (1994). Suicidal children grow up: suicidal behavior and psychiatric disorders among relatives. *Journal of the American Academy of Child and Adolescent Psychiatry*, **33**(8), 1087–1097.

Pfeffer, C. R., Normandin, L., & Kakuma, T. (1998). Suicidal children grow up: relations between family psychopathology and adolescents' lifetime suicidal behavior. *Journal of Nervous and Mental Disease*, **186**(5), 269–275.

Qin, P., Agerbo, E., & Mortensen, P. B. (2002). Suicide risk in relation to family history of completed suicide and psychiatric disorders: a nested case-control study based on longitudinal registers. *Lancet*, **360**(9340), 1126–1130.

Sorensen, H. J., Mortensen, E. L., Wang, A. G., et al. (2009). Suicide and mental illness in parents and risk of suicide in offspring: a birth cohort study. *Social Psychiatry and Psychiatric Epidemiology*, **44**(9), 748–751.

Stenager, K., & Qin, P. (2008). Individual and parental psychiatric history and risk for suicide among adolescents and young adults in Denmark: a population-based study. *Social Psychiatry and Psychiatric Epidemiology*, **43**(11), 920–926.

Wender, P. H., Kety, S. S., Rosenthal, D., et al. (1986). Psychiatric disorders in the biological and adoptive families of adopted individuals with affective disorders. *Archives of General Psychiatry*, **43**(10), 923–929.

World Health Organization. (2001). *World Health Report: new understanding, new hope*. Geneva: WHO.

World Health Organization. (2007). *Suicide Prevention (SUPRE), WHO, Geneva*.

World Health Organization, UNAIDS, & UNICEF (eds.). (2007). *Towards universal access. Scaling up priority HIV/AIDS interventions in the health sector Progress Report*. Geneva, Switzerland: WHO.

Chapter

8

Childhood adversities as risk factors for onset and persistence of suicidal behavior

Ronny Bruffaerts, Koen Demyttenaere, Laura Helena Andrade,
Guilherme Borges, Wai Tat Chiu, Ron de Graaf, Charlene A. Deming,
Irving Hwang, Nancy A. Sampson, David R. Williams, Ronald C. Kessler,
and Matthew K. Nock

Introduction

Mental disorders generally are seen as critical risk factors for subsequent suicidal behavior. Both older and more recent research indicates that the vast majority of people who die by suicide meet criteria for a mental disorder at the time of their death (Nock et al., 2008b). Mood disorders such as major depression are the disorders most often associated with suicidal behavior (Petronis et al., 1990). Using data from the World Mental Health Surveys, Nock and colleagues (Nock et al., 2008a) reported that mood disorders, even after adjusting for sociodemographic characteristics, were most strongly associated with suicidal behavior, with odds ratios (ORs) ranging between 3.4 and 5.9. Other mental disorders, although to a lesser extent, appear to be significant risk factors as well, including: impulse-control disorders, anxiety disorders, and substance use disorders (Nock et al., 2008).

Although there is an unequivocal relationship between mental disorders and the onset and persistence of suicidal behavior, most people with mental disorders generally do not manifest suicidal behavior (McHolm et al., 2003). Importantly, environmental and experiential factors also predict the onset and persistence of a range of suicidal outcomes. Moreover, these factors have a stronger relationship with adverse mental health outcomes than known genetic factors (Risch et al., 2009).

Among environmental risk factors, exposure to negative childhood experiences deserves special attention. There is consistent evidence showing a significant association between reported adversities in childhood and adolescence on the one hand and suicide ideation, plans, and attempts in adulthood on the other hand

(Wagner, 1997; Ystgaard et al., 2004). For instance, the experience of sexual or physical abuse has appeared to be highly associated with suicidal behavior (Angst et al., 1992; Bryant & Range, 1995).

An important question is how and why childhood adversities may increase the likelihood of subsequent suicidal behavior. One possibility is that childhood adversities increase the odds of developing a mental disorder, and it is this increased likelihood of having a mental disorder that increases the risk of suicidal behavior. Indeed, prior studies have shown that mental disorders partially mediate the association between childhood adversities and suicidal behavior. Mental disorders appear to be a particularly important mediator of the association between childhood sexual abuse and suicidal behavior. Indeed, recent studies have shown that after adjustment for respondents' mental disorders, the strength of the ORs were 56%–67% lower for the association between sexual abuse and lifetime suicide attempts, compared to 9%–42% lower for other adversities (Bebbington et al., 2009; Enns et al., 2006).

Taken together, studies suggest that childhood adversities may be implicated in the occurrence of suicidal behavior, but many questions about this association remain. Existing literature on this question has four important limitations. First, both population-based and clinical studies have assessed a relatively limited number of childhood adversities. The effects of a broad range of adversities on a broad range of suicidal behaviors have not yet been investigated. Second, in general, simple models have been tested that do not take into account the possible interaction between types of adversity experience or the effect of the accumulation of multiple adversities. In addition, there is no systematic research to investigate the effects

Suicide, eds. Matthew K. Nock, Guilherme Borges, and Yutaka Ono. Published by Cambridge University Press.

of childhood adversities on suicidal behavior over the course of the lifespan, despite earlier evidence for such an effect (Molnar et al., 2001). Third, the majority of earlier research shows that there is an association between adversities and suicidal behavior, but we are not aware of studies that have investigated the extent to which childhood adversities predict the persistence of suicidal behavior over time. Fourth, little is known about the association of childhood adversities and suicidal behavior in general population samples with marked differences in culture, language, and level of socioeconomic development.

In this report, we use data from the World Mental Health (WMH) Surveys. The WMH Surveys were conducted in general population samples, using lay-administered structured psychiatric interviews measuring the presence of mental disorders, and assessing, among other things, a broad range of childhood adversities and suicidal behaviors. The specific aims of the study were to investigate: (1) the associations between childhood adversities and the subsequent onset of multiple forms of suicidal behavior (i.e., suicide ideation, plans, and attempts), using separate models estimating overall (bivariate) and specific (multivariate) effects of each type and number of adversities; (2) the extent to which the associations differ over the course of the respondents' lifespan; (3) the associations between childhood adversities and the persistence of suicidal behavior over time; and (4) the extent to which these associations are observed consistently across high-, middle-, and low-income countries. This chapter represents an extension of an earlier paper using WMH data on childhood adversities and suicidal behavior (Bruffaerts et al., 2010).

Method

A detailed description of the respondent samples, study procedures, statistical analyses, and assessment of suicidal behavior is provided in Chapter 3 of this volume. Assessment and analysis of sociodemographic factors (Chapter 6) and parental psychopathology (Chapter 7), which are included as covariates in the following analyses, are described in those earlier chapters.

Assessment of childhood adversities

Respondents were classified as having experienced physical abuse when they indicated that, when they were growing up, their father or mother (includes biological, step- or adoptive parent) slapped, hit,

pushed, grabbed, shoved, or threw something at them, or that they were beaten up as a child by the people who raised them. For sexual abuse, the following questions were asked: *"The next two questions are about sexual assault. The first is about rape. We define this as someone either having sexual intercourse with you or penetrating your body with a finger or object when you did not want them to, either by threatening you or using force, or when you were so young that you didn't know what was happening. Did this ever happen to you?"*; *"Other than rape, were you ever sexually assaulted or molested?"*. Sexual abuse was the only adversity where information was not collected that would distinguish whether the perpetrator was a family member or someone else. However, previous research using a similar measure but which did allow such a distinction showed that a good indirect way to distinguish family versus non-family sexual abuse is to ask about number of instances of victimization, with cases involving one or two instances typically perpetrated by a stranger and those involving three or more instances typically perpetrated by a family member (Molnar et al., 2001). In the WMH Surveys, therefore, respondents who reported that any of these experiences occurred to them three times or more were coded as having experienced sexual abuse within the family context. The rationale for focusing on sexual abuse in the family context is that such abuse is most likely to be a chronic stressor.

For the assessment of neglect, two neglect scales were created. These were based on responses to the neglect items: *"How often were you made to do chores that were too difficult or dangerous for someone your age?"*; *"How often were you left alone or unsupervised when you were too young to be alone?"*; *"How often did you go without things you needed like clothes, shoes, or school supplies because your parents or caregivers spent the money on themselves?"*; *"How often did your parents or caregivers make you go hungry or not prepare regular meals?"*; *"How often did your parents or caregivers ignore or fail to get you medical treatment when you were sick or hurt?"*. The serious neglect scale was the sum of the number of neglect items where the respondent replied "often" or "sometimes", plus one if the respondent rated either of his/her parents as having spent little or no effort in watching over them to ensure they had a good upbringing. The severe neglect scale is the sum of the number of neglect items where respondents replied "often" plus one if the respondent rated either of his/her parents as having spent no effort in watching over them to ensure they had a good upbringing. Both the serious and severe neglect scales ranged from 0–6. For the final definition of neglect, the respondent had to have a score of at least one on the severe neglect scale and at least two on the serious neglect scale.

For parental death, parental divorce, or other parental loss, respondents were first asked whether they lived with both of their parents when they were brought up. If respondents replied in the negative, they were asked: "*Did your biological mother or father die, were they separated or divorced, or was there some other reason?*". According to their answers to these questions, respondents were classified as having experienced parental death (i.e., when they indicated that one or both parents died), parental divorce (i.e., when they indicated that their parents divorced), and other parental loss (i.e., when respondents replied that they were either adopted, went to boarding school, were in foster care, or that they left home before the age of sixteen).

Respondents were coded as having experienced family violence when they indicated that they "*Were often hit, shoved, pushed, grabbed or slapped while growing up*", or "*Witnessed physical fights at home, like when your father beat up your mother?*".

Family economic adversity was coded positive if there was a positive response to either of the two following items. Item (a) was: "*During your childhood and adolescence, was there ever a period of six months or more when your family received money from a government assistance program like Welfare, Aid to Families with Dependent Children, General Assistance, or Temporary Assistance for Needy Families?*". Item (b) was endorsed when there was no male head of the family and the female head did NOT work all or most of the time during the respondent's childhood,

or in cases when there was no female head of the family and the male head did NOT work all or most of the respondent's childhood, or in cases when there was no female head and no male head of the family.

Respondents were classified as having had a physical illness when they responded affirmatively to the question: "*Did you ever have a life-threatening illness?*". They were then asked whether they ever had or were diagnosed by a medical doctor as having cancer, epilepsy, diabetes, or AIDS. Respondents who responded affirmatively on any of these diseases prior to the age of 18 years were classified as having had a physical illness in childhood.

There were a few instances in which particular surveys did not include certain risk factors. Specifically, South Africa did not assess neglect; Shenzhen did not assess sexual abuse; ESEMeD did not assess neglect and parental divorce; Israel did not assess neglect and family violence; and New Zealand did not assess neglect, parental death, parental divorce, and other parental loss. These countries were excluded from the respective bivariate models, and coded "zero" for these variables in the multivariate models.

Results

Prevalence of childhood adversities and onset of suicidal behavior

Overall, we found that the prevalence of childhood adversities was between 3.2% and 11.1%, with death of a parent the most commonly reported adversity (11.1%), followed closely by physical abuse (10.7%), and family violence (8.6%). Parental divorce was reported by 5.7% of respondents, similar to the report of other parental loss (5.3%) (see Figure 8.1). After

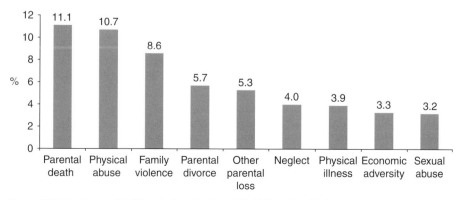

Figure 8.1. Prevalence of childhood adversities in the World Mental Health Surveys (%).

disaggregation for income categories, figures are comparable for the three income categories. However, there also are some interesting differences: physical abuse seems to be more common in middle- and low-income countries than in high-income countries (13.1% and 12.6%, respectively versus 8.6%) (see Appendix Table 8.1). By contrast, sexual abuse was more common among respondents from high- (5.0%) than those from middle- (0.9%) or low-income countries (1.2%). A last difference in the distribution of specific childhood adversities by income categories is that loss of a parent (either death of a parent or parental loss other than by death or divorce) is more common in middle- and low-income than in high-income countries.

Lifetime suicide attempt and ideation were reported by 2.7% (or n=2831) and 9.4% (or n=8382) of the respondents, respectively. Among those with suicide ideation, 34.5% (or n=3324) developed a plan, and about one in two (i.e., 55.2%) of those with a plan (or n=1894) made a suicide attempt. Alternatively, among those without a suicide plan, 15.1% (or n=937) made a suicide attempt ("unplanned attempt").

Among those with a history of suicide attempt, nearly one third (29.3%) reported physical abuse, about one in four (24.8%) reported family violence, and one in six (14.5%) reported sexual abuse. Adversities were all in the 6.0%–29.3% range among those with a lifetime suicide attempt (see Table 8.1). In both the total sample and among suicide ideators, we see that physical and sexual adversities are among the most common adversities in nearly all the suicidal outcomes studied. After disaggregation for income category, we see that prevalence estimates of childhood adversities among respondents with suicide attempts were in the 8.4%–28.8% range in high-income countries (with a median of 19.2%) (see Appendix Table 8.2), between 3.7% and 31.0% (median of 12.7%) in middle-income (see Appendix Table 8.3), and between 1.7% and 30.5% (median 11.0%) in low-income countries (see Appendix Table 8.4). Although the proportion of sexual abuse among suicide attempters may vary by income level, the predominance of physical abuse among attempters is an important finding across income categories. Physical abuse and family violence were common among those with ideation and attempt, although this finding was more explicit in high-income countries compared to middle- or low-income countries. More detailed results reported for each adversity and each type of suicidal behavior and after disaggregating for income categories are found in Table 8.2 and Appendix Tables 8.2–8.4.

Bivariate associations between childhood adversities and the onset of suicidal behavior

As shown in Table 8.2, bivariate survival models show that eight out of the nine adversities included in the analyses are significantly associated with the subsequent onset of suicide attempt and ideation, with ORs ranging from 1.2 to 5.7. The median significant OR for suicide attempt is 2.4 compared to 1.9 for suicide ideation. Regarding lifetime suicide attempts, there were five adversities that yielded ORs higher than 2.0: sexual abuse (OR=5.7), physical abuse (OR=3.7), neglect (OR=2.4); family violence (OR=2.4), and physical illness (OR=2.3). Physical and sexual abuse consistently had the highest odds for both suicide attempts and ideation (Ors=2.7–3.7 and OR=3.4–5.7, respectively). As a group, childhood adversities are less predictive of which respondents with suicide ideation go on to make a suicide plan or attempt. Indeed, sexual abuse is the only type of childhood adversity to significantly predict all five of the investigated suicide outcomes (Ors=1.3–5.7).

Multivariate associations between childhood adversities and subsequent onset of suicidal behavior: the effects of type of childhood adversities

In multivariate additive models that tested the unique associations between adversity and subsequent onset of suicidal behavior (see Table 8.3), all ORs decrease; however, 16 of the 18 ORs for suicide ideation and attempts are still greater than 1.0 and remain statistically significant, with median significant ORs of 1.5 (for suicide ideation) and 1.7 (for suicide attempts).

As shown in Table 8.3, no adversities predict all five suicidal outcomes. However, neglect predicts four of the five outcomes (ORs=1.4–2.0) and four adversities predict three suicidal outcomes: physical abuse (ORs=1.3–2.4), sexual abuse (ORs=1.2–3.8), parental divorce (ORs=1.4–1.6), and parental loss other than divorce or

Table 8.1. Prevalence of childhood adversities among those with each type of suicidal behavior (all countries combined)

Childhood adversity	Among total sample %ᵃ (SE) with adversities						Among ideators %ᵃ (SE) with adversities			
	Ideation	No ideation	Attempt	No attempt	Plan	No plan	Planned attempt	No planned attempt	Unplanned attempt	No unplanned attempt
Type of adversity										
Physical abuse	20.6 (0.6)	7.1 (0.2)	29.3 (1.2)	7.4 (0.2)	25.4 (1.0)	20.3 (1.0)	29.7 (1.5)	20.3 (1.8)	26.8 (1.8)	18.6 (1.1)
Sexual abuse	8.5 (0.3)	1.6 (0.1)	14.5 (0.8)	1.7 (0.1)	12.3 (0.7)	8.3 (0.5)	15.4 (1.0)	11.1 (1.2)	12.3 (1.1)	6.6 (0.6)
Neglect	13.1 (0.5)	5.0 (0.2)	19.3 (0.9)	5.2 (0.1)	17.5 (0.8)	12.9 (0.8)	20.8 (1.2)	14.0 (1.5)	15.4 (1.6)	11.1 (0.8)
Parental death	14.2 (0.5)	13.8 (0.2)	16.1 (0.8)	13.8 (0.2)	15.0 (0.8)	15.7 (0.8)	16.6 (1.1)	15.8 (1.7)	15.6 (1.7)	15.7 (1.0)
Parental divorce	11.7 (0.5)	5.2 (0.2)	15.6 (1.0)	5.3 (0.2)	11.9 (0.7)	10.2 (0.6)	14.7 (1.2)	9.3 (1.1)	17.8 (1.8)	9.4 (0.7)
Other parental loss	8.4 (0.4)	5.2 (0.1)	11.2 (0.7)	5.3 (0.1)	8.9 (0.7)	9.1 (0.7)	10.3 (0.9)	6.9 (1.0)	12.9 (1.3)	7.8 (0.7)
Family violence	17.6 (0.5)	6.0 (0.2)	24.8 (1.1)	6.3 (0.2)	21.5 (0.9)	17.1 (0.8)	23.3 (1.2)	18.1 (1.6)	25.4 (1.9)	14.9 (0.9)
Physical illness	6.6 (0.3)	3.4 (0.1)	8.7 (0.7)	3.5 (0.1)	7.9 (0.6)	7.3 (0.6)	9.2 (0.9)	7.4 (1.2)	8.2 (1.2)	6.3 (0.6)
Financial adversity	4.8 (0.3)	3.0 (0.1)	6.0 (0.5)	3.1 (0.1)	4.7 (0.4)	5.4 (0.5)	5.5 (0.6)	3.2 (0.6)	7.4 (0.9)	4.8 (0.5)
Number of adversitiesᵇ										
1	30.0 (0.7)	23.7 (0.3)	28.4 (1.1)	24.0 (0.3)	29.2 (1.0)	31.5 (1.2)	27.5 (1.4)	29.4 (1.9)	30.0 (1.9)	33.0 (1.4)
2	15.6 (0.5)	8.0 (0.2)	18.8 (0.9)	8.2 (0.2)	18.1 (0.9)	15.5 (0.8)	19.2 (1.2)	18.2 (1.7)	18.0 (1.5)	14.4 (0.9)
3	7.9 (0.4)	2.3 (0.1)	11.7 (0.8)	2.5 (0.1)	9.9 (0.6)	7.9 (0.6)	11.9 (0.9)	7.9 (1.3)	11.3 (1.6)	7.2 (0.7)
4	3.0 (0.2)	0.6 (0.1)	5.8 (0.6)	0.6 (0.1)	4.2 (0.4)	2.8 (0.3)	5.5 (0.6)	3.1 (0.6)	5.3 (1.0)	1.9 (0.3)
5	1.2 (0.1)	0.2 (0.0)	2.8 (0.4)	0.2 (0.0)	2.5 (0.4)	1.7 (0.2)	4.0 (0.7)	0.8 (0.2)	3.8 (0.6)	0.8 (0.1)
6+	0.4 (0.1)	0.0 (0.0)	1.2 (0.2)	0.0 (0.0)						

ᵃ % represents the percentage of people with the adversity among the cases with the outcome variable indicated in the column header. For example, the first cell is the % of those with physical abuse among those with ideation.

ᵇ For number of adversities, the last OR represents the odds for that number of adversities or more. For example, for unplanned attempt, 5 represents ≥5 (that is, 5+).

Table 8.2. Bivariate associations between type of adversities and suicidal behavior[a] (all countries combined)

Type of childhood adversity	Among total sample			Among ideators	
	Ideation	Attempt	Plan	Planned attempt	Unplanned attempt
	OR (95% CI)	OR (95% CI)	OR (95% CI)	OR (95% CI)	OR (95% CI)
Physical abuse	2.7* (2.5–3.0)	3.7* (3.2–4.2)	1.1 (0.9–1.3)	1.5* (1.2–2.0)	1.2 (0.9–1.6)
Sexual abuse	3.4* (3.0–3.8)	5.7* (5.0–6.5)	1.3* (1.0–1.5)	1.4* (1.0–1.9)	1.3* (1.0–1.8)
Neglect	1.8* (1.5–2.1)	2.4* (2.0–2.9)	1.4* (1.1–1.8)	1.6* (1.0–2.4)	1.0 (0.7–1.5)
Parental death	1.2* (1.1–1.3)	1.3* (1.1–1.5)	1.0 (0.8–1.2)	1.1 (0.8–1.6)	1.0 (0.7–1.3)
Parental divorce	1.4* (1.2–1.6)	1.7* (1.4–2.1)	0.9 (0.8–1.2)	1.6* (1.1–2.5)	1.3 (0.9–1.8)
Other parental loss	1.5* (1.3–1.8)	2.0* (1.6–2.3)	1.0 (0.8–1.2)	1.4 (1.0–1.9)	1.5* (1.1–2.0)
Family violence	1.9* (1.7–2.0)	2.4* (2.1–2.8)	1.1 (0.9–1.3)	1.3 (1.0–1.7)	1.4* (1.1–1.8)
Physical illness	1.8* (1.6–2.0)	2.3* (1.9–2.7)	1.1 (0.9–1.4)	1.3 (0.8–1.9)	1.4 (0.9–2.0)
Financial adversity	1.1 (1.0–1.3)	1.2 (1.0–1.5)	0.8 (0.6–1.0)	1.5 (0.9–2.4)	1.3 (0.9–1.9)

* Significant at the 0.05 level, two-sided test.
[a] Assessed in the Part 2 sample due to having Part 2 controls. Each row represents a separate bivariate model. Models control for person–years and country, and also include significant variables from the chapters on sociodemographics and parental psychopathology.

Table 8.3. Multivariate additive associations between type of childhood adversities and suicidal behavior[a] (all countries combined)

Type of childhood adversity	Among total sample			Among ideators	
	Ideation	Attempt	Plan	Planned attempt	Unplanned attempt
	OR (95% CI)	OR (95% CI)	OR (95% CI)	OR (95% CI)	OR (95% CI)
Physical abuse	2.1* (1.9–2.3)	2.4* (2.1–2.8)	1.0 (0.8–1.2)	1.3* (1.0–1.7)	1.1 (0.8–1.4)
Sexual abuse	2.5* (2.2–2.9)	3.8* (3.2–4.4)	1.2* (1.0–1.5)	1.3 (1.0–1.8)	1.3 (0.9–1.7)
Neglect	1.7* (1.5–1.9)	2.0* (1.7–2.4)	1.4* (1.1–1.7)	1.5* (1.1–2.1)	1.1 (0.8–1.5)
Parental death	1.2* (1.1–1.3)	1.3* (1.1–1.5)	1.1 (0.9–1.3)	1.2 (0.9–1.6)	1.0 (0.8–1.4)
Parental divorce	1.4* (1.2–1.5)	1.6* (1.4–1.9)	1.0 (0.8–1.2)	1.4 (1.0–2.1)	1.4* (1.1–1.9)
Other parental loss	1.2* (1.1–1.4)	1.3* (1.1–1.6)	0.9 (0.7–1.1)	1.2 (0.8–1.6)	1.5* (1.1–2.0)
Family violence	1.3* (1.2–1.4)	1.5* (1.2–1.7)	1.0 (0.9–1.2)	1.1 (0.8–1.4)	1.3 (1.0–1.6)
Physical illness	1.6* (1.4–1.8)	1.8* (1.5–2.2)	1.1 (0.9–1.4)	1.2 (0.8–1.8)	1.4 (0.9–2.0)
Financial adversity	1.0 (0.8–1.1)	0.9 (0.7–1.1)	0.8 (0.6–1.0)	1.2 (0.7–2.1)	1.1 (0.7–1.6)

* Significant at the 0.05 level, two-sided test.
[a] Assessed in the Part 2 sample due to having Part 2 controls. Models control for person–years, country, and significant variables from the chapters on sociodemographics and parental psychopathology.

parental death (ORs=1.2–1.5). Overall, these data suggest that although adversities are predictive of suicide ideation and attempts in the total sample, they are far less predictive of which ideators go on to make plans or attempts. Indeed, of the 27 ORs for the prediction of plans and attempts among ideators, only six are significant, yielding only moderate associations in the 1.2–1.5 range.

Multivariate associations between childhood adversities and subsequent onset of suicidal behavior: the effects of number of childhood adversities

Next we estimated the association between the number of childhood adversities a person has experienced and

Table 8.4. Multivariate associations between number of adversities and suicidal behavior[a] (all countries combined)

Number of childhood adversities[b]	Among total sample		Among ideators		
	Ideation	Attempt	Plan	Planned attempt	Unplanned attempt
	OR (95% CI)	OR (95% CI)	OR (95% CI)	OR (95% CI)	OR (95% CI)
1	1.8* (1.7–2.0)	2.3* (2.0–2.6)	1.0 (0.9–1.2)	1.2 (0.9–1.6)	1.2 (0.9–1.6)
2	2.5* (2.2–2.7)	3.7* (3.2–4.3)	1.2* (1.0–1.5)	1.4 (1.0–1.9)	1.5* (1.2–2.0)
3	3.7* (3.2–4.2)	6.4* (5.3–7.8)	1.3* (1.0–1.7)	2.0* (1.3–3.0)	1.6* (1.1–2.3)
4	5.3* (4.2–6.5)	11.3* (8.8–14.4)	1.3 (1.0–1.7)	2.5* (1.5–4.4)	2.3* (1.4–4.0)
5	5.7* (4.2–7.9)	14.8* (10.1–21.6)	1.1 (0.7–1.6)	6.0* (2.7–13.3)	2.4* (1.5–4.1)
6+	6.1* (4.1–9.1)	19.4* (12.7–29.5)			
χ^2 (p-value)	782.3 (<0.001)	742.7 (<0.001)	8.5 (0.13)	34.2 (<0.001)	22.7 (<0.001)

* Significant at the 0.05 level, two-sided test.
[a] Assessed in the Part 2 sample due to having Part 2 controls. Models control for person–years, country, and include significant variables from the chapters on sociodemographics and parental psychopathology.
[b] For number of adversities, the last OR represents the odds for that number of adversities or more. For example, for unplanned attempt, 5 represents ≥5 (that is, 5+).

the odds of subsequent suicidal behavior (see Table 8.4). The data suggest a strong dose–response relationship between the number of adversities and the majority of the suicidal outcomes in the study (i.e., attempts, ideation, planned and unplanned attempts). The dose–response effect is most pronounced for suicide attempts among the total sample, where ORs range from 2.3 (for one adversity) to 19.4 (for six or more adversities). Similar (but weaker) associations are seen for suicide ideation among the total sample (with ORs between 1.8 [for one adversity] to 6.1 [for six or more adversities]). The data also reveal that the number of adversities experienced is strongly related to unplanned attempts among ideators. Despite the fact that the associations are weaker than those found for both attempts and ideation among the total sample, these ORs range between 1.2 (for one adversity) and 2.4 (for five or more reported adversities).

When data are disaggregated by income, comparable figures are found for the association between the number of adversities and suicidal behavior. However, the dose–response relationship is strongest in high-income countries (see Appendix Table 8.5). Moreover, in middle-income (see Appendix Table 8.6) and low-income countries (see Appendix Table 8.7), the number of adversities lost its statistical significance in predicting lifetime plans, planned attempts, and unplanned attempts among ideators.

Multivariate associations between childhood adversities and subsequent onset of suicidal behavior: the effects of type and number of childhood adversities

In the next set of analyses, we tested the unique associations between the type and number of childhood adversities and each of the five suicidal outcomes. There are four notable findings in these analyses (see Table 8.5). First, all investigated adversities yield statistically significant ORs with lifetime ideation (ORs=1.3–3.4) and attempts (ORs=1.3–4.6), with median ORs of 1.7 and 2.2, respectively. Again, sexual and physical abuse are the most predictive adversities of both ideation and attempts (ORs=2.7–4.6). After disaggregation for income categories, we found less significant associations in middle- and low-income countries than in high-income countries. However, the median significant ORs between adversities and suicide ideation (median significant ORs in the 1.6–2.0 range) and between adversities suicide attempts (median OR=2.5) remain similar in the three income categories.

Second, the strong association between most adversities and suicide attempts only holds in high-income countries (see Appendix Table 8.8) where all nine adversities are associated with lifetime attempts, with a median OR of 2.5. In middle- (see Appendix

Table 8.9) and low-income countries (see Appendix Table 8.10) only physical and sexual abuse are consistently associated with suicide attempts. With regard to the association between adversities and ideation, after disaggregation for income category, of the 27 ORs (three income categories and nine adversities), 23 are significant (all in the 1.3–3.4 range). Among these, the strongest associations were found in high- and middle-income countries (8/9 and 9/9 significant ORs, respectively) with median ORs between 1.6 and 2.0, and somewhat less in low-income countries, in which 6/9 ORs were significant, with a median of 1.7.

Third, the data also point to the finding that adversities do not have consistent predictive values for suicide plans and attempts among respondents with suicide ideation. In the ideator sample (see Table 8.5), of the 27 ORs investigated, only three (i.e., neglect, parental divorce, and financial adversity) are significant. Neglect predicts planned attempts (OR=1.5) and divorce of a parent predicts unplanned attempts (OR =1.5), whereas financial adversity appears to be protective against lifetime suicide plans among respondents with suicide ideation (OR=0.7). Moreover, in the separate income categories, there is no consistency as to which adversities are predictive of plans or attempts among ideators. For example, in high-income countries (see Appendix Table 8.8), neglect is a modest predictor of plans and planned attempts among ideators (ORs 1.5–1.9), but this adversity appears to be insignificant in predicting plans or attempts among ideators in middle- (see Appendix Table 8.9) and low-income countries (see Appendix Table 8.10). Similarly, financial adversity is protective against plans among ideators (OR=0.6) only in high-income countries. In contrast, in middle-income countries, physical illness is protective (OR= 0.5). An interesting last finding here is that, in general, there are no predictors of unplanned suicide attempts, with the exception of sexual abuse in low-income countries (OR=4.0).

Fourth, the ORs for the association between the number of adversities and suicide ideation and attempt become increasingly small (less than 1.0) in this model (with all countries combined) (see Table 8.5). This finding indicates that the joint effects of having experienced multiple childhood adversities were significantly less strong than the product of the ORs of the individual adversities. This effect is not observed for suicide plans or attempts among ideators. Moreover, this effect was observed in high-income countries, existed only for

suicide ideation in middle-income countries, and was absent in low-income countries (see Appendix Tables 8.8–8.10).

Estimating the role of respondent mental disorders as a potential mediating factor

Our statistical analyses enabled us to generate estimates of the impact of respondents' lifetime mental disorders on the association between childhood adversities and each of the suicide outcomes measured. These results are shown in Table 8.6. Several important findings stand out in the comparison of the ORs with and without adjustments for lifetime mental disorders. First, after adjustment for lifetime mental disorders, ORs decrease but only some lose their statistical significance. The impact of lifetime mental disorders is only moderate, but greater in sexual and physical abuse relative to the other adversities. For example, the OR for the association between physical/sexual abuse and suicide attempt is estimated at 3.3/4.6 prior to and 2.6/3.1 after adjustment for respondents' lifetime mental disorders. In other words, the ORs decrease 21% and 33%, respectively. This also is the case for the rest of the adversities, although to a lesser extent; after adjustment for lifetime mental disorders, the ORs of the seven remaining adversities decrease by 6% to16%. A similar pattern is observed in the case of suicide ideation.

Second, this effect is more pronounced in high-income than in middle- and low-income countries (see Appendix Tables 8.11–8.13). Looking at the associations between physical/sexual abuse and suicide attempt, we see that in high-income countries ORs drop by 26/31% after adjustment for respondents' lifetime mental disorders. By comparison, in middle- and low-income countries, ORs also drop after adjustment for lifetime mental disorders, but to a lesser extent: 17/23% in middle-, and 12/19% in low-income countries. These findings suggest that lifetime mental disorders are a greater mediator of the associations between childhood adversities and suicidal outcomes in high-income countries than in middle- and low-income countries.

Differences in the observed effects across the lifespan

Examination of the differences in the observed effects across the lifespan suggests that the impact of

Table 8.5. Multivariate interactive associations between type and number of childhood adversities and suicidal behavior[a] (all countries combined)

| | Among total sample | | | Among ideators | |
| | Ideation | Attempt | Plan | Planned attempt | Unplanned attempt |
Childhood adversity	OR (95% CI)	OR (95% CI)	OR (95% CI)	OR (95% CI)	OR (95% CI)
Type of adversity					
Physical abuse	2.7* (2.4–3.0)	3.3* (2.7–4.0)	0.9 (0.7–1.2)	1.3 (0.9–1.9)	1.1 (0.8–1.6)
Sexual abuse	3.4* (2.9–4.0)	4.6* (3.7–5.7)	1.2 (0.9–1.5)	1.3 (0.9–1.9)	1.3 (0.9–1.9)
Neglect	2.3* (2.0–2.6)	2.9* (2.3–3.5)	1.3 (1.0–1.7)	1.5* (1.0–2.2)	1.1 (0.7–1.7)
Parental death	1.4* (1.3–1.6)	1.7* (1.4–2.0)	1.0 (0.8–1.2)	1.2 (0.8–1.7)	1.1 (0.7–1.5)
Parental divorce	1.7* (1.5–1.9)	2.2* (1.8–2.6)	0.9 (0.7–1.2)	1.4 (0.9–2.2)	1.5* (1.0–2.1)
Other parental loss	1.7* (1.5–1.9)	2.0* (1.6–2.5)	0.9 (0.7–1.1)	1.1 (0.7–1.7)	1.5 (1.0–2.2)
Family violence	1.7* (1.5–1.9)	2.0* (1.6–2.5)	1.0 (0.8–1.2)	1.0 (0.7–1.5)	1.3 (0.9–1.9)
Physical illness	2.0* (1.7–2.3)	2.5* (2.0–3.1)	1.1 (0.8–1.4)	1.2 (0.7–2.0)	1.4 (0.9–2.1)
Financial adversity	1.3* (1.1–1.6)	1.3* (1.0–1.7)	0.7* (0.5–1.0)	1.1 (0.6–2.2)	1.1 (0.7–1.9)
9 df χ^2 test for 9 types	528.9 (<.001)*	329.6 (<.001)*	18.9 (0.03)*	7.1 (0.63)	8.3 (0.51)
8 df χ^2 test for difference between types	267.6 (<.001)*	167.8 (<.001)*	18.6 (0.02)*	4.3 (0.83)	5.4 (0.71)
Number of adversities[b]					
2	0.7* (0.6–0.8)	0.7* (0.5–0.9)	1.2 (0.9–1.7)	0.9 (0.6–1.4)	1.0 (0.6–1.7)
3	0.5* (0.4–0.6)	0.5* (0.3–0.7)	1.3 (0.8–2.1)	1.0 (0.5–2.3)	0.9 (0.4–1.9)
4	0.3* (0.2–0.5)	0.3* (0.2–0.5)	1.3 (0.7–2.4)	1.0 (0.4–3.0)	1.0 (0.3–2.9)
5	0.2* (0.1–0.3)	0.2* (0.1–0.3)	1.1 (0.5–2.6)	2.0 (0.4–9.4)	0.8 (0.2–3.5)
6+	0.1* (0.0–0.2)	0.1* (0.0–0.2)			
χ^2 (p-value)	80.5 (<0.001)*	37.5 (<0.001)*	4.9 (0.30)	3.4 (0.49)	0.6 (0.96)

* Significant at the 0.05 level, two-sided test.
[a] Assessed in the Part 2 sample due to having Part 2 controls. Models control for person–years, country, and significant variables from the chapters on sociodemographics and parental psychopathology.
[b] For number of adversities, the last OR represents the odds for that number of adversities or more. For example, for unplanned attempt, 5 represents ≥5 (that is, 5+).

childhood adversities on the occurrence of suicidal behavior is most prominent early in life (see Table 8.7). Indeed, adversities have the strongest associations with attempts in childhood (those aged 4–12 years; median significant OR=3.8), with this effect decreasing across the teen years (those aged 13–19 years; median significant OR=2.5) and young adulthood (those aged 20–29 years; median significant OR =2.0), with a slight increase in later adult life (those aged 30+ years; median significant OR=2.3). Here too,

sexual and physical abuse are the most powerful predictors of suicide attempts among young people. The odds of suicide attempt during childhood are more than ten-fold higher (OR=10.9) among people with a history of sexual abuse than comparable people without. Again, we see a graded relationship in which the effects of sexual abuse are gradually weaker in higher age groups: suicide attempts in the teen years are 6.1-fold higher among those with sexual abuse in childhood, and in young adulthood or later adulthood are

Table 8.6. Multivariate interactive associations between type and number of childhood adversities and suicidal behavior after adjustment for respondents' lifetime mental disorders[a] (all countries combined)

	Among total sample			Among ideators	
	Ideation	Attempt	Plan	Planned attempt	Unplanned attempt
Childhood adversity	OR (95% CI)	OR (95% CI)	OR (95% CI)	OR (95% CI)	OR (95% CI)
Type of adversity					
Physical abuse	2.3* (2.0–2.5)	2.6* (2.1–3.1)	0.9 (0.7–1.1)	1.3 (0.9–1.8)	1.1 (0.7–1.6)
Sexual abuse	2.6* (2.2–3.0)	3.1* (2.5–3.9)	1.1 (0.9–1.4)	1.3 (0.9–1.9)	1.2 (0.8–1.8)
Neglect	2.1* (1.9–2.4)	2.6* (2.1–3.1)	1.3 (1.0–1.6)	1.5* (1.0–2.1)	1.1 (0.7–1.7)
Parental death	1.4* (1.3–1.6)	1.6* (1.4–1.9)	1.0 (0.8–1.2)	1.1 (0.8–1.6)	1.0 (0.7–1.5)
Parental divorce	1.7* (1.5–1.9)	2.0* (1.7–2.5)	0.9 (0.7–1.2)	1.4 (0.9–2.2)	1.5* (1.0–2.1)
Other parental loss	1.6* (1.4–1.8)	1.8* (1.5–2.3)	0.8 (0.6–1.1)	1.1 (0.7–1.8)	1.5 (0.9–2.2)
Family violence	1.5* (1.4–1.7)	1.7* (1.4–2.1)	0.9 (0.7–1.2)	1.0 (0.6–1.4)	1.2 (0.9–1.8)
Physical illness	1.8* (1.6–2.1)	2.1* (1.7–2.7)	1.1 (0.8–1.4)	1.1 (0.7–1.8)	1.4 (0.9–2.1)
Financial adversity	1.3* (1.0–1.5)	1.2 (0.9–1.5)	0.7* (0.5–1.0)	1.1 (0.6–2.1)	1.1 (0.6–1.8)
9 df χ^2 test for 9 types	372.3 (<0.001)*	197.7 (<0.001)*	17.5 (0.04)*	7.1 (0.63)	7.8 (0.56)
8 df χ^2 test for difference between types	157.4 (<0.001)*	91.5 (<0.001)*	17.2 (0.03)*	4.6 (0.79)	5.8 (0.67)
Number of adversities[b]					
2	0.7* (0.6–0.8)	0.7* (0.6–0.9)	1.2 (0.9–1.6)	0.9 (0.6–1.5)	1.0 (0.6–1.8)
3	0.5* (0.4–0.6)	0.5* (0.3–0.7)	1.3 (0.8–2.1)	1.1 (0.5–2.3)	0.9 (0.4–2.1)
4	0.4* (0.3–0.5)	0.4* (0.2–0.6)	1.3 (0.7–2.3)	1.2 (0.4–3.6)	1.1 (0.4–3.1)
5	0.2* (0.1–0.3)	0.2* (0.1–0.4)	1.1 (0.5–2.6)	1.9 (0.4–9.1)	0.9 (0.2–4.0)
6+	0.1* (0.0–0.2)	0.1* (0.0–0.2)			
χ^2 (p-value)	73.0 (<0.001)*	30.5 (<0.001)*	4.4 (0.36)	2.3 (0.67)	0.5 (0.98)

* Significant at the 0.05 level, two-sided test.
[a] Assessed in the Part 2 sample due to having Part 2 controls. Models control for person–years, country, and significant variables from the chapters on sociodemographics and parental psychopathology.
[b] For number of adversities, the last OR represents the odds for that number of adversities or more. For example, for unplanned attempt, 5 represents ≥5 (that is, 5+).

about three-fold higher in respondents with sexual abuse than in those without. Comparable figures are found for physical abuse.

After disaggregating for income categories (see Appendix Tables 8.14–8.16), the associations described above hold, but especially in high-income countries, where there is clear evidence for a lifetime influence of childhood adversities with, again, physical (ORs=3.1–6.1) and sexual abuse (ORs=3.3–8.8) as consistent significant predictors of suicide attempts

across the lifespan. We also found evidence for a subadditive effect of the number of adversities reported for suicide attempts during childhood, teen years, and later adulthood. An additional finding among respondents from high-income countries is that five out of the nine adversities significantly predict suicide attempt in childhood (ORs=2.8–8.8), whereas seven to nine of the nine adversities predict suicide attempt later than the childhood years (i.e., during the teen years, young adulthood, and later adulthood)

Table 8.7. Multivariate interactive associations between type and number of childhood adversities with subsequent onset of suicide attempt across the lifespan[a] (all countries combined)

Childhood adversity	Lifetime attempt during childhood (age 4–12 years)	Lifetime attempt during teen years (age 13–19 years)	Lifetime attempt during young adulthood (age 20–29 years)	Lifetime attempt during later adulthood (age 30+ years)
	OR (95% CI)	OR (95% CI)	OR (95% CI)	OR (95% CI)
Type of adversity				
Physical abuse	6.3* (3.1–13.0)	4.1* (3.0–5.6)	2.5* (1.8–3.5)	2.7* (1.9–3.9)
Sexual abuse	10.9* (5.0–23.7)	6.1* (4.4–8.4)	2.9* (1.9–4.3)	3.1* (2.0–4.7)
Neglect	4.6* (1.5–14.1)	2.7* (1.9–3.7)	2.1* (1.4–3.0)	3.8* (2.7–5.4)
Parental death	2.2* (1.0–4.8)	1.6* (1.2–2.2)	1.5* (1.1–2.0)	1.7* (1.3–2.3)
Parental divorce	3.2* (1.5–6.9)	2.2* (1.6–2.9)	2.0* (1.4–2.8)	2.0* (1.3–3.1)
Other parental loss	4.2* (2.0–8.8)	2.3* (1.6–3.3)	1.3 (0.9–1.9)	2.0* (1.3–2.9)
Family violence	2.6* (1.2–5.8)	2.2* (1.6–3.1)	1.6* (1.1–2.3)	2.1* (1.5–3.1)
Physical illness	3.3* (1.6–6.8)	3.0* (2.0–4.3)	1.9* (1.2–3.0)	2.4* (1.5–3.7)
Financial adversity	1.4 (0.6–2.9)	1.4 (0.9–2.1)	1.0 (0.6–1.6)	1.5 (0.8–2.7)
9 df χ² test for 9 types	62.6 (<0.001)*	197.4 (<0.001)*	77.9 (<0.001)*	77.0 (<0.001)*
8 df χ² test for difference between types	48.2 (<0.001)*	117.9 (<0.001)*	47.3 (<0.001)*	30.7 (<0.001)*
Number of adversities				
2	0.5 (0.2–1.4)	0.6* (0.4–0.8)	1.0 (0.6–1.5)	0.7 (0.5–1.1)
3	0.3 (0.1–1.4)	0.3* (0.2–0.6)	0.9 (0.4–1.7)	0.5* (0.2–1.0)
4	0.2 (0.0–1.3)	0.2* (0.1–0.5)	0.7 (0.3–1.8)	0.3* (0.1–0.7)
5	0.1* (0.0–0.9)	0.1* (0.0–0.4)	0.5 (0.1–1.6)	0.1* (0.0–0.3)
6+	0.0* (0.0–0.8)	0.0* (0.0–0.2)	0.2 (0.0–1.7)	0.0* (0.0–0.1)
χ² (p-value)	7.7 (0.18)	21.7 (<0.001)*	4.3 (0.51)	25.9 (<0.001)*

* Significant at the 0.05 level, two-sided test.
[a] Assessed in the Part 2 sample due to having Part 2 controls. Models control for person–years, country, and significant variables from the chapters on sociodemographics and parental psychopathology.

(ORs=1.6–6.6). In more detail, neglect, the death of a parent, family violence, and financial adversity do not predict suicide attempt in the childhood years, but they do predict attempt later in life. In addition, the impact of childhood adversities is more pronounced for suicide attempt in early childhood (median significant OR=5.4) than for attempt later in life (median significant ORs=2.7–3.1). All-in-all, in high-income countries, there is sufficient evidence for a lifelong impact of a broad range of childhood adversities on suicide attempts. A quite different picture emerges when we look at the influence of childhood adversities on suicide attempt in middle- and low-income countries. In middle-income countries, of the 36 associations (nine adversities by four age periods), only 12 are significantly different from 1.0. Physical abuse is the

only adversity that predicts suicide attempt across the whole lifespan (ORs=1.8–4.8). In order of importance, sexual abuse (OR=96.1), neglect (OR=6.8), and physical abuse (OR=4.8) are strongly associated with suicide attempt in childhood. An interesting finding is that respondents who reported financial adversities in their childhood are significantly less likely (OR=0.0) to have tried to kill themselves during the childhood years. The same trend we find in middle-income countries also applies to low-income countries. Indeed, of the 36 associations investigated, only nine are significantly different from 1.0. In contrast to high- and middle-income countries, there are no adversities that predict suicide attempt across the whole lifespan. However, we do find that physical abuse predicts suicide attempt during childhood (OR=3.9), during

Table 8.8. Multivariate associations between type and number of childhood adversities and persistence of suicidal behavior[a] (all countries combined)

Childhood adversity	Ideation OR (95% CI)	Plan OR (95% CI)	Attempt OR (95% CI)
Type of adversity			
Physical abuse	1.2 (1.0–1.4)	1.4* (1.1–1.9)	1.5* (1.1–2.3)
Sexual abuse	1.2 (1.0–1.4)	1.4* (1.1–1.9)	1.6* (1.1–2.3)
Neglect	1.0 (0.9–1.2)	1.0 (0.8–1.4)	1.0 (0.7–1.4)
Parental death	0.9 (0.8–1.1)	1.1 (0.8–1.4)	0.7 (0.4–1.0)
Parental divorce	0.9 (0.7–1.1)	0.9 (0.7–1.3)	0.8 (0.5–1.1)
Other parental loss	1.2 (1.0–1.5)	1.2 (0.9–1.7)	0.8 (0.5–1.3)
Family violence	1.0 (0.8–1.2)	1.2 (0.9–1.6)	1.0 (0.7–1.6)
Physical illness	1.0 (0.8–1.2)	0.9 (0.6–1.3)	1.3 (0.8–2.1)
Economic adversity	1.0 (0.8–1.4)	0.9 (0.5–1.5)	1.0 (0.6–1.6)
9 df χ^2 test for 9 types	17.2 (0.05)*	19.6 (0.02)*	52.4 (<.001)*
8 df χ^2 test for difference between types	17.1 (0.03)*	15.8 (0.05)*	49.3 (<.001)*
Number of adversities[b]			
2	1.1 (0.9–1.4)	1.1 (0.7–1.5)	1.1 (0.7–1.8)
3	1.1 (0.7–1.6)	0.9 (0.5–1.6)	0.9 (0.4–1.9)
4	1.2 (0.7–2.0)	0.9 (0.4–2.0)	1.0 (0.3–3.1)
5	0.9 (0.5–1.8)	0.9 (0.3–2.6)	0.6 (0.1–2.5)
6+	0.9 (0.3–2.3)		1.4 (0.2–8.8)
χ^2 (p-value)	3.9 (0.56)	1.7 (0.79)	8.8 (0.12)

* Significant at the 0.05 level, two-sided test.
[a] Results are based on multivariate discrete time survival models. Models control for country, age-related variables, and significant variables from the chapters on sociodemographics and parental psychopathology.
[b] For number of adversities, the last OR represents the odds for that number of adversities or more. For example, for plan, 5 represents ≥5 (that is, 5+).

young adulthood (OR=2.8), and during later adulthood (OR=2.6). Sexual abuse, by contrast, is a strong predictor of suicide attempt in childhood, the teen years, and during later adulthood (OR=10.1, 5.0, and 3.9, respectively). Four out of nine adversities are associated with suicide attempt in later adulthood: sexual abuse (OR=3.9), physical abuse (OR=2.6), neglect (OR=2.3), and the death of a parent (OR=2.0). Again, financial adversities appear to be protective against suicide attempt in early childhood (OR=0.0).

Effects of childhood adversities on persistence of suicidal behavior

In the backwards recurrence models predicting the persistence of suicidal behavior over time, physical and sexual abuse are the only adversities with significant associations, with both predicting the persistence

of suicide plans and attempts (see Table 8.8). The results of the more fine-grained logistic regression persistence models (results not reported in tables) also highlighted the importance of physical and sexual abuse in predicting the persistence of suicidal behavior over time. More specifically, physical and sexual abuse are associated with the persistence beyond two years after age of onset of suicide ideation (OR=1.3), suicide plan (OR=1.5–1.7), and suicide attempt (OR=1.8–1.9). The only other factor that predicts high persistence of suicidal behavior time is other parental loss, which is associated with the persistence of suicide ideation beyond two years after age of onset (OR=1.4) and with very high persistence of suicide plans; that is, persistence into the five (OR=2.0) and one (OR=2.1) years prior to interview.

The importance of physical and sexual abuse in predicting the persistence of suicidal behavior is apparent in the findings from the recurrence models for high-income countries, but not for middle- and low-income countries (see Appendix Tables 8.17–8.19). The only significant associations in middle-income countries are for other parental loss and economic adversity predicting the persistence of suicide ideation; and the only significant associations in low-income countries are for economic adversity predicting lower persistence of suicide ideation and plans, and other parental loss predicting lower persistence of suicide attempts (see Appendix Tables 8.18–8.19).

Discussion

There are several especially noteworthy findings in this study. First, we found that a broad range of childhood adversities are strong predictors of the subsequent onset of suicide ideation and attempts. Bodily injury-related adversities (especially sexual and physical abuse) are more predictive than other adversities, even after additional adjustments for respondents' lifetime mental disorders. Second, a strong dose–response relationship was found between the number of adversities experienced and subsequent onset of suicide ideation and attempts. Two experiences are associated with a 1.2–3.7-fold increase (median OR=2.0), three experiences a 1.3–6.4-fold increase (median OR=2.0), four experiences a 2.3–11.3-fold increase (median OR=3.9), and five or more experiences a 2.4–14.8-fold increase (median OR=6.1) of all the five suicide-related outcomes studied. Third, the adjusted ORs between the number of adversities and subsequent onset of both suicide attempt and ideation generally become increasingly smaller (and less than 1.0) in the multivariate model in which both type of adversity and the number of adversities are entered. This suggests that the joint effects of multiple adversities are significantly less than the product of the ORs associated with the individual adversities. Fourth, the childhood adversities included in this study (except parental divorce) generally do not predict unplanned suicide attempts when both type and number of adversities were taken into account in the same statistical model. However, if these variables are entered separately, both the number of adversities (i.e., two or more) and type of adversities (i.e., parental divorce and parental loss other than parental divorce or parental death) predict unplanned suicide attempts. Fifth, childhood adversities are associated with subsequent suicide attempts across the lifespan, but their influence is stronger during the childhood and adolescent years.

Sixth, the persistence of suicidal behavior is predicted by physical abuse and sexual abuse. Seventh, remarkable differences are found in the associations between childhood adversities and each of the five suicide-related outcomes when data are disaggregated by income categories. Childhood adversities are less predictive of suicide-related behavior in middle- and low-income countries compared to high-income countries. Several of these findings warrant further discussion.

Dose–response relationship between the number of childhood adversities and suicidal behavior

There was a clear dose–response relationship between the number of reported childhood experiences and each of the suicide-related outcome measures across all three income categories. This finding replicates earlier work on the graded relationship between number of adversities and lifetime suicide attempt (Chapman et al., 2004; Dube et al., 2001; Enns et al., 2006; Felitti et al., 1998), and extends it by documenting the association between childhood adversities and this more carefully defined range of suicidal behaviors. Although there is evidence for a dose–response relationship, ORs between number of adversities and subsequent suicide attempt and ideation become increasingly smaller. This suggests that joint effects of exposure to multiple adversities are significantly less than the product of the ORs associated with the individual adversities. In other words, there is a decrease in the predictive power when the number of experienced adversities in childhood gets larger. In this way, we extend existing literature by emphasizing the importance of controlling for multiple adversities. We may assume some psychological mechanisms behind this finding, but because this is the first study that investigated this effect, underlying mechanisms should be investigated in further studies.

The impact of bodily injury-related childhood adversities on subsequent onset of suicidal behavior

After rigorously controlling for the effects of multiple adversities, sociodemographics, and parental mental illness, there was at least a three-fold increase in suicide ideation and attempt among people with a history of sexual or physical abuse, a finding that also is consistent with previous studies (Bebbington et al., 2009; Dinwiddie et al., 2000; Kessler et al., 1997). Even after adjusting for respondents' lifetime mental disorders, people with a history of childhood sexual or physical abuse still had at least a 2.3-fold higher odds for subsequent suicide ideation and attempt. The comparison between the strength of the association prior to and after adjustment for respondents' mental disorder status may shed light on the mediating effect of mental disorders on the relationship between childhood adversities and suicidal behavior. After adjustment, the OR for suicide attempt decreased 6%–33%. We confirm previous reports (Bebbington et al., 2009) that the mediating effect of mental disorders is more pronounced in respondents with a history of childhood sexual abuse, compared to other adverse experiences. This is quite understandable as sexual abuse is known to be among the highest predictors of mental disorders (Green et al., 2010). Our findings also support the hypothesis (Enns et al., 2006; Molnar et al., 2001) that childhood sexual or physical abuse may be especially important risk factors for suicidal behavior that occurs at a relatively young age. Indeed, we found that sexual abuse was strongly associated with suicide attempts during childhood (between the ages of 4 and 12 years); people with a history of childhood sexual abuse were 10.9-fold more likely to have attempted killing themselves in their childhood, after the onset of the abuse. This also was the case for physical abuse, although the association was less strong (i.e., OR=6.3).

To the best of our knowledge, our study is the first to compare the consequences of more violent and bodily injury-related versus less violent childhood adversities in general population samples. Sexual and physical abuse were especially predictive of lifetime suicide ideation and attempt. Our findings are in line with psychological theories that bodily injury may lead to a loss of the positive relationship with one's own body, problematic development of personal identity and psychological integrity, which, in turn, could lead to a wide range of psychological and psychiatric problems, including mental disorders, self-injury, and suicidal behavior (Nock, 2009; Wenninger & Heiman, 1998; Young, 1992). The observed association between aggressive and or injury-related childhood adversities and lifetime suicide ideation and attempt could be explained by the stress–diathesis theory. This theory claims that early life stress may create particular vulnerable conditions for enhanced sensitivity of the hypothalamic–pituitary–adrenal (HPA) axis (Nemeroff, 1998). In stress research,

there is evidence that acute and chronic events may initiate stress responses with biological and emotional consequences. Hypersecretion of catecholamines and activation of the HPA axis are typical biological responses with emotional responses such as higher levels of anxiety, the development of posttraumatic stress disorder, relationship conflicts, or depression (Levin et al., 2001). These findings are consistent with McEwen's theory of allostasis (McEwen, 2000). This concept enables us to hypothesize that exposure to early life stressors may increase the allostatic load of an individual. It points to the cumulative biological wear and tear that occurs through chronic or repeated stress that may contribute to chronic disease in adulthood (Anda et al., 2006).

The role of childhood adversities as predictors of unplanned suicide attempts

Another interesting point of discussion pertains to the association between childhood adversities and unplanned suicide attempts. Whereas physical injury-related adversities (like sexual and physical abuse) are highly associated with suicide ideation and attempt, we did not find a clear effect for unplanned suicide attempts. Indeed, in multivariate analyses, after adjustment for a broad range of potential mediators, the strongest predictors of unplanned attempts were parental divorce, death, or other loss (e.g., being adopted, being in boarding school, or foster care). It has been shown before that parental divorce may be implicated in adolescent suicidal behavior (Ang & Ooi, 2004; Tomori et al., 2001; Wunderlich et al., 1998), but the effects of parental loss have never been investigated in relation to suicide attempts in childhood. The fact that childhood adversities predicted other suicidal outcomes but not unplanned (or "impulsive") attempts suggests that the process of making an unplanned suicide attempt is different from the processes involved in other suicidal behaviors.

The impact of childhood adversities on suicidal behavior across the lifespan

Given that adolescence and early adulthood are generally seen as periods in which there is a high risk of first onset suicidal behavior (Kessler et al., 1999; Roy, 2004), and that there are not many studies focusing on differences in the risk factors for suicidal behavior across the lifespan (Nock et al., 2008b), our data are of value because they show how an important set of risk factors (i.e., childhood adversities) differentially predict suicidal behavior over the course of a person's life. The effects of adversities are especially strong in childhood (median significant OR=3.8), but become less predictive for attempts in the teen years (median significant OR=2.5), young adulthood (median significant OR=2.0), and later adulthood (median significant OR=2.3). Our data suggest a similar decrease of the influence of adversities on suicide ideation. At this point, our data do not allow us to identify in which groups of respondents suicide attempts and ideation will decrease eventually and in which the influence of adversities will remain stable throughout the lifespan. Although these variations require further investigation, our results importantly show that, once respondents have reached a certain critical age (i.e., early adulthood), the influence of adversities systematically decrease and people tend to "mature out". Maturing out is traditionally explained as a developmental phase or transition that occurs from adolescence to adulthood, with great emphasis on acquiring more personal responsibilities or long-term commitments, leading to a significant decrease of high-risk childhood-onset behavior (McCrady & Epstein, 1999; Schulenberg et al., 1999).

Childhood adversities as predictors of persistence of suicidal behavior

Only a few adversities predict the persistence of suicidal behavior, with smaller effect sizes than those for the onset of suicidal behavior. It is important to acknowledge clinically that sexual and physical abuse were risk factors for both onset and persistence of suicidal behavior (Borges et al., 2008). No evidence was found for any subadditive interaction effect of childhood adversity on persistence of suicidal behavior.

Are childhood adversities consistent predictors of suicidal behavior in countries with differences in income?

After disaggregation for income categories, there are some points that warrant comment. First, the major conclusion is that the effects of childhood adversities on suicide attempts exist in all income levels, but are strongest and most consistent in high-income countries. Second, although the association between childhood

adversities and suicide attempts is mediated by respondents' lifetime mental disorders and is seen cross-nationally, this effect is larger in high-income than in middle- and low-income countries. Despite the cross-nationally consistent finding that most adversities are associated with subsequent suicide ideation, our data suggest that the processes leading from ideation to attempt are related to income category. Sexual and physical abuse can be interpreted as "core adversities" closely linked with a systematic increase of the likelihood of a suicide attempt. Regarding the importance of other adversities, there seems to be a graded relationship dependent upon country income categories, with a systematic increase of the importance of these adversities with increasing income. However, the results of our study only allow us to speculate upon the specific role income categories may have on the relationship between childhood adversities and suicidal behavior. In order to discern these additional potential effects, cross-national and cross-cultural studies in this matter are needed.

Limitations of the study

The results presented in this chapter should be interpreted in light of the following limitations. A first limitation is the retrospective report of childhood adversities. It has been shown that recall bias may affect the accuracy of the recalled adversity; rates of forgetting to report abusive experiences have been estimated in the 20%–33% range (Elliott & Briere, 1995; Wilsnack et al., 2002). On balance, there is evidence supporting the validity of the recall of childhood adversities (Hardt & Rutter, 2004). Second, respondents who were not able to speak the main language(s) of the country sufficiently, institutionalized respondents, and respondents without a fixed address were not included in the WMH Surveys. The latter group included mainly migrant minorities. It cannot be ruled out that different patterns of association would be found between adversities and suicidal behavior among such excluded individuals. Moreover, given that suicide risk is elevated in inpatients (Qin & Nordentoft, 2005) and that inpatients are more likely to have had a history of childhood adversities (Rosenberg et al., 2000), we might assume that the association between adversities and suicidal behavior are even stronger in psychiatric inpatients. Third, the approach in this study to persistence is an approximation of the duration of the suicidal episode and the risk of recurrence among those with a history of past suicidal episodes. Because the

WMH Surveys are cross-sectional surveys, it was not possible to calculate persistence directly from respondents' self-reported information of the duration of previous suicide episodes, the time to recurrence after offset of these previous episodes, the duration of a subsequent episode, etc. Fourth, although the list of childhood adversities used in this study is larger than in most previous studies, it is far from exhaustive and did not assess timing, sequencing, severity, or duration of any of these adversities. Fifth, despite the fact that we additionally adjusted for respondents' lifetime mental disorder, we could not rule out fully the possibility of mood-congruent recall bias in estimating the strength of the association between adversities and suicidal behavior. However, we do not consider this to be a major threat to validity as the detailed nature of the assessment for childhood adversity would have mitigated against under-recall somewhat, and any general under-reporting of childhood adversity would not have determined the pattern of results obtained, though again it may mean that the size of the effects observed is somewhat underestimated.

Implications

There are several key implications of these findings. First, clinicians should be aware of the significance of a broad range of childhood adversities that occur with some frequency in the general population, with increased rates among those experiencing suicidal behavior. The findings from this study are especially relevant to suicide attempts in childhood or the teen years because of the direct strong association between adversities and attempts. The effect adversities have on subsequent suicidal behavior also is important because suicide attempts are common reasons why people seek medical care (Pirkis et al., 2001). Second, clinicians should be aware of the influence that childhood adversities have on a wide range of behavioral risk factors including: smoking (Felitti et al., 1998), the use of illicit substances (Felitti et al., 1998), and suicidal behavior (this chapter). These findings add to the knowledge that people with childhood adversities are significantly more likely to have chronic somatic conditions (e.g., back or neck pain, obesity, asthma, arthritis) than those without such adversities (Bruffaerts & Demyttenaere, 2009a, 2009b; Scott et al., 2008; Von Korff et al., 2009). Third, because childhood adversities are so closely related to suicidal behavior, and especially in children and teenagers, more attention

may be given to the prevention of these adversities (Felitti et al., 1998). Both universal and selective prevention of childhood adversities appear to be rather difficult because both would require changes on the level of family and household environments of a common phenomenon (MacMillan et al., 1997). By contrast, indicated preventive strategies (i.e., identifying those families at risk) may be more suitable and practical (Felitti et al., 1998).

Acknowledgements

Portions of this chapter are based on Bruffaerts, R., Demyttenaere, K., Borges, E., Haro, J. M., Chiu, W. T., Hwang, I., et al. (2010). Childhood adversities as risk factors for onset and persistence of suicidal behaviour. *British Journal of Psychiatry*, **197**(1), 20–27. Copyright © 2010. The Royal College of Psychiatrists. Reproduced with permission.

References

Anda, R. F., Felitti, V. J., Bremner, J. D., et al. (2006). The enduring effects of abuse and related adverse experiences in childhood. A convergence of evidence from neurobiology and epidemiology. *European Archives of Psychiatry and Clinical Neuroscience*, **256**(3), 174–186.

Ang, R. P., & Ooi, Y. P. (2004). Impact of gender and parents' marital status on adolescents' suicidal ideation. *International Journal of Social Psychiatry*, **50**(4), 351–360.

Angst, J., Degonda, M., & Ernst, C. (1992). The Zurich Study: XV. Suicide attempts in a cohort from age 20 to 30. *European Archives of Psychiatry and Clinical Neuroscience*, **242**(2–3), 135–141.

Bebbington, P. E., Cooper, C., Minot, S., et al. (2009). Suicide attempts, gender, and sexual abuse: data from the 2000 British Psychiatric Morbidity Survey. *American Journal of Psychiatry*, **166**(10), 1135–1140.

Borges, G., Angst, J., Nock, M. K., Ruscio, A. M., & Kessler, R. C. (2008). Risk factors for the incidence and persistence of suicide-related outcomes: a 10-year follow-up study using the National Comorbidity Surveys. *Journal of Affective Disorders*, **105**(1–3), 25–33.

Bruffaerts, R., & Demyttenaere, K. (2009a). Childhood adversities and adult obesity. In M. R. V. Korff, K. M. Scott, & O. Gureje (eds.), *Global Perspectives on Mental-Physical Comorbidity in the WHO World Mental Health Surveys* (pp. 165–174). New York, NY: Cambridge University Press.

Bruffaerts, R., & Demyttenaere, K. (2009b). The role of childhood adversities in adult-onset spinal pain. In M. R. V. Korff, K. M. Scott, & O. Gureje (eds.), *Global Perspectives on Mental-Physical Comorbidity in the WHO*

World Mental Health Surveys (pp. 154–164). New York, NY: Cambridge University Press.

Bruffaerts, R., Demyttenaere, K., Borges, G., et al. (2010). Childhood adversities as risk factors for onset and persistence of suicidal behaviour. *British Journal of Psychiatry*, **197**(1), 20–27.

Bryant, S., & Range, L. (1995). Suicidality in college women who report multiple versus single types of maltreatment by parents: a brief report. *Journal of Child Sexual Abuse*, **4**, 87–94.

Chapman, D. P., Whitfield, C. L., Felitti, V. J., et al. (2004). Adverse childhood experiences and the risk of depressive disorders in adulthood. *Journal of Affective Disorders*, **82** (2), 217–225.

Dinwiddie, S., Heath, A. C., Dunne, M. P., et al. (2000). Early sexual abuse and lifetime psychopathology: a co-twin-control study. *Psychological Medicine*, **30**(1), 41–52.

Dube, S. R., Anda, R. F., Felitti, V. J., et al. (2001). Childhood abuse, household dysfunction, and the risk of attempted suicide throughout the life span: findings from the Adverse Childhood Experiences Study. *Journal of the American Medical Association*, **286**(24), 3089–3096.

Elliott, D. M., & Briere, J. (1995). Posttraumatic stress associated with delayed recall of sexual abuse: a general population study. *Journal of Traumatic Stress*, **8**(4), 629–647.

Enns, M. W., Cox, B. J., Afifi, T. O., et al. (2006). Childhood adversities and risk for suicidal ideation and attempts: a longitudinal population-based study. *Psychological Medicine*, **36**(12), 1769–1778.

Felitti, V. J., Anda, R. F., Nordenberg, D., et al. (1998). Relationship of childhood abuse and household dysfunction to many of the leading causes of death in adults. The Adverse Childhood Experiences (ACE) Study. *American Journal of Preventive Medicine*, **14**(4), 245–258.

Green, J. G., McLaughlin, K. A., Berglund, P. A., et al. (2010). Childhood adversities and adult psychiatric disorders in the national comorbidity survey replication I: associations with first onset of DSM-IV disorders. *Archives of General Psychiatry*, **67**(2), 113–123.

Hardt, J., & Rutter, M. (2004). Validity of adult retrospective reports of adverse childhood experiences: review of the evidence. *Journal of Child Psychology and Psychiatry*, **45** (2), 260–273.

Kessler, R. C., Borges, G., & Walters, E. E. (1999). Prevalence of and risk factors for lifetime suicide attempts in the National Comorbidity Survey. *Archives of General Psychiatry*, **56**(7), 617–626.

Kessler, R. C., Davis, C. G., & Kendler, K. S. (1997). Childhood adversity and adult psychiatric disorder in the US National Comorbidity Survey. *Psychological Medicine*, **27**(5), 1101–1119.

Levin, H. S., Brown, S. A., Song, J. X., et al. (2001). Depression and posttraumatic stress disorder at three months after mild to moderate traumatic brain injury. *Journal of Clinical and Experimental Neuropsychology*, **23** (6), 754–769.

MacMillan, H. L., Fleming, J. E., Trocme, N., et al. (1997). Prevalence of child physical and sexual abuse in the community. Results from the Ontario Health Supplement. *Journal of the American Medical Association*, **278**(2), 131–135.

McCrady., B. S., & EE, Epstein, E. E. (eds.). (1999). *Addictions: A comprehensive guidebook*. New York, NY: Oxford University Press.

McEwen, B. S. (2000). Allostasis and allostatic load: implications for neuropsychopharmacology. *Neuropsychopharmacology*, **22**(2), 108–124.

McHolm, A. E., MacMillan, H. L., & Jamieson, E. (2003). The relationship between childhood physical abuse and suicidality among depressed women: results from a community sample. *American Journal of Psychiatry*, **160** (5), 933–938.

Molnar, B. E., Buka, S. L., & Kessler, R. C. (2001). Child sexual abuse and subsequent psychopathology: results from the National Comorbidity Survey. *American Journal of Public Health*, **91**(5), 753–760.

Nemeroff, C. B. (1998). The neurobiology of depression. *Scientific American*, **278**(6), 42–49.

Nock, M. K. (2009). Why do people hurt themselves? New insights into the nature and functions of self-injury. *Current Directions in Psychological Science*, **18**(2), 78–83.

Nock, M. K., Borges, G., Bromet, E. J., et al. (2008a). Cross-national prevalence and risk factors for suicidal ideation, plans and attempts. *British Journal of Psychiatry*, **192**(2), 98–105.

Nock, M. K., Borges, G., Bromet, E. J., et al. (2008b). Suicide and suicidal behavior. *Epidemiologic Reviews*, **30**, 133–154.

Petronis, K. R., Samuels, J. F., Moscicki, E. K., & Anthony, J. C. (1990). An epidemiologic investigation of potential risk factors for suicide attempts. *Social Psychiatry and Psychiatric Epidemiology*, **25**(4), 193–199.

Pirkis, J. E., Burgess, P. M., Meadows, G. N., & Dunt, D. R. (2001). Suicidal ideation and suicide attempts as predictors of mental health service use. *Medical Journal of Australia*, **175**(10), 542–545.

Qin, P., & Nordentoft, M. (2005). Suicide risk in relation to psychiatric hospitalization: evidence based on longitudinal registers. *Archives of General Psychiatry*, **62**(4), 427–432.

Risch, N., Herrell, R., Lehner, T., et al. (2009). Interaction between the serotonin transporter gene (5-HTTLPR), stressful life events, and risk of depression: a meta-analysis. *Journal of the American Medical Association*, **301**(23), 2462–2471.

Rosenberg, H. J., Rosenberg, S. D., Wolford, G. L., 2nd, et al. (2000). The relationship between trauma, PTSD, and medical utilization in three high risk medical populations. *International Journal of Psychiatry in Medicine*, **30**(3), 247–259.

Roy, A. (2004). Family history of suicidal behavior and earlier onset of suicidal behavior. *Psychiatry Research*, **129**(2), 217–219.

Schulenberg, J., Maggs, J. L., & Hurrelmann, K. (eds.). (1999). *Health risks and developmental transitions during adolescence*. Boston, MA: Cambridge University Press.

Scott, K. M., Von Korff, M., Alonso, J., et al. (2008). Childhood adversity, early-onset depressive/anxiety disorders, and adult-onset asthma. *Psychosomatic Medicine*, **70**(9), 1035–1043.

Tomori, M., Kienhorst, C. W., de Wilde, E. J., & van den Bout, J. (2001). Suicidal behaviour and family factors among Dutch and Slovenian high school students: a comparison. *Acta Psychiatrica Scandinavica*, **104**(3), 198–203.

Von Korff, M., Alonso, J., Ormel, J., et al. (2009). Childhood psychosocial stressors and adult onset arthritis: broad spectrum risk factors and allostatic load. *Pain*, **143**(71–2), 76–83.

Wagner, B. M. (1997). Family risk factors for child and adolescent suicidal behavior. *Psychological Bulletin*, **121**(2), 246–298.

Wenninger, K., & Heiman, J. R. (1998). Relating body image to psychological and sexual functioning in child sexual abuse survivors. *J Trauma Stress*, **11**(3), 543–562.

Wilsnack, S. C., Wonderlich, S. A., Kristjanson, A. F., Vogeltanz-Holm, N. D., & Wilsnack, R. W. (2002). Self-reports of forgetting and remembering childhood sexual abuse in a nationally representative sample of US women. *Child Abuse and Neglect*, **26**(2), 139–147.

Wunderlich, U., Bronisch, T., & Wittchen, H. U. (1998). Comorbidity patterns in adolescents and young adults with suicide attempts. *European Archives of Psychiatry and Clinical Neuroscience*, **248**(2), 87–95.

Young, L. (1992). Sexual abuse and the problem of embodiment. *Child Abuse and Neglect*, **16**(1), 89–100.

Ystgaard, M., Hestetun, I., Loeb, M., & Mehlum, L. (2004). Is there a specific relationship between childhood sexual and physical abuse and repeated suicidal behavior? *Child Abuse and Neglect*, **28**(8), 863–875.

Chapter

9

Traumatic events and suicidal behavior

Dan J. Stein, Wai Tat Chiu, Irving Hwang, Guilherme Borges, Yueqin Huang, Herbert Matschinger, Johan Ormel, Nancy A. Sampson, Maria Carmen Viana, Ronald C. Kessler, and Matthew K. Nock

Introduction

An expanding literature has contributed to our understanding of the roles that the environment, genes, and gene–environment interactions have in the occurrence of suicidal behavior (Roy et al., 2007). The exact contribution of environmental factors and genetic variance may vary broadly, but for at least some genes it is thought that factors in the environment contribute more strongly to psychopathology (e.g., depression, suicidal behavior) than does genetic variation (Risch et al., 2009). Exposure to psychological trauma may be a particularly important environmental contributor to suicidal behavior. In this chapter we focus on the World Mental Health (WMH) Survey findings on associations between the experience of potentially traumatic events during adulthood and subsequent suicidal behavior.

An association between early childhood abuse and later suicidal behavior has been reported in several studies (Brodsky & Stanley, 2008; Bruffaerts et al., 2010; Dube et al., 2001), with approximately 20% of suicide attempts in young people thought to be attributable to exposure to childhood sexual abuse (Wilcox et al., 2009). Not all data are consistent, however. For example, a recent study found that outside of the context of posttraumatic stress disorder (PTSD), neither assaultive nor non-assaultive psychological trauma independently predict later suicide attempts (Wilcox et al., 2009).

A number of additional questions are important for understanding the nature of the association between exposure to traumatic events and suicidal behavior, and have not yet been adequately addressed in the literature. First, few studies have assessed which traumatic events are unique in predicting suicidal behavior and its persistence. In contexts characterized

by significant social disruption, a range of traumas may co-occur. For instance, a person living in a violent community may be both a witness and a victim of crimes including physical and sexual assault. Multivariate analyses, controlling for the effects of different traumatic events in a large sample may be able to show that specific traumas have a particularly high association with suicidal behavior. Presumably, various kinds of traumatic events, such as physical assault or sexual abuse, are experienced as more distressing, and so may be more strongly associated with later suicidal behavior. However, the literature to date has not rigorously tested these kinds of distinctions, or the contribution of varying traumatic events at differing periods of the lifespan.

Second, little previous work has explored the extent to which specific traumatic events predict the progression from suicide ideation to suicide plans and attempts. Exposure to traumatic events may be predictive of suicide ideation, but may not necessarily be useful in predicting which people with suicide ideation go on to make suicide plans and attempts. Recent studies have indicated that several known risk factors for suicidal behavior, such as the presence of a depressive disorder, may predict the onset of suicide ideation, but may not predict which people with ideation proceed to make a suicide attempt (Nock et al., 2009). An analogous line of research has yet to examine the specific effects of traumatic events on the onset or persistence of suicidal thoughts and behaviors. These are research areas that have clear clinical implications and are deserving of empirical attention.

Third, most studies on the association of traumatic events and suicidal behavior to date have been undertaken in high-income, developed countries. In regions where traumatic events are more prevalent

(Williams et al., 2007), or where there is a different range of traumas to which individuals are exposed, there may potentially be different associations between trauma and suicidal behavior. Recent work has suggested that PTSD is a stronger predictor of suicide attempts in developing countries (odds ratio (OR) = 5.6) than in developed countries (OR = 3.0) (Nock et al., 2009). In order to develop better screening, prevention, and intervention programs throughout the world, we need accurate information on the risk factors for suicidal behavior in both developed and developing countries.

In this chapter, we use data from the World Health Organization (WHO) World Mental Health Surveys to address these issues. The current chapter expands on a previous paper from this dataset (Stein et al., 2010) by providing a more detailed analysis of the effects of traumatic events on subsequent suicidal behavior, presenting new information about how such effects differ cross-nationally, and across the lifespan.

Method

A detailed description of the respondent samples, study procedures, statistical analyses, and assessment of suicidal behavior is provided in Chapter 3 of this volume. The assessment and analysis of sociodemographic factors (Chapter 6), parental psychopathology (Chapter 7), and childhood adversities (Chapter 8), which are included as covariates in the following analyses, is described in those earlier chapters.

Assessment of traumatic events

The WMH version of the WHO Composite International Diagnostic Interview (CIDI) Version 3.0, a fully structured diagnostic interview administered by trained lay interviewers (Kessler & Üstün, 2004), includes a screen for traumatic events as part of the module for the diagnosis of PTSD, which was used to assess traumatic events. The events in this module include those from a number of categories, including: (1) natural and man-made disasters and accidents; (2) combat, war, and refugee experiences; (3) sexual and interpersonal violence; (4) witnessing or perpetrating violence; and (5) death or trauma to a loved one. Respondent age at the time of occurrence of each event was recorded and traumatic events were treated as time-varying covariates in each statistical model except for persistence models, in which traumatic events were observed at the time of each suicide outcome and

treated as a constant throughout the respondent's life course. Only traumatic events that occurred temporally prior to each suicidal behavior being examined were tested as predictors in each model.

There were a few instances in which specific surveys did not include certain risk factors. Specifically, India and Brazil did not assess combat, exposure to war, and refugee status; Brazil also did not assess natural disaster; and Shenzhen did not assess any trauma events. These countries were excluded from the respective bivariate models, and coded "zero" for these variables in the multivariate models. For Israel, the entire sample is coded "yes" for exposure to war with the age-of-onset set to the age the respondents moved to Israel.

Results

Prevalence of traumatic events

Traumatic events are common among the samples investigated, with ranges between 2.1% and 30.5%. Most common were death of a loved one (30.5%), witnessing violence (21.8%), interpersonal violence (18.8%), accidents (17.7%), exposure to war (16.2%), and trauma to a loved one (12.5%). Other traumas are less common and occurred in less than 10% of the sample. In the pooled sample, lifetime suicide ideation and attempts are reported by 9.6% (or n = 8126) and 2.8% (or n = 2778) of respondents, respectively. Among ideators, 34.8% (or n = 3252) have a suicide plan, and 55.7% of these respondents (or n = 1871) make a suicide attempt. Among ideators (n = 8126), 65.2% (or n = 4874) do not make a suicide plan, and of these without a plan, 15.3% (or n = 907) make an attempt.

Among respondents with a history of suicide attempt, almost one in five (i.e., 20.9%) report the loss of a loved one and about one in six (i.e., 16.0%) report interpersonal violence (see Table 9.1). We find roughly comparable patterns for estimates of traumas in the other suicide-related behaviors included. More detailed results reported for each adversity and each type of suicidal behavior after disaggregating for income categories are shown in Appendix Tables 9.1–9.3.

Bivariate associations between traumatic events and suicidal behavior

Tabulation of bivariate associations (see Table 9.2) shows that the majority of traumatic events, including

Table 9.1. Prevalence of traumatic events among those with each type of suicidal behavior (all countries combined)

Traumatic events	Among total sample						Among ideators			
	%ᵃ (SE) with adversities						%ᵃ (SE) with adversities			
	Ideation	No ideation	Attempt	No attempt	Plan	No plan	Planned attempt	No planned attempt	Unplanned attempt	No unplanned attempt
Disasters/accidents										
All man-made disasters	6.4 (0.4)	3.6 (0.1)	7.0 (0.6)	3.8 (0.1)	8.1 (0.7)	9.3 (0.7)	7.4 (0.8)	13.3 (1.4)	6.9 (0.9)	9.2 (0.8)
Natural disaster	6.1 (0.4)	4.0 (0.1)	7.6 (0.7)	4.1 (0.1)	7.4 (0.6)	8.2 (0.7)	7.8 (0.8)	9.8 (1.3)	7.9 (1.3)	7.8 (0.6)
Accident	14.5 (0.6)	7.4 (0.1)	15.0 (0.9)	7.7 (0.1)	16.8 (0.9)	21.0 (1.0)	15.2 (1.2)	25.2 (2.0)	14.9 (1.6)	20.5 (1.0)
War/combat/refugee experiences										
Exposure to war	8.8 (0.4)	12.8 (0.2)	9.2 (0.8)	12.7 (0.2)	9.7 (0.7)	10.7 (0.7)	11.1 (1.1)	11.0 (1.5)	5.4 (0.9)	11.0 (0.8)
Combat	2.0 (0.2)	2.5 (0.1)	1.2 (0.2)	2.5 (0.1)	2.3 (0.3)	3.6 (0.6)	1.4 (0.3)	2.2 (0.6)	0.9 (0.3)	3.9 (0.7)
Refugee	1.2 (0.2)	2.1 (0.1)	1.4 (0.3)	2.1 (0.1)	1.3 (0.2)	1.7 (0.3)	1.6 (0.4)	1.1 (0.3)	0.9 (0.3)	1.8 (0.3)
Sexual/interpersonal violence										
Sexual violence	9.7 (0.4)	2.5 (0.1)	12.6 (0.7)	2.8 (0.1)	11.0 (0.7)	12.5 (0.8)	11.7 (0.9)	14.5 (1.5)	15.0 (1.6)	11.4 (0.8)
Interpersonal violence	16.2 (0.6)	7.5 (0.2)	16.0 (0.9)	7.9 (0.1)	17.5 (1.0)	20.7 (0.9)	15.7 (1.1)	27.3 (2.0)	17.4 (1.5)	20.6 (1.0)
Witness/perpetrator violence										
Witness violence	15.3 (0.6)	10.5 (0.2)	14.7 (0.8)	10.7 (0.2)	16.8 (0.9)	20.7 (0.9)	15.0 (1.0)	22.7 (2.0)	15.0 (1.5)	20.8 (1.0)
Perpetrator violence	2.1 (0.2)	0.8 (0.0)	2.6 (0.3)	0.9 (0.0)	3.1 (0.4)	3.1 (0.4)	2.7 (0.4)	4.5 (1.0)	2.6 (0.6)	3.2 (0.4)
Loss/trauma										
Death of loved one	20.1 (0.6)	11.8 (0.2)	20.9 (0.9)	12.1 (0.2)	22.2 (0.9)	30.0 (0.9)	21.6 (1.2)	31.1 (2.1)	20.9 (1.8)	30.1 (1.1)
Trauma to loved one	8.6 (0.4)	4.2 (0.1)	10.9 (0.8)	4.4 (0.1)	10.0 (0.7)	14.2 (0.7)	10.9 (0.9)	14.9 (1.3)	10.7 (1.3)	13.2 (0.7)
All others	8.5 (0.4)	3.3 (0.1)	10.5 (0.8)	3.6 (0.1)	10.7 (0.8)	13.0 (0.7)	10.8 (1.0)	16.1 (1.8)	10.1 (1.2)	12.3 (0.7)

Table 9.1. (cont.)

| | Among total sample | | | | Among ideators | | | | | |
| | %^a (SE) with adversities | | | | %^a (SE) with adversities | | | | | |
Traumatic events	Ideation	No ideation	Attempt	No attempt	Plan	No plan	Planned attempt	No planned attempt	Unplanned attempt	No unplanned attempt
Number of traumatic events[b]										
1	26.0 (0.7)	21.3 (0.2)	27.3 (1.1)	21.4 (0.2)	26.7 (1.0)	25.8 (0.9)	27.3 (1.4)	26.5 (1.9)	26.0 (2.0)	26.0 (1.0)
2	16.3 (0.5)	9.8 (0.1)	17.1 (0.9)	9.9 (0.1)	17.4 (0.8)	19.0 (0.8)	17.5 (1.2)	20.6 (1.5)	17.0 (1.6)	19.0 (0.8)
3	8.6 (0.4)	4.7 (0.1)	8.8 (0.6)	4.9 (0.1)	9.5 (0.6)	11.9 (0.6)	8.7 (0.8)	14.7 (1.2)	9.2 (1.2)	11.8 (0.7)
4	4.0 (0.3)	2.1 (0.1)	4.5 (0.5)	2.3 (0.1)	4.9 (0.6)	7.7 (0.6)	5.0 (0.7)	9.1 (1.1)	4.2 (0.7)	8.0 (0.6)
5	1.9 (0.2)	1.0 (0.0)	2.2 (0.3)	1.0 (0.0)	2.6 (0.4)	3.8 (0.3)	2.5 (0.4)	4.7 (0.7)	2.0 (0.6)	3.5 (0.4)
6	0.8 (0.1)	0.4 (0.0)	1.3 (0.2)	0.5 (0.0)	1.3 (0.2)	1.9 (0.3)	1.3 (0.3)	1.9 (0.5)	2.2 (0.8)	2.5 (0.3)
7	0.4 (0.1)	0.2 (0.0)	0.6 (0.2)	0.3 (0.0)	0.8 (0.2)	1.1 (0.2)	0.6 (0.2)	1.4 (0.5)		
8+	0.2 (0.1)	0.1 (0.0)								
N[c]	(8126)	(204,095)	(2778)	(211,402)	(3252)	(8035)	(1743)	(2000)	(907)	(6110)

[a] % represents the percentage of people with the adversity among the cases with the outcome variable indicated in the column header. For example, the first cell is the % of those who experienced a man-made disaster among those with suicide ideation. Because Shenzhen did not assess traumatic events, it was excluded from these prevalence estimates, so these estimates are based on N=102,245 (response rate 71.6%).

[b] For number of traumatic events, the last OR represents the odds for that number of traumatic events or more. For example, for unplanned attempt, 6 represents ≥6 (that is, 6+).

[c] Number of cases with the outcome variable; N represents the number of person–years.

Table 9.2. Bivariate models for associations between traumatic events and suicidal behavior[a] (all countries combined)

Traumatic events	Among total sample		Among ideators		
	Ideation	Attempt	Plan	Planned attempt	Unplanned attempt
	OR (95% CI)	OR (95% CI)	OR (95% CI)	OR (95% CI)	OR (95% CI)
Disasters/accidents					
All man-made disasters	1.3* (1.1–1.5)	1.3* (1.0–1.6)	1.2 (0.9–1.5)	0.9 (0.6–1.3)	1.0 (0.7–1.4)
Natural disaster	1.1 (0.9–1.3)	1.3 (1.0–1.6)	1.3* (1.1–1.6)	1.2 (0.8–1.7)	1.3 (0.9–2.0)
Accident	1.5* (1.4–1.7)	1.4* (1.2–1.7)	1.1 (0.9–1.3)	0.7* (0.5–1.0)	0.9 (0.7–1.2)
War/combat/refugee experiences					
Exposure to war	1.1 (0.9–1.2)	1.3* (1.0–1.7)	1.1 (0.9–1.4)	1.6* (1.0–2.5)	0.7 (0.4–1.1)
Combat	1.2 (1.0–1.6)	0.9 (0.6–1.3)	1.3 (0.9–1.9)	1.2 (0.6–2.6)	0.5 (0.2–1.1)
Refugee	1.1 (0.9–1.5)	1.2 (0.8–1.8)	1.0 (0.6–1.7)	1.6 (0.8–3.2)	1.2 (0.5–3.0)
Sexual/interpersonal violence					
Sexual violence	2.2* (2.0–2.4)	2.6* (2.2–3.1)	1.1 (0.9–1.3)	0.9 (0.6–1.2)	1.5* (1.1–2.0)
Interpersonal violence	1.8* (1.6–2.0)	1.9* (1.6–2.2)	1.1 (0.9–1.3)	0.7* (0.5–0.9)	1.1 (0.8–1.5)
Witness/perpetrator violence					
Witness violence	1.4* (1.2–1.5)	1.4* (1.2–1.6)	1.2 (1.0–1.4)	0.9 (0.7–1.3)	1.2 (0.9–1.6)
Perpetrator violence	1.6* (1.3–1.9)	1.5* (1.1–2.0)	1.2 (0.9–1.7)	0.6 (0.4–1.1)	1.1 (0.6–2.0)
Loss/trauma					
Death of loved one	1.2* (1.1–1.3)	1.1 (1.0–1.3)	0.9 (0.8–1.0)	0.9 (0.7–1.1)	0.8 (0.6–1.0)
Trauma to loved one	1.3* (1.1–1.4)	1.3* (1.1–1.6)	0.8* (0.7–1.0)	1.0 (0.7–1.3)	1.0 (0.7–1.3)
All others	1.5* (1.4–1.8)	1.6* (1.3–1.9)	1.0 (0.8–1.2)	0.9 (0.7–1.3)	1.0 (0.7–1.4)

* Significant at the 0.05 level, two-sided test.
[a] Assessed in the Part 2 sample due to having Part 2 controls. Models control for person–years, country, and significant variables from the chapters on sociodemographics, parental psychopathology, and childhood adversities.

those in the categories of disasters/accidents, war/combat/refugee experiences, sexual/interpersonal violence, witness/perpetrator violence, loss/trauma, and all others are significantly associated with lifetime suicide ideation and suicide attempt. The ORs are highest for sexual and interpersonal violence. Among those with suicide ideation, traumas generally are not predictive of suicide plan or either planned or unplanned attempts. However, among respondents with suicide ideation, natural disaster is positively associated with suicide plan, exposure to war is positively associated with planned attempt, and sexual violence is positively associated with unplanned attempt. Interestingly, several types of events are associated with decreased odds of suicide

plans among ideators (i.e., trauma to a loved one), and planned attempts among ideators (i.e., accident and interpersonal violence). A similar overall pattern of findings holds for disaggregation of high-, middle-, and low-income countries.

Multivariate associations of traumatic events with lifetime suicidal behavior

There are fewer significant associations between traumatic events and both suicide ideation and suicide attempt after adjusting for the effects of other traumatic events (see Table 9.3). Nevertheless, ORs remain highest for sexual violence and interpersonal violence. Disaggregation of these associations shows that they

Table 9.3. Multivariate models for associations between traumatic events and suicidal behavior[a] (all countries combined)

| Traumatic events | Among total sample | | Among ideators | | |
	Ideation OR (95% CI)	Attempt OR (95% CI)	Plan OR (95% CI)	Planned attempt OR (95% CI)	Unplanned attempt OR (95% CI)
Disasters/accidents					
All man-made disasters	1.1 (1.0–1.3)	1.1 (0.9–1.3)	1.1 (0.9–1.4)	0.9 (0.6–1.4)	1.0 (0.7–1.4)
Natural disaster	0.9 (0.8–1.1)	1.1 (0.9–1.4)	1.3* (1.0–1.6)	1.2 (0.9–1.8)	1.4 (1.0–2.0)
Accident	1.3* (1.2–1.5)	1.2* (1.0–1.4)	1.0 (0.9–1.2)	0.7 (0.5–1.0)	0.9 (0.6–1.1)
War/combat/refugee experiences					
Exposure to war	1.0 (0.8–1.1)	1.2 (0.9–1.5)	1.1 (0.8–1.4)	1.7* (1.1–2.6)	0.6 (0.4–1.1)
Combat	1.0 (0.8–1.3)	0.7* (0.5–1.0)	1.2 (0.8–1.8)	1.2 (0.5–2.7)	0.4 (0.2–1.1)
Refugee	1.0 (0.8–1.3)	1.0 (0.6–1.6)	0.9 (0.5–1.6)	1.5 (0.8–3.1)	1.5 (0.6–3.8)
Sexual/interpersonal violence					
Sexual violence	2.0* (1.8–2.2)	2.3* (2.0–2.7)	1.0 (0.8–1.3)	0.9 (0.7–1.2)	1.5* (1.1–2.1)
Interpersonal violence	1.6* (1.4–1.8)	1.6* (1.4–1.9)	1.0 (0.9–1.3)	0.7* (0.5–1.0)	1.1 (0.8–1.4)
Witness/perpetrator violence					
Witness violence	1.2* (1.0–1.3)	1.2* (1.0–1.4)	1.2 (1.0–1.4)	1.0 (0.7–1.4)	1.2 (0.9–1.7)
Perpetrator violence	1.2 (1.0–1.5)	1.2 (0.9–1.7)	1.1 (0.8–1.6)	0.7 (0.4–1.2)	1.3 (0.7–2.3)
Loss/trauma					
Death of loved one	1.1 (1.0–1.2)	1.0 (0.9–1.1)	0.9* (0.7–1.0)	0.9 (0.7–1.1)	0.8* (0.6–1.0)
Trauma to loved one	1.1 (0.9–1.2)	1.1 (0.9–1.4)	0.8* (0.7–1.0)	1.0 (0.8–1.3)	1.0 (0.7–1.3)
All others	1.3* (1.2–1.5)	1.4* (1.1–1.7)	1.0 (0.8–1.2)	1.0 (0.7–1.3)	1.0 (0.7–1.4)
χ^2 (p-value)	450.4 (<0.001)*	254.7 (<0.001)*	23.4 (0.037)*	26.6 (0.014)*	23.6 (0.036)*

* Significant at the 0.05 level, two-sided test.
[a] Assessed in the Part 2 sample due to having Part 2 controls. Each row represents a separate bivariate model. Models control for person–years, country, and significant variables from the chapters on sociodemographics, parental psychopathology, and childhood adversities.

are largely due to traumatic events predicting ideation rather than the transition from ideation to attempt. Here too, among ideators, natural disaster predicts the development of a suicide plan, exposure to war predicts planned attempt, and sexual violence predicts unplanned attempt. As in the bivariate models, several types of trauma again are associated with decreased odds of suicide plans (i.e., death and trauma to a loved one) and attempts (i.e., interpersonal violence) among ideators.

Effects of the number of traumatic events

The number of traumatic events experienced is significantly associated with the odds of subsequent suicide ideation and suicide attempt (see Table 9.4). Here too, these associations are due primarily to traumatic events predicting ideation, rather than the transition from ideation to plan or attempt. For example, the ORs for suicide attempt increase from 1.6 for those with a single traumatic event (relative to those with zero events) to 4.3 for those with six traumatic events. However, in a multivariate model including both type and number of traumatic events (see Table 9.5), the increased odds of a suicide attempt associated with more traumatic events increase at a decreasing rate (i.e., they are subadditive). That is, the effects of having multiple traumatic events is less than the sum of the individual effects due to the incremental predictive power of individual traumatic events decaying as the

Table 9.4. Associations between number of traumatic events and suicidal behavior[a] (all countries combined)

Number of traumatic events[b]	Among total sample		Among ideators		
	Ideation	Attempt	Plan	Planned attempt	Unplanned attempt
	OR (95% CI)	OR (95% CI)	OR (95% CI)	OR (95% CI)	OR (95% CI)
1	1.5* (1.4–1.6)	1.6* (1.4–1.9)	1.0 (0.9–1.2)	0.8 (0.6–1.0)	0.9 (0.7–1.2)
2	1.9* (1.8–2.1)	2.1* (1.8–2.5)	1.1 (0.9–1.4)	0.8 (0.6–1.1)	1.1 (0.8–1.5)
3	2.1* (1.8–2.4)	2.1* (1.8–2.6)	1.0 (0.8–1.3)	0.6* (0.4–0.8)	1.0 (0.7–1.4)
4	2.2* (1.8–2.6)	2.4* (1.8–3.1)	1.0 (0.7–1.3)	0.7 (0.4–1.1)	0.8 (0.5–1.3)
5	2.4* (2.0–2.9)	2.9* (2.1–4.0)	1.1 (0.8–1.6)	0.8 (0.5–1.4)	0.9 (0.5–1.6)
6	2.8* (2.0–3.8)	4.3* (2.8–6.5)	1.2 (0.7–2.0)	0.7 (0.3–1.7)	1.8 (0.8–4.0)
7	3.8* (2.2–6.6)	3.1* (1.8–5.3)	1.7 (0.9–3.2)	0.7 (0.3–1.8)	
8+	2.7* (1.4–5.2)				
χ^2 (p-value)	269.7 (<0.001)*	121.8 (<0.001)*	4.2 (0.76)	10.4 (0.17)	4.2 (0.65)

* Significant at the 0.05 level, two-sided test.
[a] Assessed in the Part 2 sample due to having Part 2 controls. Models control for person–years, country, and significant variables from the chapters on sociodemographics, parental psychopathology, and childhood adversities.
[b] For number of traumatic events, the last OR represents the odds for that number of traumatic events or more. For example, for unplanned attempt, 6 represents ≥6 (that is, 6+).

Table 9.5. Final multivariate models for associations between traumatic events and suicidal behavior[a] (all countries combined)

Traumatic events	Among total sample		Among ideators		
	Ideation	Attempt	Plan	Planned attempt	Unplanned attempt
	OR (95% CI)	OR (95% CI)	OR (95% CI)	OR (95% CI)	OR (95% CI)
Disasters/accidents					
All man-made disasters	1.4* (1.2–1.7)	1.4* (1.1–1.8)	1.2 (0.9–1.6)	0.8 (0.5–1.2)	0.9 (0.6–1.3)
Natural disaster	1.2 (1.0–1.4)	1.4* (1.1–1.9)	1.3 (1.0–1.7)	1.1 (0.7–1.6)	1.2 (0.8–1.7)
Accident	1.6* (1.4–1.8)	1.6* (1.2–2.0)	1.1 (0.8–1.4)	0.6* (0.4–1.0)	0.7 (0.5–1.1)
War/combat/refugee experiences					
Exposure to war	1.1 (1.0–1.3)	1.5* (1.2–1.9)	1.1 (0.8–1.5)	1.5 (0.9–2.5)	0.5* (0.3–1.0)
Combat	1.3* (1.0–1.8)	1.0 (0.7–1.4)	1.3 (0.8–2.0)	1.0 (0.4–2.2)	0.4* (0.2–0.9)
Refugee	1.3 (0.9–1.7)	1.3 (0.8–2.1)	0.9 (0.5–1.7)	1.2 (0.6–2.7)	1.3 (0.5–3.3)
Sexual/interpersonal violence					
Sexual violence	2.3* (2.0–2.7)	2.9* (2.3–3.6)	1.1 (0.8–1.4)	0.8 (0.6–1.2)	1.3 (0.9–2.0)
Interpersonal violence	1.9* (1.6–2.1)	2.0* (1.6–2.4)	1.1 (0.8–1.4)	0.6* (0.4–1.0)	0.9 (0.7–1.4)
Witness/perpetrator violence					
Witness violence	1.4* (1.2–1.6)	1.5* (1.2–1.8)	1.2 (0.9–1.6)	0.9 (0.6–1.3)	1.1 (0.7–1.6)
Perpetrator violence	1.6* (1.3–2.0)	1.7* (1.2–2.3)	1.2 (0.8–1.7)	0.6 (0.3–1.1)	1.0 (0.5–2.1)

Table 9.5. (cont.)

Traumatic events	Among total sample			Among ideators	
	Ideation	Attempt	Plan	Planned attempt	Unplanned attempt
	OR (95% CI)	OR (95% CI)	OR (95% CI)	OR (95% CI)	OR (95% CI)
Loss/trauma					
Death of loved one	1.3* (1.1–1.4)	1.2* (1.0–1.5)	0.9 (0.7–1.1)	0.8 (0.6–1.1)	0.7* (0.5–1.0)
Trauma to loved one	1.3* (1.1–1.6)	1.5* (1.1–1.8)	0.8 (0.6–1.1)	0.9 (0.6–1.3)	0.8 (0.6–1.2)
All others	1.7* (1.4–1.9)	1.8* (1.4–2.2)	1.0 (0.8–1.3)	0.8 (0.6–1.3)	0.9 (0.6–1.3)
13 df χ^2 test for 13 types	239.5 (<0.001)*	149.3 (<0.001)*	20.7 (0.08)	25.2 (0.02)*	23.8 (0.03)*
12 df χ^2 test for difference between types	157.4 (<0.001)*	93.9 (<0.001)*	20.1 (0.07)	22.7 (0.03)*	20.6 (0.06)
Number of traumatic events[b]					
2	0.9 (0.7–1.0)	0.8 (0.6–1.0)	1.0 (0.8–1.4)	1.3 (0.8–2.0)	1.3 (0.8–2.1)
3	0.6* (0.5–0.8)	0.5* (0.4–0.8)	0.9 (0.6–1.4)	1.1 (0.5–2.4)	1.3 (0.7–2.7)
4	0.4* (0.3–0.6)	0.4* (0.2–0.6)	0.8 (0.4–1.5)	1.6 (0.6–4.4)	1.4 (0.5–3.7)
5	0.3* (0.2–0.5)	0.3* (0.2–0.6)	0.8 (0.4–1.9)	2.4 (0.7–8.9)	1.8 (0.5–6.7)
6	0.3* (0.2–0.5)	0.3* (0.1–0.7)	0.8 (0.3–2.4)	2.7 (0.5–16.3)	3.9 (0.6–25.1)
7	0.3* (0.1–0.6)	0.1* (0.0–0.4)	0.9 (0.2–3.7)	3.3 (0.4–29.2)	
8+	0.1* (0.0–0.3)				
χ^2 (p-value)	45.5 (<0.001)*	22.6 (<0.001)*	2.7 (0.85)	5.8 (0.44)	3.6 (0.62)

* Significant at the 0.05 level, two-sided test.
[a] Assessed in the Part 2 sample due to having Part 2 controls. Models control for person–years, country, and significant variables from the chapters on sociodemographics, parental psychopathology, and childhood adversities.
[b] For number of traumatic events, the last OR represents the odds for that number of traumatic events or more. For example, for unplanned attempt, 6 represents ≥6 (that is, 6+).

number of events increases. We do not see subadditive effects in the case of suicide plan or attempt among ideators. A similar pattern of findings holds in high-, middle-, and low-income countries (see Appendix Tables 9.4–9.6).

Effects of traumatic events over the life course

We next examined whether the effect of traumatic events on suicidal behavior differs over the lifespan. Results revealed that combat and refugee experiences are associated with significantly higher odds of suicide ideation and attempts during adolescence and adulthood (i.e., 13+ years of age) relative to the earlier part of the life course (i.e., ≤12 years of age) (see Table 9.6). In contrast, experiencing sexual or interpersonal violence and witnessing violence are associated with

higher odds of suicidal behavior earlier in life (i.e., ≤12 years of age) relative to the later part of the life course (i.e., 13+ years of age). The cross-national analyses generally revealed a similar pattern of findings (see Appendix Tables 9.7–9.9)

Persistence of suicidal behavior

The results of the backwards recurrence models reveal that several specific types of traumatic events predict the persistence of suicidal behavior (see Table 9.7). The most consistent effects are for accidents and sexual violence, which predict both the persistence of ideation and attempts. The persistence of suicide ideation also is predicted by refugee status and by other trauma, whereas the persistence of attempts is predicted by man-made disasters, exposure to war, and death of a loved one. Detailed results for high-, middle-, and low-

Table 9.6. Interactions between traumatic events and suicidal behavior over the life course[a] (all countries combined)

		Among total sample						Among ideators			
		Ideation		Attempt		Plan		Planned attempt		Unplanned attempt	
Interactions		OR (95% CI)	χ² (p-value)	OR (95% CI)	χ² (p-value)	OR (95% CI)	χ² (p-value)	OR (95% CI)	χ² (p-value)	OR (95% CI)	χ² (p-value)
Disasters/accidents											
All man-made disasters	13–19	0.6 (0.3–1.5)	4.6 (0.20)	0.5 (0.1–2.0)	2.4 (0.49)	0.3 (0.0–2.0)	7.9 (0.05)*	0.3 (0.0–6.0)	5.1 (0.16)	–	–
	20–29	0.7 (0.3–1.5)		0.4 (0.1–1.8)		0.2 (0.0–1.2)		0.6 (0.0–12.3)		–	
	30+	0.5 (0.2–1.1)		0.6 (0.1–2.6)		0.4 (0.1–2.4)		1.0 (0.0–22.4)		–	
Natural disaster	13–19	1.0 (0.5–2.0)	7.6 (0.05)	0.5 (0.1–1.7)	3.1 (0.38)	4.9 (0.9–26.7)	11.3 (0.01)*	–	–	–	–
	20–29	0.7 (0.4–1.5)		0.4 (0.1–1.3)		1.6 (0.3–8.2)		–		–	
	30+	0.6 (0.3–1.2)		0.5 (0.1–1.6)		1.9 (0.4–9.5)		–		–	
Accident	13–19	1.5 (0.8–2.7)	16.2 (0.001)*	1.1 (0.4–3.4)	1.8 (0.61)	0.5 (0.1–2.8)	1.6 (0.67)	–	–	–	–
	20–29	1.1 (0.6–1.9)		0.8 (0.3–2.3)		0.4 (0.1–2.2)		–		–	
	30+	0.8 (0.4–1.4)		0.8 (0.3–2.2)		0.4 (0.1–2.5)		–		–	
War/combat/refugee experiences											
Exposure to war	13–19	0.6 (0.3–1.4)	3.2 (0.36)	1.5 (0.3–8.8)	0.5 (0.91)	0.3 (0.0–8.6)	5.8 (0.12)	–	–	–	–
	20–29	0.5 (0.2–1.2)		1.3 (0.2–7.4)		0.2 (0.0–5.4)		–		–	
	30+	0.6 (0.3–1.2)		1.6 (0.3–9.0)		0.4 (0.0–10.3)		–		–	
Combat	13–19	13.5* (3.5–51.4)	21.1 (<0.001)*	117.2* (24.4–562.3)	45.6 (<0.001)*	0.5 (0.1–3.5)	4.6 (0.10)	–	73.4 (<0.001)*	0.0* (0.0–0.0)	69.2 (<0.001)*
	20–29	14.4* (4.3–48.6)		90.0* (20.6–394.3)		0.4 (0.2–1.0)		0.9 (0.2–4.1)		0.4 (0.0–3.4)	
	30+	9.5* (2.9–30.9)		98.1* (24.2–396.9)		–		–		–	
Refugee	13–19	6.8* (2.5–18.5)	15.8 (0.001)*	161.7* (50.0–522.3)	94.1 (<0.001)*	1.1 (0.3–4.0)	0.1 (0.97)	9.9 (0.6–163.7)	103.5 (<0.001)*	0.8 (0.0–47.0)	0.2 (0.93)
	20–29	5.6* (2.0–16.0)		129.1* (38.8–430.1)		1.0 (0.3–3.1)		–		1.5 (0.2–13.0)	
	30+	4.3* (1.8–10.1)		110.6* (37.0–330.5)		–		–		–	
Sexual/interpersonal violence											
Sexual violence	13–19	0.7 (0.4–1.3)	17.4 (<0.001)*	0.5 (0.2–1.3)	7.5 (0.06)	0.2 (0.0–1.6)	6.1 (0.11)	0.4 (0.0–4.4)	1.6 (0.65)	0.1 (0.0–8.9)	1.6 (0.66)
	20–29	0.5* (0.3–0.9)		0.4* (0.2–0.9)		0.1* (0.0–1.0)		0.7 (0.1–7.1)		0.1 (0.0–6.8)	
	30+	0.4* (0.2–0.7)		0.4* (0.1–0.9)		0.1 (0.0–1.2)		0.6 (0.1–6.1)		0.1 (0.0–6.1)	
Interpersonal violence	13–19	0.4 (0.2–1.1)	22.4 (<0.001)*	0.3 (0.1–1.1)	4.0 (0.26)	0.2 (0.0–1.7)	5.8 (0.12)	2.1 (0.0–983.7)	4.9 (0.18)	–	–
	20–29	0.2* (0.1–0.6)		0.3* (0.1–1.0)		0.2 (0.0–1.4)		1.6 (0.0–754.1)		–	
	30+	0.2* (0.1–0.6)		0.3 (0.1–1.2)		0.3 (0.0–2.2)		–		–	

Table 9.6. (cont.)

		Among total sample						Among ideators			
		Ideation		Attempt		Plan		Planned attempt		Unplanned attempt	
Interactions		OR (95% CI)	χ² (p-value)	OR (95% CI)	χ² (p-value)	OR (95% CI)	χ² (p-value)	OR (95% CI)	χ² (p-value)	OR (95% CI)	χ² (p-value)
Witness/perpetrator violence											
Witness violence	13–19	0.3* (0.2–0.5)	17.6 (<0.001)*	0.2* (0.1–0.6)	10.0 (0.02)*	0.0* (0.0–0.2)	14.5 (0.002)*	0.0* (0.0–0.0)	29.3 (<.001)*	—	2.3 (0.32)
	20–29	0.3* (0.2–0.6)		0.2* (0.1–0.6)		0.0* (0.0–0.2)		0.0* (0.0–0.0)		—	
	30+	0.3* (0.2–0.6)		0.2* (0.1–0.6)		0.1* (0.0–0.3)		0.0* (0.0–0.0)		—	
Perpetrator violence	13–19	0.6 (0.2–1.7)	2.5 (0.48)	1.7 (0.2–18.3)	1.5 (0.69)	3.8 (0.3–49.7)	5.4 (0.14)	—	—	1.6 (0.2–10.8)	0.3 (0.87)
	20–29	0.6 (0.2–1.4)		1.7 (0.2–18.1)		1.2 (0.1–15.2)		—		1.3 (0.3–6.5)	
	30+	0.5 (0.2–1.2)		2.5 (0.2–25.9)		1.7 (0.1–20.3)		—		—	
Loss/trauma											
Death of loved one	13–19	0.7 (0.4–1.2)	13.1 (0.004)*	0.6 (0.2–1.7)	3.6 (0.31)	0.6 (0.1–3.0)	0.6 (0.91)	1.0 (0.0–29.3)	3.6 (0.31)	0.3 (0.0–4.0)	1.3 (0.73)
	20–29	0.6 (0.3–1.2)		0.5 (0.2–1.4)		0.6 (0.1–2.7)		0.4 (0.0–12.2)		0.2 (0.0–3.3)	
	30+	0.5* (0.2–0.8)		0.4 (0.1–1.2)		0.6 (0.1–3.0)		0.7 (0.0–19.3)		0.2 (0.0–3.2)	
Trauma to loved one	13–19	1.1 (0.5–2.1)	12.2 (0.01)*	0.4 (0.2–1.1)	9.4 (0.03)*	0.4 (0.1–1.9)	5.2 (0.16)	0.5 (0.1–4.0)	1.4 (0.70)	0.0* (0.0–0.0)	2.2 (0.34)
	20–29	0.8 (0.4–1.5)		0.3* (0.1–0.7)		0.2 (0.0–1.1)		0.4 (0.1–2.8)		0.0* (0.0–0.0)	
	30+	0.5 (0.3–1.1)		0.3* (0.1–0.8)		0.2 (0.1–1.2)		0.6 (0.1–4.0)		0.0* (0.0–0.0)	
All others	13–19	1.2 (0.6–2.5)	11.4 (0.01)*	0.6 (0.2–1.5)	2.6 (0.45)	1.5 (0.4–5.9)	9.9 (0.02)*	0.0 (0.0–14.0)	3.4 (0.34)	0.0* (0.0–0.0)	0.9 (0.63)
	20–29	1.0 (0.5–2.1)		0.5 (0.2–1.2)		0.6 (0.1–2.2)		0.0 (0.0–7.5)		0.0* (0.0–0.0)	
	30+	0.7 (0.3–1.3)		0.6 (0.2–1.4)		1.0 (0.2–3.7)		0.0 (0.0–11.7)		0.0* (0.0–0.0)	
39 df χ² test for all trauma			188.4 (<0.001)*		336.7 (<0.001)*		68.2 (0.001)*		348.8 (<0.001)*		280.4 (<0.001)*
χ² test for all trauma and dummies for number of traumas			243.9 (<0.001)*		567.5 (<0.001)*		76.6 (0.01)*		575.5 (<0.001)*		—
Number of traumatic events[b]											
2	13–19	1.1 (0.5–2.4)	52.0 (<0.001)*	6.7* (2.1–21.7)	125.1 (<0.001)*	3.8 (0.4–33.6)	17.6 (0.22)	—	41.3 (<0.001)*	—	182.5 (<0.001)*
	20–29	1.3 (0.6–2.8)		7.7* (2.4–24.7)		7.1 (0.8–62.8)		—		—	
	30+	1.5 (0.7–3.2)		6.2* (2.0–19.8)		4.3 (0.5–34.7)		—		—	
3	13–19	1.6 (0.4–6.7)		4.0 (0.6–27.9)		7.9 (0.3–183.5)		0.0* (0.0–0.0)		—	
	20–29	2.3 (0.5–9.8)		4.2 (0.6–27.6)		27.6* (1.2–649.6)		0.0* (0.0–0.0)		—	
	30+	3.5 (0.8–14.5)		2.9 (0.4–19.4)		9.7 (0.5–206.7)		0.0* (0.0–0.0)		—	
4	13–19	1.0 (0.2–5.1)		1.0 (0.1–14.6)		—		0.0* (0.0–0.0)		0.0* (0.0–0.0)	
	20–29	1.6 (0.3–8.5)		1.9 (0.1–26.2)		—		0.0* (0.0–0.0)		0.0* (0.0–0.0)	
	30+	3.5 (0.7–18.1)		1.3 (0.1–19.4)		—		0.0* (0.0–0.0)		0.0* (0.0–0.0)	

5	13–19	29.6* (1.8–475.9)	–	0.4 (0.0–3.5)	0.2 (0.0–4.3)	0.0* (0.0–0.0)
	20–29	–	–	3.1 (0.6–17.1)	6.5 (0.4–116.3)	1.2 (0.0–32.6)
	30+	–	–	–	–	–
6	13–19	0.1* (0.0–0.9)	–	2.0 (0.1–65.8)	2.4 (0.0–276.4)	–
	20–29	0.3 (0.1–1.3)	–	11.9* (1.3–105.6)	23.4 (0.5–1069.3)	1.0 (0.0–59.7)
	30+	–	–	–	–	–
7	13–19	0.1* (0.0–0.8)	0.8 (0.0–29.5)	–	–	
	20–29	0.2* (0.0–0.8)	5.2 (0.3–80.0)	20.8* (1.5–283.4)	29.3 (0.3–2496.6)	
	30+	–	–	–	–	
8+	13–19	0.0* (0.0–0.0)				
	20–29	0.5 (0.1–5.1)				
	30+	–				

*Significant at the 0.05 level, two-sided test.

0.0* (0.0–0.0) OR is ≤0.05 indicating very low risk.

– Not included due to small cell size.

[a] Assessed in the Part 2 sample. Models control for person–years, country, significant variables from the chapters on sociodemographics, parental psychopathology, childhood adversities, and interaction terms between life course intervals (4–12, 13–19, 20–29, 30+ years) and each control. Only the interaction terms between the life course intervals and PTSD variables are shown in table.

[b] For number of traumatic events or more. For example, for unplanned attempt, 6 represents ≥6 (that is, 6+).

Table 9.7. Associations between traumatic events and the persistence of suicidal behavior[a] (all countries combined)

Traumatic events	Ideation OR (95% CI)	Plan OR (95% CI)	Attempt OR (95% CI)
Disasters/accidents			
All man-made disasters	1.2 (0.9–1.5)	1.2 (0.8–1.7)	1.7* (1.0–2.8)
Natural disaster	1.1 (0.8–1.4)	0.9 (0.6–1.3)	0.9 (0.5–1.6)
Accident	1.3* (1.0–1.6)	1.3 (0.9–1.8)	1.6* (1.0–2.6)
War/combat/refugee experiences			
Exposure to war	1.1 (0.9–1.5)	1.3 (0.8–2.0)	1.7* (1.0–2.9)
Combat	1.1 (0.7–1.9)	0.5 (0.2–1.3)	1.6 (0.6–4.5)
Refugee	1.7* (1.0–2.9)	1.1 (0.5–2.4)	2.4 (1.0–6.2)
Sexual/interpersonal violence			
Sexual violence	1.3* (1.1–1.6)	1.2 (0.8–1.7)	1.6* (1.1–2.3)
Interpersonal violence	1.2 (1.0–1.4)	0.8 (0.5–1.1)	1.1 (0.7–1.8)
Witness/perpetrator violence			
Witness violence	1.1 (0.9–1.4)	0.9 (0.7–1.3)	1.4 (0.9–2.1)
Perpetrator violence	1.0 (0.7–1.5)	1.3 (0.7–2.3)	1.2 (0.6–2.5)
Loss/trauma			
Death of loved one	1.2 (1.0–1.4)	1.2 (0.9–1.6)	1.7* (1.2–2.4)
Trauma to loved one	1.1 (0.8–1.3)	1.0 (0.7–1.4)	1.5 (1.0–2.3)
All others	1.2* (1.0–1.5)	1.3 (1.0–1.8)	1.5 (1.0–2.1)
13 df χ^2 test for 13 types	16.2 (0.24)	15.4 (0.28)	20.0 (0.10)
12 df χ^2 test for difference between types	9.3 (0.68)	16.1 (0.19)	10.0 (0.62)
Number of traumatic events[b]			
1			
2	0.7* (0.6–0.9)	0.8 (0.5–1.2)	0.6* (0.4–1.0)
3	0.7* (0.5–1.0)	0.9 (0.5–1.6)	0.5 (0.2–1.1)
4	0.4* (0.2–0.7)	0.4* (0.2–0.9)	0.3* (0.1–0.7)
5	0.4* (0.2–0.9)	0.4 (0.1–1.3)	0.1* (0.0–0.5)
6	0.3* (0.1–0.7)	0.8 (0.2–3.1)	0.1* (0.0–0.6)
7+	0.3 (0.1–1.0)		
χ^2 (p-value)	11.6 (0.07)	10.2 (0.07)	10.1 (0.07)

* Significant at the 0.05 level, two-sided test.
[a] Results are based on multivariate discrete time survival models. Models control for country, age-related variables, and significant variables from the chapters on sociodemographics, parental psychopathology, and childhood adversities.
[b] For number of traumatic events, the last OR represents the odds for that number of traumatic events or more. For example, for attempt, 6 represents ≥6 (that is, 6+).

income countries are presented in Appendix Tables 9.10–9.12. The results of the more fine-grained logistic regression persistence models (results not reported in tables) do not show consistent effects for any specific types of traumatic events. The persistence of suicide ideation is predicted by prior sexual violence (OR = 1.3 for persistence beyond two years after age of onset) and witnessing violence (OR = 1.7 for persistence within the past ten years). The persistence of suicide planning is predicted by accident (OR = 2.2

for very high persistence, that is, into the five years prior to interview) and trauma to a loved one (OR = 3.0–4.5 for persistence into the year prior to interview). High persistence of suicide attempt is predicted most strongly by exposure to war (ORs = 7.6–31.0 for persistence into the 10, five, and one year prior to interview), and also by man-made disaster (OR = 5.5 into the past 10 years) and trauma to a loved one (OR = 207.6 for attempt in the past year among those with persistent attempts).

Interaction of traumatic events and PTSD

As noted earlier, some data have suggested that the association between traumatic events and suicidal behavior is seen primarily in the context of PTSD (Wilcox et al., 2009). The interactions between traumatic events and the presence of PTSD in predicting suicide ideation and attempt are presented in Table 9.8. As shown, the relative absence of significant effects suggests that the relationship between traumatic events and suicidal behavior does not occur solely in the presence of PTSD. Indeed, slightly more ORs suggest a decrease in the odds of suicidal behavior in the presence of PTSD than an increase (with 30 ORs ≥1.0 and 35 ORs <1.0). Results are similar in the data separating countries by income level (see Appendix Tables 9.13–9.15).

Discussion

Several limitations of this study require emphasis. It is important to note that the PTSD module of the WMH-CIDI does not specifically list all potential traumas throughout the globe. For example, the category of "other trauma" may include a range of crucial traumas such as human rights violations (Stein et al., 2009). Further, we did not assess the severity and duration of individual traumas. Severity and duration of trauma may be important in predicting, for example, which subjects with suicide ideation go on to make a suicide attempt. Another important limitation is that there are several differences across surveys such as variation in response rates and the fact that some of the samples are not nationally representative. We controlled for differential response using poststratification adjustments, but response rates may have been related to trauma exposure or suicidal behavior, thus limiting the generalizability of the estimates. An additional set of limitations emerges from the fact that assessment of both traumatic events and suicidal behavior is

based on retrospective self-report. The questionnaire attempted to increase the recall of respondents and decrease differences in reporting, but the data are nevertheless subject to bias at the level of individual respondents (e.g., bias in recall based on current mood), and to various kinds of bias at the level of the sites (e.g., responses to questions about trauma and suicide may be influenced by the different cultural contexts in which the surveys were given) (Alonso et al., 2008; Lopez & Guarnaccia, 2000; Schacter, 1999; Schraedley et al., 2002).

Despite these limitations, the data presented here provide a more detailed analysis of the relationship between traumatic events and suicidal behavior than has previously been possible. Thus, they extend previous data from community and clinical studies (Brodsky & Stanley, 2008; Santa Mina & Gallop, 1998; Tiet et al., 2006; Wiederman et al., 1998; Wilcox et al., 2009). There are several important findings from this study. First, we found a strong association between sexual and interpersonal violence and suicide ideation and attempt, with sexual violence also predicting the persistence of suicide ideation. Second, there is a strong dose–response relation between multiple traumatic events and suicide ideation/attempt; however, these effects are subadditive in nature with a decrease in the strength of the association among those with an increasing number of events. Third, although the experience of traumatic events predicts suicide ideation, it is less useful in predicting the progression from suicide ideation to suicide attempt. Fourth, sexual or interpersonal violence and witnessing violence are associated with higher odds of suicidal behavior earlier in life relative to the later part of the life course, whereas combat and refugee experiences are associated with significantly higher odds of suicide ideation and attempts during adolescence and adulthood relative to the earlier part of the life course. Fifth, the patterns of findings observed generally are consistent across high-, middle-, and low-income countries. Sixth and finally, in several instances, the experience of traumatic events was associated with decreased odds of suicidal behavior – a surprising finding that requires replication and future research in order to better understand the nature of these effects.

Previous work has emphasized the relationship between exposure to sexual and interpersonal violence and suicidal behavior (Brent et al., 1999; Brodsky et al., 2001; Brown et al., 1999; Dube et al., 2001; Fergusson

Table 9.8. Interactions between the occurrence of traumatic events and DSM-IV posttraumatic stress disorder in the prediction of suicidal behavior[a] (all countries combined)

	Among total sample			Among ideators	
	Ideation	Attempt	Plan	Planned attempt	Unplanned attempt
Traumatic events	OR (95% CI)	OR (95% CI)	OR (95% CI)	OR (95% CI)	OR (95% CI)
Disasters/accidents					
All man-made disasters	1.1 (0.6–1.8)	0.6 (0.3–1.2)	0.7 (0.4–1.4)	0.9 (0.2–3.4)	0.3 (0.1–1.3)
Natural disaster	1.0 (0.6–1.8)	0.9 (0.5–1.8)	0.7 (0.4–1.4)	1.1 (0.4–2.6)	0.5 (0.1–1.7)
Accident	1.1 (0.8–1.7)	0.8 (0.5–1.3)	1.3 (0.8–2.1)	1.1 (0.6–2.3)	0.4 (0.1–1.0)
War/combat/refugee experiences					
Exposure to war	1.6 (0.8–3.1)	1.8 (0.9–3.7)	1.8 (0.8–4.0)	1.0 (0.3–3.8)	2.8 (0.4–18.2)
Combat	1.6 (0.5–4.8)	0.6 (0.2–1.9)	0.6 (0.2–1.5)	0.6 (0.1–4.7)	0.0* (0.0–0.0)
Refugee	0.6 (0.3–1.4)	1.0 (0.4–2.9)	1.1 (0.3–3.5)	0.4 (0.1–2.6)	13.0 (0.6–295.2)
Sexual/interpersonal violence					
Sexual violence	0.9 (0.6–1.3)	1.1 (0.7–1.7)	0.6* (0.3–0.9)	0.8 (0.3–1.9)	0.9 (0.4–2.0)
Interpersonal violence	0.8 (0.5–1.1)	1.1 (0.7–1.6)	1.1 (0.7–1.7)	0.7 (0.3–1.5)	1.4 (0.7–3.1)
Witness/perpetrator violence					
Witness violence	1.3 (0.9–1.9)	1.3 (0.8–2.1)	0.8 (0.5–1.4)	1.7 (0.8–3.4)	0.9 (0.3–2.6)
Perpetrator violence	0.4* (0.2–0.9)	1.2 (0.6–2.3)	1.9 (0.7–4.7)	1.4 (0.4–5.0)	2.8 (0.5–14.4)
Loss/trauma					
Death of loved one	0.8 (0.6–1.0)	0.8 (0.6–1.2)	0.8 (0.5–1.3)	1.1 (0.6–1.9)	0.9 (0.4–1.8)
Trauma to loved one	0.9 (0.6–1.2)	0.7 (0.5–1.1)	0.6* (0.4–1.0)	0.8 (0.4–1.6)	2.1 (0.9–5.1)
All others	0.6* (0.4–0.9)	0.7 (0.5–1.2)	1.0 (0.6–1.6)	1.3 (0.6–2.8)	0.7 (0.3–1.6)
13 df χ^2 group test	228.3 (<0.001)*	118.1 (<0.001)*	17.2 (0.19)	24.9 (0.02)*	22.6 (0.05)*
13 df group interaction test	25.2 (0.02)*	18.9 (0.13)	21.1 (0.07)	5.5 (0.96)	224.0 (<0.001)*

* Significant at the 0.05 level, two-sided test.
0.0* (0.0–0.0) OR is ≤0.05 indicating very low risk.
[a] Assessed in the Part 2 sample due to having Part 2 controls. Models included interaction terms between DSM-IV posttraumatic stress disorder (PTSD) and each trauma event. Only interaction terms are shown in the table; however, the main effects are still controlled for. Models control for person–years, country, and significant variables from the chapters on sociodemographics, parental psychopathology, and childhood adversities.

et al., 1996). Several different mechanisms may account for these associations. First, in vulnerable people, disruptions in interpersonal relationships may play a key role in precipitating suicide. Second, exposure to sexual and interpersonal violence may be associated with a range of psychiatric disorders (including depression and PTSD), as well as with key psychological phenomena such as increased impulsivity – which, in turn, play an important role in stress–diathesis models of suicide (Brodsky et al., 2001;

Brodsky & Stanley, 2008; Dube et al., 2001; Minzenberg et al., 2008; Molnar et al., 2001; Nock et al., 2009). Our finding that sexual or interpersonal violence and witnessing violence are associated with higher odds of suicidal behavior earlier in life relative to the later part of the life course is consistent with the emphasis of much of the literature on how these traumas lead to disrupted development, with alterations in early attachments and in related psychological processes (e.g., trust).

It is notable that many traumas are associated with suicidal behavior in bivariate, but not in multivariate models. This finding emphasizes the complex pattern of relationships between traumatic events and suicidal behavior. Some types of traumatic events may be associated with suicidal behavior only because they co-occur with other events that are themselves associated with such behavior. For example, perpetrating violence against others is associated with subsequent suicide attempt in bivariate but not multivariate analyses. This may be because the association between these two variables is explained by witnessing violence (even when one is the perpetrator). Another possibility is that associations between traumatic events and suicidal behavior can be explained by the presence of some element common to all such events so that when they are all considered simultaneously the unique effect of each type of event diminishes. On balance, the fact that most events continue to significantly predict subsequent suicide attempt in the multivariate model suggests that such an explanation cannot fully explain the observed results.

The data here show that although more traumatic events are associated with increased suicidal behavior, this influence increases at a decreasing rate. These associations are in keeping with previous literature on a stress–diathesis theory of suicidal behavior, where trauma leads to a stress response with psycho-biological changes, in which multiple traumas increase the strength of the stress response, but in which multiple other factors play a role in ultimately precipitating suicide ideation and attempt. It is notable that certain kinds of trauma, namely sexual violence and accidents, are predictive of the persistence of suicide ideation. Stress–diathesis models have not commonly been elaborated on to address the complexities of severity and timing of both risk factors and suicide outcomes; data such as these may encourage such work to proceed.

These data also suggest that the relation between traumatic events and subsequent suicide attempt is due primarily to traumatic events predicting suicide ideation but not the progression from suicide ideation to suicide attempt. This overall finding notwithstanding, it is notable that in the total sample, natural disaster predicted the development of a suicide plan among those with ideation, exposure to war predicted the development of a planned attempt among ideators, and sexual violence predicted unplanned attempt among ideators. These data are consistent with prior studies on the different forms of psychopathology that follow different traumatic events. Specifically, it has been suggested that exposure to natural disasters and war may lead to survivor guilt and ultimately planned suicide, whereas exposure to sexual violence may be associated with a range of more impulsive psycho-pathology (Hendin & Haas, 1991; Minzenberg et al., 2008). However, it is notable that this pattern of findings was not consistent across high-, middle-, and low-income countries, suggesting that these findings should be interpreted with caution until they are replicated across studies.

Despite this lack of consistency in the risk factors for transitions from suicide ideation to plan/attempt, it is remarkable that across different income countries, the risk factors for suicide ideation and attempt were quite similar. This finding is in keeping with a cumulative body of work on risk factors, indicating that many appear to have some degree of universality (Nock et al., 2009). For instance, whereas the prevalence of both mental disorders and suicidal behavior differs cross-nationally, the associations between these constructs are quite consistent (Nock et al., 2009). Such consistency of findings in various parts of the world supports the validity of the patterns of association noted in our study, despite the limitations addressed above.

In contrast to data collected by Wilcox and colleagues (2009), our data indicates that the relationships between traumatic events and suicidal events held true whether or not the diagnostic criteria for PTSD were met. The Wilcox et al. study was, however, limited to a young sample of urban African American adults. In further analyses, we found that in high-income countries, exposure to war interacted with PTSD to predict increased suicide ideation, whereas exposure to man-made disasters interacted with PTSD to predict fewer suicide attempts. However, in middle-income countries, exposure to refugee trauma interacted with PTSD to predict increased suicide ideation, whereas exposure to a natural disaster interacted with PTSD to predict suicidal plans among ideators. The findings here are consistent with a view that the mechanisms that underlie the relationship between trauma exposure and suicidal behavior are multiple, and may not be explicable on the basis of any particular kind of trauma or any single psychiatric entity. Certain traumas may have different meanings and implications in different contexts, and additional research is needed to investigate in more detail the interactions between early life adversity, adult-onset traumas, and various psychobiological and psychosocial risk and resilience factors in the prediction of suicidal behavior (Makhija & Sher, 2007).

The data here have a number of implications for both mental health policy and clinical assessment and management. Mental health policy-makers need to be increasingly aware that violence and other traumas comprise a major public health problem (Krug et al., 2002) and that a range of relevant interventions are required around the world. Prevention may ultimately play an important role in reducing the burden of psychiatric disorder, including suicidal behavior, with the prevention of traumas such as sexual and interpersonal violence a particularly important goal. Clinicians should be encouraged to assess patients routinely for exposure to trauma, including multiple traumas, especially when there is concurrent psychopathology, including suicide ideation or attempts. Future research is needed to determine the impact of particular clinical and policy interventions targeting the association between traumatic events and suicidal behavior.

Acknowledgements

Portions of this chapter are based on Stein, D. J., Chiu, W. T., Hwang, I., et al. (2010). Cross-national analysis of the associations between traumatic events and suicidal behavior: findings from the WHO World Mental Health Surveys. PLoS One, 5(5), e10574. Reproduced with permission.

References

Alonso, J., Buron, A., Bruffaerts, R., et al. (2008). Association of perceived stigma and mood and anxiety disorders: results from the World Mental Health Surveys. *Acta Psychiatrica Scandinavica*, **118**(4), 305–314.

Brent, D. A., Baugher, M., Bridge, J., Chen, T., & Chiappetta, L. (1999). Age- and sex-related risk factors for adolescent suicide. *Journal of the American Academy of Child and Adolescent Psychiatry*, **38**(12), 1497–1505.

Brodsky, B. S., Oquendo, M., Ellis, S. P., et al. (2001). The relationship of childhood abuse to impulsivity and suicidal behavior in adults with major depression. *American Journal of Psychiatry*, **158**(11), 1871–1877.

Brodsky, B. S., & Stanley, B. (2008). Adverse childhood experiences and suicidal behavior. *Psychiatric Clinics of North America*, **31**(2), 223–235.

Brown, J., Cohen, P., Johnson, J. G., & Smailes, E. M. (1999). Childhood abuse and neglect: specificity of effects on adolescent and young adult depression and suicidality. *Journal of the American Academy of Child and Adolescent Psychiatry*, **38**(12), 1490–1496.

Bruffaerts, R., Demyttenaere, K., Borges, G., et al. (2010). Childhood adversities as risk factors for onset and persistence of suicidal behaviour. *British Journal of Psychiatry*, **197**(1), 20–27.

Dube, S. R., Anda, R. F., Felitti, V. J., et al. (2001). Childhood abuse, household dysfunction, and the risk of attempted suicide throughout the life span: findings from the Adverse Childhood Experiences Study. *Journal of the American Medical Association*, **286**(24), 3089–3096.

Fergusson, D. M., Lynskey, M. T., & Horwood, L. J. (1996). Childhood sexual abuse and psychiatric disorder in young adulthood: I. Prevalence of sexual abuse and factors associated with sexual abuse. *Journal of the American Academy of Child and Adolescent Psychiatry*, **35**(10), 1355–1364.

Hendin, H., & Haas, A. P. (1991). Suicide and guilt as manifestations of PTSD in Vietnam combat veterans. *American Journal of Psychiatry*, **148**(5), 586–591.

Kessler, R. C., & Üstün, T. B. (2004). The World Mental Health (WMH) Survey Initiative Version of the World Health Organization (WHO) Composite International Diagnostic Interview (CIDI). *International Journal of Methods in Psychiatric Research*, **13**(2), 93–121.

Krug, E. G., Mercy, J. A., Dahlberg, L. L., & Zwi, A. B. (2002). The world report on violence and health. *Lancet*, **360**(9339), 1083–1088.

Lopez, S. R., & Guarnaccia, P. J. (2000). Cultural psychopathology: uncovering the social world of mental illness. *Annual Review of Psychology*, **51**, 571–598.

Makhija, N., & Sher, L. (2007). Childhood abuse, adult alcohol use disorders and suicidal behaviour. *QJM*, **100**(5), 305–309.

Minzenberg, M. J., Poole, J. H., & Vinogradov, S. (2008). A neurocognitive model of borderline personality disorder: effects of childhood sexual abuse and relationship to adult social attachment disturbance. *Development and Psychopathology*, **20**(1), 341–368.

Molnar, B. E., Buka, S. L., & Kessler, R. C. (2001). Child sexual abuse and subsequent psychopathology: results from the National Comorbidity Survey. *American Journal of Public Health*, **91**(5), 753–760.

Nock, M. K., Hwang, I., Sampson, N., et al. (2009). Cross-national analysis of the associations among mental disorders and suicidal behavior: findings from the WHO World Mental Health Surveys. *PLoS Medicine*, **6**(8), e1000123.

Risch, N., Herrell, R., Lehner, T., et al. (2009). Interaction between the serotonin transporter gene (5-HTTLPR), stressful life events, and risk of depression: a meta-analysis. *Journal of the American Medical Association*, **301**(23), 2462–2471.

Roy, A., Hu, X. Z., Janal, M. N., & Goldman, D. (2007). Interaction between childhood trauma and serotonin transporter gene variation in suicide. *Neuropsychopharmacology*, **32**(9), 2046–2052.

Santa Mina, E. E., & Gallop, R. M. (1998). Childhood sexual and physical abuse and adult self-harm and suicidal behaviour: a literature review. *Canadian Journal of Psychiatry*, **43**(8), 793–800.

Schacter, D. L. (1999). The seven sins of memory. Insights from psychology and cognitive neuroscience. *American Psychologist*, **54**(3), 182–203.

Schraedley, P. K., Turner, R. J., & Gotlib, I. H. (2002). Stability of retrospective reports in depression: traumatic events, past depressive episodes, and parental psychopathology. *Journal of Health and Social Behavior*, **43**(3), 307–316.

Stein, D. J., Chiu, W. T., Hwang, I., et al. (2010). Cross-national analysis of the associations between traumatic events and suicidal behavior: findings from the WHO World Mental Health Surveys. *PLoS One*, **5**(5), e10574.

Stein, D. J., Williams, S. L., Jackson, P. B., et al. (2009). Perpetration of gross human rights violations in South Africa: association with psychiatric disorders. *South African Medical Journal*, **99**(5, Pt 2), 390–395.

Tiet, Q. Q., Finney, J. W., & Moos, R. H. (2006). Recent sexual abuse, physical abuse, and suicide attempts among male veterans seeking psychiatric treatment. *Psychiatric Services*, **57**(1), 107–113.

Wiederman, M. W., Sansone, R. A., & Sansone, L. A. (1998). History of trauma and attempted suicide among women in a primary care setting. *Violence and Victims*, **13**(1), 3–9.

Wilcox, H. C., Storr, C. L., & Breslau, N. (2009). Posttraumatic stress disorder and suicide attempts in a community sample of urban American young adults. *Archives of General Psychiatry*, **66**(3), 305–311.

Williams, S. L., Williams, D. R., Stein, D. J., et al. (2007). Multiple traumatic events and psychological distress: the South Africa stress and health study. *Journal of Traumatic Stress*, **20**(5), 845–855.

Chapter

10

Mental disorders, comorbidity, and suicidal behavior

Matthew K. Nock, Charlene A. Deming, Wai Tat Chiu, Irving Hwang, Matthias Angermeyer, Guilherme Borges, Annette Beautrais, Maria Carmen Viana, Elie G. Karam, Norito Kawakami, Nancy A. Sampson, Thatikonda Padma Sudhakar, and Ronald C. Kessler

Introduction

Over the past several decades, numerous studies have highlighted the strong association that exists between the presence of a mental disorder, particularly depression, and the subsequent onset of suicidal behavior (i.e., suicide ideation, plans, and attempts) (Harris & Barraclough, 1997; Phillips et al., 2002; Pokorny, 1983). For example, psychological autopsy studies have revealed that as many as 90%–95% of those who die by suicide have a diagnosable mental disorder (Cavanagh et al., 2003). Although this association has been demonstrated in dozens of studies, several key questions remain about how and why mental disorders predict subsequent suicidal behavior.

First, virtually all prior studies on this topic have tested only the bivariate associations between mental disorders and suicidal behavior (Bostwick & Pankratz, 2000; Harris & Barraclough, 1997; Kessler et al., 2005a; Nock et al., 2008a; Phillips et al., 2004; Sareen et al., 2005; Weissman et al., 1989). A limitation of this approach is that because most mental disorders show strong comorbidity (Kessler et al., 2005b), many of the associations observed could be attributable to the true effects of just a few key disorders. For instance, it may be that depression is a key predictor of suicidal behavior and that anxiety disorders are only associated with suicidal behavior because they tend to co-occur with depression. Teasing apart which disorders are *uniquely* associated with suicidal behavior after accounting for psychiatric comorbidity is likely to facilitate significant progress in our understanding of how and why suicidal behavior occurs.

Second, several studies recently have revealed that the strong association between mental disorders and suicide attempts is largely attributable to the fact that

such disorders predict suicide ideation, but are less useful in predicting which people with ideation go on to make a suicide attempt (Nock et al., 2010a). It would be useful to know if mental disorders differentially predict distinct parts of the pathway to suicide. It may be that disorders characterized by negative thinking (e.g., depression) are especially useful in predicting suicide ideation, whereas those characterized by impulsiveness or poor behavioral inhibition (e.g., alcohol/substance disorders) are especially predictive of acting on one's suicide ideation and making an attempt. Such models await empirical evaluation and replication.

Third, the cross-national generality of findings on the importance of mental disorders for predicting suicidal behavior has been widely debated. Studies conducted in developed countries consistently have reported this finding (Kessler et al., 1999; Moscicki, 1999; Weissman et al., 1999); however, several studies conducted in developing countries have implied that mental disorders play a smaller role in the prediction of suicidal behavior (Vijayakumar, 2004; Vijayakumar et al., 2005). Clarifying this issue is important not only for scientific purposes, but also for developing appropriate screening and prevention programs worldwide (Goldsmith et al., 2002; Vijayakumar, 2004; WHO, 2008).

The purpose of the analyses presented in this chapter is to provide a clearer understanding of the nature of the associations between mental disorders and suicidal behavior in a way that addresses each of the aforementioned limitations. Building on earlier chapters in this volume, here we examine the unique associations between mental disorders and the subsequent first onset and persistence of suicide ideation, plans, and attempts. This chapter extends earlier work on the association between mental disorders and suicidal behavior in the cross-national WMH Surveys (Nock et al., 2010a) by examining the persistence of the observed associations and by testing the extent to which these effects vary over the lifespan and across high-, middle-, and low-income countries.

Method

A detailed description of the respondent samples, study procedures, statistical analyses, and assessment of suicidal behavior is provided in Chapter 3 of this volume. Notably, many of the analyses presented in this chapter are based on the WMH Part 2 sample (n=55,299), which included assessment of correlates and disorders of secondary interest. The assessment and analysis of sociodemographic factors (Chapter 6), parental psychopathology (Chapter 7), childhood adversities (Chapter 8), and traumatic events during adulthood (Chapter 9), which are included as covariates in the following analyses, are described in earlier chapters.

There were a few instances in which specific surveys did not include certain risk factors. Specifically, Mexico did not assess intermittent explosive disorder (IED); Bulgaria, India, and Lebanon did not assess oppositional defiant disorder (ODD); China and Nigeria did not assess ODD and attention deficit hyperactivity disorder (ADHD); Japan did not assess ADHD, ODD, conduct disorder (CD), and separation anxiety disorder (SAD); New Zealand did not assess any of the impulse-control disorders (ADHD, ODD, CD, IED) or SAD; Israel did not assess any of the impulse-control disorders, SAD, and specific and social phobias; Ukraine did not assess ODD, ADHD, SAD, specific phobia, and bipolar disorder; South Africa did not assess ODD, ADHD, CD, SAD, specific phobia, or bipolar disorder; Shenzhen did not assess ODD, CD, SAD, substance disorders, and posttraumatic stress disorder (PTSD); and ESEMeD countries did not assess dysthymic and bipolar disorders, IED, and drug use disorders. These countries were excluded from the respective bivariate models, and coded "zero" for these variables in the multivariate models.

Results

Prevalence of DSM-IV mental disorders among those with suicidal behavior

Data on the prevalence of each type of mental disorder assessed among those with suicidal behavior are

presented in Table 10.1. Perhaps the most striking finding is the relatively low prevalence of a specific prior mental disorder among those with each suicidal outcome. For example, among respondents in the total sample making a suicide attempt, even the most prevalent of disorders occurs relatively infrequently. Indeed, among those making a suicide attempt, only 23.5% have a prior major depressive disorder, 21.4% have a specific phobia, 15.8% have social phobia, 13.4% have an alcohol use disorder, and all other disorders occur at even lower rates. Overall, the rates of mental disorders are even lower among those in the total sample with suicide ideation, and highest among those with ideation making a planned suicide attempt (see Table 10.1). This same pattern is seen across high-, middle-, and low-income countries – with the same four disorders occurring most commonly among high- and middle-income countries and with social phobia being replaced by intermittent explosive disorder in low-income countries (see Appendix Tables 10.1–10.3).

Bivariate and multivariate associations between DSM-IV mental disorders and suicidal behavior

Although each disorder occurs among suicidal respondents at rates that were lower than anticipated based on prior studies, they occur much more frequently among suicidal respondents than non-suicidal respondents. In bivariate models, every disorder assessed is associated with significantly increased odds of the subsequent onset of suicide ideation and attempt among the total sample (see Table 10.2). Depression is the strongest predictor of suicide ideation (OR=3.0); however, it does not predict suicide plans or attempts among ideators and, in fact, the presence of depression is associated with lower odds of suicide attempt (ORs=0.7–0.8). Instead, among those with suicide ideation, planned suicide attempts are predicted by panic disorder (OR=1.6) and bipolar disorder (OR=1.6) and unplanned suicide attempts are predicted by alcohol use disorders (OR=1.4). Similar results emerged in multivariate models with all disorders entered simultaneously as predictors of each suicide-related outcome (see Table 10.3). More specifically, ORs decrease in most cases causing some disorders to no longer meet criteria for statistical significance, but the overall pattern is the same in the prediction of suicide ideation and attempts in the total sample, as well as in the prediction of suicide attempts among ideators.

Table 10.1. Prevalence of DSM-IV mental disorders with each type of suicidal behavior^a (all countries combined)

Mental disorders	Among total sample						Among ideators			
	%^{b} (SE) with disorder						%^{b} (SE) with disorder			
	Ideation	No ideation	Attempt	No attempt	Plan	No plan	Planned attempt	No planned attempt	Unplanned attempt	No unplanned attempt
Anxiety disorders										
Panic disorder	3.2 (0.2)	0.6 (0.0)	5.5 (0.5)	0.7 (0.0)	5.0 (0.4)	4.0 (0.3)	6.4 (0.7)	5.2 (0.8)	4.3 (0.7)	3.7 (0.4)
Generalized anxiety disorder	6.3 (0.3)	1.1 (0.0)	9.4 (0.7)	1.4 (0.0)	8.7 (0.6)	11.1 (0.7)	10.3 (0.9)	15.7 (1.8)	8.3 (1.0)	10.0 (0.7)
Specific phobia	15.9 (0.5)	5.0 (0.1)	21.4 (1.0)	5.3 (0.1)	20.1 (0.9)	15.9 (0.8)	22.9 (1.2)	19.2 (1.5)	18.1 (1.5)	14.3 (0.8)
Social phobia	12.1 (0.5)	2.3 (0.1)	15.8 (0.9)	2.6 (0.1)	16.1 (0.9)	13.0 (0.7)	18.0 (1.2)	18.3 (1.6)	12.9 (1.5)	12.6 (0.9)
Posttraumatic stress	5.9 (0.3)	1.0 (0.1)	10.4 (0.7)	1.2 (0.1)	8.9 (0.6)	8.2 (0.6)	11.5 (0.9)	11.7 (1.2)	8.6 (1.1)	6.8 (0.6)
Separation anxiety disorder	4.8 (0.3)	1.0 (0.0)	7.1 (0.5)	1.1 (0.1)	6.3 (0.6)	6.0 (0.5)	6.9 (0.7)	6.0 (1.0)	7.3 (1.1)	5.1 (0.6)
Agoraphobia	2.5 (0.2)	0.7 (0.0)	3.5 (0.4)	0.7 (0.0)	3.6 (0.5)	2.5 (0.3)	3.9 (0.5)	4.0 (0.9)	2.3 (0.6)	2.3 (0.3)
Mood disorders										
Major depressive disorder	16.6 (0.5)	3.3 (0.1)	23.5 (1.0)	4.0 (0.1)	24.5 (1.0)	26.7 (0.9)	27.5 (1.4)	41.1 (2.1)	17.4 (1.4)	25.4 (1.0)
Dysthymic disorder	3.7 (0.2)	0.5 (0.0)	5.9 (0.6)	0.7 (0.0)	5.9 (0.5)	6.1 (0.4)	6.8 (0.8)	10.1 (1.4)	4.2 (0.8)	5.0 (0.4)
Bipolar disorder	2.5 (0.2)	0.3 (0.0)	4.7 (0.5)	0.4 (0.0)	3.9 (0.4)	3.6 (0.4)	5.3 (0.6)	4.3 (0.7)	3.8 (0.9)	2.8 (0.3)
Impulse-control disorders										
Oppositional defiant disorder	3.3 (0.3)	0.4 (0.0)	5.7 (0.5)	0.4 (0.0)	5.1 (0.6)	2.1 (0.2)	5.8 (0.7)	4.1 (0.8)	5.6 (0.9)	1.7 (0.3)
Conduct disorder	3.2 (0.3)	0.3 (0.0)	5.5 (0.5)	0.4 (0.0)	4.4 (0.6)	2.2 (0.3)	5.4 (0.8)	3.3 (0.8)	5.5 (0.8)	1.7 (0.3)
Attention deficit hyperactivity disorder	3.0 (0.3)	0.4 (0.0)	5.0 (0.5)	0.5 (0.0)	4.5 (0.5)	1.9 (0.2)	5.1 (0.6)	3.3 (0.8)	4.6 (0.9)	1.5 (0.2)
Intermittent explosive disorder	5.1 (0.3)	0.9 (0.0)	6.7 (0.5)	1.0 (0.0)	7.0 (0.6)	5.5 (0.5)	7.4 (0.8)	7.1 (1.0)	5.2 (0.8)	4.8 (0.5)
Substance use disorders										
Alcohol abuse or dependence	9.0 (0.4)	2.6 (0.1)	13.4 (0.8)	2.9 (0.1)	13.5 (0.8)	13.5 (0.8)	14.3 (1.1)	17.7 (1.7)	12.2 (1.4)	11.9 (0.9)
Drug abuse or dependence	4.2 (0.3)	0.6 (0.0)	6.9 (0.6)	0.7 (0.0)	7.2 (0.6)	4.9 (0.4)	8.2 (0.8)	9.8 (1.4)	4.8 (0.8)	4.5 (0.4)

Number of mental disorders[c]

1	22.9 (0.6)	9.8 (0.1)	23.5 (1.0)	10.2 (0.1)	23.6 (0.9)	23.2 (0.8)	24.0 (1.3)	22.5 (1.7)	22.3 (1.7)	23.2 (0.9)
2	11.7 (0.4)	2.7 (0.1)	14.5 (0.9)	3.0 (0.1)	15.4 (0.8)	13.8 (0.6)	16.1 (1.2)	18.0 (1.4)	12.5 (1.3)	13.1 (0.7)
3	6.5 (0.3)	0.9 (0.0)	10.0 (0.7)	1.1 (0.0)	8.4 (0.6)	7.5 (0.5)	10.7 (1.0)	11.0 (1.3)	9.2 (1.1)	7.8 (0.6)
4	3.3 (0.3)	0.4 (0.0)	5.5 (0.5)	0.5 (0.0)	5.7 (0.6)	5.2 (0.4)	5.8 (0.6)	7.4 (1.0)	4.8 (1.0)	4.1 (0.4)
5	1.9 (0.2)	0.2 (0.0)	2.9 (0.3)	0.2 (0.0)	2.8 (0.3)	2.3 (0.2)	3.4 (0.4)	3.5 (0.6)	2.2 (0.5)	1.8 (0.2)
6	1.0 (0.1)	0.1 (0.0)	2.0 (0.3)	0.1 (0.0)	2.2 (0.3)	1.5 (0.2)	2.4 (0.5)	2.8 (0.7)	1.1 (0.4)	1.3 (0.2)
7	0.4 (0.1)	0.0 (0.0)	0.6 (0.2)	0.1 (0.0)	0.8 (0.2)	0.9 (0.2)	0.5 (0.2)	1.6 (0.5)	1.7 (0.5)	1.1 (0.2)
8	0.1 (0.0)	0.0 (0.0)	0.6 (0.2)	0.0 (0.0)	0.3 (0.1)	0.5 (0.1)	0.7 (0.2)	1.3 (0.5)		
9	0.2 (0.1)	0.0 (0.0)	1.0 (0.3)	0.0 (0.0)	0.3 (0.1)	0.1 (0.1)	1.4 (0.4)	0.3 (0.1)		
10+	0.1 (0.0)	0.0 (0.0)			0.3 (0.1)	0.1 (0.0)				
N[d]	(8382)	(210,870)	(2831)	(218,419)	(3324)	(8252)	(1766)	(2064)	(937)	(6271)

[a] As all subsequent models are based on the Part 2 sample, the percentages are also all based on the Part 2 sample despite some being Part 1 disorders.

[b] % represents the percentage of people with the disorder among the cases with the outcome variable indicated in the column header. For example, the first cell is the % of those with panic disorder among those with suicide ideation.

[c] For number of mental disorders, the last OR represents the odds for that number of disorders or more. For example, for unplanned attempt, 7 represents ≥7 (that is, 7+).

[d] Number of cases with the outcome variable; N represents the number of person–years.

Table 10.2. Bivariate model for associations between DSM-IV mental disorder and each type of suicidal behavior[a] (all countries combined)

Mental disorders	Among total sample		Among ideators		
	Ideation	Attempt	Plan	Planned attempt	Unplanned attempt
	OR (95% CI)	OR (95% CI)	OR (95% CI)	OR (95% CI)	OR (95% CI)
Anxiety disorders					
Panic disorder	2.1* (1.8–2.5)	2.4* (2.0–3.1)	1.4* (1.1–1.8)	1.6* (1.0–2.5)	1.0 (0.7–1.6)
Generalized anxiety disorder	2.8* (2.4–3.2)	2.9* (2.4–3.5)	1.0 (0.8–1.2)	0.9 (0.7–1.3)	1.1 (0.8–1.6)
Specific phobia	1.8* (1.7–1.9)	2.0* (1.7–2.2)	1.3* (1.1–1.5)	1.3 (1.0–1.6)	1.1 (0.8–1.5)
Social phobia	2.3* (2.0–2.5)	2.1* (1.8–2.5)	1.3* (1.0–1.5)	1.1 (0.8–1.5)	0.9 (0.6–1.2)
Posttraumatic stress	1.8* (1.6–2.2)	2.1* (1.8–2.5)	1.2 (0.9–1.4)	1.2 (0.8–1.6)	1.4 (0.9–2.0)
Separation anxiety disorder	1.7* (1.4–2.0)	1.6* (1.3–2.0)	1.0 (0.8–1.4)	1.4 (0.9–2.3)	1.2 (0.8–1.9)
Agoraphobia	1.6* (1.3–2.0)	1.8* (1.3–2.3)	1.3 (0.9–1.9)	1.1 (0.7–1.9)	0.8 (0.4–1.6)
Mood disorders					
Major depressive disorder	3.0* (2.7–3.2)	3.2* (2.8–3.6)	1.0 (0.9–1.2)	0.8* (0.6–1.0)	0.7* (0.5–0.9)
Dysthymic disorder	2.8* (2.4–3.3)	2.5* (1.9–3.3)	1.1 (0.9–1.4)	0.8 (0.5–1.1)	0.8 (0.5–1.3)
Bipolar disorder	2.2* (1.8–2.7)	2.5* (1.9–3.3)	1.1 (0.8–1.5)	1.6* (1.1–2.4)	1.2 (0.7–2.1)
Impulse-control disorders					
Oppositional defiant disorder	2.2* (1.8–2.8)	2.6* (2.0–3.3)	1.6* (1.0–2.4)	1.0 (0.6–1.6)	1.4 (0.9–2.3)
Conduct disorder	2.2* (1.8–2.7)	2.3* (1.7–3.1)	1.3 (0.9–1.8)	1.4 (0.9–2.3)	1.1 (0.6–1.9)
Attention deficit hyperactivity disorder	1.7* (1.4–2.1)	1.9* (1.4–2.5)	1.4 (1.0–1.9)	1.0 (0.7–1.7)	1.3 (0.7–2.3)
Intermittent explosive disorder	2.5* (2.1–2.9)	2.4* (1.9–2.9)	1.2 (0.9–1.5)	1.0 (0.7–1.5)	0.9 (0.6–1.4)
Substance use disorders					
Alcohol abuse or dependence	1.9* (1.7–2.1)	2.6* (2.2–3.0)	1.4* (1.1–1.7)	1.0 (0.8–1.4)	1.4* (1.0–2.0)
Drug abuse or dependence	2.1* (1.7–2.5)	2.5* (2.0–3.0)	1.7* (1.3–2.1)	0.9 (0.6–1.4)	0.9 (0.6–1.4)

* Significant at the 0.05 level, two-sided test.
[a] Assessed in the Part 2 sample due to having Part 2 controls. Models control for person–years, country, and significant variables from the chapters on sociodemographics, parental psychopathology, childhood adversities, and traumatic events.

Table 10.3. Multivariate models for associations between DSM-IV mental disorders and each type of suicidal behavior[a] (all countries combined)

| Mental disorders | Among total sample | | Among ideators | | |
| | Ideation | Attempt | Plan | Planned attempt | Unplanned attempt |
	OR (95% CI)	OR (95% CI)	OR (95% CI)	OR (95% CI)	OR (95% CI)
Anxiety disorders					
Panic disorder	1.2 (1.0–1.4)	1.3* (1.0–1.7)	1.3 (1.0–1.7)	1.5 (0.9–2.4)	1.0 (0.6–1.7)
Generalized anxiety disorder	1.6* (1.3–1.9)	1.6* (1.3–2.0)	0.9 (0.7–1.0)	0.9 (0.7–1.3)	1.3 (0.9–1.8)
Specific phobia	1.4* (1.3–1.5)	1.5* (1.3–1.7)	1.2* (1.0–1.4)	1.2 (0.9–1.6)	1.1 (0.8–1.5)
Social phobia	1.6* (1.4–1.7)	1.3* (1.1–1.5)	1.1 (0.9–1.4)	1.0 (0.8–1.3)	0.8 (0.6–1.1)
Posttraumatic stress	1.3* (1.1–1.5)	1.4* (1.1–1.7)	1.1 (0.9–1.3)	1.2 (0.8–1.6)	1.5* (1.0–2.2)
Separation anxiety disorder	1.1 (0.9–1.3)	1.0 (0.8–1.3)	1.0 (0.7–1.3)	1.4 (0.9–2.2)	1.3 (0.8–2.0)
Agoraphobia	1.1 (0.9–1.4)	1.3 (1.0–1.6)	1.2 (0.8–1.8)	1.2 (0.7–2.0)	0.9 (0.5–1.7)
Mood disorders					
Major depressive disorder	2.3* (2.0–2.5)	2.3* (2.0–2.7)	1.0 (0.8–1.1)	0.7* (0.6–0.9)	0.6* (0.5–0.8)
Dysthymic disorder	1.1 (0.9–1.3)	0.9 (0.6–1.2)	1.1 (0.8–1.4)	0.8 (0.5–1.2)	1.0 (0.6–1.6)
Bipolar disorder	1.1 (0.9–1.4)	1.3 (0.9–1.7)	1.0 (0.7–1.3)	1.7* (1.1–2.6)	1.3 (0.7–2.2)
Impulse-control disorders					
Oppositional defiant disorder	1.4* (1.1–1.8)	1.6* (1.2–2.1)	1.3 (0.9–2.0)	0.9 (0.6–1.6)	1.5 (0.9–2.5)
Conduct disorder	1.4* (1.1–1.7)	1.4* (1.0–1.9)	1.0 (0.7–1.4)	1.4 (0.8–2.4)	0.9 (0.5–1.6)
Attention deficit hyperactivity disorder	1.0 (0.8–1.3)	1.1 (0.8–1.5)	1.2 (0.8–1.6)	1.1 (0.7–1.8)	1.1 (0.6–1.8)
Intermittent explosive disorder	1.8* (1.5–2.1)	1.6* (1.2–2.0)	1.1 (0.9–1.4)	1.0 (0.7–1.5)	0.9 (0.6–1.4)
Substance use disorders					
Alcohol abuse or dependence	1.4* (1.2–1.6)	1.9* (1.5–2.3)	1.2 (0.9–1.5)	1.1 (0.8–1.5)	1.6* (1.1–2.2)
Drug abuse or dependence	1.2 (1.0–1.5)	1.2 (0.9–1.6)	1.5* (1.2–1.9)	0.8 (0.5–1.3)	0.7 (0.4–1.2)
χ^2 (p-value)	1007.1 (<0.001)*	565.7 (<0.001)*	45.8 (<0.001)*	29.9 (0.02)*	33.7 (0.01)*

* Significant at the 0.05 level, two-sided test.
[a] Assessed in the Part 2 sample due to having Part 2 controls. Models control for person–years, country, and significant variables from the chapters on sociodemographics, parental psychopathology, childhood adversities, and traumatic events.

Associations between number of comorbid disorders and suicidal behavior

Models testing the association between the number of prior mental disorders (ignoring type of disorder) and suicidal behavior revealed a strong dose–response relationship (see Table 10.4). The OR for suicide ideation in the total sample increased from 2.3 among those with one disorder (compared to those with no disorders) up to 6.2 among those with five disorders. The odds of suicide ideation remained elevated among those with six to 10+ disorders, although it showed a slight decrease as the number of disorders increased. The OR for suicide attempt in the total sample increased from 2.9 among those with one disorder to a high of 17.1 among those with nine or more disorders. There was a general pattern of increasing odds of suicide plan among those with suicide ideation, but no such pattern in models predicting suicide attempts among ideators. A similar overall pattern also was observed across high-, middle-, and low-income countries (see Appendix Tables 10.4–10.6).

Final multivariate models testing associations between type and number of mental disorders and suicidal behavior

Final multivariate models that included both type and number of disorders simultaneously are presented in Table 10.5. The pattern of associations in these more comprehensive models is similar to those in the earlier models. Each mental disorder examined is associated with increased odds of suicide ideation and attempt in the total sample, with depression emerging as the strongest predictor. Mental disorders are less powerful in predicting which people with suicide ideation go on to have suicide plans and make suicide attempts. These transitions are not predicted by depression, but instead by anxiety, impulse-control (along with bipolar disorder), and substance use disorders. These models reveal that the ORs for the number of disorders predicting suicide ideation and attempt in the total sample increase at a decreasing rate (see bottom of Table 10.5). This is known as a subadditive interaction; that is, a situation in which the effects of comorbid disorders are less than the sum of their individual

Table 10.4. Associations between number of DSM-IV mental disorders and each type of suicidal behavior[a] (all countries combined)

Number of mental disorders[b]	Among total sample		Among ideators		
	Ideation	Attempt	Plan	Planned attempt	Unplanned attempt
	OR (95% CI)	OR (95% CI)	OR (95% CI)	OR (95% CI)	OR (95% CI)
1	2.3* (2.2–2.5)	2.9* (2.5–3.3)	1.2* (1.1–1.5)	1.2 (0.9–1.6)	1.1 (0.8–1.4)
2	3.4* (3.1–3.7)	4.6* (3.9–5.5)	1.4* (1.1–1.7)	1.0 (0.7–1.3)	1.1 (0.7–1.5)
3	4.5* (4.0–5.1)	6.4* (5.2–7.9)	1.5* (1.2–1.9)	1.0 (0.6–1.5)	1.0 (0.7–1.5)
4	4.6* (3.8–5.6)	7.6* (6.1–9.6)	1.4* (1.0–2.0)	1.0 (0.7–1.5)	1.0 (0.6–1.7)
5	6.2* (4.9–7.8)	6.7* (4.9–9.0)	1.4 (1.0–2.1)	1.5 (0.9–2.4)	1.0 (0.5–1.8)
6	6.1* (4.6–8.0)	9.4* (6.0–14.5)	2.1* (1.4–3.0)	0.9 (0.4–2.0)	0.8 (0.3–1.8)
7	5.4* (3.4–8.7)	4.7* (2.5–8.7)	1.5 (0.8–2.8)	0.4 (0.1–1.2)	1.2 (0.6–2.4)
8	3.8* (2.2–6.4)	9.6* (5.6–16.6)	0.8 (0.3–1.8)	0.9 (0.4–2.0)	
9	4.8* (2.3–10.0)	17.1* (9.2–31.7)	3.5 (0.9–13.9)	9.0* (2.3–35.8)	
10+	3.5* (1.4–8.6)		3.2* (1.1–9.3)		
χ^2 (p-value)	1114.3 (<0.001)*	616.7 (<0.001)*	33.5 (<0.001)*	17.1 (0.05)*	1.2 (0.99)

* Significant at the 0.05 level, two-sided test.
[a] Assessed in the Part 2 sample due to having Part 2 controls. Models control for person–years, country, and significant variables from the chapters on sociodemographics, parental psychopathology, childhood adversities, and traumatic events.
[b] For number of mental disorders, the last OR represents the odds for that number of disorders or more. For example, for unplanned attempt, 7 represents ≥7 (that is, 7+).

Table 10.5. Final multivariate models for associations between DSM-IV mental disorders and each type of suicidal behavior[a] (all countries combined)

Mental disorders	Among total sample		Among ideators		
	Ideation	Attempt	Plan	Planned attempt	Unplanned attempt
	OR (95% CI)	OR (95% CI)	OR (95% CI)	OR (95% CI)	OR (95% CI)
Anxiety disorders					
Panic disorder	2.3* (1.9–2.7)	3.3* (2.4–4.5)	1.5* (1.1–2.1)	1.9* (1.1–3.4)	1.2 (0.7–2.0)
Generalized anxiety disorder	2.9* (2.4–3.4)	3.5* (2.8–4.4)	1.0 (0.8–1.3)	1.2 (0.8–1.8)	1.5 (0.9–2.3)
Specific phobia	2.0* (1.8–2.2)	2.5* (2.1–2.9)	1.4* (1.1–1.7)	1.6* (1.1–2.2)	1.2 (0.9–1.7)
Social phobia	2.5* (2.2–2.9)	2.6* (2.1–3.2)	1.3* (1.0–1.7)	1.3 (0.9–1.8)	0.9 (0.6–1.3)
Posttraumatic stress	2.2* (1.8–2.6)	3.0* (2.4–3.7)	1.3 (1.0–1.7)	1.5 (1.0–2.3)	1.7* (1.1–2.8)
Separation anxiety disorder	2.0* (1.6–2.5)	2.3* (1.7–2.9)	1.1 (0.8–1.6)	1.7 (1.0–2.9)	1.4 (0.8–2.5)
Agoraphobia	1.8* (1.5–2.2)	2.4* (1.8–3.2)	1.4 (0.9–2.2)	1.5 (0.8–2.8)	1.0 (0.5–2.1)
Mood disorders					
Major depressive disorder	3.2* (2.8–3.6)	3.8* (3.1–4.6)	1.1 (0.9–1.3)	0.9 (0.6–1.3)	0.7* (0.5–0.9)
Dysthymic disorder	2.4* (2.0–3.0)	2.5* (1.8–3.5)	1.3 (1.0–1.8)	1.0 (0.6–1.6)	1.1 (0.6–2.1)
Bipolar disorder	2.5* (2.0–3.1)	3.4* (2.4–4.8)	1.2 (0.8–1.8)	2.1* (1.3–3.6)	1.4 (0.8–2.7)
Impulse-control disorders					
Oppositional defiant disorder	2.7* (2.2–3.4)	3.7* (2.7–4.9)	1.6* (1.0–2.5)	1.1 (0.6–2.1)	1.7 (1.0–2.9)
Conduct disorder	2.6* (2.1–3.2)	3.0* (2.1–4.3)	1.2 (0.8–1.7)	1.7 (0.9–3.1)	1.1 (0.6–2.0)
Attention deficit hyperactivity disorder	2.0* (1.5–2.5)	2.4* (1.7–3.3)	1.4 (1.0–2.0)	1.3 (0.7–2.2)	1.2 (0.7–2.3)
Intermittent explosive disorder	2.9* (2.5–3.4)	3.1* (2.4–4.1)	1.3 (1.0–1.7)	1.3 (0.8–2.1)	1.0 (0.6–1.6)
Substance use disorders					
Alcohol abuse or dependence	2.1* (1.8–2.4)	3.2* (2.6–4.0)	1.3 (1.0–1.7)	1.3 (0.9–2.0)	1.7* (1.1–2.7)
Drug abuse or dependence	2.5* (2.1–3.1)	3.0* (2.3–4.0)	1.8* (1.3–2.4)	0.9 (0.5–1.7)	0.8 (0.5–1.5)
13 df χ^2 test for 13 types	614.6 (<0.001)*	245.9 (<0.001)*	30.9 (0.01)*	31.1 (0.01)*	34.4 (0.01)*
12 df χ^2 test for difference between types	114.9 (<0.001)*	49.3 (<0.001)*	23.8 (0.07)	26.1 (0.04)*	35.2 (0.002)*

Table 10.5. (cont.)

	Among total sample		Among ideators		
	Ideation	Attempt	Plan	Planned attempt	Unplanned attempt
Mental disorders	OR (95% CI)	OR (95% CI)	OR (95% CI)	OR (95% CI)	OR (95% CI)
Number of mental disorders[b]					
2	0.6* (0.5–0.7)	0.5* (0.4–0.7)	0.9 (0.7–1.2)	0.6 (0.4–1.0)	0.9 (0.6–1.4)
3	0.3* (0.2–0.4)	0.2* (0.2–0.4)	0.7 (0.5–1.2)	0.5 (0.3–1.1)	0.7 (0.3–1.5)
4	0.1* (0.1–0.2)	0.1* (0.1–0.2)	0.6 (0.3–1.0)	0.4 (0.1–1.1)	0.6 (0.2–1.7)
5	0.1* (0.0–0.1)	0.0* (0.0–0.1)	0.4* (0.2–1.0)	0.5 (0.1–1.7)	0.5 (0.1–1.8)
6	0.0* (0.0–0.1)	0.0* (0.0–0.0)	0.5 (0.2–1.3)	0.3 (0.1–1.3)	0.3 (0.1–1.7)
7	0.0* (0.0–0.0)	0.0* (0.0–0.0)	0.3* (0.1–0.9)	0.1* (0.0–0.6)	0.4 (0.1–3.1)
8	0.0* (0.0–0.0)	0.0* (0.0–0.0)	0.1* (0.0–0.5)	0.1* (0.0–1.0)	
9	0.0* (0.0–0.0)	0.0* (0.0–0.0)	0.3 (0.0–2.5)	0.7 (0.0–13.3)	
10+	0.0* (0.0–0.0)		0.2 (0.0–1.5)		
χ^2 (p-value)	336.1 (<0.001)*	199.7 (<0.001)*	15.5 (0.08)	17.7 (0.02)*	2.2 (0.90)

* Significant at the 0.05 level, two-sided test.
0.0* (0.0–0.0) OR is ≤ .05 indicating very low risk.
[a] Assessed in the Part 2 sample due to having Part 2 controls. Models control for person–years, country, and significant variables from the chapters on sociodemographics, parental psychopathology, childhood adversities, and traumatic events.
[b] For number of mental disorders, the last OR represents the odds for that number of disorders or more. For example, for unplanned attempt, 7 represents ≥7 (that is, 7+).

effects due to the incremental predictive power of individual disorders decaying as the number of comorbid disorders increases. This pattern was not observed consistently in the prediction of suicide plans and attempts among ideators. This same general pattern of findings was observed across high-, middle-, and low-income countries (see Appendix Tables 10.7–10.9).

Associations between mental disorders and early-, middle-, and late-onset suicidal behavior

Models testing the associations between mental disorders and suicide attempts across the lifespan were estimated by classifying age of onset into terciles and using the lowest tercile as the reference group (see Table 10.6). Results revealed that overall, most of the ORs estimated are below 1.0 for the middle and upper terciles, meaning that, in general, mental disorders are less predictive of suicide attempt later in life. The only two significant effects observed are for social phobia (OR=0.7) and depression (OR=0.6), with the findings suggesting lower odds of suicide attempt in the

presence of these disorders in the upper tercile. This same overall pattern is observed in high-, middle-, and low-income countries; however, social phobia and depression are not significantly associated with suicide attempts in any analysis, and the only significant finding observed is a lower odds of suicide attempts in the presence of alcohol use disorders among the upper tercile in middle-income countries (notably, a similar but non-significant effect is observed in low-income countries) (see Appendix Tables 10.10–10.12).

Mental disorders and the persistence of suicidal behavior

The results from the backward recurrence models revealed that most of the disorders examined are associated with the persistence of suicide ideation. Effects are substantially weaker for the prediction of suicide plans and attempts, although several significant associations emerged, with anxiety disorders showing the strongest and most consistent associations with suicide ideation, plan, and attempt (see Table 10.7). A similar overall pattern is observed across high-, middle-, and low-income countries (see Appendix Tables 10.13–10.15).

Table 10.6. Interactions between DSM-IV mental disorders and life course intervals[a] (all countries combined)

Interactions		Attempts among total sample	
		OR (95% CI)	χ^2 (p-value)
Anxiety disorders			
Panic disorder	middle 33%	–	0.1 (0.81)
	upper 33%	0.9 (0.6–1.6)	
Generalized anxiety disorder	middle 33%	0.9 (0.6–1.6)	1.5 (0.47)
	upper 33%	0.8 (0.5–1.3)	
Specific phobia	middle 33%	0.8 (0.6–1.1)	1.6 (0.45)
	upper 33%	0.9 (0.6–1.2)	
Social phobia	middle 33%	0.8 (0.6–1.2)	4.0 (0.13)
	upper 33%	0.7* (0.5–1.0)	
Posttraumatic stress	middle 33%	0.9 (0.5–1.4)	2.1 (0.35)
	upper 33%	1.2 (0.8–1.9)	
Separation anxiety disorder	middle 33%	1.5 (0.9–2.5)	3.1 (0.21)
	upper 33%	1.5 (0.9–2.5)	
Agoraphobia	middle 33%	–	0.4 (0.54)
	upper 33%	1.2 (0.7–2.1)	
Mood disorders			
Major depressive disorder	middle 33%	0.8 (0.6–1.2)	8.0 (0.02)*
	upper 33%	0.6* (0.4–0.9)	
Dysthymic disorder	middle 33%	–	2.7 (0.10)
	upper 33%	1.6 (0.9–2.7)	
Bipolar disorder	middle 33%	–	0.0 (0.89)
	upper 33%	1.0 (0.6–1.9)	
Impulse-control disorders			
Oppositional defiant disorder	middle 33%	–	–
	upper 33%	–	
Conduct disorder	middle 33%	–	–
	upper 33%	–	
Attention deficit hyperactivity disorder	middle 33%	–	–
	upper 33%	–	
Intermittent explosive disorder	middle 33%	0.7 (0.4–1.1)	2.5 (0.28)
	upper 33%	0.7 (0.5–1.2)	
Substance use disorders			
Alcohol abuse or dependence	middle 33%	0.9 (0.5–1.8)	3.6 (0.17)
	upper 33%	0.6 (0.3–1.2)	
Drug abuse or dependence	middle 33%	0.7 (0.3–1.5)	0.9 (0.63)
	upper 33%	0.7 (0.3–1.6)	
26 df χ2 test for all chronic conditions			33.2 (0.06)
25 df χ2 test for all conditions and dummies for number of conditions			43.7 (0.02)*

Table 10.6. (cont.)

Interactions		Attempts among total sample	
		OR (95% CI)	χ^2 (p-value)
Number of mental disorders			
2	middle 33%	0.8 (0.5–1.1)	
	upper 33%	0.9 (0.6–1.2)	
3	middle 33%	0.9 (0.5–1.5)	
	upper 33%	1.0 (0.6–1.6)	
4	middle 33%	–	
	upper 33%	0.7 (0.4–1.2)	
5	middle 33%	–	
	upper 33%	–	
6	middle 33%	–	
	upper 33%	–	
7	middle 33%	–	
	upper 33%	–	
8	middle 33%	–	
	upper 33%	–	
9+	middle 33%	–	
	upper 33%	–	

* Significant at the 0.05 level, two-sided test.
– Condition not included in model due to small cell size. Small cell size determined by calculating the expected number of cases of the condition based on the % of people with the outcome and the total number of people with the condition. If the expected value was less than 5, the condition was dropped from the model.
[a] Assessed in the Part 2 sample. Models control for person–years, country, and significant variables from the chapters on sociodemographics, parental psychopathology, childhood adversities, and traumatic events. Models also included all controls and interaction terms between life course intervals (intervals determined by the 33.3% percentiles of the age-of-onset for the outcome) and each control. Only the interaction terms between the life course intervals and mental disorder variables are shown in table.

The results of the more fine-grained logistic regression persistence models (results not reported in tables) similarly show that the presence of mental disorders are most predictive of the persistence of suicide ideation, with weaker associations for the prediction of suicide plans and attempts. Mental disorders are especially predictive of the persistence of suicide ideation beyond two years (significant ORs: specific phobia = 1.4, social phobia = 1.8, agoraphobia = 1.9, depression = 1.4, ODD=1.9), but not more persistence ideation, as only one of the 64 ORs estimated in the four models for more persistent ideation is significant – with CD predicting very high persistence of ideation (i.e., into the past year; OR=4.5). In the prediction of the persistence of suicide plans, only specific phobia (OR=1.4) and social phobia (OR=2.1) predict persistence beyond two years, bipolar disorder (OR=3.8) predicts persistence into the past five years; and panic (OR=3.3), dysthymic (OR=12.0), and conduct (OR=14.2) disorders predict very high persistence (i.e., into the past year among those with persistent plans). For suicide attempts, only panic (OR=2.3), social phobia (OR=1.6), and PTSD (OR=2.1) predict persistence beyond two years, and no disorders predict persistence of suicide attempts beyond that time.

Discussion

There are several important findings from this study. First, this study documents the prevalence of prior, specific mental disorders among those in the community who engage in suicidal behavior. Psychological autopsy studies and studies among clinical samples of suicide attempters consistently have reported high rates of mental disorders among those dying by suicide and making non-lethal suicide attempts, respectively (Bostwick & Pankratz, 2000; Cavanagh et al., 2003; Nock et al., 2008b). Prior studies

Table 10.7. Associations between DSM-IV mental disorders and persistence of suicidal behavior[a] (all countries combined)

Mental disorders	Ideation OR (95% CI)	Plan OR (95% CI)	Attempt OR (95% CI)
Anxiety disorders			
Panic disorder	1.7* (1.3–2.1)	2.0* (1.3–3.0)	1.8* (1.1–3.1)
Generalized anxiety disorder	1.2 (0.9–1.5)	1.4 (1.0–2.0)	1.1 (0.7–1.6)
Specific phobia	1.4* (1.2–1.7)	1.5* (1.1–1.9)	1.3 (0.9–1.9)
Social phobia	1.6* (1.3–1.9)	1.9* (1.4–2.6)	1.6* (1.1–2.4)
Posttraumatic stress	1.2 (1.0–1.5)	1.4 (1.0–1.9)	1.7* (1.2–2.5)
Separation anxiety disorder	1.4* (1.1–1.8)	1.5 (1.0–2.3)	1.3 (0.8–2.1)
Agoraphobia	2.0* (1.5–2.6)	1.9* (1.2–2.9)	2.0* (1.2–3.5)
Mood disorders			
Major depressive disorder	1.4* (1.2–1.7)	1.3* (1.0–1.7)	1.2 (0.9–1.6)
Dysthymic disorder	1.2 (0.9–1.5)	1.4 (0.9–2.1)	1.3 (0.7–2.3)
Bipolar disorder	1.4 (1.0–2.0)	1.5 (0.9–2.4)	0.9 (0.6–1.5)
Impulse-control disorders			
Oppositional defiant disorder	1.8* (1.3–2.5)	1.5 (0.9–2.4)	1.2 (0.7–2.0)
Conduct disorder	1.0 (0.7–1.4)	1.5 (0.8–2.5)	1.7 (1.0–3.1)
Attention deficit hyperactivity disorder	1.1 (0.9–1.5)	1.1 (0.7–1.7)	0.8 (0.5–1.4)
Intermittent explosive disorder	1.3 (1.0–1.6)	1.3 (0.9–2.0)	1.2 (0.8–1.9)
Substance use disorders			
Alcohol abuse or dependence	1.1 (0.8–1.3)	1.2 (0.8–1.7)	1.0 (0.7–1.6)
Drug abuse or dependence	1.1 (0.8–1.6)	1.0 (0.6–1.6)	1.2 (0.7–2.1)
16 df χ^2 test for 16 types	75.7 (<0.001)*	38.9 (0.001)*	27.3 (0.04)*
15 df χ^2 test for difference between types	44.6 (<0.001)*	19.8 (0.18)	22.2 (0.10)
Number of mental disorders[b]			
2	0.9 (0.7–1.2)	1.0 (0.7–1.4)	1.0 (0.7–1.7)
3	0.7 (0.5–1.0)	0.5* (0.3–0.8)	0.7 (0.4–1.3)
4	0.6 (0.4–1.0)	0.4* (0.2–0.9)	0.6 (0.3–1.5)
5	0.5 (0.3–1.0)	0.3* (0.1–0.7)	0.4 (0.1–1.3)
6	0.5 (0.2–1.1)	0.2* (0.1–0.7)	0.4 (0.1–1.6)
7	0.2* (0.1–0.5)	0.2* (0.0–0.7)	0.3 (0.1–2.2)
8+	0.2* (0.1–0.8)		
χ^2 (p-value)	16.3 (0.02)*	18.3 (0.01)*	4.6 (0.59)

* Significant at the 0.05 level, two-sided test.
– Dropped because the expected value is less than 5.
[a] Results are based on multivariate discrete time survival models. Models control for country, age-related variables, and significant variables from the chapters on sociodemographics, parental psychopathology, and childhood adversities. Neither types nor number of traumatic events were significant, so they were not included as part of the control.
[b] For number of mental disorders, the last OR represents the odds for that number of disorders or more. For example, for attempt, 7 represents ≥7 (that is, 7+).

using data from the WMH Surveys have revealed lower rates of mental disorders among those in the community who experience suicide ideation (42.9%–51.8%) or make a suicide attempt (54.6%–65.7%) (Nock et al., 2010a; Nock et al., 2009). The current study provides a much more fine-grained analysis of which disorders are most prevalent among those with suicidal behavior. When examined in this way, we see that individual disorders have relatively low prevalence rates (e.g., among suicide attempters, only 23.5% have a prior history of major depression), a pattern that replicates across high-, middle-, and low-income countries. These findings force us to rethink the common perception that most suicide attempters have major depression or some other specific disorder, and highlight the need to better understand what other (i.e., non-diagnostic) factors may increase the risk of suicidal behavior.

Second, this study adds to prior research demonstrating that a wide range of mental disorders predict subsequent suicidal behavior, and that much of the observed association between mental disorders and suicide attempts is explained by the occurrence of suicide ideation (Kessler et al., 1999; Nock et al., 2008a; Nock et al., 2009). Moreover, consistent with previous studies, the current results reveal that although depression is among the strongest risk factors for suicide ideation, it does not predict which people with suicide ideation go on to make a suicide plan and/or attempt. Instead, disorders characterized by anxiety and poor impulse-control (e.g., bipolar disorder, alcohol use disorder, PTSD, panic disorder) predict this transition. This pattern also is consistent across high-, middle-, and low-income countries illustrating the robust nature of this finding. The current study also replicates prior findings showing a strong dose–response relationship between the number of prior mental disorders and the odds of suicide ideation, plans, and attempts (Kessler et al., 1999; Nock et al., 2008a; Nock et al., 2009). This result now has been replicated across several different studies and countries; however, there is not yet a clear understanding of how or why the accumulation of mental disorders increases risk. It is possible that high comorbidity is associated with increasing distress, impairment, or disease burden (Angst et al., 2002; Hawton et al., 2003), which ultimately becomes too difficult for a person to tolerate, thus leading to suicide ideation or attempts. Another possibility is that with increasing comorbidity comes the likelihood of having

combinations of disorders that interact to lead to suicide attempts (e.g., major depression leads to suicide ideation, but one or more anxiety or impulse-control disorders are needed to then push the person to act on their suicide ideation). This remains an important unanswered question for future studies in this area.

Third, a new finding in this study is that the effects of mental disorders in predicting subsequent suicidal behavior are slightly, but consistently, weaker later in life. These effects are consistent across disorders and across countries; however, few of these effects are statistically significant and so we cannot draw any firm conclusions from these data. At the very least, this finding suggests that future studies should carefully examine the extent to which mental disorders predict subsequent suicidal behavior later in life. If these effects are replicated, this would suggest a need to identify what other factors may be more useful in predicting suicidal behavior later in life. Several possible sets of risk factors are covered elsewhere in this volume, including the experience of stressful life events such as the loss of a spouse (Chapter 9) and the experience of chronic and/or severe medical conditions such as cancer or heart disease (Chapter 11).

Fourth and finally, this study also reveals that beyond predicting the subsequent onset of suicidal behavior, mental disorders also predict the *persistence* of such behaviors over time. As in the prediction of the onset of suicidal behavior, disorders were most strongly predictive of suicide ideation and effects generally decreased in the prediction of the persistence of plans and attempts. Interestingly, anxiety disorders showed the strongest and most consistent effects in predicting the persistence of suicidal behavior, followed by impulse-control disorders. This pattern of findings may be due to the more persistent nature of anxiety disorders, and to some extent impulse-control disorders, compared to depression, which generally is more episodic in nature. That is, anxiety disorders may be associated with a more persistent pattern of distress that leads a person to repeatedly consider using suicide as a means of escaping this continual distress. It also was observed that mental disorders have the strongest effect in predicting the short-term persistence of suicidal behavior (i.e., over the two years after onset), but are weaker predictors of the long-term persistence. Although the reason for the association between the persistence of suicidal behavior and the occurrence of mental disorders is not yet known, this is a new and important finding that should be the focus of additional investigation in future studies.

Several key limitations should be kept in mind when interpreting these results. First, although the WMH data are from large representative surveys conducted in 21 different countries, several were not nationally representative, an important factor in trying to make inferences about the populations from which these samples were drawn. Moreover, participating countries are not representative of all countries in the world, further limiting the generality of these findings. A related limitation is that survey response rates varied across participating countries. We controlled for differential response using poststratification adjustments; however, it is possible that response rates are related to the occurrence of mental disorders or suicidal behavior – a fact that could bias cross-national comparisons. These study limitations affect the results presented in each chapter of the book and should be borne in mind when interpreting all results of this study.

Second, the retrospective self-report nature of these data introduces potential problems such as under-reporting of mental disorders and suicidal behavior and biased recall of such problems, especially for disorders of childhood and adolescence (Angold et al., 1996). We attempted to limit this latter concern by focusing only on the diagnosis of such disorders among those <44 years old at the time of their interview, but this does not completely eliminate this concern. On the other hand, systematic reviews have proposed that people are able to recall prior experiences accurately enough to provide useful information (Brewin et al., 1993; Hardt & Rutter, 2004). Moreover, retrospective data are especially valuable when prospective data are unavailable, such as in the current study (Schlesselman, 1982). Another potential limitation regarding the nature of these self-report data is that cultural factors could have affected respondents' willingness to report on suicidal behavior and the occurrence of mental disorders (Alonso et al., 2008) along with their interpretation of interview questions assessing these constructs (Lopez & Guarnaccia, 2000; Thakker & Ward, 1998).

Third, although the WMH Survey assesses several different forms of suicidal behavior (i.e., suicide ideation, plans, attempts) and a range of different mental disorders and their comorbidity, this study did not include the full range of possible suicidal behaviors (e.g., did not assess suicide gestures, preparatory acts)

or mental disorders (e.g., psychotic disorders, obsessive compulsive disorder, personality disorders). In addition, although we examined the persistence of suicidal behavior, we did not examine here the effects of the persistence of mental disorders, nor did we test the effects of factors such as the severity or complexity of each disorder. This could have led to an underestimate of the effects of mental disorders on suicidal behavior. For example, disorder persistence and/or severity may be strong predictors of the transition from suicide ideation to plans or attempts, or of the persistence of suicidal behavior. Research questions such as these can be examined in future studies using the WMH data and await empirical focus in future studies.

Future directions

The results of this study highlight important directions for future work in the domains of science, practice, and policy that have the potential to improve the understanding and prevention of suicide. Scientifically, this study demonstrates the usefulness of examining a range of suicidal outcomes (including the persistence of suicidal behavior), controlling for diagnostic comorbidity when testing the effects of mental disorders on suicidal outcomes, and of considering how effects may differ across time (i.e., life course) and space (i.e., cross-nationally). Additional large-scale studies of suicidal behavior are needed to more carefully and precisely study how and why mental disorders may increase the risk of suicidal behavior.

Clinically, this study highlights the importance of assessing not only for depression among those who may be at risk for suicidal behavior, but also for the broader range of mental disorders and for diagnostic comorbidity. Clinicians should assess for risk of suicide whenever presented with patients with multimorbidity, and also should be aware of the significant associations among mental disorders and the persistence of suicidal behavior. Finally, the fact that mental disorders are somewhat less predictive of suicidal behavior in older adults suggests that clinicians working with older patients should weight these factors accordingly, and perhaps assess for other factors that may increase suicide risk, such as the loss of a loved one (Chapter 9) or the experience of a significant medical condition (Chapter 11).

Finally, these findings have important implications for public health efforts aimed at suicide prevention.

Specifically, these findings show that a wide range of mental disorders are significant risk factors for suicidal behavior, which suggests that cross-national prevention aimed at screening and treating mental disorders may help to reduce suicidal behavior worldwide. There is growing evidence that such programs can indeed have an impact on the rates of suicidal behavior (Hampton, 2010; Mann et al., 2005). Unfortunately, resources devoted to such programs are lacking around the world, especially in low-income countries (Vijayakumar, 2004; Wang et al., 2007; WMH Consortium, 2004). Taken together, the available data suggest that mental disorders are strongly predictive of suicidal behavior and that enhancing screening and treatment efforts focused on depression can reduce suicidal behavior; however, such programs are simply not disseminated or used around the world. Serious efforts are needed to address this enormous gap.

Importantly, focusing only on the presence of mental disorders would be insufficient, as our results show that many people with suicidal behavior do not meet criteria for any prior mental disorder. This makes identifying those at risk much more difficult and underscores the need for new methods of suicide risk assessment (e.g., Nock & Banaji, 2007; Nock et al., 2010b). Despite the identification of risk factors for suicidal behavior in this chapter and throughout this volume, there remains much work to be done before we are able to accurately identify those at risk and intervene in a way that decreases their likelihood of suicidal behavior and suicide death. The results of the current study provide another small step in the right direction, but significant future efforts are needed to better prevent the enormous loss of life resulting from suicide.

Acknowledgements

Portions of this chapter are based on Nock, M. K., Hwang, I., Sampson, N., Kessler, R. C., Angermeyer, M., Beautrais, A., et al. (2009). Cross-national analysis of the associations among mental disorders and suicidal behavior: findings from the WHO World Mental Health Surveys. *PLoS Med.*, 6(8), e1000123. doi.10.1371/journal. pmed.1000123. Reproduced with permission.

References

Alonso, J., Buron, A., Bruffaerts, R., et al. (2008). Association of perceived stigma and mood and anxiety disorders: results from the World Mental Health Surveys. *Acta Psychiatrica Scandinavica*, 118(4), 305–314.

Angold, A., Erkanli, A., Costello, E. J., & Rutter, M. (1996). Precision, reliability and accuracy in the dating of symptom onsets in child and adolescent psychopathology. *Journal of Child Psychology and Psychiatry*, 37(6), 657–664.

Angst, J., Sellaro, R., & Ries Merikangas, K. (2002). Multimorbidity of psychiatric disorders as an indicator of clinical severity. *European Archives of Psychiatry and Clinical Neuroscience*, 252(4), 147–154.

Bostwick, J. M., & Pankratz, V. S. (2000). Affective disorders and suicide risk: a reexamination. *American Journal of Psychiatry*, 157(12), 1925–1932.

Brewin, C. R., Andrews, B., & Gotlib, I. H. (1993). Psychopathology and early experience: a reappraisal of retrospective reports. *Psychological Bulletin*, 113(1), 82–98.

Cavanagh, J. T., Carson, A. J., Sharpe, M., & Lawrie, S. M. (2003). Psychological autopsy studies of suicide: a systematic review. *Psychological Medicine*, 33(3), 395–405.

Goldsmith, S. K., Pellmar, T. C., Kleinman, A. M., & Bunney, W. E. (eds.). (2002). *Reducing suicide: A national imperative*. Washington, DC: The National Academies Press.

Hampton, T. (2010). Depression care effort brings dramatic drop in large HMO population's suicide rate. *Journal of the American Medical Association*, 303(19), 1903–1905.

Hardt, J., & Rutter, M. (2004). Validity of adult retrospective reports of adverse childhood experiences: review of the evidence. *Journal of Child Psychology and Psychiatry*, 45(2), 260–273.

Harris, E. C., & Barraclough, B. (1997). Suicide as an outcome for mental disorders. A meta-analysis. *British Journal of Psychiatry*, 170, 205–228.

Hawton, K., Houston, K., Haw, C., Townsend, E., & Harriss, L. (2003). Comorbidity of Axis I and Axis II disorders in patients who attempted suicide. *American Journal of Psychiatry*, 160(8), 1494–1500.

Kessler, R. C., Berglund, P., Borges, G., Nock, M. K., & Wang, P. S. (2005a). Trends in suicide ideation, plans, gestures, and attempts in the United States, 1990–1992 to 2001–2003. *Journal of the American Medical Association*, 293(20), 2487–2495.

Kessler, R. C., Borges, G., & Walters, E. E. (1999). Prevalence of and risk factors for lifetime suicide attempts in the National Comorbidity Survey. *Archives of General Psychiatry*, 56(7), 617–626.

Kessler, R. C., Chiu, W. T., Demler, O., Merikangas, K. R., & Walters, E. E. (2005b). Prevalence, severity, and comorbidity of 12-month DSM-IV disorders in the National Comorbidity Survey Replication. *Archives of General Psychiatry*, 62(6), 617–627.

Lopez, S. R., & Guarnaccia, P. J. (2000). Cultural psychopathology: uncovering the social world of mental illness. *Annual Review of Psychology*, **51**, 571–598.

Mann, J. J., Apter, A., Bertolote, J., et al. (2005). Suicide prevention strategies: a systematic review. *Journal of the American Medical Association*, **294**(16), 2064–2074.

Moscicki, E. K. (1999). Epidemiology of suicide. In D. G. Jacobs (ed.), *The Harvard Medical School guide to suicide assessment and intervention*, pp. 40–51. San Francisco, CA: Jossey-Bass.

Nock, M. K., & Banaji, M. R. (2007). Prediction of suicide ideation and attempts among adolescents using a brief performance-based test. *Journal of Consulting and Clinical Psychology*, **75**(6), 707–715.

Nock, M. K., Borges, G., Bromet, E. J., et al. (2008a). Cross-national prevalence and risk factors for suicidal ideation, plans, and attempts in the WHO World Mental Health Surveys. *British Journal of Psychiatry*, **192**(2), 98–105.

Nock, M. K., Borges, G., Bromet, E. J., et al. (2008b). Suicide and suicidal behavior. *Epidemiologic Reviews*, **30**, 133–154.

Nock, M. K., Hwang, I., Sampson, N., & Kessler, R. C. (2010a). Mental disorders, comorbidity, and suicidal behaviors: results from the National Comorbidity Survey Replication. *Molecular Psychiatry*, **15**(8), 868–876.

Nock, M. K., Hwang, I., Sampson, N., et al. (2009). Cross-national analysis of the associations among mental disorders and suicidal behavior: findings from the WHO World Mental Health Surveys. *PLoS Medicine*, **6**(8), e1000123.

Nock, M. K., Park, J. M., Finn, C. T., et al. (2010b). Measuring the suicidal mind: implicit cognition predicts suicidal behavior. *Psychological Science*, **21**(4), 511–517.

Phillips, M. R., Yang, G., Li, S., & Li, Y. (2004). Suicide and the unique prevalence pattern of schizophrenia in mainland China: a retrospective observational study. *Lancet*, **364**(9439), 1062–1068.

Phillips, M. R., Yang, G., Zhang, Y., et al. (2002). Risk factors for suicide in China: a national case-control psychological autopsy study. *Lancet*, **360**(9347), 1728–1736.

Pokorny, A. D. (1983). Prediction of suicide in psychiatric patients. Report of a prospective study. *Archives of General Psychiatry*, **40**(3), 249–257.

Sareen, J., Cox, B. J., Afifi, T. O., et al. (2005). Anxiety disorders and risk for suicidal ideation and suicide attempts: a population-based longitudinal study of adults. *Archives of General Psychiatry*, **62**(11), 1249–1257.

Schlesselman, J. J. (1982). *Case-control Studies: Design, Conduct, and Analysis*. New York, NY: Oxford University Press.

Thakker, J., & Ward, T. (1998). Culture and classification: the cross-cultural application of the DSM-IV. *Clinical Psychology Review*, **18**(5), 501–529.

Vijayakumar, L. (2004). Suicide prevention: the urgent need in developing countries. *World Psychiatry*, **3**(3), 158–159.

Vijayakumar, L., John, S., Pirkis, J., & Whiteford, H. (2005). Suicide in developing countries (2): risk factors. *Crisis*, **26**(3), 112–119.

Wang, P. S., Aguilar-Gaxiola, S., Alonso, J., et al. (2007). Use of mental health services for anxiety, mood, and substance disorders in 17 countries in the WHO World Mental Health Surveys. *Lancet*, **370**(9590), 841–850.

Weissman, M. M., Bland, R. C., Canino, G. J., et al. (1999). Prevalence of suicide ideation and suicide attempts in nine countries. *Psychological Medicine*, **29**(1), 9–17.

Weissman, M. M., Klerman, G. L., Markowitz, J. S., & Ouellette, R. (1989). Suicidal ideation and suicide attempts in panic disorder and attacks. *New England Journal of Medicine*, **321**(18), 1209–1214.

WHO. (2008). *World Health Organization: Suicide Prevention (SUPRE)*. Retrieved June 20, 2008, from http://www.who.int/mental_health/prevention/suicide/suicideprevent/en/.

WMH Consortium. (2004). WHO World Mental Health Consortium. Prevalence, severity, and unmet need for treatment of mental disorders in the World Health Organization World Mental Health Surveys. *Journal of the American Medical Association*, **291**(21), 2581–2590.

Chapter

11

Chronic physical conditions and the onset of suicidal behavior

Kate M. Scott, Wai Tat Chiu, Irving Hwang, Guilherme Borges, Silvia Florescu, Daphna Levinson, Josep Maria Haro, Nancy A. Sampson, Ronald C. Kessler, and Matthew K. Nock

Introduction

Does the experience of a debilitating chronic physical condition place the sufferer at an increased risk of suicide? To clinicians, who witness the disability and pain their patients experience, and to the lay public, who either experience such conditions themselves or have family members who do so, the answer may seem to be self-evident. The impression that physical conditions are associated with suicide is borne out by the research, at least for some conditions (see Harris & Barraclough, 1994; Quan et al., 2002; Stenager & Stenager, 2000 for reviews). Although the methodology and results from these studies vary considerably, collectively they suggest that cancer, HIV/AIDS, renal disease, and some neurological conditions (e.g., Huntington's disease, stroke, epilepsy, multiple sclerosis, spinal cord lesions) are associated with completed suicides.

Yet there remains an important unanswered research question, which is at the heart of the debate over euthanasia, and of clinical concern: to what extent do those who contemplate or complete suicide when experiencing chronic physical conditions do so with judgment unimpaired by depression or other mental disorders? Most of the studies on suicide mortality have not determined whether these associations are independent of mental disorders (Harris & Barraclough, 1994; Stenager & Stenager, 2000), and, indeed, some researchers have assumed that mental disorders are the link between physical conditions and suicide (Bebbington et al., 1991). There are a small number of suicide mortality studies that have measured and, therefore, been able to control for mental disorders, and some of these have found cancer to be independently associated with suicide (Quan et al., 2002; Rockett et al.,

2007; Waern et al., 2002), though not all studies have shown this association (Henriksson et al., 1995). For other physical conditions, the findings are conflicting (see Quan et al., 2002; Waern et al., 2002), and in general, mortality studies that have controlled for mental disorders are too few in number to determine whether there are reliable associations between physical conditions and suicide independent of mental disorders.

This chapter concerns suicide attempts rather than suicide mortality, with the data drawn from general population samples. The use of general population samples offers two related methodological advantages over many of the mortality studies. First, it provides an appropriate general population comparison group, the lack of which has been a problem for many of the mortality studies (Stenager & Stenager, 2000). Second, the fact that the group with physical conditions also are drawn from the general population means that the associations we observe are not biased either by the greater severity of hospitalized patients, or by the experience of hospitalization itself.

Compared to studies on the association of physical conditions with suicide mortality, there have been relatively few studies using suicidal behavior as the outcome of interest, and the studies that have been done in this area vary greatly in methodology. For example, some studies have focused on ideation and others on attempts (Fairweather et al., 2006; Goodwin et al., 2003a; Goodwin et al., 2003b); the age range of study participants varies (Druss & Pincus, 2000; Lawrence et al., 2000); and studies also vary in the type(s) of physical conditions included (Beautrais, 2002; Brennan Braden & Sullivan, 2008; Goodwin et al., 2003a; Gupta et al., 1997; Rasic et al., 2008; Tang & Crange, 2006). This

Suicide, eds. Matthew K. Nock, Guilherme Borges, and Yutaka Ono. Published by Cambridge University Press.
© World Health Organization 2012.

degree of methodological variability, especially when it is among a relatively small number of studies, makes it virtually impossible to arrive at conclusions about the associations between physical conditions and suicidal behavior from the extant literature. One finding of interest though, which is fairly consistent among these studies of suicidal behavior, is that although several physical conditions have been found to be associated with suicidal behavior, once mental disorders are included in the models (where such data has been collected), few physical conditions remain significantly associated with the outcomes, and there is little consistency in which conditions those are (Druss & Pincus, 2000; Goodwin et al., 2003a; Goodwin et al., 2003b).

This chapter presents analyses investigating the association of a range of *temporally prior* physical conditions with the subsequent *first onset* of suicide ideation, plans, and attempts. These analyses are novel in a number of respects. We adjust for a much wider range of psychosocial, demographic, and socioeconomic covariates than has been included in prior research, in addition to adjustment for mental disorders. We investigate the association between *number* and *type* of physical condition and suicide outcomes, and take their mutual influence into account in final estimates. We also examine whether associations between physical conditions and suicidal behavior differ according to when in the life course the suicidal behavior occurs. Lastly, we provide the first investigation of whether associations vary across lower- and higher-income countries, prompted by the suggestion that in developing countries factors other than mental disorders (such as physical illness) may more strongly predict suicidal behavior (Maselko & Patel, 2008). This chapter represents an extension of an earlier paper using the same data (Scott et al., 2010) by providing a much greater level of detail regarding the associations between physical conditions and suicidal behavior, including the results from the analyses of how these effects vary across the lifespan, the extent to which they are consistent across high-income, and lower-income countries, and whether chronic physical conditions are associated with the persistence of suicidal behavior.

Method

A detailed description of the respondent samples, study procedures, statistical analyses, and assessment of suicidal behavior is provided in Chapter 3 of this volume. The assessment and analysis of

sociodemographic factors (Chapter 6), parental psychopathology (Chapter 7), childhood adversities (Chapter 8), traumatic events during adulthood (Chapter 9), and mental disorders (Chapter 10), which are included as covariates in the following analyses, are described in those earlier chapters. One notable difference from the earlier chapters is that this chapter uses data from only 14 of the 22 World Mental Health (WMH) Surveys because not all surveys collected information on the age-of-onset of the physical conditions. The surveys included here are: Colombia, Mexico, United States, Shenzhen (China), Japan, New Zealand, Belgium, France, Germany, Italy, the Netherlands, Romania, Spain, and Israel (Part 1 n = 72,181; Part 2 n = 37,915; response rate = 69.0%). The World Bank (2008) classifies Belgium, France, Germany, Israel, Italy, Japan, the Netherlands, New Zealand, Spain, and the United States as high-income countries, and classifies Mexico, Romania, China, and Colombia, as middle- or low-income countries (hereafter referred to as lower-income countries).

Assessment of physical conditions

Physical conditions were assessed using a checklist adapted from the U.S. Health Interview Schedule. Respondents were asked: "*Have you ever had . . . arthritis or rheumatism; chronic back or neck problems; frequent or severe headaches; any other chronic pain; seasonal allergies like hay fever; a stroke; a heart attack?*". They were then asked: "*Did a doctor or other health professional ever tell you that you had . . . heart disease; high blood pressure; asthma; tuberculosis; any other chronic lung disease (like COPD or emphysema); diabetes or high blood sugar; an ulcer in the stomach or intestine; HIV infection or AIDS; epilepsy or seizures; cancer?*". Additionally, respondents were asked how old they were when they were first diagnosed with the condition or first had the condition. For these analyses, heart attack and stroke were collapsed into one category, as were respiratory conditions (i.e., asthma, COPD, emphysema, tuberculosis). HIV/AIDS could not be included due to small numbers.

Results

Prevalence of physical conditions among those with suicidal behavior

The prevalence of each physical condition among those with each suicidal behavior is shown in Table 11.1.

Table 11.1. Prevalence of physical conditions in those with suicidal behavior (all countries combined)

Physical conditions	Among total sample — %[a] (SE) with chronic condition						Among ideators — %[a] (SE) with chronic condition			
	Ideation	No ideation	Attempt	No attempt	Plan	No plan	Planned attempt	No planned attempt	Unplanned attempt	No unplanned attempt
Cancer	0.7 (0.1)	0.8 (0.1)	1.0 (0.2)	0.7 (0.1)	1.0 (0.2)	2.2 (0.3)	1.2 (0.3)	2.7 (0.6)	0.7 (0.3)	1.6 (0.3)
Cardiovascular										
Heart disease	2.0 (0.2)	1.7 (0.1)	1.6 (0.3)	1.7 (0.1)	1.8 (0.4)	3.6 (0.4)	1.1 (0.3)	3.7 (0.8)	2.5 (0.8)	3.7 (0.5)
High blood pressure	4.6 (0.3)	4.5 (0.1)	4.9 (0.7)	4.6 (0.1)	5.2 (0.6)	9.5 (0.6)	4.3 (0.7)	9.3 (1.3)	6.2 (1.3)	9.4 (0.6)
Heart attack or stroke	1.2 (0.2)	1.0 (0.1)	1.3 (0.3)	0.9 (0.1)	1.2 (0.3)	2.4 (0.2)	1.2 (0.3)	1.5 (0.4)	1.2 (0.5)	2.2 (0.3)
Diabetes	0.8 (0.1)	1.0 (0.0)	0.7 (0.2)	1.0 (0.0)	0.5 (0.2)	2.1 (0.2)	0.5 (0.2)	2.8 (0.8)	1.0 (0.4)	2.2 (0.3)
Ulcer	4.1 (0.3)	2.6 (0.1)	4.0 (0.5)	2.7 (0.1)	4.5 (0.5)	6.9 (0.6)	4.2 (0.7)	7.8 (1.3)	3.6 (1.0)	6.4 (0.6)
Musculoskeletal										
Arthritis	7.6 (0.4)	7.0 (0.1)	7.2 (0.7)	7.0 (0.1)	8.1 (0.7)	14.4 (0.8)	6.8 (0.9)	17.3 (1.7)	7.6 (1.4)	14.3 (0.8)
Back and neck pain	15.6 (0.6)	10.2 (0.2)	14.4 (1.0)	10.6 (0.2)	16.7 (1.0)	26.9 (0.9)	13.4 (1.1)	30.6 (2.2)	15.5 (1.9)	27.7 (1.0)
Headache	18.2 (0.6)	8.1 (0.2)	19.9 (1.2)	8.6 (0.2)	20.1 (1.1)	25.2 (1.0)	20.1 (1.5)	28.3 (2.3)	19.3 (1.8)	24.9 (1.1)
Other chronic pain	5.8 (0.4)	2.9 (0.1)	7.3 (0.7)	3.1 (0.1)	7.1 (0.7)	9.9 (0.6)	6.1 (0.8)	12.8 (1.6)	8.6 (1.6)	8.4 (0.7)
Respiratory										
Allergies	15.4 (0.6)	9.2 (0.2)	16.1 (1.1)	9.5 (0.2)	16.4 (1.1)	20.7 (0.9)	15.0 (1.3)	23.2 (1.9)	18.2 (2.1)	20.6 (1.0)
Other respiratory	10.7 (0.5)	5.1 (0.1)	12.0 (0.9)	5.2 (0.1)	12.7 (1.0)	11.6 (0.7)	11.4 (1.1)	14.7 (1.8)	12.9 (1.7)	10.7 (0.7)
Epilepsy	0.4 (0.1)	0.1 (0.0)	0.7 (0.3)	0.1 (0.0)	0.5 (0.2)	0.8 (0.2)	0.7 (0.4)	0.4 (0.2)	0.8 (0.4)	0.8 (0.3)
Number of physical conditions										
1	27.2 (0.7)	18.3 (0.2)	27.0 (1.2)	18.5 (0.2)	26.8 (1.1)	26.8 (0.8)	28.3 (1.6)	24.2 (1.7)	24.9 (2.0)	28.0 (1.0)
2	12.2 (0.5)	7.9 (0.1)	13.3 (1.0)	8.2 (0.1)	13.7 (0.9)	17.3 (0.7)	12.7 (1.1)	19.0 (1.4)	15.1 (1.8)	17.9 (0.8)
3	5.1 (0.3)	3.2 (0.1)	5.5 (0.6)	3.3 (0.1)	6.4 (0.6)	10.3 (0.5)	5.1 (0.7)	13.2 (1.3)	6.0 (1.0)	9.8 (0.6)
4	2.6 (0.3)	1.4 (0.0)	1.9 (0.3)	1.4 (0.0)	2.5 (0.4)	5.5 (0.4)	2.0 (0.4)	6.5 (0.9)	1.8 (0.6)	5.5 (0.5)
5+	1.7 (0.2)	0.9 (0.0)	2.4 (0.5)	0.9 (0.0)	2.2 (0.4)	3.9 (0.3)	1.5 (0.4)	4.9 (0.8)	3.4 (1.2)	3.2 (0.4)
N[b]	(6320)	(144,575)	(207.2)	(150,737)	(2369)	(6709)	(1271)	(1552)	(710)	(5165)

[a] % represents the percentage of people with the chronic condition among the cases with the outcome variable indicated in the column header. For example, the first cell is the % of those with cancer among those with ideation.

[b] Number of cases with the outcome variable; N represents the number of person–years.

The difference in prevalence among the physical conditions for any given outcome (e.g., among attempters in the total sample, 1.6% for heart disease; 4.9% for high blood pressure; 14.4% for back/neck pain) reflects the differing prevalence of the physical conditions in the general population. The differences in prevalence between those with and without each suicide outcome (e.g., 1.6% heart disease prevalence among attempters in the total sample versus 1.7% among those not making an attempt) do not meaningfully reflect associations between the physical condition and the outcome because these prevalence rates are not adjusted for age, which is positively associated with physical conditions but negatively associated with suicidal behavior.

Association between type of physical condition and suicidal behavior

The bivariate associations between individual types of physical condition and the five suicide outcomes are shown in Table 11.2. These associations are adjusted for sociodemographics, parental psychopathology, childhood adversities, and traumatic events, but not for other physical conditions. Most physical conditions are significantly associated with suicide ideation in the total sample, and several physical conditions (i.e., high blood pressure, heart attack/stroke, arthritis, headache, other chronic pain, respiratory conditions) are associated with attempts in the total sample. These latter associations are presumably

Table 11.2. Bivariate models for associations between physical conditions and suicidal behavior[a] (all countries combined)

	Among total sample		Among ideators		
	Ideation	Attempt	Plan	Planned attempt	Unplanned attempt
Physical conditions	OR (95% CI)	OR (95% CI)	OR (95% CI)	OR (95% CI)	OR (95% CI)
Cancer	0.9 (0.6–1.4)	1.4 (0.8–2.4)	0.9 (0.5–1.6)	1.8 (0.9–3.8)	1.3 (0.5–3.1)
Cardiovascular					
Heart disease	1.4* (1.1–1.9)	1.2 (0.7–1.8)	0.8 (0.5–1.4)	0.6 (0.3–1.3)	1.5 (0.8–3.0)
High blood pressure	1.2* (1.0–1.5)	1.5* (1.1–2.0)	1.0 (0.8–1.4)	1.1 (0.7–1.7)	1.6 (1.0–2.6)
Heart attack or stroke	1.8* (1.3–2.5)	1.9* (1.2–3.2)	0.9 (0.6–1.5)	2.0 (0.8–5.0)	1.4 (0.5–4.0)
Diabetes	1.1 (0.8–1.6)	1.2 (0.7–2.1)	0.7 (0.4–1.2)	0.9 (0.4–2.2)	1.9 (0.8–4.5)
Ulcer	1.3* (1.1–1.6)	1.2 (0.9–1.6)	1.1 (0.8–1.4)	1.0 (0.5–1.8)	1.1 (0.6–2.1)
Musculoskeletal					
Arthritis	1.4* (1.2–1.6)	1.4* (1.1–1.8)	1.0 (0.8–1.3)	0.9 (0.6–1.3)	1.2 (0.8–1.8)
Back and neck pain	1.3* (1.2–1.5)	1.1 (0.9–1.3)	0.9 (0.8–1.1)	0.6* (0.4–0.9)	0.9 (0.7–1.3)
Headache	1.7* (1.5–1.8)	1.4* (1.2–1.7)	0.9 (0.8–1.1)	0.8 (0.6–1.1)	0.9 (0.7–1.3)
Other chronic pain	1.4* (1.2–1.7)	1.6* (1.3–2.1)	1.0 (0.8–1.3)	0.8 (0.5–1.1)	1.8* (1.2–2.9)
Respiratory					
Allergies	1.0 (0.9–1.1)	1.0 (0.8–1.2)	0.9 (0.7–1.0)	0.7 (0.5–1.0)	1.1 (0.8–1.5)
Other respiratory	1.3* (1.1–1.5)	1.3* (1.1–1.6)	1.1 (0.9–1.4)	0.9 (0.7–1.3)	1.4 (1.0–2.0)
Epilepsy	2.6* (1.4–5.1)	–	1.2 (0.5–2.8)	3.5* (1.1–11.2)	–

* Significant at the 0.05 level, two-sided test.
– Condition not included in model due to small cell size. Small cell size determined by calculating the expected number of cases of the condition based on the % of people with the outcome and the total number of people with the condition. If the expected value was less than 5, the condition was dropped from the model.
[a] Models estimate one physical condition at a time and control for person–years, country, and significant variables from the chapters on sociodemographics, parental psychopathology, childhood adversities, and traumatic events.

Table 11.3. Multivariate models for associations between each type of physical condition and suicidal behavior, controlling for other types[a] (all countries combined)

Physical conditions	Among total sample		Among ideators		
	Ideation	Attempt	Plan	Planned attempt	Unplanned attempt
	OR (95% CI)	OR (95% CI)	OR (95% CI)	OR (95% CI)	OR (95% CI)
Cancer	0.9 (0.6–1.3)	1.3 (0.8–2.2)	0.9 (0.5–1.6)	1.9 (0.9–4.1)	1.2 (0.5–2.9)
Cardiovascular					
Heart disease	1.2 (0.8–1.6)	0.9 (0.6–1.4)	0.8 (0.5–1.4)	0.6 (0.3–1.2)	1.3 (0.7–2.5)
High blood pressure	1.1 (0.9–1.3)	1.3 (1.0–1.8)	1.0 (0.8–1.4)	1.1 (0.7–1.8)	1.5 (0.9–2.4)
Heart attack or stroke	1.5* (1.1–2.1)	1.7* (1.0–2.9)	1.0 (0.6–1.7)	2.0 (0.8–5.3)	1.1 (0.4–3.0)
Diabetes	1.0 (0.7–1.4)	0.9 (0.5–1.7)	0.6 (0.4–1.2)	0.8 (0.3–2.1)	1.6 (0.7–4.0)
Ulcer	1.2 (1.0–1.4)	1.0 (0.8–1.4)	1.1 (0.8–1.4)	1.0 (0.6–1.9)	1.1 (0.6–2.0)
Musculoskeletal					
Arthritis	1.2* (1.1–1.5)	1.3 (1.0–1.6)	1.0 (0.8–1.3)	1.0 (0.7–1.5)	1.1 (0.7–1.6)
Back and neck pain	1.2* (1.1–1.3)	0.9 (0.8–1.2)	0.9 (0.8–1.1)	0.7* (0.5–0.9)	0.9 (0.6–1.2)
Headache	1.6* (1.4–1.7)	1.4* (1.1–1.6)	1.0 (0.8–1.1)	0.9 (0.7–1.2)	0.9 (0.6–1.1)
Other chronic pain	1.2* (1.0–1.4)	1.5* (1.2–1.9)	1.0 (0.8–1.3)	0.9 (0.6–1.3)	1.9* (1.2–3.0)
Respiratory					
Allergies	0.9 (0.8–1.0)	0.9 (0.8–1.1)	0.8 (0.7–1.0)	0.7 (0.5–1.0)	1.0 (0.7–1.4)
Other respiratory	1.3* (1.1–1.5)	1.3* (1.0–1.6)	1.2 (1.0–1.5)	1.1 (0.7–1.5)	1.4 (0.9–2.0)
Epilepsy	2.1* (1.1–4.1)	–	1.2 (0.5–2.8)	3.3* (1.1–10.4)	–
χ^2 (p-value)	176.5 (<0.001)*	49.1 (<0.001)*	10.1 (0.69)	22.1 (0.05)	14.5 (0.27)

* Significant at the 0.05 level, two-sided test.
– Condition not included in model due to small cell size. Small cell size determined by calculating the expected number of cases of the condition based on the % of people with the outcome and the total number of people with the condition. If the expected value was less than 5, the condition was dropped from the model.
[a] Models include all physical conditions and control for person–years, country, and significant variables from the chapters on sociodemographics, parental psychopathology, childhood adversities, and traumatic events.

largely a function of the association of physical conditions with ideation, as only epilepsy is positively associated with attempts once ideation is taken into account.

Table 11.3 presents the results from an additive multivariate model that estimates associations between each type of physical condition and the suicide outcomes, adjusting for controls and for other physical conditions. The significant chi-square values for ideation (176.5) and attempts (49.1) in the total sample indicate that there are significant differences among types of physical conditions in their associations with the outcomes. Most of the physical conditions are associated with ideation,

with epilepsy being the most strongly associated (OR = 2.1), but most conditions are not associated with predicting which ideators make plans or attempts. Exceptions to this are that epilepsy is associated with increased odds of planned attempt among ideators, other chronic pain with increased odds of unplanned attempt among ideators, and back and neck pain with decreased odds of planned attempt among ideators. The ORs generally are smaller in this model than in the bivariate model, reflecting correction for over-estimation of effects of individual physical condition types in the bivariate model, which does not take physical condition comorbidity into account.

Table 11.4. Model for associations between number of physical conditions and suicidal behavior[a] (all countries combined)

Number of physical conditions	Among total sample		Among ideators		
	Ideation	Attempt	Plan	Planned attempt	Unplanned attempt
	OR (95% CI)	OR (95% CI)	OR (95% CI)	OR (95% CI)	OR (95% CI)
1	1.5* (1.4–1.7)	1.5* (1.3–1.7)	1.0 (0.8–1.2)	1.1 (0.8–1.5)	0.9 (0.7–1.2)
2	1.5* (1.3–1.7)	1.4* (1.2–1.8)	0.9 (0.8–1.2)	0.7 (0.5–1.0)	1.2 (0.9–1.7)
3	1.7* (1.5–2.0)	1.5* (1.2–2.0)	0.9 (0.7–1.2)	0.6* (0.4–1.0)	1.1 (0.7–1.7)
4	2.0* (1.6–2.7)	1.3 (0.9–2.0)	0.8 (0.6–1.2)	0.6 (0.4–1.1)	0.8 (0.4–1.6)
5+	2.5* (1.8–3.7)	2.9* (1.7–4.9)	1.0 (0.7–1.4)	0.7 (0.4–1.4)	3.6* (1.7–7.7)
χ^2 (p-value)	124.3 (<0.001)*	37.5 (<0.001)*	1.4 (0.92)	12.8 (0.03)*	13.5 (0.02)*

*Significant at the 0.05 level, two-sided test.
[a] Model controls for person–years, country, and significant variables from the chapters on sociodemographics, parental psychopathology, childhood adversities, and traumatic events.

Association between number of physical conditions and suicidal behavior

The next model (see Table 11.4) considers the association between number of physical conditions and suicidal behavior. It appears that the risk of ideation and attempts in the total sample increases as the number of physical conditions increases. However, this model does not take into account the type of condition, and it assumes an additive relationship between number of conditions and the suicide outcome. The next model, which does take type into account, and which removes the additive assumption, gives a different perspective on the association between number of conditions and suicide outcomes.

Associations between physical conditions and suicidal behavior, controlling for number and type

The final multivariate model shown in Table 11.5 is a non-additive model that includes both type and number of physical conditions and considers their independent associations with the outcomes. This model is a better fit than the previous models, which consider only type or only number of physical conditions. Physical condition type remains significantly associated with suicide ideation after allowing for the number of physical conditions ($\chi^2 = 145.2$, p<0.001), and it is also the case that there is significant variability among physical condition types in their associations with ideation ($\chi^2 = 64.1$, p<0.001). Most physical conditions are associated with ideation in the total sample, and it is notable that epilepsy remains the most strongly associated with both ideation (OR = 2.6) and planned attempts among ideators (OR = 4.5). Cancer and heart attack/stroke also are significantly associated with planned attempts among ideators (ORs = 2.5 and 2.7, respectively).

The number of physical conditions remains significantly associated with ideation in the total sample after allowing for type ($\chi^2 = 27.4$, p<0.001). However, in contrast to the model shown in Table 11.4, this model indicates that although the odds of suicide ideation and attempts increase with an increasing number of physical conditions, the added risk becomes smaller with each additional condition.

The magnitude of associations between specific physical condition types and the suicidal behavior outcomes shown in Table 11.5 is somewhat greater than that shown in Table 11.3. This reflects the fact that the estimates in Table 11.5 take the subadditive effect of number of conditions into account.

Table 11.5. Final multivariate models for associations between each type of physical condition and suicidal behavior, controlling for other types, and number of physical conditions; unadjusted for mental disorder[a] (all countries combined)

Physical conditions	Among total sample		Among ideators		
	Ideation	Attempt	Plan	Planned attempt	Unplanned attempt
	OR (95% CI)	OR (95% CI)	OR (95% CI)	OR (95% CI)	OR (95% CI)
Cancer	1.1 (0.7–1.7)	1.6 (1.0–2.6)	0.9 (0.5–1.6)	2.5* (1.1–5.4)	0.9 (0.3–2.2)
Cardiovascular					
Heart disease	1.5* (1.1–2.0)	1.0 (0.6–1.7)	0.9 (0.5–1.6)	0.7 (0.3–1.5)	1.0 (0.5–2.1)
High blood pressure	1.3* (1.1–1.7)	1.6* (1.2–2.3)	1.1 (0.8–1.6)	1.5 (0.9–2.4)	1.2 (0.7–2.2)
Heart attack or stroke	1.9* (1.3–2.7)	2.1* (1.2–3.7)	1.0 (0.6–1.7)	2.7* (1.0–7.4)	0.8 (0.3–2.3)
Diabetes	1.3 (0.9–1.8)	1.1 (0.6–2.1)	0.7 (0.4–1.2)	1.1 (0.4–2.7)	1.3 (0.5–3.3)
Ulcer	1.5* (1.2–1.8)	1.2 (0.8–1.8)	1.2 (0.9–1.6)	1.3 (0.7–2.5)	0.9 (0.5–1.8)
Musculoskeletal					
Arthritis	1.6* (1.3–1.9)	1.5* (1.1–2.0)	1.1 (0.8–1.5)	1.3 (0.8–2.1)	0.8 (0.5–1.3)
Back and neck pain	1.5* (1.3–1.7)	1.2 (0.9–1.5)	1.0 (0.8–1.3)	0.9 (0.6–1.4)	0.7 (0.5–1.2)
Headache	1.9* (1.6–2.1)	1.6* (1.3–2.0)	1.0 (0.8–1.3)	1.2 (0.8–1.7)	0.7 (0.5–1.1)
Other chronic pain	1.5* (1.3–1.9)	1.8* (1.4–2.4)	1.1 (0.8–1.5)	1.1 (0.7–1.8)	1.5 (0.9–2.4)
Respiratory					
Allergies	1.1 (1.0–1.2)	1.1 (0.8–1.3)	0.9 (0.7–1.1)	0.9 (0.6–1.4)	0.9 (0.6–1.3)
Other respiratory	1.6* (1.4–1.9)	1.5* (1.2–2.0)	1.3 (1.0–1.7)	1.4 (0.9–2.3)	1.1 (0.7–1.7)
Epilepsy	2.6* (1.3–5.1)	–	1.2 (0.5–3.0)	4.5* (1.3–15.2)	–
13 df χ^2 test for 13 types	145.2 (<.001)*	55.4 (<.001)*	10.0 (0.69)	22.2 (0.05)	12.2 (0.43)
12 df χ^2 test or difference between types	64.1 (<0.001)*	24.2 (0.01)*	8.9 (0.71)	20.2 (0.06)	12.0 (0.36)
Number of physical conditions					
2	0.7* (0.6–0.8)	0.8 (0.6–1.0)	0.9 (0.7–1.2)	0.6* (0.3–1.0)	1.5 (0.9–2.7)
3	0.5* (0.4–0.7)	0.6* (0.4–0.9)	0.9 (0.5–1.4)	0.4 (0.2–1.0)	1.4 (0.6–3.3)
4	0.4* (0.3–0.6)	0.3* (0.2–0.6)	0.7 (0.4–1.4)	0.3* (0.1–0.9)	1.1 (0.3–4.0)
5+	0.3* (0.1–0.5)	0.4 (0.2–1.1)	0.8 (0.3–2.0)	0.3 (0.1–1.4)	5.1 (1.0–26.6)
χ^2 (p-value)	27.4 (<0.001)*	13.7 (0.01)*	1.4 (0.84)	6.4 (0.17)	8.9 (0.06)

* Significant at the 0.05 level, two-sided test.
– Condition not included in model due to small cell size. Small cell size determined by calculating the expected number of cases of the condition based on the % of people with the outcome and the total number of people with the condition. If the expected value was less than 5, the condition was dropped from the model.
[a] Assessed in the Part 2 sample due to having Part 2 controls. Models control for person–years, country, and significant variables from the chapters on sociodemographics, parental psychopathology, childhood adversities, and traumatic events.

Table 11.6. Final multivariate models for associations between each type of physical condition and suicidal behavior, controlling for other types, and number of physical conditions; adjusted for mental disorder[a] (all countries combined)

Physical conditions	Among total sample		Among ideators		
	Ideation	Attempt	Plan	Planned attempt	Unplanned attempt
	OR (95% CI)	OR (95% CI)	OR (95% CI)	OR (95% CI)	OR (95% CI)
Cancer	1.1 (0.7–1.6)	1.2 (0.6–2.5)	0.9 (0.5–1.6)	2.3 (1.0–5.2)	0.8 (0.3–2.2)
Cardiovascular					
Heart disease	1.4* (1.0–1.9)	1.0 (0.6–1.8)	0.9 (0.5–1.6)	0.8 (0.4–1.6)	1.0 (0.5–2.0)
High blood pressure	1.3* (1.0–1.5)	1.5* (1.1–2.1)	1.1 (0.8–1.6)	1.4 (0.9–2.3)	1.2 (0.7–2.2)
Heart attack or stroke	1.9* (1.3–2.8)	1.9* (1.1–3.5)	1.0 (0.6–1.6)	2.7 (0.9–8.0)	0.9 (0.3–2.3)
Diabetes	1.3 (0.9–1.8)	1.1 (0.6–2.1)	0.6 (0.3–1.2)	1.0 (0.4–2.5)	1.4 (0.6–3.3)
Ulcer	1.4* (1.1–1.7)	1.2 (0.8–1.7)	1.1 (0.8–1.5)	1.2 (0.6–2.3)	1.0 (0.5–2.0)
Musculoskeletal					
Arthritis	1.5* (1.3–1.8)	1.5* (1.1–1.9)	1.1 (0.8–1.5)	1.3 (0.8–2.1)	0.8 (0.5–1.3)
Back and neck pain	1.4* (1.2–1.6)	1.0 (0.8–1.3)	1.0 (0.8–1.2)	0.8 (0.5–1.3)	0.7 (0.5–1.2)
Headache	1.6* (1.5–1.9)	1.4* (1.1–1.7)	1.0 (0.8–1.2)	1.1 (0.8–1.7)	0.8 (0.5–1.1)
Other chronic pain	1.3* (1.1–1.7)	1.6* (1.2–2.0)	1.0 (0.8–1.4)	1.1 (0.6–1.8)	1.5 (0.9–2.4)
Respiratory					
Allergies	1.1 (0.9–1.2)	1.0 (0.8–1.3)	0.9 (0.7–1.1)	0.9 (0.6–1.3)	0.8 (0.6–1.3)
Other respiratory	1.5* (1.3–1.8)	1.5* (1.2–1.9)	1.3 (1.0–1.6)	1.4 (0.9–2.3)	1.1 (0.7–1.7)
Epilepsy	2.2* (1.2–4.3)	–	1.3 (0.5–3.0)	4.4* (1.2–16.2)	–
13 df χ^2 test for 13 types	100.5 (<0.001)*	39.5 (<0.001)*	10.9 (0.62)	22.2 (0.05)	12.2 (0.43)
12 df χ^2 test for difference between types	50.1 (<0.001)*	22.1 (0.02)*	9.8 (0.63)	21.7 (0.04)*	12.3 (0.34)
Number of physical conditions					
2	0.7* (0.6–0.8)	0.8 (0.6–1.0)	0.9 (0.7–1.2)	0.6 (0.4–1.0)	1.5 (0.8–2.6)
3	0.5* (0.4–0.7)	0.6* (0.4–0.9)	0.9 (0.5–1.4)	0.5 (0.2–1.1)	1.4 (0.6–3.3)
4	0.4* (0.3–0.6)	0.3* (0.2–0.6)	0.7 (0.4–1.4)	0.3* (0.1–0.9)	1.0 (0.3–3.8)
5+	0.3* (0.2–0.5)	0.5 (0.2–1.3)	0.8 (0.3–1.9)	0.4 (0.1–1.7)	4.9 (0.9–25.5)
χ^2 (p-value)	25.8 (<0.001)*	14.9 (0.01)*	1.3 (0.86)	5.8 (0.22)	9.1 (0.06)

* Significant at the 0.05 level, two-sided test.
– Condition not included in model due to small cell size. Small cell size determined by calculating the expected number of cases of the condition based on the % of people with the outcome and the total number of people with the condition. If the expected value was less than 5, the condition was dropped from the model.
[a] Assessed in the Part 2 sample due to having Part 2 controls. Models control for person–years, country, and significant variables from the chapters on sociodemographics, parental psychopathology, childhood adversities, traumatic events, and mental disorders.

Table 11.7. Interactions between physical conditions and life course interval during which the suicide attempt was made[a] (all countries combined)

Interactions		Attempts among total sample	
		OR (95% CI)	χ^2 (p-value)
Cancer	middle 33%	–	0.7 (0.42)
	upper 33%	0.5 (0.1–2.4)	
Cardiovascular			
Heart disease	middle 33%	–	3.9 (0.05)*
	upper 33%	0.4* (0.1–1.0)	
High blood pressure	middle 33%	–	1.8 (0.18)
	upper 33%	0.6 (0.3–1.3)	
Heart attack or stroke	middle 33%	–	0.1 (0.82)
	upper 33%	1.2 (0.3–4.6)	
Diabetes	middle 33%	–	6.9 (0.01)*
	upper 33%	0.1* (0.0–0.6)	
Ulcer	middle 33%	–	0.9 (0.33)
	upper 33%	0.7 (0.3–1.5)	
Musculoskeletal			
Arthritis	middle 33%	0.5 (0.2–1.4)	3.7 (0.16)
	upper 33%	0.5 (0.2–1.0)	
Back and neck pain	middle 33%	0.8 (0.4–1.6)	3.6 (0.16)
	upper 33%	0.6 (0.3–1.1)	
Headache	middle 33%	0.7 (0.4–1.1)	7.1 (0.03)*
	upper 33%	0.5* (0.3–0.8)	
Other chronic pain	middle 33%	0.9 (0.4–2.2)	0.3 (0.85)
	upper 33%	1.1 (0.5–2.5)	
Respiratory			
Allergies	middle 33%	0.4* (0.2–0.7)	26.1 (<0.001)*
	upper 33%	0.3* (0.2–0.5)	
Other respiratory	middle 33%	1.0 (0.6–1.7)	0.7 (0.70)
	upper 33%	0.8 (0.5–1.4)	
Epilepsy	middle 33%	–	–
	upper 33%	–	
26 df χ^2 test for all chronic conditions			43.4 (<0.001)*
25 df χ^2 test for all conditions and dummies for number of conditions			59.4 (<0.001)*
Number of physical conditions			
2	middle 33%	1.4 (0.7–2.6)	
	upper 33%	1.8 (0.9–3.9)	
3	middle 33%	0.9 (0.3–2.6)	
	upper 33%	1.8 (0.6–5.0)	
4	middle 33%	–	
	upper 33%	3.2 (0.9–11.1)	

Table 11.7. (cont.)

Interactions		Attempts among total sample	
		OR (95% CI)	χ^2 (p-value)
5+	middle 33%	–	
	upper 33%	8.6* (1.2–63.7)	
χ^2 (p-value)			6.7 (0.35)

* Significant at the 0.05 level, two-sided test.
– Condition not included in model due to small cell size. Small cell size determined by calculating the expected number of cases of the condition based on the % of people with the outcome and the total number of people with the condition. If the expected value was less than 5, the condition was dropped from the model.
[a] Assessed in the Part 2 sample. Models included all controls listed for prior analyses and interaction terms between life course intervals (intervals determined by the 33.3% percentiles of the age-of-onset for the outcome) and each control.

Adjustment for mental disorders in associations between physical conditions and suicidal behavior, controlling for number and type

Adjustment for a wide range of lifetime anxiety, mood, substance use, and impulse-control DSM-IV mental disorders makes little substantive difference to the associations between physical conditions and suicidal behavior (see Table 11.6). All physical conditions that are significantly associated with attempts and ideation in the total sample in the final multivariate model shown in Table 11.5 remain significant after including mental disorders in the model. However, of the three conditions that are significantly associated with planned attempts among ideators prior to adjustment for mental disorders, only epilepsy remains significant after adjustment for mental disorders; cancer and heart attack/stroke drop to marginal significance.

Interactions between physical conditions and when in the life course the suicidal behavior occurs

The results of analyses that tested for interactions between each physical condition and when in the life course the suicide outcome occurred (in terms of tectiles of the outcome distribution) are shown in Table 11.7 for attempts in the total sample (not adjusted for mental disorders). The table shows a common pattern across most physical conditions of the association being smaller in magnitude in the oldest or older groups relative to the youngest third. For example, in the first column of data in Table 11.7, which shows the interaction between physical conditions and life course for suicide attempts, the interaction OR of 0.4 for heart disease among the oldest third of those attempting suicide indicates that the association in this group is only 40% of the magnitude of the association in the reference group (those in the youngest third of suicide attempters). Owing to low power, this pattern is only significant for some conditions. A similar pattern is evident for suicide ideation in the total sample (data not shown), though it is only significant for the pain conditions.

Associations between physical conditions and persistence of suicidal behavior

Results from the backward recurrence models show that physical conditions are less strongly associated with persistence of suicidal behavior relative to their associations with first onset of suicidal behavior (Table 11.8). Only diabetes and headache are significantly associated with persistent ideation (ORs = 2.3 and 1.2, respectively), and ulcer (OR = 2.8) is the only condition to be associated with persistent attempts in the total sample.

The results of the more fine-grained logistic regression persistence models (results not reported in tables) show that several physical conditions are associated with the persistence of suicidal behavior over time. Specifically, high blood pressure is associated with very high persistence of suicide ideation (i.e., into the past year among those with high persistence; OR = 13.4); ulcer is associated with persistence of ideation into the past five years (OR = 2.7), and with suicide attempts beyond two

Table 11.8. Physical conditions and persistence of suicidal behavior[a] (all countries combined)

Physical conditions	Ideation OR (95% CI)	Plan OR (95% CI)	Attempt OR (95% CI)
Cancer	0.9 (0.4–1.9)	–	–
Cardiovascular			
Heart disease	0.7 (0.4–1.2)	1.3 (0.6–2.8)	1.2 (0.5–2.8)
High blood pressure	1.1 (0.8–1.5)	0.7 (0.4–1.2)	0.5 (0.2–1.3)
Heart attack/stroke	0.9 (0.5–1.7)	1.7 (0.6–4.8)	2.4 (0.7–8.2)
Diabetes	2.3* (1.1–4.9)	–	–
Ulcer	1.1 (0.8–1.6)	1.5 (0.8–2.7)	2.8* (1.2–6.6)
Musculoskeletal			
Arthritis	0.9 (0.7–1.3)	0.9 (0.5–1.5)	0.9 (0.5–1.6)
Back and neck pain	1.2 (1.0–1.4)	1.2 (0.8–1.7)	1.2 (0.8–2.0)
Headache	1.2* (1.0–1.5)	1.2 (0.9–1.6)	1.3 (0.9–1.9)
Other chronic pain	0.9 (0.7–1.2)	1.3 (0.8–2.0)	1.4 (0.8–2.4)
Respiratory			
Allergies	0.9 (0.7–1.1)	1.1 (0.8–1.5)	1.2 (0.8–1.9)
Other respiratory	1.0 (0.8–1.2)	0.9 (0.6–1.3)	1.0 (0.7–1.5)
Epilepsy	0.3 (0.1–1.0)	–	–
13 df χ^2 test for 13 types	23.1 (0.04)*	13.3 (0.21)	15.9 (0.10)
12 df χ^2 test for difference between types	20.7 (0.05)	11.9 (0.22)	14.8 (0.10)
Number of physical conditions			
2	0.9 (0.7–1.2)	0.8 (0.5–1.2)	0.6 (0.3–1.0)
3	1.0 (0.6–1.5)	0.9 (0.5–1.8)	0.8 (0.3–1.9)
4	1.1 (0.6–2.0)	0.7 (0.2–2.0)	0.7 (0.2–2.6)
5+	1.7 (0.7–4.3)	2.2 (0.6–8.2)	0.4 (0.1–2.0)
χ^2 (p-value)	3.8 (0.43)	11.9 (0.02)*	5.1 (0.28)

* Significant at the 0.05 level, two-sided test.
– Dropped because the expected value is less than 5.
[a] Results are based on multivariate discrete time survival models. Models control for country, age-related variables, and significant variables from the chapters on sociodemographics, parental psychopathology, childhood adversities, and mental disorders. None of the types and number of traumatic events are significant, so they were not included as part of the control.

years (OR = 3.6) and into the past five (OR = 8.0) and one (OR = 18.9) years; arthritis is associated with persistence of ideation into the past 10 (OR = 3.0) and five (OR = 1.9) years, and with suicide plans into the past five (OR = 4.1) and one (OR = 3.5) years; and headache is associated with persistence of ideation beyond two years (OR = 1.3), suicide plans (OR = 4.7) and attempts (OR = 18.0) into the past year among those with high persistence.

Consistency of results by country income level

First, it is notable that the prevalence of each physical condition among those with each suicidal behavior tends to be higher in high-income countries than in lower-income countries; this is especially notable with respiratory diseases, but is apparent with most other conditions as well. This is to be expected given the older age structure of high-income countries (see Appendix Tables 11.1–11.2). When the final multivariate models (not adjusted for mental disorders) for these two sets of countries are compared, physical conditions are, generally speaking, more consistently associated with the suicide outcomes in the high-income countries (see Appendix Tables 11.3–11.4). For example, in high-income countries, all three of the cardiovascular conditions are significantly associated with suicide ideation in the final multivariate model, but in lower-income countries, none of them are significantly associated with ideation. However, there is one exception to this general pattern: arthritis is more strongly associated with ideation (OR = 2.3) and attempts (OR = 3.4) in lower-income countries than in high-income countries (OR = 1.4 for ideation and OR = 1.2 for attempts).

The next two tables (see Appendix Tables 11.5–11.6) attempt to determine the cross-national consistency of the finding noted previously in the pooled analyses that chronic conditions more strongly predict suicide attempts among younger age groups. Owing to small numbers, this could only be consistently assessed for a small number of physical conditions: the pain conditions and high blood pressure. It is apparent that this general pattern holds for high-income countries but not for lower-income countries. However, for ulcer, the pattern only holds for lower-income countries.

The final two appendix tables (see Appendix Tables 11.7–11.8) suggest that there is little consistency across high- and lower-income countries in terms of the association between physical conditions and persistence of suicidal behavior, but comparisons are made difficult by the restricted number of conditions that could be considered in lower-income countries. It is notable that several conditions (high blood pressure, ulcer, back/neck pain, and allergies) are associated with persistent suicide ideation in lower-income countries, but not in high-income countries (see Appendix Tables 11.7–11.8).

Discussion

To summarize our findings from this extensive set of analyses, we found that after taking account of both type and number of physical conditions, most physical conditions were associated with suicide ideation in the total sample. In addition, several conditions were associated with attempts in the total sample (high blood pressure, heart attack/stroke, arthritis, chronic headache, other chronic pain, and respiratory conditions), and epilepsy, cancer, and heart attack/stroke were associated with planned attempts among ideators. Considering differences among physical conditions in their strength of association with suicidal behavior, we found that of those conditions included here, epilepsy was the physical condition most strongly associated with suicidal behavior. Having a greater number of physical conditions was associated with increased risk of suicidal outcomes but at a decreasing rate. In general, we did not find associations between physical conditions and suicidal behavior to be stronger in lower-income countries as has been suggested by previous research, although there was one exception to this trend (i.e., arthritis). Physical conditions were more strongly associated with suicide attempts among the younger age groups; a pattern that was most evident in high-income countries. We found that physical conditions were more predictive of first-onset suicidal behavior, rather than persistence of suicidal behavior, although some conditions (especially ulcers and headaches) did predict persistence of suicidal behavior. Finally, adjustment for mental disorders did not greatly alter our findings, although the associations between cancer and heart attack/stroke and planned attempts among ideators dropped to marginal significance.

This last finding is perhaps the most surprising; despite the fact that we adjusted for a wider range of diagnosed mental disorders than any prior study, this made little difference to the associations between physical conditions and suicidal behavior. This is surprising as prior studies on the association of physical conditions with suicidal behavior, although variable in methodology, have been consistent in finding that adjustment for mental disorders has markedly reduced the number of physical conditions significantly associated with the suicidal outcome (Druss & Pincus, 2000; Goodwin et al., 2003a; Goodwin et al., 2003b; Lawrence et al., 2000; Rasic et al., 2008). There are many methodological differences between the current study and these prior studies; however, three differences in particular may best account for this discrepancy in results.

First, most of these analyses concern *first*-onset suicidal behavior as the outcome variable. This contrasts with other cross-sectional studies where the measure of suicidal behavior represents a mix of first onset and persistent suicidal behavior. As we show here, the associations between physical conditions and first-onset suicidal behavior are considerably stronger than associations between physical conditions and persistent suicidal behavior.

The second key methodological feature of these analyses is that our analyses concern *temporally prior* physical conditions. This contrasts with the usual measure of physical conditions used in cross-sectional surveys and represents an aggregate of physical conditions that occur before, and those that occur after, the onset of the suicidal behavior. It is probable that aggregating physical conditions that can plausibly predict suicidal behavior (because they precede the suicidal outcome) with those that cannot predict suicidal behavior (because they follow the outcome), and where reverse causality is unlikely (suicidal behavior does not obviously lead to physical condition onset), will weaken the associations between physical conditions and suicidal outcomes.

The third way in which this study departs from earlier general population studies is in its larger sample size. It has been suggested that some prior studies may have been too underpowered to detect associations (Rollman & Shear, 2003).

We found that many physical conditions were risk factors for suicide ideation and attempts, regardless of whether they were comorbid with mental disorders. This is an important finding from a clinical point of view because it indicates that concern over the possibility of suicide should not be restricted to those with mental disorders. However, from a practical point of view, given the low base-rate of suicide attempts and the high base-rate of chronic physical conditions, it is perhaps most important for clinicians to note that it is those individuals with both chronic physical conditions and comorbid mental disorders who are the highest risk of suicidal behavior, and that this combination in a younger person is of particular concern.

We need to note several limitations of these data. The key limitation is that the information on the occurrence and timing of suicidal behavior, mental disorders, and covariates such as childhood adversity was collected retrospectively. Comprehensive reviews (Brewin et al., 1993; Hardt & Rutter, 2004) of the validity of retrospective reports have drawn the conclusion that the retrospective reports of clearly operationalized past events are reasonably valid, although there is a considerable degree of under-reporting and possibly some bias. Bias can result from current mental state influencing recall (Williams et al., 1997), but this is less of an issue in these analyses as we report associations with and without mental disorder adjustment.

A second limitation is sample selection bias, either through the survey participants being healthier than non-participants, or through differential selection out of the population due to early mortality (e.g., because of suicide completion or a physical condition). These kinds of sample selection biases would generally be expected to lead to downward bias in estimates of the strength of the associations between predictors and physical conditions. These biases will, consequently, make the results we find conservative for the most part. A third limitation is that the medical conditions were assessed on the basis of self-report of diagnoses rather than independent verification by a medical practitioner, although this limitation is mitigated by the generally good agreement between self-report of medical diagnoses and physician or medical record confirmation of those diagnoses (Baumeister et al., 2010; Kehoe et al., 1994; Kriegsman et al., 1996; NCHS, 1994). With regard to the symptomatic pain conditions, self-report is generally regarded as the preferred method of case ascertainment, but there is greater potential for the influence of mood on symptom reporting. Finally, it is also a limitation that only 13 physical conditions could be examined and that some conditions had to be aggregated into single categories.

In conclusion, in this first comprehensive, cross-national analysis of this topic, many physical conditions were found to be associated with the subsequent first onset of suicide ideation and some were found to be associated with the subsequent first onset of suicide attempts and with planned attempts among ideators. Most of these associations remained significant after adjustment for mental disorders. Of all the conditions we studied, epilepsy was the most strongly associated with suicidal behavior. In clinical settings, the combination of a chronic physical condition with comorbid mental disorder in a young person should raise concern as to the possibility of suicidal behavior.

Acknowledgements

Portions of this chapter are based on Scott, K. M., Hwang, I., Chiu, W. T., et al. (2010). Chronic physical conditions and their association with first onset of suicidal behavior in the World Mental Health Surveys. Psychosomatic Medicine, 72(7), 712–719. Reproduced with permission.

References

Baumeister, H., Kriston, L., Bengel, J., & Harter, M. (2010). High agreement of self-report and physician-diagnosed somatic conditions yields limited bias in examining mental-physical comorbidity. *Journal of Clinical Epidemiology* **63**(5), 558–565.

Beautrais, A. L. (2002). A case control study of suicide and attempted suicide in older adults. *Suicide and Life-Threatening Behavior*, **32**(1), 1–9.

Bebbington, P. E., Hurry, J., & Tennant, C. (1991). The Camberwell Community Survey: a summary of results. *Social Psychiatry and Psychiatric Epidemiology*, **26**(5), 195–201.

Brennan Braden, J., & Sullivan, M. D. (2008). Suicidal thoughts and behavior among adults with self-reported pain conditions in the National Comorbidity Survey Replication. *Journal of Pain*, **9**(12), 1106–1115.

Brewin, C. R., Andrews, B., & Gotlib, I. H. (1993). Psychopathology and early experience: a reappraisal of retrospective reports. *Psychological Bulletin*, **113**(1), 82–98.

Druss, B., & Pincus, H. (2000). Suicide ideation and suicide attempts in general medical illnesses. *Archives of Internal Medicine*, **160**(10), 1522–1526.

Fairweather, A. K., Anstey, K. J., Rodgers, B., & Butterworth, P. (2006). Factors distinguishing suicide attempters from suicide ideators in a community sample: social issues and physical health problems. *Psychological Medicine* **36**(9), 1235–1245.

Goodwin, R., Kroenke, K., Hoven, C., & Spitzer, R. L. (2003a). Major depression, physical illness, and suicidal ideation in primary care. *Psychosomatic Medicine*, **65**(4), 501–505.

Goodwin, R., Marusic, A., & Hoven, C. (2003b). Suicide attempts in the United States: the role of physical illness. *Social Science and Medicine*, **56**(8), 1783–1788.

Gupta, L., Ward, J., & D'Este, C. (1997). Differential effectiveness of telephone prompts by medical and nonmedical staff in increasing survey response rates: a randomised trial. *Australian and New Zealand Journal of Public Health*, **21**(1), 98–99.

Hardt, J., & Rutter, M. (2004). Validity of adult retrospective reports of adverse childhood experiences: review of the evidence. *Journal of Child Psychology and Psychiatry*, **45**(2), 260–273.

Harris, E. C., & Barraclough, B. M. (1994). Suicide as an outcome for medical disorders. *Medicine*, **73**(6), 281–296.

Henriksson, M. M., Isometsa, E. T., Hietanen, P. S., Aro, H. M., & Lonnqvist, J. K. (1995). Mental disorders in cancer suicides. *Journal of Affective Disorders*, **36**(1–2), 11–20.

Kehoe, R., Wu, S.-Y., Leske, M. C., & Chylack, L. T. (1994). Comparing self-reported and physician reported medical history. *American Journal of Epidemiology*, **139**(8), 813–818.

Kriegsman, D. M., Penninx, B. W., Van Eijk, J. T., Boeke, A. J., & Deeg, D. J. (1996). Self-reports and general practitioner information on the presence of chronic diseases in community dwelling elderly. *Journal of Clinical Epidemiology*, **49**(12), 1407–1417.

Lawrence, D., Almeida, O. P., Hulse, G. K., Jablensky, A. V., & D'Arcy Holman, C. (2000). Suicide and attempted suicide among older adults in Western Australia. *Psychological Medicine*, **30**(4), 813–821

Maselko, J., & Patel, V. (2008). Why women attempt suicide: the role of mental illness and social disadvantage in a community cohort study in India. *Journal of Epidemiology and Community Health*, **62**(9), 817–822.

NCHS. (1994). Evaluation of National Health Interview Survey diagnostic reporting. *Vital and Health Statistics 2*, **120**, 1–116.

Quan, H., Arboleda-Florez, J., Fick, G. H., Stuart, H. L., & Love, E. J. (2002). Association between physical illness and suicide among the elderly. *Social Psychiatry and Psychiatric Epidemiology*, **37**(4), 190–197.

Rasic, D. T., Belik, S.-L., Bolton, J. M., Chochinov, H. M., & Sareen, J. (2008). Cancer, mental disorders, suicidal ideation and attempts in a large community sample. *Psychooncology* **17**(7), 660–667.

Rockett, I. R., Wang, S., Lian, Y., & Stack, S. (2007). Suicide-associated comorbidity among US males and females: a multiple cause of death analysis. *Injury Prevention*, **13**(5), 311–315.

Rollman, B. L., & Shear, M. K. (2003). Depression and medical comorbidity: red flags for current suicidal ideation in primary care. *Psychosomatic Medicine*, **65**(4), 506–507.

Scott, K. M., Hwang, I., Chiu, W. T., et al. (2010). Chronic physical conditions and their association with first onset of suicidal behavior in the World Mental Health Surveys. *Psychosomatic Medicine*, **72**(7), 712–719.

Stenager, E. N., & Stenager, E. (2000). Physical illness and suicidal behaviour. In K. Hawton, & K. Van Heeringen (eds.), *The International Handbook of Suicide and Attempted Suicide*. London, England: John Wiley & Sons, Ltd.

Tang, N. K. Y., & Crange, C. (2006). Suicidality in chronic pain: a review of the prevalence, risk factors and psychological links. *Psychological Medicine*, **36**(5), 575–586.

Waern, M., Rubenowitz, E., Runeson, B., et al. (2002). Burden of illness and suicide in elderly people: case-control study. *British Medical Journal*, **324**(7350), 1355.

Williams, J. M. G., Watts, F. N., MacLeod, C., & Mathews, A. (eds.). (1997). *Cognitive Psychology and Emotional Disorders*, second edition. Chichester, England: John Wiley and Sons.

World Bank. (2008). *Data and Statistics*. Accessed September 17, 2008 at: <http://go.worldbank.org/D7SN0B8YU0>.

Chapter

12

Integrative models of suicidal behavior

Matthew K. Nock, Jordi Alonso, Guilherme Borges, Somnath Chatterji,
Charlene A. Deming, Wai Tat Chiu, Irving Hwang, Yutaka Ono, and
Nancy A. Sampson

Introduction

Prior chapters in this volume examine the extent to which individual risk factor domains (e.g., parental psychopathology, childhood adversity, mental disorders) predict the subsequent onset and persistence of suicidal behavior (i.e., suicide ideation, plans, and attempts). Each of these chapters provides valuable and previously unavailable information about a wide range of risk factors for suicidal behavior. An important next step not addressed in these earlier chapters or in the research literature more broadly, is to carefully examine the relative contribution of each of these different risk factor domains. It is highly unlikely that the risk factors examined in this volume, and those that exist more broadly, operate in isolation. It is much more plausible to assume that risk factors cluster together and influence one another in various ways. For instance, parental psychopathology, childhood adversity, traumatic life events, the presence of mental disorders, and chronic physical conditions all are associated with suicidal behavior (as outlined in Chapters 7–11, respectively); however, we know from decades of research that these factors are themselves interrelated. Teasing apart the "causal thicket" of correlates, confounds, and causal mechanisms leading to suicidal behavior will require the completion of a great many studies beyond this one (Kendler, 2008; Nock, 2009; Wimsatt, 1994). Indeed, the correlational design of the World Mental Health (WMH) Survey Initiative does not allow us even to test simple causal relations between risk factors and suicidal behavior. However, an examination of the relative associations between each domain and suicidal behavior, controlling for all others, will bring us a step closer to understanding the unique association between each risk factor domain and suicidal behavior. In this way, the data can provide a clearer understanding of the magnitude of the potential causal effects of each domain.

Understanding the relative associations between individual risk factor domains and suicidal behavior is important not only for scientific reasons, but also for more applied clinical and public policy work. For instance, earlier findings have revealed that childhood adversity is significantly associated with suicidal behavior later in life. This suggests that interventions aimed at decreasing childhood adversities may be useful for preventing suicidal behavior. However, examining risk factor domains in concert may reveal that childhood adversity is only associated with suicidal behavior because it is a marker for some other risk factor domain, such as parental psychopathology, and when that domain is taken into account, the effects of childhood adversity are diminished or completely negated. Prior research has provided some support for this idea (e.g., Rind et al., 1998); however, such questions remain hotly debated (Lilienfeld, 2002). The size and scope of the WMH initiative provides a unique opportunity to carefully and comprehensively examine an integrative risk factor model for suicidal behavior that considers the unique effects of each risk factor domain.

The analyses and results presented here complement previous chapters by providing a clearer understanding of the unique associations between each risk factor domain and the subsequent onset of suicidal behavior. The results presented in each of the prior chapters describe odds ratios (ORs) that represent the individual-level associations between risk factor and outcome; however, they do not take into account either the prevalence of each risk factor or the overlap among risk factor domains. The prevalence of the risk factors being examined is important because it provides information about the overall impact of that factor on the

Table 12.1. Population attributable risk proportions of risk factors predicting the subsequent first occurrence of suicide ideation[a] (all countries combined)

Conditions cured	Model				
	1	2	3	4	5
	PARP	PARP	PARP	PARP	PARP
Parental psychopathology	11.29%	6.19%	5.22%	5.15%	3.43%
Childhood adversity	–	28.36%	25.86%	24.79%	18.60%
Trauma	–	–	17.82%	16.51%	10.02%
Chronic conditions	–	–	–	7.54%	4.82%
Mental disorders	–	–	–	–	31.08%
All conditions	–	–	–	–	62.37%

PARP, population attributable risk proportions.
[a] Assessed in the Part 2 sample. All models control for countries and person–years.

occurrence of the outcome. For instance, impulse-control disorders are more strongly associated with suicide attempt than are anxiety disorders (i.e., the ORs are higher for impulse-control disorders); however, because anxiety disorders have a higher prevalence, more cases of suicidal behavior can be attributed to anxiety than to impulse-control disorders. To address the gaps in this earlier work, in the current chapter we estimate population attributable risk proportions (PARPs) to examine the unique population-level effects of each risk factor domain. PARPs represent the proportion of observed cases of each suicidal behavior that would be prevented if each set of risk factors were prevented, assuming that the associations between a risk factor and outcome are causal. As such, these results provide valuable information about the possible public health implications of targeting each risk factor domain. Consistent with prior chapters, we examine the onset of multiple forms of suicidal behavior (i.e., suicide ideation and attempt) and estimate models in the total sample as well as separately for high-, middle-, and low-income countries.

Method

A detailed description of the respondent samples, study procedures, statistical analyses, and assessment of suicidal behavior is provided in Chapter 3 of this volume. The assessment and analysis of sociodemographic factors (Chapter 6), parental psychopathology (Chapter 7), childhood adversities (Chapter 8), traumatic life events (Chapter 9), mental disorders (Chapter 10), and physical conditions (Chapter 11), which are included as covariates in the following analyses, are described in those earlier chapters.

Following the analysis plan outlined in Chapter 3, we estimated PARPs for each risk factor domain in five different models for suicide ideation, five for suicide attempt, and five for suicide attempt among ideators. In each series of models, we began by examining the PARPs for the most distal risk factor domain (parental psychopathology) and in each subsequent model added what we believed to be the next most proximal risk factor domain for suicidal behavior. More specifically, the first model included only parental psychopathology. The second model included parental psychopathology and childhood adversity. The third model added traumatic events during adulthood. The fourth added chronic physical conditions. The fifth and final model added mental disorders. All models included controls for country, person–years, and sociodemographic factors (respondent age, gender, education, and marital status). As in prior chapters, the analyses were conducted first on the total sample, and were replicated separately for high-, middle-, and low-income countries.

Results

Risk factors for suicide ideation

Results reveal that 11.29% of cases of first onset of suicide ideation is associated with the presence of psychopathology among respondents' parents (see

Table 12.1, Model 1). However, when childhood adversity is entered into the model (Model 2), the effect of parental psychopathology drops substantially (6.19%) and is much smaller than the PARP for childhood adversity (28.36%). This means that much of the effect of parental psychopathology on the onset of suicide ideation is explained by the occurrence of childhood adversity. The effects of these risk factor domains decrease slightly in Models 3–5 when traumatic events, chronic physical conditions, and mental disorders, respectively, are taken into consideration. The final model predicting suicide ideation in the total sample (Model 5) shows that overall all risk factor domains combined account for 62.37% of cases of suicide ideation, with the largest proportion of cases attributed to the occurrence of prior mental disorders (31.08%), followed by childhood adversity (18.60%), traumatic events (10.02%), chronic physical conditions (4.82%), and parental psychopathology (3.43%).

Overall, a similar pattern of results is observed across high-, middle-, and low-income countries (see Appendix Tables 12.1–12.3). The only notable differences are that in low-income countries, the effects of parental psychopathology are relatively stronger, the effects of childhood adversity and mental disorders are weaker, and the overall proportion of cases explained by these risk factor domains is smaller.

Risk factors for suicide attempt in the total sample

The results from models predicting suicide attempt are similar to those for suicide ideation; however, the effects are stronger in the prediction of suicide attempt for all risk factor domains with the exception of chronic physical conditions. More specifically, results reveal that 21.13% of cases of suicide attempt is associated with the presence of psychopathology among respondents' parents, when entered alone (see Table 12.2, Model 1). When childhood adversity is entered into the model (Model 2), the effect of parental psychopathology again drops substantially (to 9.84%) and is much smaller than the PARP for childhood adversity (at 54.59%). The effects of these risk factor domains decrease slightly in Models 3–5. The final model for the total sample (Model 5) shows that, overall, these risk factors account for 80.32% of cases of suicide attempt, with the largest proportion of cases again attributed to the occurrence of prior mental

disorders (52.01%), followed by childhood adversity (41.33%), traumatic events (11.44%), parental psychopathology (4.96%), and chronic physical conditions (3.05%).

Overall, a similar pattern of results is observed across high-, middle-, and low-income countries (see Appendix Tables 12.4–12.6). The only notable differences again are for low-income countries, where the effects are smaller for all predictors as well as for the overall proportion of cases explained by these risk factor domains.

Risk factors for suicide attempt among ideators

In models predicting suicide attempts among those with prior suicide ideation, the effects of each risk factor domain are greatly diminished. More specifically, in this model only 1.86% of cases would be eliminated with the curing of parental psychopathology (see Table 12.3, Model 1). When childhood adversity enters the model (Model 2), the effect of parental psychopathology is essentially erased (0.39%), whereas the effect of childhood adversity is more substantial (10.41%). The effects of traumatic events, chronic physical conditions, and mental disorders in Models 3–5 are not useful in predicting suicide attempts among ideators. Interestingly, however, in the final model for attempts among ideators, which accounts for only 7.05% of cases, effects remain strongest for childhood adversity (9.75%), with the PARPs for all other factors ≤3.00%.

Cross-nationally, a similar general pattern emerged in which childhood adversity has the strongest effects on attempts among ideators (see Appendix Tables 12.7–12.9). Notably, however, the effects of all risk factors are strongest in high-income countries, diminished somewhat in middle-income countries, and are virtually absent in low-income countries.

Discussion

This chapter tested several integrative models that incorporated each of the risk factor domains examined in earlier chapters. Doing so provides an initial picture of the relative contribution of each set of risk factors identified earlier in this volume. Several key findings from these analyses warrant additional comment.

First, overall, these analyses revealed that if we were able to cure the currently known risk factors for lifetime

Table 12.2. Population attributable risk proportions of risk factors predicting the subsequent first occurrence of suicide attempt[a] (all countries combined)

	Model				
	1	2	3	4	5
Conditions cured	PARP	PARP	PARP	PARP	PARP
Parental psychopathology	21.13%	9.84%	8.23%	8.06%	4.96%
Childhood adversity	–	54.59%	52.40%	51.53%	41.33%
Trauma	–	–	22.60%	21.68%	11.44%
Chronic conditions	–	–	–	6.84%	3.05%
Mental disorders	–	–	–	–	52.01%
All conditions	–	–	–	–	80.32%

PARP, population attributable risk proportions.
[a] Assessed in the Part 2 sample. All models control for country and person–years.

Table 12.3. Population attributable risk proportions of sociodemographic factors predicting the subsequent first occurrence of suicide attempt among ideators[a] (all countries combined)

	Model				
	1	2	3	4	5
Conditions cured	PARP	PARP	PARP	PARP	PARP
Parental psychopathology	1.86%	0.39%	0.40%	0.40%	0.10%
Childhood adversity	–	10.41%	10.62%	10.80%	9.75%
Trauma	–	–	-3.56%	-3.24%	-4.34%
Chronic conditions	–	–	–	-1.22%	-1.55%
Mental disorders	–	–	–	–	3.00%
All conditions	–	–	–	–	7.05%

PARP, population attributable risk proportions.
[a] Assessed in the Part 2 sample. All models control for country and person–years.

suicidal behavior assessed in the WMH Surveys and outlined in these chapters, assuming that the observed associations are causal (a point to which we will return later), we would prevent 62% of cases of suicide ideation, 80% of cases of suicide attempt, and 7% of suicide attempts among ideators. On one hand, these findings are quite encouraging because they suggest that by intervening upon known risk factors, we may be able to begin to decrease the rate of suicidal behavior. On the other hand, it is important to note that many causes of suicidal behavior remain unexplained; this is especially true for suicide ideation and even more so for the prediction of

suicide attempts among ideators. The higher PARPs for suicide attempt (relative to ideation and attempts among ideators) may seem surprising at first glance; however, it is representative of the fact that most of these risk factors occur at a higher rate among suicide attempters than among suicide ideators and have stronger ORs in predicting attempt than ideation. Unfortunately, in practice it is the prediction of suicide ideation and attempts among ideators that hold the most promise for prevention, given that suicide ideators are greater in numbers, more easily identifiable, and working with them provides an opportunity to intervene earlier in the pathway to suicide. Gaining a better understanding of the risk factors for suicide ideation, and especially for those factors predicting which ideators will go on to make a suicide attempt, is arguably the greatest priority for suicide research moving forward.

Second, these findings highlight the fact that it is tremendously important that researchers and clinicians begin to consider risk factors for suicidal behavior in concert. Indeed, in virtually every case, the PARPs for each risk factor domain dropped significantly from the time that they were added to the time that they appeared in the final model. Using the final model predicting suicide attempt in the total sample as an example, the PARPs for parental psychopathology decreased from their point of entry to their effect in this model by approximately 75%, whereas the PARPs for traumatic events and chronic physical conditions each dropped by 50%. This suggests that models that include individual risk factors, or even entire risk factor domains, are likely to over-estimate the causal effects of such domains if they do not consider other factors at the same time. Moreover, a failure to include a broader range of risk factors precludes any opportunity for learning about how these factors may work together to predict suicidal behavior, an important next step in this line of research.

Third, although the results presented here cannot speak to the direction or potential causal nature of these associations, they do reveal several interesting pieces of information. As one example, it is notable that the greatest decrease in the PARPs for parental psychopathology occurs when childhood adversity is added to the model, and to a lesser extent when respondent mental disorders are added. This pattern of findings suggests that much of the association observed between parental psychopathology and suicidal behavior may be explained by childhood adversities (and to a lesser extent by respondent psychopathology). Moreover, the PARPs for childhood adversities do not decrease much at all with the addition to the model of traumatic events during adulthood or chronic physical conditions. It is only when respondent mental disorders are added that a decrease in the PARPs for childhood adversity is observed. This suggests that the association between childhood adversity and suicidal behavior is explained in part by the development of mental disorders in the respondent. This pattern is observed across both suicide ideation and attempt, and is seen across high-, middle-, and low-income countries, suggesting that this is a fairly robust pattern of findings. Thus, although we

did not simultaneously test the web of associations among the different risk factor domains and each suicidal outcome (e.g., via structural equation modeling), this initial study provides a first look at the ways in which these risk factors may together contribute to the development of suicidal behavior.

There are several major limitations of the work presented in this chapter. Several of these limitations apply to studies presented in each chapter of this volume and will not be reviewed in detail here. These include: the varied response rates across countries, the fact that we only included data from 21 countries and so these findings should not be considered global estimates, the use of retrospective self-report data, and the potential differences across cultures/countries in the interpretation of questions or tendency to respond in a certain way (e.g., varying levels of stigma around suicide).

Several additional limitations of the current analyses also should be noted. First, although the analyses presented in this chapter included each of the risk factor domains examined in prior chapters, we did not organize our analyses in a way that allowed us to test any falsifiable, theoretical models of suicidal behavior. Instead, our analyses tested the combined effects of each risk factor domain organized chronologically (e.g., first risk factors associated with one's parents, then childhood, then adulthood). Our intent for this chapter, and this volume, was to map out several key risk factor domains believed to be associated with suicidal behavior and to study the nature of these associations in fine detail in order to inform future work in this area. An important next step will be to begin to better understand how to integrate these, and other factors in a way that explains how and why suicidal behavior occurs.

A second and related limitation is that many factors known to play a role in the occurrence of suicidal behavior (e.g., genetic factors, brain functioning, the presence of psychological traits such as hopelessness and impulsiveness) were not considered in this model. All research projects are constrained in the number of constructs that can be included at one time, and although the WMH Surveys assessed a broad range of risk factors, many important factors simply could not be included. Therefore, an important direction for future research is the illumination of how different types of risk factors (e.g., genetic, environmental, psychological) interact to produce suicidal behavior.

Third, the design of this study and the resulting nature of these analyses do not allow us to even begin to untangle the complex causal associations among these factors. This is an obvious point but one worth noting, especially given that the PARP estimates assume causal associations among variables. Because we do not know the extent to which the observed associations are causal, the PARP estimates can only provide a glimpse of what could be done to prevent suicidal behavior: (1) if the associations were causal, and (2) if we had some method of modifying each set of risk factors. As a field, unfortunately we currently fall short in both regards. Therefore, although on one hand it is encouraging to see that if we were able to modify this known set of risk factors, we could prevent 80% of suicide attempts, it is important, and humbling, to remind ourselves of these two points. Analyses like the ones presented in this chapter provide an essential next step in our understanding of which factors predict suicidal behavior and provide an encouraging picture of what is possible, but ultimately remind us of the long road ahead to accurately predicting and preventing suicidal behavior.

References

Kendler, K. S. (2008). Explanatory models for psychiatric illness. *American Journal of Psychiatry*, **165**(6), 695–702.

Lilienfeld, S. O. (2002). When worlds collide. Social science, politics, and the Rind et al. (1998). Child sexual abuse meta-analysis. *The American Psychologist*, **57**(3), 176–188.

Nock, M. K. (2009). Suicidal behavior among adolescents: correlates, confounds, and (the search for) causal mechanisms. *Journal of the American Academy of Child & Adolescent Psychiatry*, **48**(3), 237–239.

Rind, B., Tromovitch, P.,& Bauserman, R. (1998). A meta-analytic examination of assumed properties of child sexual abuse using college samples. *Psychological Bulletin*, **124**(1), 22–53.

Wimsatt, W. C. (1994). The ontology of complex systems: levels of organization, perspectives, and causal thickets. In M. Matthen, & R. Ware (eds.), *Biology and society: Reflections on methodology*, Vol. 20 (Supplement), pp. 207–274.

Chapter

13

Prevalence and identification of groups at risk for twelve-month suicidal behavior in the WHO World Mental Health Surveys

Guilherme Borges, Josep Maria Haro, Wai Tat Chiu, Irving Hwang, Giovanni de Girolamo, Maria Elena Medina-Mora, Nancy A. Sampson, David R. Williams, and Matthew K. Nock

Introduction

Suicide is a leading cause of death worldwide, with approximately one million suicide deaths per year around the globe (WHO, 2009a). Efforts to prevent suicide include: education of physicians, restricting access to lethal means, public education, screening programs, and media education (Mann et al., 2005). Screening programs to detect those at risk for suicide are particularly appealing, usually focusing on detecting those with mental disorders and those with a prior suicide attempt (Nock et al., 2008b; Suominen et al., 2004), both of which are associated with an elevated risk for subsequent suicide. Nevertheless, it also could be argued that preventive efforts should start even earlier and more actions should be focused on detecting those at risk for a first suicide attempt given that approximately half of people attempting suicide die at their first attempt (Isometsa & Lonnqvist, 1998).

If we want to detect those at risk for a suicide attempt, a logical step is to focus on individuals reporting suicide ideation, a phenomenon that is quite common with lifetime prevalence of suicide ideation varying from 2.6% (Romania) to 15.9% (New Zealand), in the general populations in samples across the world (Nock et al., 2008a)(see Chapter 4 of this book). In fact, in clinical settings, it is after evidence of suicide ideation that most suicide risk assessments begin (Cooper-Patrick et al., 1994). Previous research has shown that suicide ideation is a persistent problem, with 35% of those who report suicide ideation still reporting it 10 years later (Borges et al., 2008) and up to 20% of ideators making a suicide attempt during the same year the ideation first began (Kessler et al., 2005;

Kuo et al., 2001). Given that approximately one-third of those with suicide ideation go on to make a suicide attempt (Nock et al., 2008a), the identification of risk factors for the transition from ideation to attempt may be useful in solving the problem of the low base-rates of suicide and suicide attempt in the general population, a problem that has obstructed previous attempts of constructing risk indices for these behaviors (Pokorny, 1983).

Prior studies have identified risk factors for suicidal behavior (i.e., suicide ideation, suicide plan, suicide attempt) (Cooper-Patrick et al., 1994; Mann et al., 1999; Pokorny, 1983). However, for several reasons, efforts to develop accurate suicide prediction models have not yet yielded useful clinical indices. First, most prior studies have used relatively small samples of selected psychiatric patients or college students. Second, most studies have focused on the long-term prediction of suicidal behavior rather than short-term prediction – the focus of the current study. Third, as stated above, most efforts have focused on the prediction of suicide death rather than the earlier transition from suicide ideation to a suicide attempt during which there is still time to intervene. Moreover, prior studies have sometimes used rating scales that may be infeasible to administer in some clinical settings due to their length and scoring requirements, whereas others have focused on a limited set of possible risk factors, such as a single psychiatric disorder or a single negative life event, ignoring the evidence that suicidal behaviors are the result of a wide group of determinants. Overall, although previous studies have identified numerous risk factors, a method for

Suicide, eds. Matthew K. Nock, Guilherme Borges, and Yutaka Ono. Published by Cambridge University Press.
© World Health Organization 2012.

combining these risk factors in a single index has only recently been proposed (Borges et al., 2006, 2010). Finally, new evidence from cross-cultural research on suicidal behavior (Nock et al., 2008a, 2009) has pointed to the fact that there is some variation in the roles of specific disorders on suicidal behavior across nations (e.g., differences in the roles played by mood disorders and substance use disorders in developed and developing nations). These results suggest that we may need risk indices that are more country specific if they are to be useful for clinicians in different parts of the world.

In this chapter, we focus on developing a method of measuring and combining risk factors for suicide attempt into a brief index that clinicians can use in actual practice. We used a large and representative cross-national epidemiological survey database that estimates the 12-month prevalence of suicidal behavior, identifies risk factors for suicide attempts in several different domains, and combines these factors to create a risk index for 12-month planned and unplanned suicide attempts separately for high-income, middle-income, and low-income countries. The current study extends earlier work by Borges et al. (2006) using data from the National Comorbidity Survey Replication (NCS-R) and a prior extension of this work using data from the World Mental Health (WMH) Survey Initiative (Borges et al., 2010), both on the construction of indices for 12-month suicide attempt. The consolidation of the World Mental Health Survey dataset allows us to explore these data further and tailor our risk index for the three groups of nations (i.e., high-income, middle-income, and low-income), thereby widening the application of the risk indices previously reported.

Method

A detailed description of the respondent samples, study procedures, statistical analyses, and assessment of suicidal behavior is provided in Chapter 3 of this volume. The assessment and analysis of sociodemographic factors (Chapter 6), parental psychopathology (Chapter 7), childhood adversities (Chapter 8), traumatic events (Chapter 9), mental disorders (Chapter 10), and physical conditions (Chapter 11), which are included as covariates in the following analyses, are described in those earlier chapters. One notable difference between this chapter and earlier ones in

this volume is that here we focus on the prediction of suicidal behavior that occurred in the 12 months prior to interview, whereas all earlier chapters focused on the prediction of suicidal behavior occurring anytime in the respondents' lifetime.

All data analytical procedures used in this chapter are outlined in Chapter 3, with the exception of the procedures used to create an index of risk factors that predict 12-month suicidal behavior. To do so, we began by combining the predictors that had odds ratios (ORs) over 2 or under 0.5 in the earlier bivariate models into new multivariate models. The predictors that continued to have ORs above 2 or below 0.5 in the multivariate models were used to create the index by constructing a predicted probability of the outcome from a version of the multivariate model that contained only these predictors. This distribution of predicted probabilities was then inspected and divided into strata using the logic of stratum-specific likelihood ratios (SSLRs) (Guyatt & Rennie, 2001). That is, we divided the distribution into strata large enough to find statistically significant monotonic relationships between all contiguous pairs of strata. Three measures of screening scale performance were then calculated for each stratum: positive predictive value (PPV; the proportion of the respondents in the stratum who made an attempt), sensitivity (SENS; the proportion of all attempters who were in the stratum), and specificity (SPEC; the proportion of all non-attempters who were in the stratum). We also calculated the area under the receiver operator characteristic curve (AUC) (Hanley & McNeil, 1982), a summary measure of prediction accuracy that, unlike the more familiar Cohen's (Cohen, 1960), is not influenced by marginal distributions (Kraemer et al., 2003).

Results

Prevalence

For the total sample, 2.0% of respondents report suicide ideation in the past 12 months, 0.6% report a plan, and 0.4% report an attempt (see Table 13.1). Each type of suicidal behavior assessed occurs at a slightly higher rate in middle- or low-income countries than in high-income countries. Estimates of the 12-month prevalence of suicide ideation, plans, and attempts are: 1.9%, 0.6%, and 0.3%, respectively, for high-income countries; 2.1%, 0.8%, and 0.4% for middle-income countries; and 2.0%, 0.6%, and 0.4%

Table 13.1. Twelve-month prevalence of suicide ideation, plan, and attempt in the World Mental Health Surveys (all countries combined)

| | Among total sample | | | Among ideators | | | |
| | Ideation | Plan | Attempt | Plan | Attempt | Planned attempt | Unplanned attempt |
Categories	% (SE)	% (SE)	% (SE)	% (SE)	% (SE)	% (SE)	% (SE)
All countries							
Female	2.3 (0.1)	0.7 (0.0)	0.4 (0.0)	30.7 (1.5)	17.0 (1.1)	38.6 (2.6)	7.5 (1.0)
Male	1.6 (0.1)	0.5 (0.0)	0.3 (0.0)	33.0 (2.1)	18.8 (1.9)	36.7 (4.0)	10.1 (1.7)
Total	2.0 (0.1)	0.6 (0.0)	0.4 (0.0)	31.6 (1.2)	17.7 (1.0)	37.8 (2.3)	8.5 (0.9)
(numerator /	(2265 /	(742 /	(409 /	(742 /	(409 /	(286 /	(123 / 1523)
denominator N)[a]	109,377)	109,377)	109,377)	2265)	2265)	742)	
High-income countries							
Female	2.2 (0.1)	0.6 (0.1)	0.3 (0.0)	27.2 (2.1)	14.4 (1.5)	34.4 (3.8)	6.9 (1.4)
Male	1.7 (0.1)	0.5 (0.1)	0.3 (0.0)	30.9 (3.0)	15.7 (2.3)	30.0 (5.3)	9.4 (1.8)
Total	1.9 (0.1)	0.6 (0.0)	0.3 (0.0)	28.7 (1.8)	15.0 (1.4)	32.5 (3.3)	7.9 (1.1)
(numerator /	(1071 /	(328 /	(173 /	(328 /	(173 /	(110 / 328)	(63 / 743)
denominator N)[a]	52,484)	52,484)	52,484)	1071)	1071)		
Middle-income countries							
Female	2.7 (0.2)	1.0 (0.1)	0.6 (0.1)	36.5 (3.2)	22.6 (2.6)	47.5 (5.5)	8.3 (2.0)
Male	1.5 (0.2)	0.5 (0.1)	0.3 (0.1)	35.9 (4.3)	17.7 (4.5)	41.1 (10.2)	4.5 (1.4)
Total	2.1 (0.1)	0.8 (0.1)	0.4 (0.1)	36.3 (2.4)	20.9 (2.1)	45.4 (4.9)	7.0 (1.4)
(numerator /	(555 /	(207 /	(122 /	(207 /	(122 /	(93 / 207)	(29 / 348)
denominator N)[a]	25,666)	25,666)	25,666)	555)	555)		
Low-income countries							
Female	2.3 (0.1)	0.7 (0.1)	0.4 (0.1)	30.9 (2.6)	15.9 (2.0)	34.5 (4.3)	7.6 (2.1)
Male	1.7 (0.1)	0.6 (0.1)	0.4 (0.1)	34.2 (3.7)	24.7 (3.8)	43.1 (6.5)	15.1 (4.8)
Total	2.0 (0.1)	0.6 (0.0)	0.4 (0.0)	32.2 (2.0)	19.6 (2.0)	38.3 (4.0)	10.6 (2.3)
(numerator /	(639 /	(207 /	(114 /	(207 /	(114 /	(83 / 207)	(31 / 432)
denominator N)[a]	31,227)	31,227)	31,227)	639)	639)		

[*] Significant gender difference at the 0.05 level, two-sided test.
[a] Numerator N refers to the number of cases with each suicide outcome, denominator N refers to the number of cases in the total sample or in the conditional sample among ideators, ideators with a plan and ideators without a plan.

for low-income countries. About a third (31.6%) of ideators reported a plan and less than a fifth (17.7%) of ideators reported an attempt. These transitions are more frequent in low- and middle-income countries than in high-income countries. Among ideators with a plan, the presence of an attempt is much more common (37.8%) than among those ideators without a plan (8.5%), and this pattern replicates for all countries. Unplanned (impulsive) attempts are not common but still make up to 36% of all attempts in high-income countries, 24% of all attempts in

middle-income countries, and 27% of all attempts in low-income countries.

Demographic risk factors

Bivariate associations consistently show that females and those younger than 50 years of age have increased odds of suicide ideation in all three groups of nations (see Table 13.2 for total sample and Appendix Tables 13.1–13.3 for results separated by income level). The bivariate ORs of these significant

Table 13.2. Bivariate associations of sociodemographic variables with 12-month suicide ideation, plan and attempt[a] (all countries combined)

Categories	Among total sample		Among ideators	
	Ideation	Plan	Planned attempt	Unplanned attempt
	OR (95% CI)	OR (95% CI)	OR (95% CI)	OR (95% CI)
4-Category age (years)				
Less than 35	2.7 (2.2–3.3)	1.6 (0.9–2.6)	1.5 (0.5–4.4)	14.5 (2.0–107.1)
35–49	2.0 (1.6–2.5)	1.5 (0.9–2.5)	1.0 (0.3–2.9)	14.7 (2.0–107.5)
50–64	1.4 (1.2–1.8)	1.5 (0.9–2.5)	0.8 (0.3–2.4)	6.7 (0.9–52.2)
65 or older	1.0 (1.0–1.0)	1.0 (1.0–1.0)	1.0 (1.0–1.0)	1.0 (1.0–1.0)
χ^2_3 (p-value)	124.4 (<0.001)*	2.8 (0.43)	6.6 (0.09)	11.6 (0.01)*
Dichotomized age (years)				
Less than 50	1.9 (1.6–2.1)	1.2 (0.9–1.5)	1.5 (0.9–2.4)	2.9 (1.5–5.7)
50 or older	1.0 (1.0–1.0)	1.0 (1.0–1.0)	1.0 (1.0–1.0)	1.0 (1.0–1.0)
χ^2_1 (p-value)	98.8 (<0.001)*	1.1 (0.30)	2.6 (0.11)	9.9 (0.002)*
Gender				
Female	1.4 (1.3–1.6)	0.9 (0.7–1.1)	1.1 (0.8–1.7)	0.8 (0.5–1.2)
Male	1.0 (1.0–1.0)	1.0 (1.0–1.0)	1.0 (1.0–1.0)	1.0 (1.0–1.0)
χ^2_1 (p-value)	38.8 (<0.001)*	1.9 (0.17)	0.4 (0.53)	1.4 (0.24)
Education				
Low	1.7 (1.4–2.0)	1.5 (1.0–2.2)	1.0 (0.5–2.1)	1.0 (0.4–2.2)
Low-average	1.5 (1.3–1.8)	1.4 (1.0–2.0)	1.2 (0.6–2.3)	1.2 (0.6–2.7)
High-average	1.5 (1.2–1.7)	1.6 (1.1–2.4)	1.3 (0.6–2.7)	1.0 (0.5–2.3)
High	1.0 (1.0–1.0)	1.0 (1.0–1.0)	1.0 (1.0–1.0)	1.0 (1.0–1.0)
χ^2_3 (p-value)	33.1 (<0.001)*	7.2 (0.07)	1.2 (0.76)	0.6 (0.91)
Income level[b]				
Low	2.0 (1.6–2.4)	1.6 (1.1–2.2)	1.7 (0.9–2.9)	0.8 (0.4–1.7)
Low-average	1.7 (1.5–2.1)	1.2 (0.8–1.7)	1.2 (0.6–2.1)	0.6 (0.3–1.2)
High-average	1.3 (1.0–1.6)	0.9 (0.6–1.3)	1.0 (0.5–1.8)	0.6 (0.3–1.3)
High	1.0 (1.0–1.0)	1.0 (1.0–1.0)	1.0 (1.0–1.0)	1.0 (1.0–1.0)
χ^2_3 (p-value)	60.8 (<0.001)*	14.7 (0.002)*	5.6 (0.13)	2.8 (0.43)
Marital status				
Married or cohabitating	1.0 (1.0–1.0)	1.0 (1.0–1.0)	1.0 (1.0–1.0)	1.0 (1.0–1.0)
Separated, widowed, or divorced	1.7 (1.5–2.0)	1.2 (0.9–1.6)	1.1 (0.7–1.9)	0.9 (0.5–1.7)
Never married	1.7 (1.5–1.9)	1.1 (0.9–1.4)	1.3 (0.8–2.0)	1.0 (0.6–1.8)
χ^2_2 (p-value)	102.1 (<0.001)*	2.2 (0.33)	1.3 (0.53)	0.2 (0.91)
Employment				
Working	1.0 (1.0–1.0)	1.0 (1.0–1.0)	1.0 (1.0–1.0)	1.0 (1.0–1.0)
Student	1.4 (1.1–1.9)	0.8 (0.5–1.2)	2.1 (0.8–5.4)	2.1 (0.8–5.2)
Homemaker	1.4 (1.2–1.6)	1.1 (0.8–1.5)	1.0 (0.6–1.6)	0.4 (0.2–0.8)
Retired	0.7 (0.5–0.8)	0.8 (0.5–1.3)	1.1 (0.4–2.8)	0.3 (0.1–1.3)
Other	2.7 (2.3–3.1)	1.6 (1.1–2.1)	2.9 (1.8–4.9)	1.0 (0.6–1.9)
χ^2_4 (p-value)	220.5 (<0.001)*	12.2 (0.02)*	20.4 (<0.001)*	11.2 (0.02)*
(numerator / denominator N)[c]	(2265 / 109,377)	(742 / 2265)	(286 / 742)	(123 / 1523)

* Significant at the 0.05 level, two-sided test.
[a] Based on logistic regression analysis controlling for country.
[b] Family income classified into four categories based on the ratio of income to number of family members: less than or equal to the official Department of Labor federal poverty line (defined in the table as families living in poverty), 1–3, 3–6, and 6+ times the poverty line.
[c] Numerator N refers to the number of cases with each suicide outcome, denominator N refers to the number of cases in the total sample or in the conditional sample among ideators, ideators with a plan and ideators without a plan.

predictors range from 1.3 to 1.7 for females and 1.2 to 2.5 for those <50 years. Less consistent associations are apparent for educational and income levels. In high-income countries and less so in middle-income countries, those with lower education and lower income have increased odds of suicide ideation compared to those with the highest education and income levels, but these associations are not apparent in low-income countries. In all countries, people who are separated, divorced, or widowed have significantly higher odds of suicide ideation relative to those who are married/cohabitating. Those who have never been married have increased odds only in high-income countries. Finally, a consistent finding regarding employment status is that, compared to those currently working, those placed in the "other" employment category (consisting mainly of unemployed persons) have significantly higher odds of suicide ideation in all countries. All other employment groups show inconsistent associations across our three groups of nations. Overall, few sociodemographic variables are associated with suicide attempts among ideators. Specifically, in high-income countries, younger age (i.e., <50 years old) predicts planned and unplanned attempts among ideators, and unemployment (i.e., "other") predicts planned attempts among ideators. In middle-income countries, having a high-average/high educational level predicts planned attempts among ideators as does unemployment. In low-income countries, unemployment again predicts planned attempts among ideators and being a student predicts unplanned attempts among ideators.

Childhood adversity-related risk factors

With only a few exceptions parental psychopathology, parental adversities, maltreatment, and other childhood adversities are significant predictors of 12-month suicide ideation in the total sample (see Table 13.3) and in all three income level groups of countries (see Appendix Tables 13.4–13.6). However, few of these measures significantly predict either planned or unplanned suicide attempts among ideators and there is no consistent predictor of planned or unplanned attempts across countries. In high-income countries, childhood physical abuse predicts both planned and unplanned attempts, whereas sexual abuse predicts only planned suicide attempts, and childhood neglect and family violence predict unplanned attempts. In middle-income countries,

none of the 16 parental psychopathologies or childhood adversities considered in the analysis predict planned or unplanned attempts. In low-income countries, family violence predicts planned attempt; parental panic and parental generalized anxiety disorder increase the odds of unplanned attempt, and parental divorce and other parental loss decrease the odds of unplanned attempts. The bivariate ORs of these significant predictors are in the range of 0.1–8.7.

Respondent mental disorders as risk factors

Respondent 12-month DSM-IV disorders are strong predictors of 12-month suicide ideation in all countries (see Table 13.4). Nearly all 16 disorders predicted ideation in all three groups of countries (see Appendix Tables 13.7–13.9). Few disorders predict suicide plans or attempts among ideators. In the total sample, panic, conduct disorders, and illicit drug abuse/dependence increase the odds of a planned attempt, whereas major depression and conduct disorders increase the odds of an unplanned attempt. No single disorder, or even the number of disorders, is consistently associated with planned or unplanned attempt across the three groups of countries. In high-income countries, specific phobia (OR=2.5) and conduct disorder (OR=16.3) are the only disorders that predict planned suicide attempts, while none predict unplanned attempts. In middle-income countries, bipolar disorder is associated with a significantly *reduced* risk of making a planned attempt (OR=0.3) and illicit drug abuse/dependence (OR=7.7) and any substance use disorder (OR=3.1) with increased risk of making a planned attempt. No disorders predict unplanned attempts, with several ORs estimated at 0.0 likely due to the small cell sizes for these analyses. In low-income countries, panic disorder (OR=9.0) and illicit drug abuse/dependence (OR=6.8) are associated with increased risk of making a planned attempt, and are the only disorders that predict planned attempts.

History of suicidal behavior

Risk factors for 12-month suicide ideation include history of prior suicidal behavior in the total sample (see Table 13.5) and in all groups of countries (see Appendix Tables 13.10–13.12), with bivariate ORs in the range of 24.3–51.8. These ORs are less extreme and also more varied in predicting suicide attempts among ideators. Several findings are especially noteworthy. First, 12-month ideators with a past history of ideation

Table 13.3. Bivariate associations of parental psychopathology and other childhood adversities[a] with 12-month suicide ideation, plan, and attempt[a] (all countries combined)

Risk factors	Among total sample		Among ideators	
	Ideation	Plan	Planned attempt	Unplanned attempt
	OR (95% CI)	OR (95% CI)	OR (95% CI)	OR (95% CI)
Parental psychopathology				
Parental suicidal behavior	3.1* (2.3–4.2)	1.6 (1.0–2.8)	1.0 (0.4–2.5)	0.9 (0.2–3.4)
Parental depression	3.3* (2.4–4.5)	1.5 (0.9–2.6)	1.4 (0.7–2.8)	1.8 (0.7–5.0)
Parental panic disorder	2.8* (2.2–3.4)	1.9* (1.3–2.7)	1.7 (0.9–3.4)	1.6 (0.7–3.8)
Parental generalized anxiety disorder	3.5* (2.7–4.7)	1.3 (0.8–2.2)	1.2 (0.5–2.9)	2.4 (0.9–6.2)
Parental substance abuse	2.3* (1.9–2.9)	0.9 (0.6–1.2)	0.8 (0.5–1.4)	0.7 (0.3–1.6)
Parental antisocial personality disorder	3.0* (2.3–3.8)	0.9 (0.5–1.7)	1.3 (0.6–2.9)	0.7 (0.3–1.7)
Other childhood adversities				
Parental death	1.3* (1.1–1.6)	1.0 (0.7–1.4)	1.1 (0.7–1.9)	0.8 (0.3–2.0)
Parental divorce	1.5* (1.2–1.8)	0.9 (0.6–1.4)	1.7 (0.8–3.6)	0.6 (0.2–1.3)
Other parental loss	2.2* (1.7–2.8)	0.9 (0.6–1.4)	0.8 (0.3–1.9)	0.8 (0.3–2.2)
Parental criminal behavior	2.5* (2.0–3.1)	0.9 (0.5–1.6)	1.4 (0.6–3.2)	1.6 (0.6–4.2)
Physical abuse	3.6* (3.1–4.2)	1.4* (1.0–1.9)	1.5 (0.9–2.4)	1.5 (0.9–2.5)
Sexual abuse	4.2* (3.5–5.2)	1.7* (1.1–2.5)	2.1* (1.1–4.0)	1.9 (0.8–4.4)
Neglect	2.5* (2.0–3.1)	2.0* (1.2–3.2)	1.0 (0.5–2.1)	1.8 (0.7–4.3)
Physical illness	1.8* (1.4–2.3)	1.1 (0.7–1.7)	1.6 (0.7–3.3)	1.8 (0.8–4.0)
Family violence	2.6* (2.2–3.0)	1.6* (1.1–2.1)	1.6 (1.0–2.5)	1.8 (1.0–3.3)
Economic adversity	1.7* (1.3–2.2)	1.5 (0.9–2.5)	0.8 (0.4–2.0)	1.2 (0.4–3.8)
(numerator / denominator N)[b]	(2010 / 55,299)	(730 / 2010)	(282 / 730)	(119 / 1280)

* Significant at the 0.05 level, two-sided test.
[a] Based on logistic regression analysis controlling for country.
[b] Numerator N refers to the number of cases with each suicide outcome, denominator N refers to the number of cases in the total sample or in the conditional sample among ideators, ideators with a plan and ideators without a plan.

in the absence of a lifetime plan or attempt are significantly *less* likely to make a first attempt in the 12 months before interview than are 12-month ideators with no prior history of suicide ideation. This pattern is found in all countries, but is significant only in planned and unplanned attempts in high-income countries and planned attempts in low-income countries. Next, 12-month ideators with a prior history of a suicide plan but no prior attempt are significantly *more* likely to make a planned and an unplanned attempt in the 12 months before the interview than are 12-month ideators with no prior plan. This pattern is found in all countries, but is significant only in unplanned attempts in high-income countries, unplanned attempts in middle-income countries, and planned attempts in low-income countries. In all

countries, 12-month ideators with a history of prior unplanned (i.e., impulsive) attempts have significantly lower odds of planned attempt (ORs=0.1–0.2) than those with no prior history. Finally, 12-month ideators with a history of prior planned attempts have modestly elevated odds of planned attempts in high-income countries (OR=1.8), planned attempts in middle-income countries (OR=3.5), and unplanned attempts in low-income countries (OR=3.6).

Summary risk index for 12-month suicide attempt among ideators

Summary risk indices based on these results (see Appendix Table 13.13 for a list of risk factors included in each index) have AUCs in the range of 54.1–81.0

Table 13.4. Bivariate associations of 12-month DSM-IV/CIDI disorders with 12-month suicide ideation, plan, and attempt[a] (all countries combined)

12-month DSM-IV disorders[b]	Among total sample		Among ideators	
	Ideation	Plan	Planned attempt	Unplanned attempt
	OR (95% CI)	OR (95% CI)	OR (95% CI)	OR (95% CI)
Anxiety disorders				
Panic disorder	9.1* (7.5–11.1)	2.0* (1.3–3.0)	2.2* (1.3–4.0)	0.8 (0.4–1.9)
Agoraphobia without panic	5.7* (4.3–7.5)	1.7* (1.1–2.8)	1.1 (0.6–2.2)	0.7 (0.3–1.8)
Generalized anxiety disorder	7.4* (6.0–9.1)	1.2 (0.8–1.8)	0.7 (0.4–1.4)	0.4 (0.2–1.0)
Specific phobia	3.9* (3.4–4.4)	1.7* (1.3–2.2)	1.5 (0.9–2.4)	1.0 (0.5–1.8)
Social phobia	6.9* (5.9–8.0)	1.8* (1.3–2.5)	0.9 (0.5–1.5)	1.0 (0.5–2.0)
Posttraumatic stress disorder	7.5* (6.1–9.2)	1.2 (.8–1.7)	1.6 (0.9–3.1)	0.9 (0.4–1.9)
Adult separation anxiety disorder	10.0* (7.4–13.6)	2.0* (1.1–3.4)	1.2 (0.5–2.6)	2.6 (1.0–6.7)
Any anxiety disorder	6.3* (5.5–7.1)	1.6* (1.3–2.1)	1.5 (1.0–2.3)	1.2 (0.7–1.9)
Mood disorders				
Major depressive disorder	11.0* (9.7–12.3)	1.7* (1.3–2.1)	1.0 (0.6–1.4)	1.6* (1.0–2.6)
Dysthymic disorder	8.8* (6.7–11.4)	2.3* (1.4–3.8)	1.0 (0.4–2.5)	0.8 (0.3–2.3)
Bipolar disorder	8.7* (7.0–10.7)	2.0* (1.3–2.9)	1.0 (0.6–1.8)	0.8 (0.4–1.9)
Any mood disorder	12.0* (10.7–13.5)	1.9* (1.5–2.4)	1.1 (0.7–1.6)	1.5 (1.0–2.4)
Impulse-control disorders				
Attention deficit hyperactivity disorder	3.7* (2.4–5.7)	1.8 (0.9–3.7)	0.9 (0.3–2.6)	0.8 (0.2–3.4)
Oppositional defiant disorder	9.9* (6.1–16.2)	2.0 (0.8–5.4)	2.0 (0.6–6.9)	2.7 (0.6–11.6)
Conduct disorder	3.9* (2.3–6.5)	2.3 (0.7–7.2)	11.3* (1.7–74.8)	4.8* (1.0–21.7)
Intermittent explosive disorder	5.4* (4.3–6.8)	1.7* (1.2–2.6)	1.2 (0.7–2.3)	1.6 (0.7–3.7)
Any impulse-control disorder	4.8* (3.8–6.1)	1.4 (0.9–2.2)	1.3 (0.7–2.4)	1.3 (0.7–2.5)
Substance use disorders				
Alcohol abuse or dependence	4.6* (3.8–5.6)	2.1* (1.4–3.0)	1.6 (0.9–2.8)	0.5 (0.2–1.3)
Illicit drug abuse or dependence	11.1* (8.4–14.8)	1.9* (1.1–3.2)	3.3* (1.4–7.7)	0.7 (0.3–2.1)
Any substance use disorder	5.8* (4.9–7.0)	2.0* (1.4–2.9)	2.2* (1.3–4.0)	0.7 (0.3–1.4)
Number of disorders				
Any	8.8* (7.6–10.1)	1.8* (1.4–2.4)	1.8* (1.1–3.2)	1.3 (0.8–2.3)
1[b]	5.1* (4.3–6.0)	1.3 (0.9–1.8)	1.5 (0.8–2.8)	1.3 (0.7–2.6)
2[b]	13.7* (11.3–16.5)	1.9* (1.3–2.6)	2.6* (1.4–4.9)	1.2 (0.5–2.6)
3+[b]	29.2* (24.0–35.5)	3.1* (2.2–4.5)	1.7 (0.9–3.3)	1.5 (0.7–2.9)
χ^2_2 (p-value)	1372.9 (<0.001)*	42.8 (<0.001)*	8.7 (0.03)*	1.4 (0.71)
(numerator / denominator N)[c]	(2265 / 109,377)	(742 / 2265)	(286 / 742)	(123 / 1523)

* Significant at the 0.05 level, two-sided test.
[a] Based on logistic regression analysis controlling for country.
[b] Rows based on multivariate regression analysis controlling for country (no disorder is the reference category).
[c] Numerator N refers to the number of cases with each suicide outcome, denominator N refers to the number of cases in the total sample or in the conditional sample among ideators, ideators with a plan and ideators without a plan.

Table 13.5. Multivariate associations between respondent history of suicidal behavior and 12-month suicide ideation, plan, and attempt[a] (all countries combined)

History of suicidal behavior prior to current year	Among total sample		Among ideators	
	Ideation	Plan	Planned attempt	Unplanned attempt
	OR (95% CI)	OR (95% CI)	OR (95% CI)	OR (95% CI)
History of ideation only	29.5* (25.4–34.1)	0.2* (0.1–0.3)	0.2* (0.1–0.4)	0.4* (0.2–0.8)
History of ideation and plan but no attempt	29.4* (22.8–37.8)	0.7 (0.5–1.1)	2.0* (1.0–4.0)	7.6* (4.2–13.9)
History of ideation with unplanned attempt	46.1* (37.8–56.2)	6.0* (4.1–8.6)	0.2* (0.1–0.3)	1.6 (0.7–3.9)
History of ideation with planned attempt	44.7* (37.2–53.6)	4.8* (3.5–6.7)	1.8* (1.1–2.8)	1.2 (0.5–3.0)
X^2_4 (p-value)	2878.6 (<0.001)*	297.2 (<0.001)*	81.8 (<0.001)*	95.3 (<0.001)*
(numerator / denominator N)[b]	(2265 / 109,377)	(742 / 2265)	(286 / 742)	(123 / 1523)

* Significant at the 0.05 level, two-sided test.
[a] Based on multivariate logistic regression analysis controlling for countries, age, age squared.
[b] Numerator N refers to the number of cases with each suicide outcome, denominator N refers to the number of cases in the total sample or in the conditional sample among ideators, ideators with a plan and ideators without a plan.

across the six outcomes (i.e., planned and unplanned attempts in high-income, middle-income, and low-income countries; see Table 13.6). This means that a randomly selected suicide attempter could be distinguished from a randomly selected non-attempter with 54.1%–81.0% accuracy based on their comparative scores on these risk indices – demonstrating a moderate to high level of precision. The three indices for planned attempts are consistent across countries in that roughly half of planned attempts (sensitivity: 44.3%–61.6%) were made by the roughly one-third to one-fourth of respondents classified as in the two highest ("severe" and "very severe") risk categories, whereas fewer than 10% of planned attempts were made by the roughly one-third to one-fourth of respondents classified as having low risk ("mild" category). Notably, roughly nine in ten of the respondents classified by the risk indices as having the highest ("very severe") risk made attempts (positive predictive value: 91.7%–96.7%). The indices for unplanned attempts have smaller proportions of respondents classified into the two highest risk categories than the indices for planned attempts, lower proportions of attempts made by people in these categories (i.e., "severe" and "very severe") (31.4%–67.8%), and smaller proportions of respondents classified at highest risk who made attempts (10.4%–50.4%).

Even with a dataset as large as the one used here, the low 12-month prevalence of suicide attempts made it impossible to develop stable risk indices separately for each participating country. However, in order to get a rough indication of the performance of the summary risk indices in particular countries, we calculated AUCs to assess concordance between predicted probability of an attempt and actual attempts. The predicted probability estimates were generated from separate equations for planned and unplanned attempts in high-, middle-, and low-income countries. The AUC estimates were substantial (>0.80) for nearly 40% of the replications, moderate (>0.70–0.80) for an additional 32.5%, and fair for another 27.5% of replications. However, prediction accuracy was considerably greater in high-income countries (nearly 43% substantial and 86% either moderate or substantial) than middle-income (42% and 75%) and low-income countries (40% and 70%) and somewhat greater for planned than unplanned attempts (see Appendix Table 13.14).

Discussion

The results of this study are limited in four important ways. First, our analysis was based on retrospective self-reports (Angold et al., 1996). Variables that can

Table 13.6. Performance of summary risk indices for 12-month suicide attempt (all countries combined)

Country group	PPV[a] (SE)	Sensitivity[b] (SE)	Specificity[c] (SE)	OR[d] (95% CI)	(n)[e]
All countries					
Attempt planned					
Mild	10.3 (2.1)	9.1 (1.8)	49.5 (2.8)	1.0 (1.0–1.0)	(237)
Moderate	38.2 (3.4)	38.2 (3.4)	38.6 (2.6)	4.9* (2.9–8.3)	(303)
Severe	66.0 (4.6)	34.1 (3.5)	11.0 (1.6)	16.8* (8.8–31.9)	(147)
Very severe	92.4 (3.4)	18.6 (3.9)	1.0 (0.4)	106.7* (36.0–316.6)	(43)
Total	38.4 (2.4)	100.0 (0.0)	100.0 (0.0)	χ^2_4=108.4 (<0.001)*	(730)
	AUC=79.0				
Attempt unplanned					
Mild	3.2 (1.0)	12.2 (3.5)	34.9 (1.9)	1.0 (1.0–1.0)	(447)
Moderate	7.7 (1.2)	39.4 (5.5)	44.4 (2.1)	2.6* (1.2–5.5)	(539)
Severe	16.0 (3.2)	34.8 (5.7)	17.0 (1.5)	6.6* (2.8–15.5)	(231)
Very severe	25.9 (7.5)	13.5 (4.4)	3.6 (0.5)	7.1* (2.2–23.4)	(63)
Total	8.5 (1.0)	100.0 (0.0)	100.0 (0.0)	χ^2_4=23.4 (<0.001)*	(1280)
	AUC=68.0				
High-income countries					
Attempt planned					
Mild	7.3 (2.5)	9.6 (3.3)	59.2 (4.0)	1.0 (1.0–1.0)	(122)
Moderate	38.4 (5.3)	38.6 (5.9)	30.1 (3.6)	7.9* (3.2–19.1)	(118)
Severe	65.7 (6.7)	41.7 (6.5)	10.5 (2.3)	23.4* (8.8–62.7)	(72)
Very severe	96.7 (3.8)	10.0 (6.1)	0.2 (0.2)	353.2* (31.3–3982.1)	(6)
Total	32.7 (3.5)	100.0 (0.0)	100.0 (0.0)	χ^2_4=51.1 (<0.001)*	(318)
	AUC=81.0				
Attempt unplanned					
Mild	1.8 (0.9)	11.8 (5.3)	53.0 (2.8)	1.0 (1.0–1.0)	(314)
Moderate	7.5 (2.4)	22.4 (6.3)	23.1 (2.5)	4.2 (1.0–18.5)	(147)
Severe	18.4 (3.5)	59.6 (7.5)	22.3 (2.3)	11.5* (4.6–28.9)	(184)
Very severe	25.1 (13.7)	6.2 (2.9)	1.6 (0.9)	26.7* (5.6–127.4)	(9)
Total	7.8 (1.2)	100.0 (0.0)	100.0 (0.0)	χ^2_4=33.4 (<0.001)*	(654)
	AUC=75.8				
Middle-income countries					
Attempt planned					
Mild	7.2 (3.0)	4.2 (1.7)	44.9 (5.9)	1.0 (1.0–1.0)	(57)
Moderate	43.6 (7.2)	34.2 (6.6)	37.2 (5.7)	9.3* (3.3–26.0)	(76)
Severe	63.2 (8.5)	32.0 (6.1)	15.6 (4.1)	19.1* (6.3–57.9)	(52)
Very severe	91.7 (6.3)	29.6 (8.0)	2.3 (1.7)	135.1* (21.6–843.0)	(20)
Total	45.6 (4.7)	100.0 (0.0)	100.0 (0.0)	χ^2_4=41.6 (<0.001)*	(205)
	AUC=80.7				
Attempt unplanned					
Mild	7.9 (6.1)	15.1 (11.2)	14.4 (2.3)	1.0 (1.0–1.0)	(49)
Moderate	6.8 (2.1)	53.6 (11.0)	60.8 (3.5)	1.2 (0.2–6.7)	(170)
Severe	9.2 (3.5)	22.8 (8.6)	18.6 (2.4)	1.7 (0.2–12.0)	(66)
Very severe	10.4 (6.3)	8.6 (4.7)	6.1 (2.3)	3.7 (0.3–38.4)	(18)
Total	7.6 (1.7)	100.0 (0.0)	100.0 (0.0)	χ^2_4=1.6 (0.67)*	(303)
	AUC=54.1				

Table 13.6. (cont.)

Country group	PPV^a (SE)	Sensitivity^b (SE)	Specificity^c (SE)	OR^d (95% CI)	(n)^e
Low-income countries					
Attempt planned					
Mild	9.9 (4.5)	6.5 (3.0)	38.0 (5.3)	1.0 (1.0–1.0)	(51)
Moderate	37.8 (5.6)	49.2 (6.5)	52.1 (5.1)	5.9* (2.0–17.6)	(107)
Severe	65.0 (9.0)	27.1 (5.4)	9.4 (2.7)	14.5* (3.8–55.0)	(36)
Very severe	95.1 (4.8)	17.2 (4.0)	0.6 (0.6)	139.3* (13.9–1397.2)	(13)
Total	39.1 (4.0)	100.0 (0.0)	100.0 (0.0)	χ^2_4=24.0 (<0.001)*	(207)
	AUC=75.6				
Attempt unplanned					
Mild	3.1 (1.6)	8.6 (4.9)	34.6 (4.2)	1.0 (1.0–1.0)	(89)
Moderate	6.0 (2.3)	25.1 (9.3)	49.6 (4.1)	2.4 (0.6–10.0)	(160)
Severe	30.1 (9.7)	44.4 (12.7)	13.1 (2.0)	23.9* (3.9–148.1)	(59)
Very severe	50.4 (18.2)	21.9 (12.0)	2.7 (0.9)	65.6* (5.8–745.8)	(15)
Total	11.3 (2.7)	100.0 (0.0)	100.0 (0.0)	χ^2_4=14.0 (0.003)*	(323)
	AUC=78.2				

* Significant at the 0.05 level, two-sided test.
^{a} Percent with attempts among each row category.
^{b} Sensitivity: out of those that had an attempt, % of each row category.
^{c} Specificity: out of those that did not have an attempt, % of each row category.
^{d} Significance tests control for countries, predicting 12-month attempt with categorical risk factor levels.
^{e} Number of cases in each row category.

change over time (e.g., educational attainment, marital status) or that are based on long-term recall (e.g., parental psychopathology, childhood adversities) are of special concern. Even though our risk index performed extremely well under this circumstance, our results should be considered preliminary and we need to cross-validate these indices prospectively. Second, we used a comparable set of methods and procedures to collect information in all countries, but still there could have been cross-cultural differences in the interpretation and the willingness to report suicidal behavior and our risk factors. In addition, we have not considered here any measure of suicide intent or the severity of the suicide attempt that may present variation across our surveys and may have affected the construction of these indices. Significant efforts were dedicated to carefully translating and back-translating the WHO-CIDI used in this study in order to minimize such concerns (Kessler & Üstün, 2004); however, differences in factors such as the stigma about suicide are likely to persist cross-nationally, despite these efforts. Third, although the overall response rate was

at an acceptable level, response rates varied across countries and, in some cases, were below commonly accepted standards. We controlled for differential response using poststratification adjustments, but it is possible that response rates were related to the presence of suicidal behavior or mental disorders, which could have biased cross-national comparisons. Fourth, although this study considered a larger than usual series of risk factor domains to build a risk index, some psychiatric disorders such as schizophrenia were not considered, nor did we consider the level of severity and chronicity of psychiatric disorders assessed by the surveys. Other psychological constructs, such as hopelessness or personality traits, biological markers or other short-term negative events, also were not considered.

With these limitations in mind, several points are worth mentioning. We found the 12-month prevalence of suicidal behavior among adults (18+ years old) in 21 countries to be, for the total sample, 2.0% for reporting suicide ideation, 0.6% for reporting a plan, and 0.4% for reporting an attempt. These rates did not vary meaningfully across our three groups of nations. Similarly to our prior report on lifetime suicidal behavior (Nock et al., 2008a), we found no differences in 12-month suicidal behavior between high-, middle-, and low-income countries, in contrast with what has been suggested by others (Vijayakumar et al., 2005). Most estimates of the prevalence of suicidal behavior in the general population are lifetime estimates as 12-month suicidal behavior is a rare phenomenon that requires large sample sizes to obtain stable estimates. One recent example is the work of Blackmore et al. (2008) that surveyed 36,984 Canadians and found only 222 cases of "suicidal acts," for a 12-month prevalence rate of 0.6%, which is a little above our own estimate for suicide attempts. This is probably because, compared to the Blackmore et al. (2008) study and other more limited surveys (Nock et al., 2008b), we used conservative items for the assessment of each suicidal behavior (e.g., presence of suicide ideation required that a person have "seriously" thought about committing suicide rather than have merely "thoughts of death" as in some prior studies). Further, we used large representative samples of respondents from the general population (i.e., rather than small selective samples that may be at higher risk for suicidal behavior, such as young adults or those in a clinical setting).

Our large and representative dataset and the use of standard definitions and methodology have allowed us, for the first time, to be able to produce meaningful estimates of the ratio of suicide attempt and completed suicide. Using our figures of 12-month suicide attempt and the WHO database on mortality (WHO, 2009b), we estimate that across the countries examined here, there are approximately 14.6 suicide attempts for every one suicide death (median ratio: 14.6; IQR: 9.1–53.7). It is not clear at this point why there is such a large variation in completed suicides across nations while the variation in 12-month attempts is so small, or why there is such large variation in the number of attempts by each suicide across the nations surveyed here. These are clearly important points for future research that reach beyond our goals in this report.

The main goal was to find potential risk factors for a suicide attempt that clinicians can assess quickly using fully structured assessments. In this regard, we successfully developed risk factor indices for 12-month suicide attempts tailored for planned versus unplanned attempts and with versions available for

high-, middle-, and low-income countries. Even though the indices differed somewhat across countries, all summary risk indices using these factors showed good discrimination (as evidenced by moderate to substantial AUCs of 54.1–81.0) in the total sample. These values are within the range of results reported to predict recent and remote attempts in a much more homogenous sample of psychiatric patients from two institutions in the United States, with ROCs of 0.80 and 0.65 (Mann et al., 2008). Our indices performed quite well when applied to most high-income countries and to a substantial minority of middle- and low-income countries. These indices tend to perform better for planned attempts than unplanned attempts, the latter of which are especially difficult to predict. Interestingly, in all groups of countries, no psychiatric disorders were associated with unplanned attempts among suicide ideators. Much more attention should be placed on finding significant predictors of unplanned attempts (Conner, 2004), which represent approximately a quarter to a third of all attempts.

An important next step is to test the usefulness of these indices in prospective studies among large clinical samples, such as those presenting to a general practice or outpatient psychiatric clinic. Patients reporting suicide ideation could receive some version of this risk index and be followed over time to test the prediction of subsequent suicide attempts. Analyses could evaluate more refined coding of the current risk factors as well as risk factors not studied here (e.g., a broader set of disorders, measures of disorder severity or chronicity). Our risk indices could be viewed as an important initial step toward bridging the gap between the science and practice of suicide risk assessment, an issue of great interest because of questions on the effectiveness of detecting and intervening with people at high risk for suicide attempts (Gaynes et al., 2004; Kessler et al., 2005). It is important to note that these indices are not intended to serve as a comprehensive suicide assessment by themselves, but instead may be best used to identify those at high risk for suicide attempt so that such individuals can receive a more focused, in-depth assessment of current risk for suicidal behavior.

Very few population-based surveys address risk factors for current suicidal behavior and much of what is known comes from studies on lifetime suicidal behavior. Therefore, our results on 12-month suicidal behavior are unique in this regard. It is notable that we were able to replicate the results of prior studies showing that female gender, younger age, lower education and income, unmarried status, unemployment, parental psychopathology, childhood adversities, the presence of every mental disorder assessed, and psychiatric comorbidity all emerged as significant risk factors for suicidal behavior in this study (Blackmore et al., 2008; Borges et al., 2008; Kessler et al., 1999; Moscicki, 1999; Nock & Kessler, 2006). As reported by a prior study (Kessler et al., 1999), the considerably weaker associations of most mental disorders with subsequent attempts than with ideation suggest that the effects of mental disorders on suicidal behavior are largely mediated by suicide ideation, and that the determinants of the transition from ideation to attempts are controlled by other factors. Importantly, and consistent with a prior study on lifetime suicidal behavior (Nock et al., 2008a), the main group of disorders associated with suicide attempt included conduct disorder followed by anxiety and substance use disorders, with some exceptions. This suggests that disorders characterized by impulse-control and anxiety may be most important in predicting the transition from suicide thoughts to suicide attempts. An inspection of the mental disorders that formed our risk indices for 12-month suicide attempt in all countries for planned attempts also showed panic disorder, oppositional defiant and conduct disorder, and drug use disorders to be among the most important.

Our results also support and extend the well-documented findings among both adults (Borges et al., 2008; Brown et al., 2000; Goldstein et al., 1991; Joiner et al., 2005; Mann et al., 2008) and adolescents (Brezo et al., 2007; Nock & Kazdin, 2002) that the strongest predictor of suicidal behavior is a past history of the same outcomes. In this research, we took advantage of our large sample size and were able to further specify the role of prior ideation, plan, and attempt in the occurrence of a planned and unplanned attempt, something that has not been done before. With these specifications, our data revealed that a history of unplanned (i.e., impulsive) suicide attempts predicts subsequent unplanned attempts (but may reduce planned ones), while a history of planned attempts predicts subsequent planned attempts (but not unplanned ones). It is clear that we were only able to elicit very limited information about the presence of a suicide plan in our surveys and future research should investigate this issue by debriefing "unplanned" attempters about the sequence of thoughts and decisions that led up to their attempts (Conner et al., 2004). We also found that risk of the transition from suicidal thoughts to attempts was significantly *lower* among those who had thought of suicide in the past but who never made a suicide plan or an attempt than among those who had never had suicidal thoughts before the past 12 months. These results should also be integrated with the results presented in Chapter 4 of this book, which suggest that the presence of a suicide plan among ideators is a key mediator. Among those ideators with a plan, the longer the period of ideation the greater the risk of attempt, but among impulsive attempters that was not the case. At this moment, it is unknown what the psychological mechanisms are that could help to explain why the risk of attempt would decrease as time passes by since the first ideation and why, among those with a plan, the inverse would occur. An important next step is to study people with a history of ideation who never made a suicide attempt in greater detail, in an effort to understand what characterizes such people (e.g., good impulse-control, low severity of suicide ideation) and what strategies they use to resist the urge to make a suicide attempt.

Future directions

This study is one of the few available that documents the prevalence of current (12-month) suicidal behavior among representative samples of adults in the general population. Even though it is reassuring that most of our risk factors are quite consistent with research based on lifetime suicidal behavior, clearly new research with protocols different from the WMH Surveys are needed to confirm our basic findings. For the first time it is possible to study the global distribution of lifetime and 12-month suicidal behavior and suicide death. New studies in this area are needed to understand the transitions among suicidal behaviors, including completed suicide. Although our risk indices resulted in satisfactory performance indicators, they need to be replicated. Ideally this replication should be done in longitudinal research among a mixed sample of general and psychiatric patients. Whether these indices, or a variation of them, will be clinically appealing is a matter of future work as well. The results of this chapter as well as others from this book highlight the need to obtain data on other factors that may contribute to our understanding of why some individuals will remain ideators (sometimes for long periods of time), while others will start making suicide plans, and still others will make a suicide attempt. Although we had a large list of risk factors from multiple domains, overall they turn out to be insufficient to understanding these transitions. Additional research is needed in this area that, ideally, should be done in tandem with research on how prior suicidal behavior is related to a current state of suicide ideation and behaviors.

Acknowledgements

Portions of this chapter are based on Borges, G., Nock, M. K., Haro Abad, J. M., et al. (2010). Twelve-month prevalence of and risk factors for suicide attempts in the WHO World Mental Health Surveys. *Journal of Clinical Psychiatry*, 71(12), 1617–1628. Copyright © 2010. Physicians Postgraduate Press, Inc. Reproduced with permission.

References

Angold A., Erkanli A., Costello E. J., & Rutter M. (1996). Precision, reliability and accuracy in the dating of symptom onsets in child and adolescent psychopathology. *Journal of Child Psychology and Psychiatry*, **37**(**6**), 657–664.

Blackmore, E. R., Munce, S., Weller, I., et al. (2008). Psychosocial and clinical correlates of suicidal acts: results from a national population survey. *British Journal of Psychiatry*, **192**(4), 279–284.

Borges, G., Angst, J., Nock, M. K., et al. (2006). A risk index for 12-month suicide attempts in the National Comorbidity Survey Replication (NCS-R). *Psychological Medicine*, **36**(12), 1747–1757.

Borges, G., Angst, J., Nock, M. K., Ruscio, A. M., & Kessler, R. C. (2008). Risk factors for the incidence and persistence of suicide-related outcomes: a 10-year follow-up study using the National Comorbidity Surveys. *Journal of Affective Disorders*, **105**(1–3), 25–33.

Borges, G., Nock, M. K., Haro Abad, J. M., et al. (2010). Twelve-month prevalence of and risk factors for suicide attempts in the WHO World Mental Health Surveys. *Journal of Clinical Psychiatry*, **71**(12), 1617–1628.

Brezo, J., Paris, J., Barker, E. D., et al. (2007). Natural history of suicidal behaviors in a population-based sample of young adults. *Psychological Medicine*, **37**(11), 1563–1574.

Brown, G. K., Beck, A. T., Steer, R. A., & Grisham, J. R. (2000). Risk factors for suicide in psychiatric outpatients: a 20-year prospective study. *Journal of Consulting and Clinical Psychology*, **68**(3), 371–377.

Cohen, J. (1960). A coefficient of agreement for nominal scales. *Educational and Psychological Measurement*, **20**, 37–46.

Conner, K. R. (2004). A call for research on planned vs. unplanned suicidal behavior. *Suicide and Life-Threatening Behavior*, **34**(2), 89–98.

Cooper-Patrick, L., Crum, R. M., & Ford, D. E. (1994). Identifying suicidal ideation in general medical patients. *Journal of the American Medical Association*, **272**(22), 1757–1762.

Gaynes, B. N., West, S. L., Ford, C. A., et al. (2004). Screening for suicide risk in adults: a summary of the evidence for the U.S. Preventive Services Task Force. *Annals of Internal Medicine*, **140**(10), 822–835.

Goldstein, R. B., Black, D. W., Nasrallah, A., & Winokur, G. (1991). The prediction of suicide. Sensitivity, specificity, and predictive value of a multivariate model applied to suicide among 1906 patients with affective disorders. *Archives of General Psychiatry*, **48**(5), 418–422.

Guyatt, G., & Rennie, D. (2001). *User's Guide to the Medical Literature: A Manual for Evidence-Based Clinical Practice.* Chicago, IL: AMA Press.

Hanley, J. A., & McNeil, B. J. (1982). The meaning and use of the area under a receiver operating characteristic (ROC) curve. *Radiology*, **143**(1), 29–36.

Isometsa, E. T., & Lonnqvist, J. K. (1998). Suicide attempts preceding completed suicide. *British Journal of Psychiatry*, **173**, 531–535.

Joiner, T. E. Jr., Conwell, Y., Fitzpatrick, K. K., et al. (2005). Four studies on how past and current suicidality relate even when "everything but the kitchen sink" is covaried. *Journal of Abnormal Psychology*, **114**(2), 291–303.

Kessler, R. C., Berglund, P., Borges, G., Nock, M., & Wang, P. S. (2005). Trends in suicide ideation, plans, gestures, and attempts in the United States, 1990–1992 to 2001–2003. *Journal of the American Medical Association*, **293**(20), 2487–2495.

Kessler, R. C., Borges, G., & Walters, E. E. (1999). Prevalence of and risk factors for lifetime suicide attempts in the National Comorbidity Survey. *Archives of General Psychiatry*, **56**(7), 617–626.

Kessler, R. C., & Üstün, T. B. 2004 The World Mental Health (WMH) Survey Initiative Version of the World Health Organization (WHO) Composite International Diagnostic Interview (CIDI). *International Journal of Methods in Psychiatric Research*, **13**(2), 93–121.

Kraemer, H. C., Morgan, G. A., Leech, N. L., et al. (2003). Measures of clinical significance. *Journal of the American Academy of Child and Adolescent Psychiatry*, **42**(12), 1524–1529.

Kuo, W. H., Gallo, J. J., & Tien, A. Y. (2001). Incidence of suicide ideation and attempts in adults : the 13-year follow-up of a community sample in Baltimore, Maryland. *Psychological Medicine*, **31**(7), 1181–1191.

Mann, J. J., Apter, A., Bertolote, J., et al. (2005). Suicide prevention strategies: a systematic review. *Journal of the American Medical Association*, **294**(16), 2064–2074.

Mann, J. J., Ellis, S. P., Waternaux, C. M., et al. (2008). Classification trees distinguish suicide attempters in major psychiatric disorders: a model of clinical decision making. *Journal of Clinical Psychiatry*, **69**(1), 23–31.

Mann, J. J., Waternaux, C., Haas, G. L., & Malone, K. M. (1999). Toward a clinical model of suicidal behavior in psychiatric patients. *American Journal of Psychiatry*, **156**(2), 181–189.

Moscicki, E. K. (1999). Epidemiology of suicide. In D. G. Jacobs (ed.). *The Harvard Medical School Guide to Suicide Assessment and Intervention*. San Francisco, CA: Jossey-Bass, 40–51.

Nock, M. K., Borges, G., Bromet, E. J., et al. (2008a). Cross-national prevalence and risk factors for suicidal ideation, plans and attempts. *British Journal of Psychiatry*, **192**(2), 98–105.

Nock, M. K., Borges, G., Bromet, E. J., et al. (2008b). Suicide and suicidal behaviors. *Epidemiologic Reviews*, **30**(1), 133–154.

Nock, M. K., Hwang, I., Sampson, N., et al. (2009). Cross-national analysis of the associations among mental disorders and suicidal behavior: findings from the WHO World Mental Health Surveys. *PLoS Medicine*, **6**(8), e1000123.

Nock, M. K., & Kazdin, A. E. (2002). Examination of affective, cognitive, and behavioral factors and suicide-related outcomes in children and young adolescents. *Journal of Clinical Child and Adolescent Psychology*, **31**(1), 48–58.

Nock, M. K., & Kessler, R. C. (2006). Prevalence of and risk factors for suicide attempts versus suicide gestures: analysis of the National Comorbidity Survey. *Journal of Abnormal Psychology*, **115**(3), 616–623.

Pokorny, A. D. (1983). Prediction of suicide in psychiatric patients. *Report of a prospective study. Archives of General Psychiatry*, **40**(3), 249–257.

Suominen, K., Isometsä, E., Suokas, J., et al. (2004). Completed suicide after a suicide attempt: a 37-year follow-up study. *American Journal of Psychiatry*, **161**(3), 562–563.

Vijayakumar, L., Nagaraj, K., Pirkis, J., & Whiteford, H. (2005). Suicide in developing countries (1): frequency, distribution, and association with socioeconomic indicators. *Crisis*, **26**(3), 104–111.

WHO. (2009a). Suicide prevention and special programmes, Available from: http://www.who.int/mental_health/prevention/en/. Accessed December 12, 2009.

WHO. (2009b). Mortality Database: Tables. Available from: http://www.who.int/healthinfo/morttables/en/. Accessed December 24, 2009.

Chapter

14

Treatment of suicidal persons around the world

Ronny Bruffaerts, Koen Demyttenaere, Guilherme Borges, Wai Tat Chiu, Viviane Kovess-Masféty, Oye Gureje, Irving Hwang, Carmen Lara, Nancy A. Sampson, Maria Carmen Viana, and Matthew K. Nock

Introduction

Suicidal behavior is a persistent and lethal public health problem (Hawton & van Heeringen, 2009; Nock et al., 2008). Death by suicide is among the leading causes of death worldwide (Murray & Lopez, 1996). Prevention programs have been established over the years (Hu, 2003; World Health Organization, 2005), of which several have shown to be effective in their ability to decrease suicide risk. In their systematic review on the effectiveness of prevention programs, Mann and colleagues (2005) concluded that physician education (targeted at depression recognition and treatment), means restriction (e.g., firearms, pesticides, or detoxification of domestic gas), and gatekeeper education (e.g., pharmacists, geriatric caregivers, schools) were three promising interventions for the prevention of suicide. Moreover, several psychological treatments (e.g., Brown et al., 2005; Linehan et al., 2006) have demonstrated an ability to reduce suicidal behavior. In an interesting but relatively small study, Chesley and Loring-McNulty (2003) investigated reasons that prevented suicidal persons from progressing to a subsequent suicide attempt. They found that ongoing treatment with a healthcare professional (i.e., primary or mental healthcare) was the most commonly endorsed reason for not attempting suicide *now*. Other social contacts (e.g., with significant others like family or friends) also were important reasons for not attempting suicide.

Although prevention and treatment programs may have a major public health impact, such as through better identification, assessment, and management of suicidal persons or the suicidal process (Hirschfeld & Russell, 1997; Luoma et al., 2002) that could lead to a reduction of suicidal acts and deaths by suicide,

available data suggest that only up to half of suicidal persons make a treatment contact in the year the suicidal behavior occurs (Rhodes et al., 2006). Stigma and financial barriers are among the most commonly reported barriers to treatment for mental disorders or emotional problems (Angermeyer & Matschinger, 2003). First, stigma may increase suicidal risk because suicidal persons may have difficulty disclosing their suicidal thoughts or plans, even when they enter formal treatment (Goldsmith et al., 2002). Moreover, persons with a history of suicide attempt also may suffer from stigma and isolation following their attempt (Knieper, 1999); the act of attempting suicide may be complicated by a societal perception that suicide represents a failure by the victim and his or her surroundings in dealing with problematic emotional issues (Cvinar, 2005). Second, financial problems are other commonly reported barriers to care for suicidal problems. Analyses of the utilization of healthcare facilities for emotional problems or mental disorders have demonstrated that the use of services often decreases when the cost increases (Simon et al., 1996).

Taken together, there is sufficient evidence to conclude that intervening in suicidal behavior may be achieved by treatment. Aiming for adequate treatment for suicidal persons is a far-reaching and complicated process that must follow several steps. Because there are limited data on the treatment of suicidal persons worldwide, a first step is to document how many suicidal persons enter treatment. Second, among those who do not enter treatment, a precise documentation of reasons why suicidal persons did not enter healthcare is essential to identify unmet needs and to take a first step toward prevention programs. Prior research has been limited in two important ways.

First, there are no studies using cross-national population-based samples investigating treatment of suicidal persons in both developed and developing countries. Second, most prior studies focus on the characteristics of treatment for suicidal behavior among those who actually enter treatment. Barriers to receiving any mental health treatment for suicidal persons have never been investigated in prior research.

The design of the World Mental Health (WMH) Surveys addresses each of these shortcomings. The WMH Surveys are general population surveys that use state-of-the art structured psychiatric interviews to measure the presence of mental disorders and suicidal behavior, as well as the receipt of treatment and barriers to care. The current study builds on earlier WMH studies reporting on the cross-national treatment of mental disorders (Wang et al., 2007) and the 12-month prevalence of suicidal behavior (Borges et al., 2010), and addresses each of the aforementioned limitations by conducting comprehensive cross-national analyses of the treatment of suicidal persons in a given 12-month period. The specific aims of the study were to investigate: (1) the proportion of respondents who entered treatment; (2) multivariate predictors of treatment; (3) barriers to treatment; (4) multivariate predictors of barriers to treatment, and (5) variations in treatment and its barriers in high-, middle-, and low-income countries worldwide.

Method

A detailed description of the respondent samples, study procedures, statistical analyses, and assessment of suicidal behavior is provided in Chapter 3 of this volume. The assessment and analysis of sociodemographic factors (Chapter 6), parental psychopathology (Chapter 7), childhood adversities (Chapter 8), traumatic life events (Chapter 9), mental disorders (Chapter 10), and physical conditions (Chapter 11), which are included as covariates in the following analyses, are described in those earlier chapters.

Assessment of treatment and barriers to care

Receipt of treatment in the prior 12 months was assessed by asking respondents if they saw any type of professional, either as an outpatient or inpatient, for problems with emotions, nerves, mental health, or use of alcohol or drugs (Wang et al., 2007). Included

were mental health professionals (e.g., psychiatrist, psychologist), general medical professionals (e.g., family doctor, occupational therapist), and other non-health professionals (e.g., religious counselors, traditional healers, complementary and alternative medicine [CAM]). Examples of these types of providers were presented in a Respondent Booklet as a visual recall aid and varied somewhat across countries, dependent on local circumstances. Respondents who reported no use of mental health services were asked whether there was a time in the past 12 months when they felt that they might have needed to see a professional for problems with their emotions, nerves, or mental health. Those who answered affirmatively were then asked to endorse reasons why they did not see a professional from a list that included three barriers to enter treatment (see Table 14.1): *low perceived need for treatment* (i.e., the problem went away on its own and they did not really need help), *structural barriers* (i.e., lack of financial means, available treatments, personnel, or

Table 14.1. Barriers to treatment assessed in the World Mental Health Surveys

Low perceived need
The problem went away by itself, and I did not really need help.

Structural barriers
My health insurance would not cover this type of treatment.
I was concerned about how much money it would cost.
I was unsure about where to go or who to see.
I thought it would take too much time or be inconvenient.
I could not get an appointment.
I had problems with things like transportation, childcare, or scheduling that would have made it hard to get to treatment.

Attitudinal barriers
I thought the problem would get better by itself.
I didn't think treatment would work.
I was concerned about what others might think if they found out I was in treatment.
I wanted to handle the problem on my own.
I was scared about being put into a hospital against my will.
I was not satisfied with available services.
I received treatment before and it did not work.
The problem didn't bother me very much.

transportation, or the presence of other inconveniences), and *attitudinal barriers* (i.e., presence of stigma, low perceived efficacy of treatments, or the desire to handle the problem on their own). Respondents who reported that they had no need of treatment in the past 12 months (i.e., endorsed the statement "*The problem went away by itself, and I did not really need help.*" as a reason for not seeking treatment) were not asked about structural or attitudinal barriers and were coded as respondents with low perceived need.

Statistical approach

Two statistical approaches were used in this chapter. First, descriptive statistics were used to document the prevalence estimates of 12-month treatment among respondents with any of the four suicidal outcomes and for respondents with any suicidal behavior. Prevalence estimates are provided using raw numbers (n), weighted proportions (%), and standard errors (SE) per mental and general medical healthcare sector. A similar analytical approach was used for the description of barriers to care among respondents who did not use services in the past 12 months. Second, multivariate logistic regression models were used to examine variation in treatment associated with sociodemographic characteristics, history of suicidal behavior, history of prior treatment, and history of lifetime mental disorders. Four main effect models were run, one for each of the three healthcare sectors (any mental healthcare, general medical healthcare, and any non-healthcare) and one for the entire sample. A similar approach was followed for barriers to treatment.

Results

Twelve-month treatment of suicidal persons

Receipt of any treatment among suicidal persons

Thirty-nine percent of respondents who experienced any suicidal behavior in the past 12 months received some treatment in the past year (between 1.8% in Nigeria and 67.9% in the U.S.) (see Table 14.2 and Appendix Table 14.1). The more severe cases access treatment at higher rates: 34.4% of respondents with only suicide ideation receive treatment, compared to 42.3% of those with both suicide ideation and plan, 49.0% of those with ideation, plan, and attempt, and 55.7% of respondents with both ideation and attempt

(without plan). More severe cases also are more likely to receive treatment from each treatment sector: mental healthcare, general medical healthcare, and even non-healthcare (i.e., human service, CAM) (see also Appendix Tables 14.2–14.4).

After disaggregation for income, two major findings stand out. First, treatment receipt is systematically lower in middle-income (between 18.5% and 49.1% of those with suicidal behavior receive treatment) and low-income countries (between 13.6% and 48.1% receive treatment) than in high-income countries (between 51.9% and 70.3% receive treatment). Second, an interesting unexpected finding is the low rate of treatment of respondents with a planned suicide attempt in low-income countries: 14.8% of these respondents report contact with any treatment provider in the previous year. Comparable figures for middle- and high-income countries are 49.1% and 70.3%, respectively. More data are available in Appendix Tables 14.5–14.7.

Predictors of treatment receipt

Multivariate models estimated the independent predictors of treatment among respondents with suicide ideation (see Table 14.3). First, higher access is associated with higher education and higher income. Second, we found a significant association between suicidal severity and the odds of receiving treatment: those with more severe suicidal behavior (e.g., attempt vs. ideation only) have higher odds of receiving treatment. In addition, respondents who meet criteria for a lifetime mood or anxiety disorder have a nearly two-fold increase in the odds of receiving treatment. A shorter time since onset of the suicide ideation also is associated with higher odds of treatment receipt (albeit moderately). Previously being in treatment yields the highest odds of treatment in the past 12 months: respondents who have been treated before for emotional reasons or mental disorders have about a six-fold increase in the odds of accessing healthcare in the past 12 months.

After disaggregation for income categories, we do not see a consistent pattern of predictors for treatment (see Appendix Tables 14.8–14.10). Nonetheless, a few notable findings stand out. First, the role of sociodemographic variables is somewhat unclear, with higher education increasing treatment in low-income countries, and being a homemaker increasing treatment in low- and middle-income countries. Further, being retired or never married decreases the likelihood of treatment in high-income countries. Second, suicidal severity predicts higher odds of treatment receipt,

Table 14.2. Twelve-month treatment of people with suicidal behavior (all countries combined)

Twelve-month treatment	Suicide ideation only (n=1161)			Suicide plan (n=448)			Unplanned suicide attempt (n=119)			Planned suicide attempt (n=282)			Any suicidal behavior (n=2010)		
	%	SE	n	%	SE	n	%	SE	n	%	SE	n	%	SE	n
Any healthcare	31.1	1.7	391	38.1	2.8	172	52.1	5.8	60	40.6	3.5	118	34.8	1.3	741
Any mental healthcare	19.4	1.4	240	24.0	2.5	111	41.6	6.1	47	31.5	3.4	90	23.1	1.1	488
Psychiatrist	11.5	1.1	139	16.4	2.2	76	22.8	4.7	31	27.3	3.3	73	15.1	1.0	319
Other mental healthcare	12.5	1.2	153	14.3	2.0	68	33.5	6.0	36	19.3	3.1	56	14.9	1.0	313
General medical healthcare	20.3	1.5	257	25.1	2.3	116	30.3	5.3	36	20.1	2.8	70	21.8	1.1	479
Any non-healthcare	9.6	1.1	114	10.5	2.0	45	11.7	4.0	14	18.9	3.2	41	11.0	0.9	214
Human service	5.1	0.8	62	5.5	1.5	22	8.2	3.8	8	10.2	2.2	26	6.0	0.7	118
CAM	5.4	0.8	63	6.6	1.6	28	3.4	1.5	6	12.7	2.9	23	6.5	0.7	120
Any of the above	34.4	1.8	432	42.3	2.8	189	55.7	5.8	66	49.0	3.7	136	39.0	1.4	823

but this is only the case in middle- and low-income countries. In more detail, respondents from middle- and low-income countries who report suicide ideation and attempt (without a plan) have approximately a four- to six-fold increase in the odds of receiving treatment. Third, being treated before is the variable with the strongest predictive value toward treatment: those with a history of treatment have a five- to 10-fold increase in the odds of receiving treatment. Fourth, lifetime mood or anxiety disorders are associated with higher odds of being treated in high-income countries: respondents from these countries who meet criteria for a DSM-IV lifetime anxiety or mood disorder have a two- to 2.6-fold increase in the odds of receiving treatment. If we look at multivariate predictors of treatment in the three income groups separately, in low-income countries, there is a trend for socio-demographic variables (i.e., education, employment type) to be more predictive toward treatment access. By contrast, treatment in middle- and high-income countries is more consistently predicted by factors related to suicidal severity, prior treatment, and lifetime mental disorders.

Rate of treatment in different sectors

Among suicidal respondents, the two most frequently accessed treatment sectors are mental healthcare (with

an average of 23.1%; between 0% in Nigeria and 50.9% in Belgium) and general medical healthcare (with an average of 21.8%; between 1.8% in Nigeria and 58.5% in Belgium), followed by non-healthcare (with an average of 11%; between 0% in China, Romania, and Bulgaria and 24.6% in the U.S.) (see Table 14.2 and Appendix Tables 14.2–14.4). Although the overall proportion of respondents entering mental healthcare is comparable to that entering general medical healthcare, a closer comparison between the number of treated cases in either general medical or mental healthcare reveals that the more severe cases are somewhat more likely to be treated in the mental healthcare sector than in the general medical healthcare sector. For example, in respondents *without* a history of suicide attempt, treatment rates are in the 19%–24% range for mental healthcare and in the 20%–25% range for general medical healthcare. By comparison, in respondents *with* a history of suicide attempt, comparable rates are in the 32%–42% range for mental healthcare and in the 20%–30% range for general medical healthcare. The role of non-healthcare as a treatment sector for suicidal behavior remains somewhat limited, with approximately one in ten respondents treated in this sector. However, among respondents with a planned suicide attempt, one in five report having contact with a non-healthcare sector. Another notable finding is that still a significant proportion of suicidal persons receive treatment from the complementary or alternative medicine sector (CAM), especially those respondents with a planned attempt (12.7%).

After disaggregation for income categories, most of the conclusions of descriptive analyses from the entire sample hold (see Appendix Tables 14.5–14.7): the proportion of respondents treated in any health-care and mental healthcare is comparable in every income category studied. This also is the situation for the more severe cases. For example, in high-income countries, among respondents *without* a history of suicide attempt, treatment rates are in the 31%–38% range for mental healthcare and in the 32%–38% range for general medical healthcare. By comparison, in respondents *with* a history of suicide attempt, rates are in the 44%–52% range for mental healthcare and in the 36%–40% range for general medical healthcare.

Comparable figures are seen in middle- and low-income countries. Interestingly, the proportion of planned suicide attempter respondents treated in complementary or alternative sectors (CAM) is considerably higher in high- (16.6%) and middle- (16.0%) than in low-income (1.0%) countries.

Predictors of treatment in different sectors

In multivariate models predicting treatment in specific sectors (see Table 14.3), clinical characteristics (i.e., suicidal severity, time since onset of the suicide ideation, or lifetime mental disorders) or being treated before do not predict entering specific healthcare sectors. Of the total of 27 investigated associations, only one is statistically significant: respondents with a history of treatment have 2.4-fold higher odds of being treated in the non-healthcare sector. By contrast, sociodemographic variables are much more predictive: higher education (OR = 1.2), having a

Table 14.3. Multivariate predictors of the treatment of people with suicidal behavior[a] (all countries combined)

Category/ sub-category	Among 12-month respondents with any suicidal behavior (n=2010)	Among respondents with any suicidal behavior who received treatment (n=823)		
	Any 12-month treatment	Any mental healthcare	General medical healthcare	Any non-healthcare
	OR (95% CI)	OR (95% CI)	OR (95% CI)	OR (95% CI)
Age				
Continuous (divided by 10)	1.1 (1.0–1.3)	0.9 (0.7–1.1)	1.3* (1.0–1.6)	1.0 (0.8–1.3)
χ^2_1 (p-value)	2.2 (0.14)	1.0 (0.32)	4.7 (0.03)*	0.0 (0.96)
Gender				
Female	0.9 (0.6–1.2)	0.8 (0.5–1.2)	1.3 (0.9–2.0)	1.9* (1.2–3.0)
Male				
χ^2_1 (p-value)	0.5 (0.48)	1.4 (0.24)	1.5 (0.22)	6.6 (0.01)*
Education				
Continuous	1.2* (1.0–1.4)	1.2* (1.0–1.5)	0.8* (0.7–1.0)	1.2 (1.0–1.5)
χ^2_1 (p-value)	5.3 (0.02)*	4.3 (0.04)*	4.0 (0.05)*	3.3 (0.07)
Marital status				
Never married	0.7* (0.5–1.0)	1.9* (1.1–3.3)	0.4* (0.3–0.8)	1.8 (1.0–3.3)
Previously married	1.0 (0.7–1.4)	0.9 (0.6–1.4)	1.0 (0.6–1.7)	1.2 (0.7–2.1)
Married/cohabiting				
χ^2_2 (p-value)	5.1 (0.08)	7.3 (0.03)*	9.7 (0.01)*	3.4 (0.19)

Table 14.3. (cont.)

Category/ sub-category	Among 12-month respondents with any suicidal behavior (n=2010)	Among respondents with any suicidal behavior who received treatment (n=823)		
	Any 12-month treatment	Any mental healthcare	General medical healthcare	Any non- healthcare
	OR (95% CI)	OR (95% CI)	OR (95% CI)	OR (95% CI)
Income				
Continuous	1.1* (1.0–1.1)	1.2* (1.1–1.4)	0.9 (0.8–1.0)	0.8* (0.6–1.0)
χ^2_1 (p-value)	5.2 (0.02)*	10.3 (0.001)*	2.9 (0.09)	4.4 (0.04)*
Employment				
Student	2.1 (0.8–5.5)	1.9 (0.7–5.1)	0.7 (0.3–1.8)	1.1 (0.4–3.3)
Homemaker	1.6 (1.0–2.5)	1.4 (0.8–2.5)	0.7 (0.4–1.3)	0.8 (0.4–1.5)
Retired	0.5 (0.3–1.1)	1.5 (0.5–4.9)	0.8 (0.2–2.8)	0.2* (0.0–0.8)
Other	1.0 (0.7–1.6)	1.8* (1.1–2.9)	0.8 (0.5–1.3)	0.8 (0.4–1.5)
Working				
χ^2_4 (p-value)	9.4 (0.05)	8.1 (0.09)	2.1 (0.72)	5.9 (0.21)
Severity of 12-month suicidal behavior				
Suicide plan	1.4 (1.0–2.0)	1.0 (0.6–1.5)	1.1 (0.7–1.8)	1.1 (0.6–1.9)
Unplanned suicide attempt	2.7* (1.5–4.9)	2.2 (1.0–5.1)	1.5 (0.7–3.4)	0.6 (0.2–1.7)
Planned suicide attempt	2.1* (1.4–3.2)	1.5 (0.9–2.6)	0.6 (0.3–1.0)	1.5 (0.8–2.8)
Ideation only				
χ^2_3 (p-value)	19.7 (<0.001)*	6.1 (0.11)	5.7 (0.13)	3.7 (0.30)
Time since ideation				
Continuous (divided by 10)	0.9* (0.7–1.0)	1.1 (0.9–1.3)	0.9 (0.7–1.1)	1.0 (0.8–1.2)
χ^2_1 (p-value)	4.0 (0.04)*	0.7 (0.40)	1.5 (0.22)	0.2 (0.68)
History of treatment				
Yes	6.2* (4.5–8.7)	1.1 (0.7–1.9)	0.8 (0.5–1.4)	2.4* (1.3–4.4)
χ^2_1 (p-value)	114.3 (0.00)*	0.2 (0.64)	0.5 (0.48)	8.6 (0.003)*
Lifetime disorder				
Any anxiety	1.9* (1.4–2.5)	1.3 (0.8–2.0)	1.3 (0.8–2.0)	1.0 (0.6–1.7)
Any mood	1.8* (1.3–2.4)	1.5 (0.9–2.3)	1.0 (0.7–1.5)	1.1 (0.7–1.9)
Any impulse	0.9 (0.6–1.3)	0.9 (0.5–1.7)	1.1 (0.6–1.8)	0.8 (0.4–1.4)
Any substance	0.9 (0.6–1.3)	1.2 (0.8–1.8)	1.1 (0.7–1.7)	1.2 (0.7–2.0)
χ^2_3 (p-value)	38.4 (<0.001)*	5.0 (0.28)	1.7 (0.78)	1.8 (0.78)
χ^2_{19} (p-value)	244.4 (<0.001)*	52.1 (<0.001)*	49.5 (<0.001)*	42.0 (0.002)*

* Significant at the 0.05 level, two-sided test.
[a] Results are based on multivariate logistic regression models controlling for country.

higher income (OR = 1.2), and other employment (OR = 1.8) are associated with higher odds of treatment in mental healthcare; whereas higher age (OR = 1.3) is associated with higher odds of treatment in general medical healthcare. Both education and having never been married are associated with lower odds of treatment in the general medical sector (ORs 0.8 and 0.4, respectively). Lastly, being female (OR = 1.9), having a lower income (OR = 0.8), and being retired (OR = 0.2) are associated with treatment in the non-healthcare sector.

Multivariate predictors of treatment in specific sectors are different for the three income groups compared (see Appendix Tables 14.8–14.10). The most important finding from these multivariate models is that, on average, in all income countries studied, clinical characteristics do not differentiate in which sectors respondents receive treatment. Sociodemographic characteristics best predict treatment in different sectors. For example, respondents from low-income countries who have never been married have lower odds of treatment in the non-healthcare sector, but comparable respondents from middle- and high-income countries have higher odds of treatment in this sector. Three sociodemographic variables predicting mental healthcare treatment are: having never been married (OR = 6.8) in low-income countries, higher education (OR = 4.2) in middle-income countries, and having a higher income (OR = 1.2) and other employment status (OR = 1.7) in high-income countries.

Barriers to treatment among suicidal respondents

Suicidal persons not receiving treatment

Sixty-one percent of respondents with suicide ideation were not treated for emotional reasons in the previous 12 months (43.9% in high-, 72.4% in middle-, and 82.8% in low-income countries) (see Appendix Tables 14.5–14.7). Among those who do not receive treatment, 42.2% report that they might have needed to see a professional for mental health or emotional problems (see Table 14.4). This perceived need for treatment is highest in high-income countries (55.2%), followed by middle- (37.7%) and low-income (32.7%) countries (see Appendix Tables 14.11–14.13). Further analyses reveal that the need for treatment is most pronounced (in the 43%–60% range) in respondents with more severe forms of suicidal

behavior (i.e., those with suicidal attempt in the past year). This is especially the case in high-income countries where, among those with a suicide attempt in the past year, between 59.5% and 74.8% report that they might have needed to see a professional for their problems despite the fact that they did not receive any treatment.

Barriers to treatment

Among those who engaged in suicidal behavior in the past year but did not receive treatment, low perceived need is consistently the most common barrier reported (57.8% of respondents with any suicidal outcome) (see Table 14.4 and Figure 14.1). This is the most prominent barrier among respondents with ideation (57.6%) and a plan (62.6%), as well as those with planned (57.0%) and unplanned (40.0%) suicide attempts. The next most common barriers are specific attitudes about seeking treatment: 26.7% mention that they wanted to handle the problem on their own, 11.5% believe the problem will get better without treatment, 8.6% report that the problem is not that severe, 8.2% believe that treatment will not be effective, and only 6.7% report stigma as the reason for not seeking treatment. The least frequently endorsed barriers are structural, including: limited finances (11.7%), lack of availability of treatment (10.9%), problems with transportation (4.1%), and the inconvenience of attending treatment (3.5%).

In high-income countries, attitudinal barriers are the most common barriers to treatment (53.5%), especially the wish to handle the problem alone (endorsed by about one in three respondents) (see Appendix Table 14.11). Low perceived need is the second most common barrier to care (44.8%). A different picture emerges in middle- (see Appendix Table 14.12) and low-income countries (see Appendix Table 14.13) where low perceived need is the most commonly endorsed barrier to care, seen in 62.3% and 67.3% of the cases, respectively. The second most important barriers in middle- and low-income countries are attitudinal barriers (endorsed by 34.6% and 31.7%, respectively). Among this set of barriers, the wish to handle the problem alone is consistently the most important reason for not seeking care. This specific reason is commonly endorsed by respondents with suicide ideation and a suicide attempt in all three income categories. This suggests that, even when people have made an attempt to end their life, they still wish to handle the problem on their own. Lastly, we

Table 14.4. Barriers to the treatment of people with suicidal behavior (all countries combined)

Reasons for not seeking 12-month treatment	Ideation only (n=723)			Suicide plan (n=253)			Unplanned suicide attempt (n=52)			Planned suicide attempt (n=142)			Any suicidal behavior (n=1170)		
	%	SE	n	%	SE	n	%	SE	n	%	SE	n	%	SE	n
Low perceived need for treatment	57.6	2.8	403	62.6	3.8	155	40.0	8.1	26	57.0	5.4	77	57.8	2.2	661
Any structural barrier	15.4	2.5	114	12.0	2.1	38	16.7	6.8	7	19.5	3.9	34	15.3	1.9	193
Financial	11.9	2.5	82	8.9	1.9	27	11.1	6.1	4	15.8	3.6	27	11.7	1.9	140
Availability	10.6	2.4	77	8.3	1.9	24	11.5	5.4	5	17.4	3.8	28	10.9	1.8	134
Transportation	3.6	0.7	36	6.1	1.6	15	0.0	0.0	0	5.5	2.0	11	4.1	0.6	62
Inconvenient	3.7	0.8	33	2.5	0.9	10	2.9	2.9	1	4.9	2.1	9	3.5	0.6	53
Any attitudinal barrier	41.1	2.8	310	34.2	3.8	87	57.1	8.4	25	39.6	5.4	58	40.3	2.2	480
Wanted to handle on own	27.1	2.2	202	21.9	3.2	59	41.7	8.5	19	27.3	5.5	37	26.7	1.8	317
Perceived ineffectiveness	7.5	1.1	85	9.4	2.2	21	9.3	5.1	6	10.4	2.8	19	8.2	0.9	131
Stigma	6.5	1.3	55	5.0	1.3	15	4.5	2.8	3	11.9	2.8	21	6.7	0.9	94
Thought would get better	12.8	2.4	83	8.9	2.2	20	8.6	4.8	4	8.9	2.7	18	11.5	1.8	125
Problem was not severe	8.1	1.3	61	10.0	2.2	26	13.8	8.6	4	7.3	2.5	11	8.6	1.1	102

Table 14.5. Multivariate predictors of barriers to the treatment of people with suicidal behavior[a] (all countries combined)

Category/subcategory	Among respondents with any suicidal behavior who did not receive treatment (n=1170)		
	Low perceived need for treatment OR (95% CI)	Any structural barrier OR (95% CI)	Any attitudinal barrier OR (95% CI)
Age			
Continuous (divided by 10)	1.0 (0.8–1.3)	0.7* (0.6–0.9)	1.0 (0.8–1.2)
χ^2_1 (p-value)	0.0 (0.89)	6.8 (0.01)*	0.1 (0.76)
Gender			
Female	0.8 (0.5–1.4)	1.5 (0.8–2.6)	1.1 (0.7–1.7)
Male			
χ^2_1 (p-value)	0.5 (0.47)	1.8 (0.19)	0.1 (0.81)
Education			
Continuous	0.9 (0.8–1.2)	0.8 (0.6–1.0)	1.1 (0.9–1.3)

Table 14.5. (cont.)

Category/subcategory	Among respondents with any suicidal behavior who did not receive treatment (n=1170)		
	Low perceived need for treatment OR (95% CI)	Any structural barrier OR (95% CI)	Any attitudinal barrier OR (95% CI)
χ^2_1 (p-value)	0.4 (0.52)	2.9 (0.09)	0.5 (0.46)
Marital status			
Never married	1.0 (0.6–1.7)	0.8 (0.4–1.3)	0.9 (0.6–1.6)
Previously married	0.9 (0.5–1.6)	1.1 (0.6–2.0)	1.1 (0.7–1.9)
Married/cohabiting			
χ^2_2 (p-value)	0.1 (0.95)	1.0 (0.61)	0.3 (0.85)
Income			
Continuous	1.0 (0.9–1.1)	1.1 (1.0–1.2)	1.0 (0.9–1.2)
χ^2_1 (p-value)	0.3 (0.59)	1.9 (0.17)	0.3 (0.56)
Employment			
Student	1.5 (0.4–5.8)	0.8 (0.2–2.9)	0.7 (0.2–2.6)
Homemaker	1.2 (0.7–2.2)	1.4 (0.7–2.8)	0.9 (0.5–1.6)
Retired	1.3 (0.5–3.4)	2.3 (0.7–7.1)	0.6 (0.2–1.5)
Other	0.6 (0.3–1.1)	1.3 (0.7–2.4)	1.6 (0.9–2.8)
Working			
χ^2_4 (p-value)	5.3 (0.26)	3.2 (0.53)	6.0 (0.20)
Severity of 12-month suicidal behavior			
Suicide plan	1.1 (0.6–1.9)	0.7 (0.4–1.3)	0.8 (0.5–1.4)
Unplanned suicide attempt	0.5* (0.2–1.0)	1.0 (0.3–3.1)	1.9 (0.9–4.2)
Planned suicide attempt	0.7 (0.4–1.2)	1.1 (0.6–2.2)	1.2 (0.7–2.2)
Ideation only			
χ^2_3 (p-value)	5.0 (0.18)	1.3 (0.73)	3.5 (0.32)
Time since ideation			
Continuous (divided by 10)	1.1 (0.9–1.3)	0.9 (0.7–1.1)	1.0 (0.8–1.2)
χ^2_1 (p-value)	0.4 (0.51)	0.9 (0.33)	0.2 (0.64)
History of treatment			
Yes	0.5* (0.3–0.9)	2.2* (1.4–3.6)	1.6 (1.0–2.7)
χ^2_1 (p-value)	6.1 (0.01)*	11.8 (0.001)*	3.8 (0.05)
Lifetime disorder			
Any anxiety	0.7 (0.5–1.1)	1.4 (0.8–2.2)	1.3 (0.8–2.0)
Any mood	0.8 (0.5–1.3)	1.5 (0.9–2.5)	1.3 (0.8–1.9)
Any impulse	1.0 (0.6–1.7)	1.0 (0.6–1.8)	0.9 (0.5–1.5)
Any substance	1.0 (0.6–1.8)	1.3 (0.8–2.4)	1.1 (0.6–1.8)
χ^2_3 (p-value)	3.6 (0.47)	4.6 (0.33)	3.3 (0.52)
χ^2_{19} (p-value)	31.6 (0.03)*	48.9 (<.001)*	25.8 (0.14)

*Significant at the 0.05 level, two-sided test.
[a] Results are based on multivariate logistic regression models controlling for country.

could not find evidence for a consistent effect of stigma as a barrier to treatment. The proportion of respondents endorsing stigma as an important reason for not seeking help remains fairly stable across income categories (all in the 6.2%–7.6% range) and across suicidal severity levels (all in the 0.0%–17.3% range).

Multivariate predictors of barriers to treatment

In multivariate prediction models of barriers to treatment (see Table 14.5), no clear pattern of predictors of barriers to care is observed. Indeed, only four associations are statistically significant. Prior treatment for mental disorders or emotional problems is associated with lower odds of reporting low perceived need (OR = 0.5), but with higher odds of reporting structural barriers to treatment (OR = 2.2). Further, increasing age is associated with lower odds of reporting structural barriers (OR = 0.7). Lastly, respondents with an unplanned suicide attempt are less likely to endorse low perceived need as a reason for not seeking treatment (OR = 0.5).

Among respondents from high-income countries (see Appendix Table 14.14), those with either a comorbid lifetime anxiety disorder or a history of treatment are more likely to endorse structural barriers (ORs 2.7–4.1). By comparison, among respondents from middle-income countries (Appendix Table 14.15), a history of treatment predicts both attitudinal (OR = 3.4) and structural barriers (OR = 3.0). In low-income countries, respondents with a planned suicide attempt and those with lifetime substance abuse disorder have higher odds of reporting attitudinal barriers (ORs 4.0–4.1). Those with lifetime substance abuse

disorders also have higher odds of reporting structural barriers (OR = 4.3) (see Appendix Table 14.16).

Discussion

There are five especially important findings in this study. First, the proportion of suicidal people receiving treatment across each of these 21 nationally representative samples around the world is unacceptably low: only 39% of suicidal respondents received treatment in the past year, with consistently lower proportions having received treatment in low- (17%) and middle-income countries (28%) than in high-income countries (56%). Treatment receipt was higher in respondents with more severe suicidal behavior and among those with mood and anxiety disorders. Second, a comparable number of respondents received treatment in general medical (22%) and mental healthcare (23%) sectors. Third, among those not receiving treatment, 42% thought that they might have needed professional help. Fourth, among those not receiving treatment, low perceived need for care was the most common reason for not seeking help, followed by attitudinal, and structural barriers. Remarkably, stigma or financial concerns were not major barriers that prevented respondents from seeking treatment. Fifth, interesting differences were found in treatment of suicidal respondents and their barriers to care when findings were disaggregated by income categories. Treatment rates were especially low in middle- and low-income countries, and in these countries, low perceived need was the most common barrier to treatment whereas

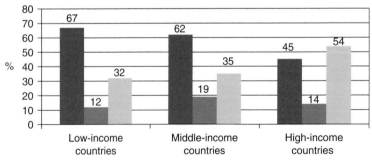

Figure 14.1. Barriers to treatment in the World Mental Health Surveys.

- Low perceived need for treatment
- Structural barriers
- Attitudinal barriers

attitudinal barriers were the highest barriers to care in high-income countries.

Treatment of suicidal persons

Our study points to the high levels of unmet need for care among those with suicidal behavior worldwide. This unmet need is more dramatic in low- and middle-income countries, where less than one in four suicidal respondents is treated for emotional reasons in a given year. Treatment rates are infrequently reported in the literature, but our data are in line with earlier reports (De Leo et al., 2005). If we draw a comparison between the treatment of persons with mental disorders and persons with suicidal behavior, our data suggest that those who are suicidal are more likely than persons with mental disorders to receive treatment. Indeed, 12-month treatment rates of persons with mental disorders vary significantly worldwide but are all within a 1%–15% range (with a median of 5%; Demyttenaere et al., 2004), compared to a 2%–68% range in our study (with a median of 32%).

Our finding that treatment rates are related to suicidal severity – the more severe cases (i.e., those where respondents have made an attempt to end their lives) were more likely to receive treatment – is in line with existing studies (e.g., De Leo et al., 2005; Pirkis et al., 2001). Remarkably, this was only the case in low- and middle-income countries; we could not find any evidence for such an effect in high-income countries. By contrast, in high-income countries, lifetime mental disorders increased the odds of receiving treatment. This is in line with the contribution from Rhodes et al. (2006) using data from the Canadian Community Health Survey Cycle 1.2 *Mental Health and Mental Wellbeing* survey (n=36,984). They found that about 29% of respondents with suicidal behavior but without depression sought professional help in the past 12 months. Interestingly, in respondents with both suicidal behavior and depression, the proportion of respondents who actually made contact with healthcare providers doubled.

The low rate of treatment revealed in this study is particularly concerning, because prior studies have documented the availability of effective treatments for suicidal behavior (Brown et al., 2005; Linehan et al., 2006). Randomized controlled trials suggest that cognitive and behavioral treatment approaches are quite effective in reducing suicidal behavior (Brown et al., 2005; Linehan et al., 2006; McLeavey

et al., 1994; Salkovskis et al., 1990). These treatments focus on the identification of thoughts, beliefs, and specific problem-solving skills to deal with the common pessimistic views of future life expectancies, and difficulties in conceptualizing a positive evaluation of oneself in the future (MacLeod & Tarbuck, 1994; Mann et al., 1999). Adding further concern to the low rate of treatment revealed in this study is the fact that it is unlikely that many of those in the current study who reported receiving treatment actually received proven effective interventions (i.e., cognitive behavioral interventions), given that only 23.1% of respondents received care from a mental health specialist. Instead, large percentages of respondents received treatment in the general medical field (21.8%) or non-healthcare settings (11.0%), where such treatments are unlikely to be available.

The role of general medical healthcare in the treatment of suicidal behavior is important as physical illness is a strong risk factor for suicidal behavior (Maris et al., 2000; Scott et al., 2010). This implies that general medical healthcare clinicians have a relatively high probability of seeing persons at risk for suicidal behavior. Despite the large cross-national differences in the structure and organization of healthcare systems, our findings suggest that general practitioners and other non-mental health providers may serve as gatekeepers for suicidal patients worldwide (Isaac et al., 2009). This suggests that there is a strong need to guarantee adequate screening and treatment of suicidal behavior in general medical healthcare. Attention must be given to sufficient training in basic recognition and management of suicidal behavior in general medical healthcare settings worldwide (Sudak et al., 2007).

A last notable finding was that in some severe forms of suicidal behavior (especially in high- and middle-income countries), up to 17% of the respondents received treatment from complementary or alternative medicine. Apart from the question of to what extent these treatment sectors provide adequate and effective treatment against suicidal problems, these data suggest a trend toward a higher use of these sectors by suicidal persons than by persons with mental disorders (Wang et al., 2007).

The predictors of treatment in the current study generally are consistent with those from previous work, with higher education and income and greater clinical severity serving as core predictors of treatment (Rhodes et al., 2006; Wang et al., 2007). However, greater severity of suicidal behavior was unrelated to the use of the mental healthcare over other forms of treatment. This suggests that although those who make actual suicide attempts are more likely to be treated than those who only think about suicide, attempters are no more likely to be referred to a mental health specialist for treatment than are non-attempters.

Barriers to treatment in suicidal persons

Our findings suggest that the help-seeking process of suicidal persons is complex, with a significant proportion of suicidal persons not receiving any treatment for emotional problems and not perceiving any need for care either. Once people have decided that they should seek treatment, they seem to wait to see whether the problem goes away by itself and whether they can deal with the suicidal behavior on their own. Suicidal thoughts and behaviors typically are transient in nature, coming and going repeatedly over time. As a result, those experiencing a suicidal crisis may simply try to "ride it out" until the crisis abates. In addition, those experiencing suicidal thoughts and behaviors typically feel pessimistic and hopeless and so may not have positive expectations that treatment will help them (Jorm, 2000). Indeed, cognitions of suicidal persons were found to be more pessimistic regarding current or future experiences, and suicidal persons had a significantly higher tendency to try to deal with problems on their own (Tousignant & Hanigan, 1993).

The findings that six out of 10 people with suicidal behavior report a low perceived need for treatment and four out of 10 people with suicidal behavior report attitudinal barriers (especially the wish to try to solve the problem on their own) are critically important ones, as these attitudes may delay access to healthcare and, thus, contribute to a progression of suicidal behavior. Moreover, such barriers may place considerable limits on implementation strategies of evidence-based mental health treatment and prevention programs (Jorm, 2000). One way to address this issue is to educate the broader public about appropriate available treatments for suicidal behavior. Indeed, there is extensive literature demonstrating the relationship between insight in emotional problems and acceptance of and compliance with treatment (Jorm et al., 2000), as well as between educational programs and suicide prevention (Mann et al., 2005). These areas represent important directions for future work.

The predominance of attitudinal barriers (in high-income countries) and low perceived need for treatment (in middle- and low-income countries) is especially interesting because it contradicts the widely accepted view that both stigma and financial concerns are among the most important barriers that prevent suicidal persons from seeking treatment (Arboleda-Flórez, 2003; Corrigan, 2004; Kohn et al., 2004). Indeed, a common belief is that many suicidal persons never pursue treatment because of the enduring effects of stigma or the high costs of mental healthcare (Goldsmith et al., 2002). Our findings challenge this conventional wisdom and show that across income categories, stigma and financial barriers are reported by a minority of suicidal people (less than one-fifth of all conditions studied). This particular finding points to the idea that stigma may not be of crucial importance in the process of seeking treatment, and that prevention efforts targeting other attitudinal barriers may be most effective. As this is the first study to address this question, future studies should focus on possible interactions between different kinds of barriers.

Implications

In an era where great emphasis lies on the prevention of suicide, our data hold important implications. Clinicians, policy makers, and healthcare planners worldwide should be aware of the significance of the large proportions of suicidal persons who do not receive any treatment for emotional problems, and of the broad range of barriers (not only stigma or financial barriers) that are frequently reported as factors that prevented suicidal persons from seeking treatment. In order to decrease the large proportions of untreated persons with suicidal behavior, specific interventions are needed to expand or reallocate treatment resources, especially in those countries with lower access to treatment. By acknowledging that it may not be feasible to provide treatment to everyone who needs it in every country, more efficient strategies (perhaps implemented in tandem with increased treatment resources) may target barriers that are preventing people from receiving available care. The current study suggests that barriers to treatment are generally not structural/financial or stigma-related, but instead concern attitudes (especially in high-income countries) and low perceived need (especially in middle- and low-income countries) that people hold toward seeking treatment for suicidal behavior.

Limitations

Our results should be interpreted in the light of several important limitations. First, our study had a moderate response rate (72.1%). Non-responders in population surveys are likely to have higher rates of mental disorders than respondents (de Graaf et al, 2000). Second, respondents who did not speak the primary language(s) of the country sufficiently, those institutionalized, and those without a fixed address were not included in this study. It may be that such persons are more likely to be suicidal. Moreover, against the background that suicide risk is elevated in inpatients or specific respondent groups (e.g., those with psychotic disorders or borderline personality disorder), we might assume that the prevalence of suicidal behavior is higher among psychiatric inpatients than non-institutionalized persons (Qin & Nordentoft, 2005). Third, the CIDI-3.0 treatment module asks about treatment for emotional or substance abuse problems but not suicidal behavior per se. Although we did control for country differences, suicidal behavior may not always be considered as an emotional or psychological problem and, therefore, not a behavior for which to seek help in the mental healthcare sector. Moreover, the information on treatment access did not include information about the adequacy or effectiveness of the treatment received. Future studies, therefore, may focus in more detail on received treatment for suicidal behavior or criteria defining treatment adequacy/effectiveness. Fourth, because we used a 12-month time frame, we were unable to examine delays in the help-seeking process in the current study. Fifth, responses to the survey may have been biased by the use of retrospective self-report. Previous studies have shown that the validity of the assessment of service use could be biased, dependent upon recall time periods (Simon & VonKorff, 1995), salience of service, or frequency of service use, all leading to a modest underestimation of recent service use (Petrou et al., 2002).

Acknowledgements

Portions of this chapter are based on Bruffaerts, R., Demyttenaere, K., Hwang, I., et al. (2011). Treatment of suicidal persons around the world. *British Journal of Psychiatry*, **199** 64–70. [Epub ahead of print, January 24.]. Copyright © 2011. The Royal College of Psychiatrists. Reproduced with permission.

References

Angermeyer, M. C., & Matschinger, H. (2003). The stigma of mental illness: effects of labelling on public attitudes towards people with mental disorder. *Acta Psychiatrica Scandinavica*, **108**(4), 304–309.

Arboleda-Flórez, J. (2003). Considerations on the stigma of mental illness. *Canadian Journal of Psychiatry*, **48**(10), 645–650.

Borges, G., Nock, M. K., Haro Abad, J. M., et al. (2010). Twelve-month prevalence of and risk factors for suicide attempts in the World Health Organization World Mental Health Surveys. *Journal of Clinical Psychiatry*, **71**(12), 1617–1628.

Brown, G. K., Ten Have, T., Henriques, G. R., et al. (2005). Cognitive therapy for the prevention of suicide attempts: a randomized controlled trial. *Journal of the American Medical Association*, **294**(5), 563–570.

Bruffaerts, R., Demyttenaere, K., Hwang, I., et al. (2011). Treatment of suicidal persons around the world. *British Journal of Psychiatry*, **199** 64–70. [Epub ahead of print, January 24.]

Chesley, K., & Loring-McNulty, N. E. (2003). Process of suicide: perspective of the suicide attempter. *Journal of the American Psychiatric Nurses Association*, **9**(2), 41–45.

Corrigan, P. (2004). How stigma interferes with mental health care. *American Psychologist*, **59**(7), 614–625.

Cvinar, J. G. (2005). Do suicide survivors suffer social stigma?: A review of the literature. *Perspectives in Psychiatric Care*, **41**(1), 14–21.

de Graaf, R., Bijl, R. V., Smit, F., Ravelli, A., & Vollebergh, W. A. M. (2000). Psychiatric and sociodemographic predictors of attrition in a longitudinal study: The Netherlands Mental Health Survey and Incidence Study (NEMESIS). *American Journal of Epidemiology*, **152**(11), 1039–1047.

De Leo, D., Cerin, E., Spathonis, K., & Burgis, S. (2005). Lifetime risk of suicide ideation and attempts in an Australian community: prevalence, suicidal process, and help-seeking behaviour. *Journal of Affective Disorders*, **86**(2–3), 215–224.

Demyttenaere, K., Bruffaerts, R., Posada-Villa, J., et al. (2004). Prevalence, severity, and unmet need for treatment of mental disorders in the World Health Organization World Mental Health Surveys. *Journal of the American Medical Association*, **291**(21), 2581–2590.

Goldsmith, S. K., Pellmar, T. C., Kleinman, A. M., & Bunney, W. E. (2002). *Reducing suicide: A national imperative*. Washington, DC: National Academy Press.

Hawton, K., & van Heeringen, K. (2009). Suicide. *Lancet*, **373**(9672), 1372–1381.

Hirschfeld, R. M., & Russell, J. M. (1997). Assessment and treatment of suicidal patients. *New England Journal of Medicine*, 337(13), 910–915.

Hu, T. W. (2003). Financing global mental health services and the role of WHO. *Journal of Mental Health Policy and Economics*, 6(3), 145–147.

Isaac, M., Elias, B., Katz, L. Y., et al. (2009). Gatekeeper training as a preventative intervention for suicide: a systematic review. *Canadian Journal of Psychiatry*, 54(4), 260–268.

Jorm, A. F. (2000). Mental health literacy: public knowledge and beliefs about mental disorders. *British Journal of Psychiatry*, 177, 396–401.

Jorm, A. F., Angermeyer, M., & Katschnig, H. (2000). Public knowledge of and attitudes to mental disorders: a limiting factor in the optimal use of treatment services. In G. Andrews, & S. Henderson (eds.). *Unmet Need in Psychiatry*, pp. 399–413. Cambridge, England: Cambridge University Press.

Knieper, A. J. (1999). The suicide survivor's grief and recovery. *Suicide and Life-Threatening Behavior*, 29(4), 353–364.

Kohn, R., Saxena, S., Levav, I., & Saraceno, B. (2004). The treatment gap in mental health care. *Bulletin of the World Health Organization*, 82(11), 858–866.

Linehan, M. M., Comtois, K. A., Murray, A. M., et al. (2006). Two-year randomized controlled trial and follow-up of dialectical behavior therapy vs. therapy by experts for suicidal behaviors and borderline personality disorder. *Archives of General Psychiatry*, 63(7), 757–766.

Luoma, J. B., Martin, C. E., & Pearson, J. L. (2002). Contact with mental health and primary care providers before suicide: a review of the evidence. *American Journal of Psychiatry*, 159(6), 909–916.

MacLeod, A. K., & Tarbuck, A. F. (1994). Explaining why negative events will happen to oneself: parasuicides are pessimistic because they can't see any reason not to be. *British Journal of Clinical Psychology*, 33 (3), 317–326.

Mann, J. J., Apter, A., Bertolote, J., et al. (2005). Suicide prevention strategies: a systematic review. *Journal of the American Medical Association*, 294(16), 2064–2074.

Mann, J. J., Waternaux, C., Haas, G. L., & Malone, K. M. (1999). Toward a clinical model of suicidal behavior in psychiatric patients. *American Journal of Psychiatry*, 156(2), 181–189.

Maris, R. W., Berman, A. L., Silverman, M. M., & Bongar, B. M. (2000). *Comprehensive textbook of suicidology*. New York, NY: Guilford Press.

McLeavey, B. C., Daly, R. J., Ludgate, J. W., & Murray, C. M. (1994). Interpersonal problem-solving skills training in the treatment of self-poisoning patients. *Suicide and Life-Threatening Behavior*, 24(4), 382–394.

Murray, C. J. L., & Lopez, A. D. (1996). *Global health statistics: A compendium of incidence, prevalence, and mortality estimates for over 200 conditions*. Cambridge, MA: Harvard University Press.

Nock, M. K., Borges, G., Bromet, E. J., et al. (2008). Suicide and suicidal behavior. *Epidemiologic Reviews*, 30, 133–154.

Petrou, S., Murray, L., Cooper, P., & Davidson, L. L. (2002). The accuracy of self-reported healthcare resource utilization in health economic studies. *International Journal of Technology Assessment in Health Care*, 18(3), 705–710.

Pirkis, J. E., Burgess, P. M., Meadows, G. N., & Dunt, D. R. (2001). Suicidal ideation and suicide attempts as predictors of mental health service use. *Medical Journal of Australia*, 175(10), 542–545.

Qin, P., & Nordentoft, M. (2005). Suicide risk in relation to psychiatric hospitalization: evidence based on longitudinal registers. *Archives of General Psychiatry*, 62(4), 427–432.

Rhodes, A. E., Bethell, J., & Bondy, S. J. (2006). Suicidality, depression, and mental health service use in Canada. *Canadian Journal of Psychiatry*, 51(1), 35–41.

Salkovskis, P. M., Atha, C., & Storer, D. (1990). Cognitive-behavioural problem solving in the treatment of patients who repeatedly attempt suicide: A controlled trial. *British Journal of Psychiatry*, 157, 871–876.

Scott, K. M., Hwang, I., Chiu, W. T., et al. (2010). Chronic physical conditions and their association with first onset of suicidal behavior in the world mental health surveys. *Psychosomatic Medicine*, 72(7), 712–719.

Simon, G. E., Grothaus, L., Durham, M. L., Von Korff, M., & Pabiniak, C. (1996). Impact of visit copayments on outpatient mental health utilization by members of a health maintenance organization. *American Journal of Psychiatry*, 153(3), 331–338.

Simon, G. E., & VonKorff, M. (1995). Recall of psychiatric history in cross-sectional surveys: implications for epidemiologic research. *Epidemiologic Reviews*, 17(1), 221–227.

Sudak, D., Roy, A., Sudak, H., et al. (2007). Deficiencies in suicide training in primary care specialties: a survey of training directors. *Academic Psychiatry*, 31(5), 345–349.

Tousignant, M., & Hanigan, D. (1993). Crisis support among suicidal students following a loss event. *Journal of Community Psychology*, 21(2), 83–96.

Wang, P. S., Aguilar-Gaxiola, S., Alonso, J., et al. (2007). Use of mental health services for anxiety, mood, and substance disorders in 17 countries in the WHO world mental health surveys. *Lancet*, 370(9590), 841–850.

World Health Organization. (2005). *WHO resource book on mental health, human rights and legislation*. Geneva: World Health Organization.

Chapter 15

Research, clinical, and policy implications of the World Mental Health Survey findings on suicidal behavior

Evelyn J. Bromet

Introduction

Death by suicide is one of the leading causes of mortality worldwide. According to the World Health Organization, one million people die by suicide every year. Suicide attempt is the strongest risk factor for completed suicide. A recent U.S. report found an annual rate of emergency department visits for suicide attempts or self-inflicted injury of 1.5 per 1000 visits (Doshi et al., 2005). This volume takes a comprehensive, lifespan approach to investigating the risk and protective factors for suicidal behavior and the transitions among these states in countries throughout the world.

Many findings are striking. First and foremost, as with suicide mortality, the prevalence of suicidal behavior showed considerable variation across the countries participating in the World Mental Health (WMH) Surveys, with lifetime rates of ideation ranging from <5% (Italy, Spain, Lebanon, Nigeria, and China) to >10% (Colombia, U.S., France, Japan, and New Zealand) and lifetime rates of attempts ranging from <1% (Italy, Nigeria) to almost 5% (Colombia, New Zealand). These results parallel an earlier cross-national report (Weissman et al., 1999) and underscore the importance and complexity of understanding the determinants of this behavior in a cross-cultural perspective. Second, consistent with the targets of ongoing primary prevention programs, suicidal behavior was linked to female gender, early childhood adversities, and early onset depression, anxiety, substance abuse, and impulse-control disorders, with multiple comorbidities being especially powerful risk factors. Third, the effects of comorbid physical disorders were as important in predicting suicidal behavior as comorbid psychiatric disorders. Given that primary care providers are the most frequent treatment contact for suicidal patients, these findings have important policy implications for both primary and secondary interventions. Fourth, and what is perhaps most extraordinary about the findings presented in this volume, the significant risk factors for suicidal behavior were largely consistent across the diverse cultural settings in the low-, middle-, and high-income countries in the WMH Surveys, in spite of differences in prevalence and the constraints inherent in applying a common interview schedule and nomenclature in these very different settings. Lastly, although we do not know the specific reason for seeking help in the WMH samples, the rates of treatment from a professional provider among those who made a suicide attempt in the past 12 months varied enormously, ranging from 0% (Bulgaria, Italy, Nigeria) to 100% (the Netherlands, Spain).

The WMH Surveys Initiative is one of the few international studies to address suicidal behavior in the general population together with a comprehensive set of personal, familial, and environmental risk factors. Compared to previous international studies, the WMH initiative has the broadest coverage with respect to countries, age range, number of psychiatric, substance, and physical disorders, and most importantly, depth of information about suicidal behavior. Not only did the results confirm previous findings from clinical and community studies, but the new results provide important extensions to the search for the causes of suicidal behavior in the general population. The limitations of the WMH Surveys are discussed throughout this volume. Mindful of these issues, we consider how, in the context of epidemiological field studies, we can further our understanding of the epidemiology of suicidal behavior and contribute meaningfully to ongoing scientific, clinical, and policy efforts. We begin with potential extensions of analyses of the WMH Surveys data and then consider new approaches for field studies, particularly longitudinal research and the integration of biological specimens to evaluate more comprehensive conceptual models.

Further analyses of World Mental Health data on suicidal behavior

How do childhood adversities increase the risk of suicidal behavior?

An important set of analyses in this book focused on the relationships between childhood risk factors and suicidal behavior. The importance of early childhood adversities was underscored a decade ago in a retrospective study of HMO (Health Maintenance Organization) enrollees showing that children exposed to adverse events had an increased risk of suicide attempts throughout the life span (Dube et al., 2001). A recent study from Sweden found that child welfare clients who were removed from their homes before age 13 years had a four to five times greater risk of being hospitalized in adulthood for a suicide attempt relative to their peers (Vinnerljung et al., 2006). The WMH data extends this line of research by its inclusion of a broader array of childhood adversities, careful dating of the first occurrence of suicidal behavior, as well as careful dating of important risk factors such as onset of anxiety, depression, and substance use disorders. In high-, middle-, and low-income countries in the WMH Surveys, close to 40% of respondents reported at least one childhood adversity. In all countries, death of a parent exceeded 10%, while family violence ranged from 5% to 8%. Early life adversities typically occurred in clusters. Multiple adversities, especially those involving childhood physical and sexual abuse, had a dose–response relationship to suicidal behavior. It is important that future WMH analyses explore whether childhood abuse is also associated with the number and lethality of suicide attempts, including whether the attempt required medical attention.

Curiously, childhood physical and sexual abuses were least likely to be reported in low-income countries, and the predictive relationships with suicidal behavior were weakest for these countries as well. This suggests that an important next step is to move "upstream" to understand the role of the larger environments in which these "individual level" adversities took place. Epidemiologists have increasingly recognized the

importance of considering multiple levels in causal analyses, from the macro-level to the individual level. In the context of this survey, this analysis could take the form of considering individual deviations from local norms derived from aggregated, geographically clustered variables. Some countries may have relevant census and small area indicators that could be put to use in placing early family adversities in the context of the larger injustices occurring to children in those regions.

What factors protect against suicide risk among those at risk?

Similarly, the WMH interview included many protective factors that could buffer the effects of childhood adversities on suicidal behavior. The key here is to understand why some individuals were resilient in the face of horrific and dangerous circumstances while others succumbed. For example, prior studies have shown that a stable, loving parental figure moderates the effects of early life adversities (Werner, 1989). The WMH data included information on whether the respondent's mother died or left the home during childhood and whether the mother was free of psychiatric, substance, and antisocial disorders. Did these factors cushion the impact of severe childhood adversities with respect to suicidal behavior, or were the conditions so harsh that protective factors played little role in diminishing their impact? Were these factors protective in some countries, or subpopulations of some countries, but not others? Ideally, addressing this question would mean formulating and testing a theoretical model that places the first onset of suicidal behavior in the context of negative childhood exposures, protective aspects of the family environment, onset of disorders, other personal vulnerability and resilience characteristics, lifespan-specific achievements, and adversities later in life (e.g., relationship discord and aggression).

What is the role of sexual orientation?

Another variable collected in some of the WMH sites is sexual orientation. Several studies have shown that the risk of suicide is considerably higher in non-heterosexual populations (Garofalo et al., 1999; McDaniel et al., 2001; Paul et al. 2002). Paul et al. (2002) also showed that among gay and bisexual men, suicide attempts cluster early in life. An important strength of the WMH dataset is the careful dating of age-of-onset of depression and anxiety. These analyses could examine whether the risk period for first suicide attempt is earlier in gay and bisexual compared to heterosexual individuals or whether this apparent finding results from earlier onset of depression and anxiety or greater exposure to childhood adversities in these youths. These analyses could also examine whether gay respondents made more lethal attempts and more often needed medical attention for the attempts than matched heterosexual controls.

How and why do externalizing disorders increase suicide risk?

Adolescents are a major focus of suicide prevention programs. For the most part, these programs focus on restricting access to guns and other lethal means and to predispositional factors, particularly depression and anxiety, that elevate the risk of suicidal behavior and suicide itself (Mann et al., 2005). Yet, the WMH data and other studies (e.g., Caspi et al., 1996; Verona et al., 2004) show that suicide attempts also are associated with youth externalizing psychopathology. In addition, externalizing disorders predicted attempts not just in the general population but also among respondents with suicide ideation. Which youths with impulse-control problems go on to make a suicide attempt? Do their characteristics vary by gender, country, parental mental health, parental divorce, socioeconomic circumstances, urbanicity, or comorbid depression and anxiety? A full exploration of problems of impulse-control could be extremely valuable as prevention programs are redesigned in the twenty-first century. In this regard, a focused analysis of the WMH cohort who were under 30 years old at the time of interview would enhance the reliability of the childhood reports about childhood externalizing disorders.

Need for a lifespan developmental perspective

Early onset physical disorder and adverse health behaviors (smoking, drug use) should be included routinely in risk models as this volume shows their importance for increasing the risk of suicidal behavior and other studies show their direct links to repeated attempts in adulthood. There may indeed be synergism between aspects of environmental exposures and early onset mental disorders when considered from this perspective. From a lifespan developmental

perspective, it is critical to understand the sequencing of diverse, inter-related risk factors rather than, as most studies to date, to estimate the effects of a single risk factor as if it were acting in isolation of other factors.

Given the high rate of suicide ideation and attempts in adolescence, another opportunity afforded by the WMH data is to identify a healthy cohort from which to observe and better understand adult-onset suicidal behavior. Specifically, it is possible in each country to identify a subsample of healthy individuals who, for example, reached the age of 21 years with no evidence of psychiatric or medical disorders or suicidal behavior. In effect, these individuals could be considered a "historical cohort" that is then followed forward in time to observe the onset of suicidal behavior, the factors associated with the occurrence and lethality of suicidal behavior, and the consequences for role functioning, including timing and number of marriages and occupational satisfaction.

Another issue is to better understand suicidal behavior in older adults, who are the highest risk group for completed suicide. One way to accomplish this is to create a nested "case control" study of respondents aged 45 years and older. Cases could be defined as those with a prior history of suicidal behavior or a history of mental health or substance use disorders; controls could be composed of respondents without a history of suicide, mental health, or substance problems. The subsequent risk of suicide ideation and attempts, particularly first-onset attempts in the controls, and their distal (childhood exposures, smoking) and proximal (loss of spouse; onset of chronic illness) risk factors could be examined. This approach could provide evidence about suicidal behavior in older adults that is directly accessible and useful to clinicians.

Need to address methodological limitations of self-report data

A criticism often leveled at the CIDI (Composite International Diagnostic Interview) is that the specific ages of onset recalled by respondents are inaccurate. However, the general periods (e.g., adolescence vs. adulthood) may be more reliable for dating not only suicidal behavior and other disorders but also risk factors such as smoking and exposure to threatening life events outside of childhood. While stratification cannot replace the prospective cohort design, such analyses would be of value for furthering our knowledge about the antecedents and evolution of suicidal behavior in adults.

An important methodological opportunity is to investigate the factors associated with the reliability of suicidal reports among respondents with major depression. This could be explored in two ways. First, responses to the CIDI depression module item on thoughts of death could be compared with endorsements in the CIDI suicide module. Second, for respondents participating in clinical reappraisal studies, the CIDI depression item on thoughts of death could be compared with the clinical interview rating. One issue is to establish the consistency of responses. The more important issue, as we know from many studies that respondents are not consistent even within an interview, is to identify the factors associated with inconsistency. These would include respondent characteristics (mental or physical health, concentration and attention problems, age, antisocial behaviors), family characteristics (family history of mental disorders, family violence when growing up), and the context of the interview itself (privacy, interruptions, noise, time of day).

Need for further exploration of the associations between specific disorders and suicidal behavior

The lifespan developmental perspective articulated in this volume provides a useful conceptual framework for organizing WMH research on suicidal behavior by integrating vulnerability factors (parental mental health), early childhood risk factors, early/late adolescence risk factors, subsequent life course events (marital, work, and family events and traumatic experiences), health and mental health, environmental supports, treatment experiences, stigma, and social role disabilities within a single model. One of the most intriguing findings, in this regard, pertains to the role of parental psychopathology. Granted that reports about parental disorders came from the respondents themselves, the findings are nonetheless fascinating. Specifically, not only was parental disorder associated with suicide ideation and attempts, but parental depression and generalized anxiety disorder were predictive of the onset and persistence of suicide ideation and plans, whereas parental panic and antisocial personality disorder predicted which people with suicide ideation went on to make an

attempt. Although more research is needed to clarify the underlying mechanisms of the risk for onset and persistence, the next steps for the WMH initiative might be to consider how familial disorders influenced the early childhood environment that, in turn, increased the likelihood of suicidal behavior in the offspring.

Although depression, anxiety, and schizophrenia have long been known to increase the risk of completed suicide, there is growing awareness of the link with posttraumatic stress disorder (PTSD) (e.g., Gradus et al., 2010). While this volume underscores the importance of early life trauma, future analyses should also evaluate the specific associations of PTSD with suicidal thoughts and behaviors. The attributable risk associated with PTSD in different countries and for different age groups should be compared. In addition, and perhaps of more importance, the protective factors that prevent respondents with PTSD from attempting suicide also need to be elucidated. Examples of resilience and protective factors that were not fully analyzed in the WMH Surveys include religiosity, personality characteristics, job satisfaction, marital cohesion, and the presence of young children in the household.

Need for further information about treatment and barriers to care

Lastly, it is important to understand the subsequent mental health and role functioning trajectories of respondents who did and did not seek help for suicide ideation or attempts. From a clinical perspective, the trajectories of the cases that sought help provide useful prognostic information. From a public health perspective, the trajectories of the cases that did not seek help offer clues for designing new interventions.

This volume represents the first steps in a comprehensive approach to understanding suicidal behavior around the globe. The findings to date are consistent with previous studies and informative for public health policy. More substantive and methodological studies can be conducted to further strengthen the value of the WMH initiative, and it is hoped that the new research will clearly show the clinical value of the findings. Indeed, despite significant advances in scientific understanding of suicidal behavior over the years, the rates of suicidal behavior have remained unchanged (Kessler et al., 2005). This statistic highlights the need for greater efforts to: (1) develop and test clinically meaningful conceptual models, and (2) translate the findings from the WMH Surveys into a form that can be readily understood by and adapted into the work of front-line clinicians working with suicidal patients.

Considerations for new epidemiological research beyond the World Mental Health Surveys

The rate-limiting steps of the WMH investigation into suicidal behavior are country-specific differences in the meaning and cultural acceptance of the questions, the reliance on self-report, the absence of longitudinal data, and cross-national differences in life expectancy, extent of the population living in abject poverty, and availability of health and mental health treatment. These are limitations of all international cross-sectional surveys. The WMH improved upon prior epidemiological studies by instituting and monitoring comparable sampling and interview methods and including a separate CIDI module on suicidal behavior, independent of mental health, containing questions about ideation, plans, and attempts. As we move forward in epidemiology, there is little doubt that cross-sectional and case control designs involving general population samples and psychiatric patients will continue to be implemented, and each generation of studies will build constructively on the strengths and limitations of its predecessors.

Inclusion of under-represented and vulnerable segments of the population

Epidemiology has many purposes. One is to provide data on prevalence and identify high risk groups. In this regard, the WMH approach covers a broad sweep of countries and demographic groups. Yet a number of high-risk groups were under-represented in the WMH Surveys, biasing the prevalence estimates downward. Some vulnerable populations were excluded from the surveys, such as the homeless, alcoholics in rehabilitation programs, incarcerated populations, the elderly living in nursing homes or other institutions, psychiatric patients in mental hospitals, and armed forces personnel. Other vulnerable subgroups were under-represented, including adults raised in foster care or orphanages, gay and lesbian populations, people with HIV/AIDS and other life threatening diagnoses, returning veterans, survivors of war and torture and their family members, indigenous groups (native

Americans, aboriginals), alcoholics who were too drunk to be interviewed, and the offspring of parents who committed suicide. Future epidemiological studies need to fill the gaps in our understanding of the rates and risk factors for these vulnerable groups.

Concerns have also been raised about the uneven response rates across the various WMH countries and its effects on findings about rates of disorder. The concern here is that individuals with suicidal thoughts might be under-represented in some countries because they were embarrassed and reluctant to participate at all. Conceivably, rather than a monetary incentive, some vulnerable individuals, especially in poor countries, might be more willing to participate if offered a different incentive, such as a free physical check-up (Guey et al., 2008). If this is not feasible, interviewers could be trained to perform basic vision, hearing, or dental checks, or to calculate body mass index, thus providing respondents with meaningful feedback about their health.

Inclusion of a wider range of potential risk factors

A related use of epidemiology is to identify the risk factors for suicidal behavior and the transitions across ideation, plans, and attempts. The WMH Surveys included a wealth of indicators encompassing demographic characteristics, early life exposures, parental history, physical and mental health, recent life events, and traumatic experiences. In clinical studies of suicidal behavior, a number of other important predictors have emerged, including access to the means of committing suicide (guns in the U.S.; pesticides in Asia), head injury, alienation, hopelessness, immigration, neighborhood incongruence, and diminished social interaction. These variables could be included in future surveys addressing the causes and evolution of suicidal behavior in community samples. In addition, given the rich literature that already exists, new studies should be designed to test an explicit conceptual model, such as a diathesis–stress model or a gene–environment interaction model, so that we can move beyond exploratory research and begin testing hypotheses about causal pathways.

Capturing of temporal trends given world events

Another function of epidemiology is to examine temporal trends. The WMH Surveys were conducted for the most part before the worldwide recession hit.

Thus, consistent with prior studies, the WMH rates of suicide ideation and attempts declined with age in developed countries. Job loss in mid-life is often accompanied by subsequent under-employment or outright unemployment. New studies need to monitor whether age-related findings about suicidal behavior change across the globe as we continue in, and hopefully emerge from, the current economic recession.

Completing the clinical picture

Another purpose of epidemiology is to complete the clinical picture. In schizophrenia research, considerable effort has gone into distinguishing between the premorbid period, the prodrome, the onset of first overt symptoms, and the point at which the symptoms reached a diagnosable threshold. Future studies of suicidal behavior need to consider whether nonsuicidal self-injury is part of the spectrum of suicidal behavior, and if so, whether non-suicidal self-injury constitutes the prodrome for suicide attempts and whether such behaviors serve to hasten the onset of suicidal behavior (Whitlock & Knox, 2007). These surveys should also take into account the type of self-injury that occurred. As most people reporting suicidal behavior do not seek help, either because of stigma or because they do not perceive the need, or in some countries, because care is unavailable, this progression is best examined in community samples.

In the WMH Surveys, suicidal behavior was treated as a categorical variable. Other aspects of mental health measured in the CIDI included symptom severity scales, such as the Quick Inventory of Depressive Symptoms and the Panic Disorder Severity Scale. Given the focus of DSM-V on incorporating a dimensional perspective along with categorical diagnosis, future studies of suicidal behavior should include severity measures that rate the intensity and duration of ideation and level of control in making an attempt, such as the Columbia Suicide Severity Scale. Although the reliability of such scales for lifetime reports may not be optimal, these scales could be applied in individuals with recent suicidal thoughts or behaviors.

The CIDI included a separate module to assess suicidal behavior. In some countries, it is culturally unacceptable and even sinful to acknowledge such thoughts, and the samples therefore contained an unknown number of false negatives. Conceivably, embedding these questions in the context of physical health might lessen the stigma and negative valence of these questions. It is also possible that better information would be obtained by asking respondents about "other people your age" rather than only about the respondents themselves. The placement and wording of these items is an important issue for research aimed at identifying risk groups for suicide around the globe. It may well be that in some countries, a separate module or different strategy will yield a more accurate estimate, while in other countries, the current approach is quite reliable.

Conversely, in some countries, there were an unknown number of false positives (e.g., highly distressed respondents with fleeting ideation who had not in fact "seriously" thought about suicide). It would be useful for future studies to include a formal clinical reappraisal study of the cases endorsing suicide ideation. A further check on the reliability of reports about suicidal behavior and a way to get timely in-depth information would be to hire a cadre of trained clinical interviewers who would be "on call" during the field work. Thus, if a respondent endorses suicide ideation, the lay interviewer (or his/her computer!) would alert the on-call clinical interviewer to follow-up with the respondent straight away. Thus, a more extensive assessment of suicidal behavior could be conducted immediately following the CIDI assessment.

Collection of prospective data on suicidal behavior

The transitions among suicidal behaviors and the validity of the risk index cannot be fully evaluated in the absence of prospective data. Because suicide ideation and suicide attempts are relatively low base-rate behaviors, a cost effective method for conducting longitudinal research in community-based samples is to identify high-risk groups either *a priori* or nested within a cohort study. One example is to identify cases having their first episode of suicidal behavior in the prior 12 months and matched controls, building in re-contact information and informed consents so that future follow-ups can readily take place. The matching criteria for the controls would be decided by the hypotheses to be tested and the established risk factors that the investigators wish not to study. For example, the WMH and other community surveys repeatedly find that women are at substantially increased risk of suicidal behavior than men. Matching on gender could, therefore, be an important feature of the design. In effect, this would mean designing a two-phase study in advance of the field work. A complementary sample of psychiatric or emergency room patients with first onset of suicidal behavior would enrich such a study as well. It bears repeating that future prospective studies should be based on a conceptual model of the factors associated with the onset and persistence of suicidal behavior.

Incorporation of laboratory measures

Fifteen years ago, Anthony et al. (1995) made a number of suggestions about the future of psychiatric epidemiology. One suggestion was to incorporate laboratory measures (e.g., brain imaging, molecular biology) as an integral part of the scope of epidemiological field studies. For suicidal behavior, this could be accomplished by case control studies designed in collaboration with basic scientists. The beginnings of such research are being undertaken. As just one example, the recently initiated study of suicide in the U.S. Army (Army Study to Assess Risk and Resilience in Service members [STARRS]) is an epidemiological study aimed at identifying modifiable risk and protective factors among >400,000 soldiers. In addition to the collection of self-report data, the study will include the collection of biological (e.g., blood and saliva samples) and behavioral (e.g., performance-based psychological tests) data in collaboration with basic scientists who have used such laboratory measures among much smaller samples of suicidal participants. Efforts such as these are expected to significantly advance understanding of the ways in which factors from different domains (biological, behavioral, psychological) may interact to lead to the development of psychiatric disorders and suicidal behavior.

Another opportunity is to identify samples from medical facilities that have electronic medical records. Suicidal behavior and other risk factors gathered by self-report, either from the internet, phone interviews, or face-to-face interviews, could be linked directly to diagnoses in the medical records, emergency room visits, and laboratory findings. One model for this is an ongoing study of PTSD in U.S. veterans' hospitals in which selected patients complete risk factor questionnaires on the internet and diagnostic interviews by telephone, and diagnoses and laboratory results in the medical records are exported into the dataset. Moreover, in this example, the medical records are monitored over time.

Clinical policy implications

The WMH data support the importance of training general medical providers around the world in the recognition and treatment of suicidal problems (Mann et al., 2005). Evidence that such suicide prevention programs reduce suicide rates is accumulating. Yet in many countries, physicians have no training in the detection and treatment of depression, anxiety, or suicide ideation and attempts. Unless a patient presents with an obvious injury and admits that it was self-inflicted, physicians will not necessarily be aware that the injury was caused by a suicidal act. Given the public health urgency of suicide, governments need to invest in education programs for primary care physicians, nurse practitioners, and allied health professionals to improve their recognition of suicidal behavior and their knowledge about the factors that put people at risk, such as prior attempts, depression, alcoholism, and increased social withdrawal. Taken in isolation, these signs might not intuitively be linked to suicidal behavior; however, clustered together, they should serve as red flags for the possibility that a patient might have or develop suicidal thoughts.

Second, as Bruffaerts and colleagues noted in Chapter 14, a broad range of barriers prevents suicidal persons from seeking treatment. These include stigma, financial barriers, and the lack of perceived need for care. Awareness programs need to be developed for the general population to improve their knowledge about the value of treatment. Public campaigns could be mounted, depending on the country, in which community members reach out to friends and neighbors, and using a snowball approach, information about detection and treatment of suicidal behavior can be disseminated. Given the availability of television and the internet in many countries, these programs could also utilize these media.

Clearly, population prevention programs need to address the cluster of conditions that accompany suicidal behavior, as discussed in this chapter. In developed countries, this would include depression, anxiety, and domestic violence, especially malevolent acts toward children (Bernal et al., 2007). In former Soviet countries, alcohol consumption and alcoholism are critical risk factors for suicide (Levi et al., 2003; Nemtsov, 2003) and suicidal behavior (Bromet et al., 2007). Indeed, Sher (2006) noted that all alcoholics should be evaluated for suicide risk. In almost all countries, men have higher rates of suicide, and women have a greater risk of ideation and attempts. It may well be that gender-specific prevention efforts would be more effective than the more general programs offered to date.

The WMH Survey findings point to some other important directions for policy makers. The young age at which suicide ideation and attempt first appears suggest that schools should remain an active setting for prevention and intervention programs. Moreover, as controversial as high school suicide prevention programs were a decade ago, it is important to consider incorporating suicide issues into middle school health education curricula and reaching out to families as well. Similarly, the powerful effects of childhood adversities suggest that child welfare agencies have an important role to play in the prevention of suicidal behavior. As Aguilar-Gaxiola (2009) stated, investment in educational and community services and supports that strengthen the ability of families to raise healthy, happy children may reduce deleterious, long-term effects of childhood psychosocial stressors. We need better coordination between child welfare, education, primary healthcare, juvenile justice, substance abuse, and mental health programs.

There are examples of successful interventions with high-risk groups, such as the multilayered intervention designed for Air Force personnel (Knox et al., 2003) and support letters mailed to a vulnerable patient population (Motto & Bostrom, 2001). As noted by the latter, however, the long-term benefits of short-term interventions are dubious. Given that suicidal behavior is complex and often persistent, sustained intervention efforts rather than short-term trials are warranted. The findings from recent clinical interventions using cognitive therapy (Brown et al., 2005) and dialectical behavior therapy (Linehan et al., 2006) suggest that, for patients referred for suicidal behavior, sustained treatment can be effective in reducing or preventing suicide attempts.

Each year on September 10, the International Association for Suicide Prevention together with the World Health Organization organizes World Suicide Prevention Day. The theme of the 2009 program was "Suicide Prevention in Different Cultures." A number of practical initiatives were encouraged to promote awareness of suicide and suicidal behavior, including organizing public events, training gate-keepers, creating and fostering support groups, and publicizing the importance of prevention through various media outlets and direct contact with policy makers. Ideally, the effectiveness of this and similar programs could be examined so that future programs are more specifically tailored to the needs of different populations.

References

Aguilar-Gaxiola, S. (2009). Policy implications. In M. R. Von Korff, K. M. Scott, & O. Gureje. (eds.). *Global Perspectives on Mental-Physical Comorbidity in the WHO World Mental Health Surveys*. New York, NY: Cambridge University Press, pp. 302–311.

Anthony, J. C., Eaton, W. W., Henderson, A. S. (1995). Looking to the future in psychiatric epidemiology. *Epidemiologic Reviews*, **17**(1), 240–243.

Bernal, M., Haro, J. M., Bernert, S., et al. (2007). Risk factors for suicidality in Europe: results from the ESEMED study. *Journal of Affective Disorders*, **101**(1–3), 27–34.

Bromet, E. J., Havenaar, J. M., Tintle, N., et al. (2007). Suicide ideation, plans, and attempts in Ukraine: Findings from the Ukraine-World Mental Health Survey. *Psychological Medicine*, **37**(6), 807–819.

Brown, G. K., Have, T. T., Henriques, G. R., et al. (2005). Cognitive therapy for the prevention of suicide attempts: a randomized controlled trial. *Journal of the American Medical Association*, **294**(5), 563–570.

Caspi, A., Moffitt, T. E., Newman, D. L., Silva, P. A. (1996). Behavioral observations at age 3 years predict adult psychiatric disorders. *Archives of General Psychiatry*, **53**(11), 1033–1039.

Doshi, A., Bourdreaux, E. D., Wang, N., Pelletier, A. J., Camargo, C. A. (2005). National study of US emergency department visits for attempted suicide and self-inflicted injury, 1997–2001. *Annals of Emergency Medicine*, **46**(4), 369–375.

Dube, S. R., Anda, R. F., Felitti, V. J., et al. (2001). Childhood abuse, household dysfunction, and the risk of attempted suicide throughout the life span: findings from the Adverse Childhood Experiences Study. *Journal of the American Medical Association*, **286**(24), 3089–3096.

Garofalo, R., Wolf, C., Wissow, L. S., Woods, E. R., Goodman, E. (1999). Sexual orientation and risk of suicide attempts among a representative sample of youth. *Archives of Pediatric and Adolescent Medicine*, **153**(5), 487–493.

Gradus, J. L., Qin, P., Lincoln, A. K., et al. (2010). Posttraumatic stress disorder and completed suicide. *American Journal of Epidemiology*, **171**(6), 721–727.

Guey, L. T., Bromet, E. J., Gluzman, S., Zakhozha, V., Paniotto, V. (2008). Determinants of participation in a longitudinal two-stage study of the health consequences of the Chernobyl accident. *BMC Medical Research Methodology*, **8**, 27.

Kessler, R. C., Berglund, P., Borges, G., Nock, M. K., Wang, P. S. (2005). Trends in suicide ideation, plans, gestures, and attempts in the United States, 1990–1992 to 2001–2003. *Journal of the American Medical Association*, **293**(20), 2487–2495.

Knox, K. L., Litts, D. A., Talcott, G. W., et al. (2003). Risk of suicide and related adverse outcomes after exposure to a suicide prevention programme in the US Air Force: cohort study. *British Medical Journal*, **327**(7428), 1376.

Levi, F., Vecchia, C., Saraceno, B. (2003). Global suicide rates. *European Journal of Public Health*, **13**(2), 97–98.

Linehan, M. M., Comtois, K. A., Murray, A. M., et al. (2006). Ten-year randomized controlled trial and follow-up of dialectical behavior therapy vs. therapy by experts for suicidal behaviors and borderline personality disorder. *Archives of General Psychiatry*, **63**(7), 757–766.

Mann, J. J., Apter, A., Bertolote, J., et al. (2005). Suicide prevention strategies: a systematic review. *Journal of the American Medical Association*, **294**(16), 2064–2074.

McDaniel, J. S., Purcell, D., D'Augelli, A. R. (2001). The relationship between sexual orientation and risk for suicide: research findings and future direction for research and prevention. *Suicide and Life-Threatening Behavior*, **31**, 84–104.

Motto, J. A., & Bostrom, A. G. (2001). A randomized controlled trial of postcrisis suicide prevention. *Psychiatric Services*, **52**(6), 828–833.

Nemtsov, A. (2003). Suicides and alcohol consumption in Russia, 1965–1999. *Drug and Alcohol Dependence*, **71**(2), 161–168.

Paul, J. P., Catania, J., Pollack, L., et al. (2002). Suicide attempts among gay and bisexual men: lifetime prevalence and antecedents. *American Journal of Public Health*, **92**(8), 1338–1345.

Sher, L. (2006). Alcoholism and suicidal behavior: a clinical overview. *Acta Psychiatrica Scandinavica*, **113**(1), 13–22.

Verona, E., Sachs-Ericsson, N., Joiner, T. E. Jr., (2004). Suicide attempts associated with externalizing psychopathology in an epidemiological sample. *American Journal of Psychiatry*, **161**(3), 444–451.

Vinnerljung, B., Jhern, A., Lindblad, F. (2006). Suicide attempts and severe psychiatric morbidity among former child welfare clients – a national cohort study. *Journal of Child Psychology and Psychiatry*, **47**(7), 723–733.

Weissman, M. M., Bland, R. C., Canino, G., J., et al. (1999). Prevalence of suicide ideation and suicide attempts in nine countries. *Psychological Medicine*, **29**(1), 9–17.

Werner, E. E. (1989). High-risk children in young adulthood: a longitudinal study from birth to 32 years. *American Journal of Orthopsychiatry*, **59**(1), 72–81.

Whitlock, J., & Knox, K. L. (2007). The relationship between self-injurious behavior and suicide in a young adult population. *Archives of Pediatric and Adolescent Medicine*, **161**(7), 634–640.

Conclusions and future directions

Matthew K. Nock, Guilherme Borges, and Yutaka Ono

Suicide has perplexed scholars, scientists, clinicians, and society more generally for thousands of years. Although we continue to lack a firm understanding of why, when, and among whom suicidal behavior will occur, the information presented in this volume provides a significant step forward in solidifying our understanding of this problem. The primary contribution of this book is its comprehensive documentation of the characteristics of suicidal behavior and several of its key risk factors among a worldwide community sample. It is our hope that this information provides a strong foundation on which to build future investigations.

What have we learned from the World Mental Health findings on suicidal behavior?

The previous chapter by Evelyn Bromet provides a wonderful summary of some of the most exciting findings of this project to date, as well as some thought provoking discussion of the most important scientific, clinical, and policy implications of this work. These will not be revisited here, but we would like to highlight several additional and more general conclusions from this project.

The WMH suicide study has helped to develop several novel areas of research on suicidal behavior. Although there have been many studies of suicidal behavior, very few have gone beyond the identification of correlates or risk factors for suicide ideation and/or attempt. This study has provided voluminous information about the onset and persistence of suicide ideation, plans, and attempts and about the probability and timing of transitioning from suicide ideation to plans and attempts. We hope that this

study will help to motivate researchers to pursue further these neglected areas of inquiry. This study also reported on the persistence of suicidal behavior over time – an outstandingly important but previously ignored aspect of suicidal behavior. In addition, this study has provided extensive documentation of how suicidal people are (or, more aptly, are not) treated around the world. The measurement and analysis methods used in this study, as well as the initial data reported in each area, provide a strong foundation on which to build in future studies that include these outcomes.

Beyond introducing novel methods for studying suicidal behavior, this study yielded new and interesting findings in several areas that have been the focus of prior suicide research. New, and replicated, findings were reported on the effects of sociodemographic factors, parental psychopathology, childhood adversities, traumatic experiences during adulthood, mental disorders, and chronic medical conditions in the prediction of suicidal outcomes. This volume also presented data on the interactions of factors from these different domains, and on the relative contribution of each. Moreover, work presented in this book documented the usefulness of combining risk factors into indices that can be used for the short-term prediction of both planned and unplanned suicide attempts. Research on suicidal behavior is most valuable if it can actually help us to predict and prevent such behaviors from occurring – and this research provides a very big step in that important direction and hopefully serves as a point of departure for future research in this direction. We hope that these are the first of many studies aimed at translating the results of risk and protective factor analyses into clinically useful risk indices.

Suicide, eds. Matthew K. Nock, Guilherme Borges, and Yutaka Ono. Published by Cambridge University Press.
© World Health Organization 2012.

Where do we go from here? Future research on suicidal behavior

The work presented in this volume advances our understanding of suicidal behavior, but leaves many important questions unanswered. Many of the limitations of the WMH Surveys have been reviewed in prior chapters, and some important directions for future work were outlined in Chapter 15. Here we offer several final thoughts on some key directions for future work in this area.

Broaden the focus geographically

This volume presents data on suicidal behavior from 21 countries around the world. Although this represents the largest, most representative study of suicidal behavior ever conducted with countries included from six continents and a wide range of cultures, this means that we have captured information from only about 10% of the countries in the world. The full WMH Survey Initiative includes 28 countries, including surveys currently being fielded in a diversity of countries such as Brazil, Nepal, Portugal, and Saudi Arabia; however, this still falls well short of achieving a truly global perspective. An important direction for future research is to continue to field studies such as the WMH Surveys in a broader range of countries/cultures, while making a special effort to learn about suicidal behavior in regions currently under-represented in the literature. For instance, data are largely unavailable for countries in Africa and the Middle East. The current project includes some countries from these regions, but only a small minority. There also is a great need to incorporate culturally informed explanations for how suicidal behavior develops and is effectively prevented around the globe.

Broaden the focus developmentally

The WMH Surveys include respondents who are 18+ years of age, with most between the ages of 18 and 65 years. As highlighted in this volume, the risk of suicidal behavior increases dramatically during adolescence (i.e., 12–18 years), and the risk of suicide death does so after age 65 years, especially among men. There is a tremendous need to better understand why these increases occur, and one valuable direction is to increase the focus on the risk of suicidal behavior during these critical periods. Several WMH countries have data specifically from adolescent samples

(Colombia, Mexico, Shanghai (China), and the United States), and so a very important next step will be to use these (and similar) data to study the characteristics, and risk and protective factors for suicidal behavior during this developmental period.

Increased focus on the transition from suicidal thoughts to behaviors

The WMH Surveys document clearly that most risk factors for suicide attempt actually predict suicide ideation, but not which people with suicide ideation go on to make a suicide attempt. Indeed, the current set of known risk factors are quite limited in their power to predict those with a suicide ideation that will pass to further attempt suicide. Future research must identify the factors that predict the transition from suicide ideation to suicide attempt. Candidate factors include: acute life events, poor impulse-control, and a lack of social support and access to prevention and intervention services. The identification of factors that better predict this transition will be important for understanding the pathway to suicide, and will be especially valuable information for clinicians who work with suicidal patients.

Increased focus on integrative and interactive models

Virtually every major theory of suicidal behavior suggests that it is the end result of the combination and interaction of a wide range of factors. However, most models tested in prior research consider only one factor at a time, or a small range of risk factors. The work presented in this volume begins to test the unique contribution of different risk factors, and in some cases their interactions, in predicting suicidal behavior. Much more work is needed toward this end. Prior, smaller studies have demonstrated that considering the interaction of risk factors can improve the prediction of suicidal behavior. For instance, Dour and colleagues (2011) showed that adolescents with both high emotion reactivity and poor problem-solving skills are at especially high risk for suicide attempt. Caspi and colleagues (2003) have shown that people with both a specific polymorphism on the serotonin transporter gene and the experience of childhood adversities are at especially high risk for subsequent suicide attempt. The WMH Surveys include assessment of a very wide range of risk and protective factors that could be used to test such theoretically derived interactive models. Interestingly, genetic data will soon be available from more than 20,000 respondents across several countries. Therefore, these data provide further unique opportunities to conduct another generation of studies on the interactions of environmental, genetic, and psychological factors that may increase the risk of suicidal behavior.

More fine-grained studies of suicidal behavior

The data from this study provide something of a long-distance view of suicidal behavior in that respondents report on their lifetime history of the occurrence of suicide ideation, plans, and attempts. Although this study considered a wide range of suicide-related outcomes, because of the measurement strategy used we were unable to study suicidal thoughts and behaviors in very fine detail as they occurred in real-time. For instance, recent studies have used ecological momentary assessment approaches to assess suicidal thoughts and behaviors as they occur in real-time (e.g., Nock et al., 2009). Such approaches can provide novel data on the frequency, severity, and duration of suicidal thoughts as well as on the environmental and psychological factors that trigger such outcomes. Other studies have used objective behavioral tests to measure suicidal thoughts. As one example, brief, computerized tests have been used to measure suicidal thinking by considering how long it takes suicidal people to respond to certain types of visual stimuli (e.g., suicide related words) (Cha et al., 2010; Nock & Banaji, 2007; Nock et al., 2010). Tests such as these provide new insight into the cognitive processes associated with suicidal behavior. Future studies can combine the efforts of these different approaches, such as by using large-scale surveys to identify those with suicidal behavior and then using real-time and objective measurement approaches to better understand the nature of suicidal thinking and behavior.

Qualitative studies of suicidal behavior

All of the data presented in this volume are based on quantitative analysis of people's responses to structured interview questions. We have learned a great deal through this process, but one thing that is lacking is an explanation *in their own words* of why people tried to kill themselves. Future studies that include semi-structured interviews with suicidal people that assess their reasons for trying to kill themselves, the factors leading to their decision to kill themselves, and the reasons that people who considered killing themselves did not do so, would be extremely useful for shedding light on these important questions. Many qualitative studies have been conducted with suicidal people (e.g., Kraft et al., 2010; Mugisha et al., 2011); however, these typically have been relatively small in scope and have not provided a clear picture of what leads people all around the world to try to end their lives. Such studies have the potential to offer insights into the nature of suicidal behavior that fully structured, quantitative studies cannot and represent a valuable direction for future research.

Intervention and prevention studies

The goal of this entire endeavor is to understand suicidal behavior so that we can better prevent it. Currently, there are no evidence-based psychological or pharmacological treatments that have proven effective in decreasing the likelihood of suicidal behavior among those at risk. Several prevention programs have shown promise (Mann et al., 2005), but require replication and broader tests of their effectiveness. The research presented in this volume, and all related research on suicidal behavior, is most valuable if it can be used to prevent the suffering and loss of life resulting from suicidal behavior. As such, perhaps the most important direction for future research is the translation of findings on the characteristics, risk factors, and protective factors for suicidal behavior into new intervention and prevention strategies.

References

Caspi, A., Sugden, K., Moffitt, T. E., *et al.* (2003). Influence of life stress on depression: moderation by a polymorphism in the 5-HTT gene. *Science*, **301**(5631), 386–389.

Cha, C. B., Najmi, S., Park, J. M., Finn, C. T., & Nock, M. K. (2010). Attentional bias toward suicide-related stimuli predicts suicidal behavior. *Journal of Abnormal Psychology*, **119**(3), 616–622.

Dour, H. J., Cha, C. B., & Nock, M. K. (2011). Evidence for an emotion-cognition interaction in the statistical prediction of suicide attempts. *Behaviour Research and Therapy*, **49**(4), 294–298.

Kraft, T. L., Jobes, D. A., Lineberry, T. W., Conrad, A., & Kung, S. (2010). Brief report: why suicide? Perceptions of suicidal inpatients and reflections of clinical researchers. *Archives of Suicide Research*, **14**(4), 375–382.

Mann, J. J., Apter, A., Bertolote, J., et al. (2005). Suicide prevention strategies: a systematic review. *Journal of the American Medical Association*, **294**(16), 2064–2074.

Mugisha, J., Knizek, B. L., Kinyanda, E., & Hjelmeland, H. (2011). Doing qualitative research on suicide in a developing country. *Crisis*, **32**(1), 15–23.

Nock, M. K., & Banaji, M. R. (2007). Prediction of suicide ideation and attempts among adolescents using a brief performance-based test. *Journal of Consulting and Clinical Psychology*, **75**(5), 707–715.

Nock, M. K., Park, J. M., Finn, C. T., et al. (2010). Measuring the suicidal mind: implicit cognition predicts suicidal behavior. *Psychological Science*, **21**(4), 511–517.

Nock, M. K., Prinstein, M. J., & Sterba, S. K. (2009). Revealing the form and function of self-injurious thoughts and behaviors: a real-time ecological assessment study among adolescents and young adults. *Journal of Abnormal Psychology*, **118**(4), 816–827.

Appendices

Appendix Table 3.1. Design effects of 12-month prevalence estimates of suicide ideation, plans, and attempts in the WMH Surveys[a]

Country specific	In the total sample			Among 12-month ideators			
	Ideation	Plan	Attempt	Plan	Attempt	Attempt among planners	Attempt among non-planners
I. Low- and lower-middle-income countries							
Colombia	2.2	1.2	2.2	0.9	1.8	1.2	2.9
India-Pondicherry	1.3	0.6	1.1	0.6	1.2	1.5	1.5
Nigeria	1.7	1.2	0.5	1.7	0.8	1.2	–
China-Beijing, China-Shanghai	2.1	2.2	1.1	1.8	1.2	0.8	1.0
China-Shenzhen	2.2	1.0	2.4	1.1	2.1	1.0	2.8
China (total)	2.2	1.9	1.5	1.9	1.4	1.0	1.7
Ukraine	1.3	1.5	1.7	1.2	1.5	1.3	1.0
II. Upper-middle-income countries							
Brazil	1.2	1.9	1.2	2.1	1.5	2.6	1.0
Bulgaria	2.0	1.9	1.5	1.4	1.1	1.0	0.3
Lebanon	1.7	1.4	1.3	1.5	1.7	1.3	0.8
Mexico	3.7	2.7	3.2	1.0	1.7	2.4	0.9
Romania	1.1	1.0	1.1	0.9	1.1	1.0	–
South Africa	1.6	1.3	1.3	1.1	1.2	1.1	1.2
III. High-income countries							
Belgium	1.8	1.3	1.2	1.0	1.6	0.9	1.1
France	1.2	1.1	1.2	1.1	1.1	1.4	–
Germany	1.0	1.0	0.9	1.1	0.8	1.1	0.7
Israel	1.1	1.2	1.2	1.1	1.2	1.1	1.1
Italy	0.8	1.0	–	1.0	–	–	–
Japan	1.5	1.2	0.9	1.0	0.8	0.4	1.1
Netherlands	1.8	0.8	0.8	1.2	1.1	1.1	1.1
New Zealand	2.0	1.9	1.8	2.2	1.8	2.0	1.1
Spain	1.4	1.3	0.9	1.7	0.9	0.7	0.6
United States	0.8	1.1	1.6	1.4	2.0	1.6	1.5
IV. Cross-national combination of countries							
Low-income countries	1.7	1.1	1.7	1.2	1.6	1.4	2.4
Middle-income countries	2.0	1.9	1.9	1.4	1.5	2.0	1.0
High-income countries	1.5	1.5	1.5	1.7	1.6	1.6	1.2
Total	1.7	1.5	1.7	1.5	1.6	1.7	1.6

– Estimated prevalence was 0.0%.
[a] As described in more detail in the text, the design effect (DE) is the square of the ratio of the standard error of the prevalence estimate using design-based methods divided by the standard error of the prevalence estimate assuming a simple random sample. DE represents the extent to which the design-based sample would have to increase in size to obtain the same standard error as that obtained in a simple random sample of the observed size. For example, the DE of 2.2 in Colombia means that the Part 2 sample of 2381 respondents would have to be 5238 (i.e., 2.2 × 2381) to achieve a design-based standard error equal in size to the standard error in a simple random sample of 2381 respondents.

Appendix Table 5.1. Associations of age-of-onset and time between age-of-onset and interview with persistence of suicide ideation among respondents with lifetime ideation (n = 10,018)

Age-of-onset	Years since ideation started																	
	03–07			08–12			13–17			18–22			23–27			28+		
	%	(SE)	(n)ᵃ	%	(SE)	(n)ᵃ	%	(SE)	(n)ᵃ	%	(SE)	(n)ᵃ	%	(SE)	(n)ᵃ	%	(SE)	(n)ᵃ
I. The percentage of lifetime ideation that continued to the year of interview																		
≤12	41.9	(12.1)	(29)	23.6	(5.0)	(128)	30.1	(5.4)	(124)	16.9	(4.5)	(100)	21.2	(4.9)	(83)	17.0	(2.8)	(222)
13–15	33.2	(3.3)	(283)	20.5	(3.2)	(249)	18.1	(3.0)	(198)	18.6	(3.3)	(171)	14.4	(3.4)	(130)	16.3	(2.7)	(264)
16–19	23.0	(2.5)	(464)	19.6	(2.8)	(284)	16.8	(2.9)	(259)	19.3	(3.2)	(234)	14.7	(4.0)	(170)	16.7	(2.3)	(391)
20–24	21.9	(3.0)	(322)	24.2	(3.4)	(258)	19.4	(3.3)	(194)	12.0	(2.9)	(164)	16.3	(4.6)	(99)	12.1	(2.5)	(267)
25–29	20.0	(3.1)	(243)	14.1	(3.1)	(219)	17.3	(3.4)	(169)	14.9	(4.0)	(115)	12.4	(3.8)	(90)	8.5	(2.4)	(164)
30–34	21.6	(3.2)	(225)	19.2	(3.8)	(172)	22.1	(4.6)	(100)	12.0	(3.5)	(108)	14.0	(5.9)	(52)	9.5	(2.7)	(131)
35+	21.0	(1.7)	(714)	18.3	(2.4)	(410)	15.9	(2.8)	(263)	10.1	(2.4)	(195)	7.5	(2.6)	(125)	11.0	(2.7)	(158)
II. The percentage of lifetime ideation that continued within two years of interview																		
≤12	46.3	(12.0)	(29)	27.4	(5.1)	(128)	32.0	(5.4)	(124)	18.9	(4.6)	(100)	26.3	(5.0)	(83)	19.3	(3.0)	(222)
13–15	41.0	(3.4)	(283)	28.0	(3.5)	(249)	19.9	(3.1)	(198)	19.9	(3.3)	(171)	17.7	(3.6)	(130)	21.2	(3.2)	(264)
16–19	32.0	(2.7)	(464)	23.5	(2.9)	(284)	20.5	(3.1)	(259)	23.4	(3.5)	(234)	17.7	(4.0)	(170)	19.1	(2.5)	(391)
20–24	27.6	(3.5)	(322)	27.6	(3.5)	(258)	21.4	(3.4)	(194)	14.1	(3.1)	(164)	16.3	(4.6)	(99)	13.2	(2.5)	(267)
25–29	24.5	(3.5)	(243)	16.1	(3.3)	(219)	18.7	(3.6)	(169)	16.0	(4.1)	(115)	15.5	(4.1)	(90)	9.5	(2.5)	(164)
30–34	25.4	(3.5)	(225)	20.9	(3.9)	(172)	22.1	(4.6)	(100)	12.8	(3.4)	(108)	14.0	(5.9)	(52)	10.7	(2.8)	(131)
35+	26.1	(1.8)	(714)	21.1	(2.5)	(410)	16.9	(2.9)	(263)	11.5	(2.5)	(195)	9.8	(3.0)	(125)	12.2	(2.8)	(158)
III. The percentage of lifetime ideation that continued to within five years of interview																		
≤12	57.0	(11.7)	(29)	45.7	(5.5)	(128)	48.4	(5.5)	(124)	30.1	(5.7)	(100)	39.1	(6.1)	(83)	27.9	(3.6)	(222)
13–15	52.6	(3.7)	(283)	42.3	(3.9)	(249)	34.7	(3.9)	(198)	27.0	(3.6)	(171)	27.1	(4.3)	(130)	25.3	(3.4)	(264)
16–19	40.6	(3.1)	(464)	34.2	(3.3)	(284)	29.0	(3.6)	(259)	32.8	(3.8)	(234)	24.9	(4.9)	(170)	22.8	(2.6)	(391)
20–24	31.3	(3.5)	(322)	34.9	(3.7)	(258)	27.7	(3.8)	(194)	22.3	(4.0)	(164)	23.1	(5.1)	(99)	16.4	(2.7)	(267)
25–29	31.6	(3.6)	(243)	25.4	(3.9)	(219)	23.1	(3.9)	(169)	24.9	(5.3)	(115)	20.5	(4.6)	(90)	11.6	(2.7)	(164)
30–34	33.8	(3.7)	(225)	27.8	(4.2)	(172)	27.0	(5.1)	(100)	19.9	(4.2)	(108)	16.5	(6.3)	(52)	14.1	(3.2)	(131)
35+	30.7	(2.0)	(714)	26.6	(2.7)	(410)	20.2	(3.1)	(263)	16.1	(3.1)	(195)	11.0	(3.2)	(125)	12.2	(2.8)	(158)
IV. The percentage of lifetime ideation that continued to within ten years of interview																		
≤12	0.0	(0.0)	(29)	37.3	(4.9)	(128)	60.6	(5.4)	(124)	39.5	(6.0)	(100)	52.1	(6.5)	(83)	37.6	(3.8)	(222)
13–15	0.0	(0.0)	(283)	40.1	(3.8)	(249)	44.9	(4.2)	(198)	42.7	(4.6)	(171)	33.9	(4.6)	(130)	33.1	(3.4)	(264)
16–19	0.0	(0.0)	(464)	34.5	(3.4)	(284)	40.0	(3.8)	(259)	42.1	(3.8)	(234)	30.8	(5.0)	(170)	28.4	(2.8)	(391)
20–24	0.0	(0.0)	(322)	35.8	(3.5)	(258)	35.8	(4.1)	(194)	30.1	(4.4)	(164)	29.2	(5.4)	(99)	19.9	(2.9)	(267)
25–29	0.0	(0.0)	(243)	41.4	(4.1)	(219)	33.5	(4.4)	(169)	29.6	(5.5)	(115)	33.7	(6.0)	(90)	13.7	(2.9)	(164)
30–34	0.0	(0.0)	(225)	32.8	(4.8)	(172)	34.1	(5.8)	(100)	23.5	(4.3)	(108)	20.9	(6.7)	(52)	16.6	(3.4)	(131)
35+	0.0	(0.0)	(714)	40.0	(3.2)	(410)	30.5	(3.5)	(263)	20.2	(3.2)	(195)	11.7	(3.2)	(125)	13.8	(3.0)	(158)

Appendix Table 5.1. (cont.)

	Years since ideation started																	
	03–07			08–12			13–17			18–22			23–27			28+		
Age-of-onset	%	(SE)	(n)[a]	%	(SE)	(n)[a]	%	(SE)	(n)[a]	%	(SE)	(n)[a]	%	(SE)	(n)[a]	%	(SE)	(n)[a]
V. The percentage of lifetime ideation that did *not* continue beyond AOO																		
≤12	43.0	(11.7)	(29)	43.8	(5.3)	(128)	32.4	(5.5)	(124)	37.3	(5.9)	(100)	25.4	(5.3)	(83)	36.6	(4.0)	(222)
13–15	48.7	(3.5)	(283)	39.9	(3.7)	(249)	45.1	(4.2)	(198)	38.4	(4.5)	(171)	41.6	(4.7)	(130)	38.2	(3.7)	(264)
16–19	63.8	(2.7)	(464)	56.8	(3.5)	(284)	49.2	(3.7)	(259)	45.6	(3.7)	(234)	49.3	(4.8)	(170)	48.2	(2.9)	(391)
20–24	71.3	(3.5)	(322)	56.6	(3.8)	(258)	59.3	(4.1)	(194)	57.8	(4.8)	(164)	62.5	(5.7)	(99)	60.1	(3.7)	(267)
25–29	71.7	(3.6)	(243)	65.8	(4.2)	(219)	61.2	(4.6)	(169)	60.8	(5.6)	(115)	42.1	(6.0)	(90)	66.6	(4.1)	(164)
30–34	69.6	(3.6)	(225)	65.9	(4.8)	(172)	62.2	(5.9)	(100)	66.0	(4.9)	(108)	53.5	(9.8)	(52)	65.1	(5.0)	(131)
35+	72.7	(1.9)	(714)	67.4	(2.9)	(410)	65.4	(3.6)	(263)	67.2	(3.8)	(195)	67.6	(4.8)	(125)	65.5	(4.4)	(158)
VI. The percentage of lifetime ideation that did *not* continue beyond five years after AOO																		
≤12	58.1	(12.1)	(29)	62.0	(5.2)	(128)	43.4	(5.5)	(124)	46.8	(6.1)	(100)	33.7	(5.7)	(83)	41.8	(4.1)	(222)
13–15	88.8	(2.1)	(283)	63.8	(3.9)	(249)	60.1	(4.1)	(198)	48.5	(4.5)	(171)	54.7	(4.7)	(130)	48.9	(3.7)	(264)
16–19	93.7	(1.4)	(464)	68.9	(3.2)	(284)	61.5	(3.8)	(259)	51.3	(3.8)	(234)	58.3	(5.0)	(170)	55.7	(2.9)	(391)
20–24	92.9	(2.1)	(322)	68.0	(3.6)	(258)	68.6	(4.0)	(194)	62.4	(4.4)	(164)	68.0	(5.6)	(99)	65.3	(3.6)	(267)
25–29	95.6	(1.3)	(243)	78.9	(3.7)	(219)	69.4	(4.3)	(169)	70.4	(5.5)	(115)	57.9	(6.3)	(90)	71.6	(3.7)	(164)
30–34	93.9	(1.9)	(225)	74.7	(4.3)	(172)	68.7	(5.5)	(100)	71.4	(4.7)	(108)	59.6	(10.0)	(52)	68.2	(4.7)	(131)
35+	95.7	(0.9)	(714)	76.0	(2.7)	(410)	73.7	(3.3)	(263)	73.6	(3.5)	(195)	80.0	(4.0)	(125)	73.4	(4.0)	(158)

AOO, age-of-onset.

[a] The entries in this column represent the unweighted number of respondents with a history of ideation in this segment of the sample. The percentages are weighted percentages of these respondents. For example, the 128 respondents with AOO ≤ 12 and 8–12 years between AOO and interview represent the denominator in the calculations of the percentages in this subsample. 43.8% of these 128, for example, did not continue to have ideation beyond their AOO.

Appendix Table 5.2. Associations of age-of-onset and time between age-of-onset and interview with persistence of suicide plans among respondents with lifetime plans (n=3424)

| | Years since ideation started | | | | | | | | | | | | | | | | | |
| | 03–07 | | | 08–12 | | | 13–17 | | | 18–22 | | | 23–27 | | | 28+ | | |
Age-of-onset	%	(SE)	(n)ᵃ	%	(SE)	(n)ᵃ	%	(SE)	(n)ᵃ	%	(SE)	(n)ᵃ	%	(SE)	(n)ᵃ	%	(SE)	(n)ᵃ
I. The percentage of lifetime plans that continued to the year of interview																		
≤12	31.4	(13.8)	(15)	27.8	(11.3)	(42)	14.8	(7.2)	(28)	13.1	(5.7)	(32)	20.9	(9.8)	(23)	10.0	(4.7)	(56)
13–15	20.6	(4.6)	(96)	15.8	(5.2)	(79)	10.5	(4.4)	(62)	16.8	(5.7)	(49)	11.0	(5.3)	(42)	18.3	(5.2)	(87)
16–19	15.2	(3.1)	(153)	15.2	(4.1)	(107)	17.2	(4.5)	(117)	11.3	(3.9)	(90)	11.2	(4.1)	(65)	14.5	(3.8)	(108)
20–24	15.8	(4.5)	(121)	18.4	(6.0)	(91)	14.2	(4.8)	(65)	6.5	(3.4)	(52)	17.2	(6.8)	(39)	13.1	(4.4)	(95)
25–29	18.1	(4.5)	(83)	6.0	(2.3)	(76)	22.0	(6.9)	(47)	19.6	(8.2)	(29)	0.0	(0.0)	(36)	9.2	(4.9)	(55)
30–34	24.9	(6.0)	(79)	13.5	(5.6)	(61)	12.9	(5.4)	(36)	14.3	(6.5)	(36)	0.0	(0.0)	(19)	5.6	(3.9)	(33)
35+	20.6	(3.0)	(229)	18.4	(3.6)	(154)	7.3	(3.3)	(66)	4.1	(2.3)	(52)	0.0	(0.0)	(34)	12.4	(6.0)	(45)
II. The percentage of lifetime plans that continued to within two years of interview																		
≤12	40.9	(14.4)	(15)	32.6	(11.2)	(42)	16.8	(7.5)	(28)	14.7	(6.0)	(32)	25.1	(10.5)	(23)	10.0	(4.7)	(56)
13–15	30.6	(5.6)	(96)	23.8	(6.9)	(79)	12.1	(4.6)	(62)	17.6	(5.7)	(49)	11.0	(5.3)	(42)	21.2	(5.6)	(87)
16–19	24.2	(4.2)	(153)	19.8	(4.3)	(107)	18.4	(4.5)	(117)	12.7	(4.0)	(90)	11.2	(4.1)	(65)	17.1	(4.1)	(108)
20–24	25.0	(5.4)	(121)	24.1	(6.2)	(91)	15.2	(4.9)	(65)	8.3	(3.9)	(52)	18.7	(6.9)	(39)	14.9	(4.6)	(95)
25–29	19.3	(4.6)	(83)	7.8	(2.8)	(76)	26.7	(7.9)	(47)	19.6	(8.2)	(29)	0.7	(0.8)	(36)	12.2	(5.2)	(55)
30–34	34.0	(6.5)	(79)	15.0	(5.7)	(61)	14.5	(5.6)	(36)	14.3	(6.5)	(36)	0.0	(0.0)	(19)	5.6	(3.9)	(33)
35+	25.0	(3.2)	(229)	21.0	(3.6)	(154)	7.8	(3.4)	(66)	6.0	(3.0)	(52)	0.0	(0.0)	(34)	12.4	(6.0)	(45)
III. The percentage of lifetime plans that continued to within five years of interview																		
≤12	59.3	(16.6)	(15)	36.4	(11.2)	(42)	41.7	(11.3)	(28)	34.9	(10.6)	(32)	43.1	(14.0)	(23)	15.0	(5.5)	(56)
13–15	48.2	(6.3)	(96)	39.0	(7.0)	(79)	21.2	(5.7)	(62)	21.3	(6.4)	(49)	23.7	(7.9)	(42)	23.8	(5.7)	(87)
16–19	41.3	(5.4)	(153)	27.6	(5.0)	(107)	25.6	(5.1)	(117)	15.7	(4.4)	(90)	20.3	(5.9)	(65)	22.2	(4.4)	(108)
20–24	22.0	(4.4)	(121)	27.2	(6.2)	(91)	20.6	(5.4)	(65)	20.4	(7.2)	(52)	25.2	(8.2)	(39)	22.0	(5.1)	(95)
25–29	41.1	(6.7)	(83)	12.2	(3.6)	(76)	27.0	(7.9)	(47)	25.4	(9.5)	(29)	7.3	(4.7)	(36)	15.1	(5.8)	(55)
30–34	29.8	(6.1)	(79)	17.1	(6.0)	(61)	14.5	(5.6)	(36)	19.9	(7.9)	(36)	11.4	(8.1)	(19)	5.6	(3.9)	(33)
35+	30.8	(3.6)	(229)	28.8	(4.6)	(154)	18.5	(5.3)	(66)	13.5	(6.2)	(52)	3.5	(3.5)	(34)	14.5	(6.3)	(45)
IV. The percentage of lifetime plans that continued to within ten years of interview																		
≤12	0.0	(0.0)	(15)	31.7	(8.7)	(42)	55.9	(10.7)	(28)	36.4	(10.7)	(32)	51.3	(13.5)	(23)	30.4	(7.0)	(56)
13–15	0.0	(0.0)	(96)	45.5	(7.2)	(79)	28.7	(6.5)	(62)	32.0	(7.4)	(49)	31.7	(7.3)	(42)	30.1	(6.4)	(87)
16–19	0.0	(0.0)	(153)	34.8	(5.7)	(107)	35.6	(5.4)	(117)	30.2	(5.9)	(90)	25.5	(6.4)	(65)	29.4	(4.9)	(108)

Appendix Table 5.2. (cont.)

Age-of-onset	Years since ideation started																	
	03–07			08–12			13–17			18–22			23–27			28+		
	%	(SE)	(n)ᵃ	%	(SE)	(n)ᵃ	%	(SE)	(n)ᵃ	%	(SE)	(n)ᵃ	%	(SE)	(n)ᵃ	%	(SE)	(n)ᵃ
20–24	0.0	(0.0)	(121)	30.1	(5.4)	(91)	27.7	(6.2)	(65)	26.2	(7.5)	(52)	25.2	(8.2)	(39)	23.1	(5.1)	(95)
25–29	0.0	(0.0)	(83)	45.2	(6.5)	(76)	33.9	(8.7)	(47)	32.8	(10.4)	(29)	31.1	(9.2)	(36)	16.7	(5.9)	(55)
30–34	0.0	(0.0)	(79)	35.3	(9.2)	(61)	24.0	(8.2)	(36)	22.7	(8.1)	(36)	13.2	(8.2)	(19)	10.1	(5.0)	(33)
35+	0.0	(0.0)	(229)	44.1	(5.1)	(154)	22.0	(5.8)	(66)	15.0	(6.4)	(52)	4.2	(3.5)	(34)	15.7	(6.4)	(45)
V. The percentage of lifetime plans that did *not* continue beyond AOO																		
≤12	40.7	(16.6)	(15)	53.1	(11.0)	(42)	32.1	(9.9)	(28)	35.9	(11.8)	(32)	32.1	(12.1)	(23)	33.0	(7.4)	(56)
13–15	59.2	(5.8)	(96)	40.4	(6.7)	(79)	61.0	(7.3)	(62)	46.3	(8.0)	(49)	42.7	(7.7)	(42)	44.7	(6.8)	(87)
16–19	68.9	(4.6)	(153)	60.5	(6.1)	(107)	55.5	(5.5)	(117)	55.0	(6.4)	(90)	53.2	(7.6)	(65)	59.5	(5.4)	(108)
20–24	74.6	(5.1)	(121)	67.1	(6.5)	(91)	67.3	(6.6)	(65)	70.4	(7.5)	(52)	65.8	(8.8)	(39)	64.4	(5.5)	(95)
25–29	68.0	(6.4)	(83)	83.5	(4.5)	(76)	63.1	(8.9)	(47)	67.2	(10.4)	(29)	48.2	(9.9)	(36)	66.6	(7.0)	(55)
30–34	65.5	(6.5)	(79)	78.5	(6.0)	(61)	76.0	(8.2)	(36)	71.9	(8.4)	(36)	82.6	(9.1)	(19)	70.7	(8.8)	(33)
35+	75.7	(3.2)	(229)	65.2	(5.2)	(229)	76.1	(6.0)	(66)	77.7	(7.8)	(52)	83.3	(6.6)	(34)	75.3	(7.4)	(45)
VI. The percentage of lifetime plans that did *not* continue beyond five years after AOO																		
≤12	68.6	(13.8)	(15)	63.6	(11.2)	(42)	50.5	(11.0)	(28)	45.9	(11.7)	(32)	36.5	(12.5)	(23)	39.7	(8.1)	(56)
13–15	94.7	(2.4)	(96)	65.3	(7.1)	(79)	73.8	(6.2)	(62)	58.1	(7.5)	(49)	55.3	(8.2)	(42)	48.9	(6.5)	(87)
16–19	94.7	(2.0)	(153)	72.7	(5.0)	(107)	66.5	(5.3)	(117)	58.6	(6.2)	(90)	63.8	(7.2)	(65)	60.7	(5.4)	(108)
20–24	96.4	(1.9)	(121)	72.8	(6.2)	(91)	75.5	(5.8)	(65)	73.8	(7.5)	(52)	73.1	(8.3)	(39)	67.3	(5.5)	(95)
25–29	95.8	(2.0)	(83)	89.8	(3.3)	(76)	69.1	(8.3)	(47)	67.2	(10.4)	(29)	68.9	(9.2)	(36)	71.2	(6.7)	(55)
30–34	98.7	(1.0)	(79)	82.9	(6.0)	(61)	76.0	(8.2)	(36)	75.4	(8.2)	(36)	82.6	(9.1)	(19)	70.7	(8.8)	(33)
35+	94.9	(1.6)	(229)	73.7	(4.5)	(229)	81.5	(5.3)	(66)	85.0	(6.4)	(52)	89.4	(5.0)	(34)	75.3	(7.4)	(45)

AOO, age-of-onset.

ᵃ The entries in this column represent the unweighted number of respondents with a history of ideation in this segment of the sample. The percentages are weighted percentages of these respondents. For example, the 42 respondents with AOO ≤ 12 and 8–12 years between AOO and interview represent the denominator in the calculations of the percentages in this subsample. 53.1% of these 42, for example, did not continue to have plans beyond their AOO.

Appendix Table 5.3. Associations of age-of-onset and time between age-of-onset and interview with repetition of suicide attempts among respondents with a history of prior lifetime attempts (n=2928)

Years since ideation started

I. The percentage of lifetime attempters who made a repeat attempt in the year of interview

Age-of-onset	03–07 %	(SE)	(n)[a]	08–12 %	(SE)	(n)[a]	13–17 %	(SE)	(n)[a]	18–22 %	(SE)	(n)[a]	23–27 %	(SE)	(n)[a]	28+ %	(SE)	(n)[a]
≤12	0.0	(0.0)	(7)	10.1	(4.2)	(36)	10.4	(6.9)	(29)	9.6	(7.0)	(27)	16.5	(8.8)	(28)	9.3	(4.8)	(56)
13–15	21.8	(5.5)	(95)	8.5	(3.4)	(73)	8.0	(3.9)	(65)	9.6	(4.0)	(64)	6.8	(4.7)	(37)	8.9	(4.0)	(85)
16–19	12.3	(3.8)	(144)	7.9	(3.1)	(97)	14.3	(4.9)	(107)	10.2	(4.4)	(82)	16.6	(8.3)	(70)	6.1	(2.7)	(109)
20–24	15.8	(4.6)	(107)	11.8	(5.9)	(81)	8.5	(3.8)	(65)	2.1	(2.1)	(57)	0.0	(0.0)	(32)	0.0	(0.0)	(98)
25–29	11.2	(5.4)	(68)	4.2	(2.5)	(54)	6.5	(3.5)	(46)	8.8	(4.7)	(32)	0.0	(0.0)	(32)	4.6	(4.4)	(45)
30–34	14.5	(5.0)	(69)	9.5	(6.6)	(42)	4.1	(2.9)	(30)	0.0	(0.0)	(24)	0.0	(0.0)	(11)	2.8	(2.8)	(33)
35+	10.6	(2.6)	(155)	5.4	(2.2)	(98)	6.3	(3.8)	(48)	0.0	(0.0)	(50)	0.0	(0.0)	(26)	2.4	(2.5)	(29)

II. The percentage of lifetime attempters who made a repeat attempt within two years of interview

Age-of-onset	03–07 %	(SE)	(n)[a]	08–12 %	(SE)	(n)[a]	13–17 %	(SE)	(n)[a]	18–22 %	(SE)	(n)[a]	23–27 %	(SE)	(n)[a]	28+ %	(SE)	(n)[a]
≤12	0.0	(0.0)	(7)	10.1	(4.2)	(36)	13.4	(7.4)	(29)	9.6	(7.0)	(27)	16.5	(8.8)	(28)	12.0	(5.2)	(56)
13–15	27.3	(6.0)	(95)	17.8	(7.3)	(73)	8.4	(3.9)	(65)	9.6	(4.0)	(64)	9.3	(5.2)	(37)	11.3	(4.3)	(85)
16–19	19.4	(4.5)	(144)	9.7	(3.4)	(97)	14.8	(4.9)	(107)	10.2	(4.4)	(82)	17.8	(8.2)	(70)	8.3	(2.9)	(109)
20–24	24.0	(5.5)	(107)	11.8	(5.9)	(81)	8.5	(3.8)	(65)	2.1	(2.1)	(57)	0.0	(0.0)	(32)	1.6	(1.1)	(98)
25–29	14.7	(5.8)	(68)	8.2	(3.8)	(54)	8.7	(3.8)	(46)	8.8	(4.7)	(32)	0.0	(0.0)	(32)	6.0	(4.6)	(45)
30–34	17.4	(5.2)	(69)	9.5	(6.6)	(42)	4.1	(2.9)	(30)	0.0	(0.0)	(24)	0.0	(0.0)	(11)	2.8	(2.8)	(33)
35+	12.9	(2.8)	(155)	7.6	(2.9)	(98)	6.3	(3.8)	(48)	0.9	(0.9)	(50)	0.0	(0.0)	(26)	2.4	(2.5)	(29)

III. The percentage of lifetime attempters who made a repeat attempt within five years of interview

Age-of-onset	03–07 %	(SE)	(n)[a]	08–12 %	(SE)	(n)[a]	13–17 %	(SE)	(n)[a]	18–22 %	(SE)	(n)[a]	23–27 %	(SE)	(n)[a]	28+ %	(SE)	(n)[a]
≤12	0.0	(0.0)	(7)	10.1	(4.2)	(36)	29.6	(9.4)	(29)	20.0	(8.7)	(27)	27.4	(11.8)	(28)	17.3	(6.1)	(56)
13–15	37.9	(6.4)	(95)	27.8	(7.6)	(73)	15.6	(5.0)	(65)	13.8	(4.9)	(64)	16.7	(6.4)	(37)	13.3	(4.6)	(85)
16–19	31.4	(4.9)	(144)	13.5	(4.1)	(97)	19.9	(5.3)	(107)	11.7	(4.5)	(82)	17.8	(8.2)	(70)	9.0	(3.0)	(109)
20–24	19.4	(4.5)	(107)	13.8	(6.0)	(81)	15.4	(4.7)	(65)	6.7	(3.9)	(57)	1.3	(1.3)	(32)	4.9	(2.5)	(98)
25–29	33.5	(6.8)	(68)	12.3	(4.8)	(54)	18.3	(6.3)	(46)	11.9	(5.5)	(32)	0.0	(0.0)	(32)	9.3	(5.5)	(45)
30–34	24.5	(6.2)	(69)	12.7	(7.1)	(42)	4.1	(2.9)	(30)	0.0	(0.0)	(24)	0.0	(0.0)	(11)	5.3	(3.7)	(33)
35+	31.5	(4.4)	(155)	11.6	(3.7)	(98)	11.5	(4.7)	(48)	3.2	(2.5)	(50)	4.8	(4.7)	(26)	5.4	(3.9)	(29)

IV. The percentage of lifetime attempters who made a repeat attempt within ten years of interview

Age-of-onset	03–07 %	(SE)	(n)[a]	08–12 %	(SE)	(n)[a]	13–17 %	(SE)	(n)[a]	18–22 %	(SE)	(n)[a]	23–27 %	(SE)	(n)[a]	28+ %	(SE)	(n)[a]
≤12	0.0	(0.0)	(7)	26.1	(8.4)	(36)	36.3	(9.3)	(29)	28.6	(9.5)	(27)	40.9	(12.2)	(28)	24.4	(6.8)	(56)
13–15	0.0	(0.0)	(95)	27.3	(7.5)	(73)	25.2	(6.2)	(65)	23.0	(6.2)	(64)	20.4	(7.0)	(37)	19.5	(5.3)	(85)
16–19	0.0	(0.0)	(144)	28.7	(5.2)	(97)	31.5	(5.8)	(107)	19.4	(5.5)	(82)	20.3	(8.3)	(70)	13.1	(3.5)	(109)
20–24	0.0	(0.0)	(107)	19.9	(4.9)	(81)	20.7	(5.2)	(65)	10.9	(4.4)	(57)	1.3	(1.3)	(32)	5.9	(2.6)	(98)
25–29	0.0	(0.0)	(68)	37.5	(7.4)	(54)	24.9	(7.4)	(46)	21.8	(7.6)	(32)	9.8	(5.9)	(32)	10.5	(5.6)	(45)
30–34	0.0	(0.0)	(69)	25.2	(8.2)	(42)	5.9	(3.4)	(30)	0.0	(0.0)	(24)	0.0	(0.0)	(11)	12.5	(6.3)	(33)
35+	0.0	(0.0)	(155)	28.8	(5.3)	(98)	17.5	(6.3)	(48)	11.5	(4.8)	(50)	8.1	(5.6)	(26)	5.4	(3.9)	(29)

Appendix Table 5.3. (cont.)

Age-of-onset	Years since ideation started																	
	03–07			08–12			13–17			18–22			23–27			28+		
	%	(SE)	(n)[a]	%	(SE)	(n)[a]	%	(SE)	(n)[a]	%	(SE)	(n)[a]	%	(SE)	(n)[a]	%	(SE)	(n)[a]
V. The percentage of lifetime attempters who never made a repeat attempt after AOO																		
≤12	100.0	(0.0)	(7)	79.1	(6.5)	(36)	60.8	(9.6)	(29)	56.6	(11.3)	(27)	43.0	(10.9)	(28)	57.9	(7.6)	(56)
13–15	64.8	(6.1)	(95)	54.3	(7.9)	(73)	61.8	(7.1)	(65)	55.7	(7.2)	(64)	56.0	(9.0)	(37)	59.7	(6.3)	(85)
16–19	79.2	(4.5)	(144)	81.1	(4.7)	(97)	60.6	(5.8)	(107)	63.4	(6.5)	(82)	57.4	(8.2)	(70)	63.0	(5.6)	(109)
20–24	78.7	(4.9)	(107)	80.5	(6.7)	(81)	75.8	(5.8)	(65)	81.4	(5.8)	(57)	86.8	(6.0)	(32)	78.9	(5.3)	(98)
25–29	82.5	(6.4)	(68)	83.4	(5.4)	(54)	73.6	(7.5)	(46)	74.8	(8.1)	(32)	67.9	(11.8)	(32)	77.4	(6.8)	(45)
30–34	83.8	(5.2)	(69)	84.3	(7.4)	(42)	90.7	(4.2)	(30)	96.9	(3.1)	(24)	91.7	(8.1)	(11)	78.7	(8.0)	(33)
35+	85.7	(3.0)	(155)	85.6	(3.6)	(98)	82.0	(6.3)	(48)	78.3	(7.9)	(50)	87.6	(6.4)	(26)	89.9	(5.2)	(29)
VI. The percentage of lifetime attempters who never made a repeat attempt beyond five years after AOO																		
≤12	100.0	(0.0)	(7)	89.9	(4.2)	(36)	63.7	(9.3)	(29)	60.7	(11.2)	(27)	56.2	(12.2)	(28)	59.4	(7.5)	(56)
13–15	91.4	(5.1)	(95)	75.9	(7.4)	(73)	81.9	(5.2)	(65)	72.2	(6.5)	(64)	70.9	(7.8)	(37)	71.6	(5.8)	(85)
16–19	97.6	(1.1)	(144)	88.6	(3.7)	(97)	68.4	(5.8)	(107)	72.2	(6.2)	(82)	69.7	(8.3)	(70)	72.2	(4.9)	(109)
20–24	97.8	(1.3)	(107)	86.5	(6.0)	(81)	79.7	(5.2)	(65)	85.9	(4.9)	(57)	96.5	(2.5)	(32)	85.5	(4.2)	(98)
25–29	96.9	(2.0)	(68)	91.8	(3.8)	(54)	81.7	(6.3)	(46)	78.2	(7.6)	(32)	87.8	(6.3)	(32)	77.4	(6.8)	(45)
30–34	98.3	(1.2)	(69)	87.0	(7.1)	(42)	92.8	(3.6)	(30)	100.0	(0.0)	(24)	91.7	(8.1)	(11)	78.7	(8.0)	(33)
35+	96.6	(1.6)	(155)	90.4	(3.4)	(98)	84.1	(6.1)	(48)	87.1	(5.0)	(50)	89.1	(6.2)	(26)	92.3	(4.5)	(29)

AOO, age-of-onset.

[a] The entries in this column represent the unweighted number of respondents with a history of ideation in this segment of the sample. The percentages are weighted percentages of these respondents. For example, the 36 respondents with AOO ≤ 12 and 8–12 years between AOO and interview represent the denominator in the calculations of the percentages in this subsample. 79.1% of these 36, for example, did not make another attempt after AOO.

Appendix Table 5.4. Joint associations of age-of-onset, age at interview, and time between age-of-onset and interview with persistence of suicide ideation in the overall backward recency model and logistic regression models for components of recency

| | Backward recency model[a] | Logistic regression models | | | | |
| | | M1[b] | M2[c] | M3[d] | M4[e] | M5[f] |
	OR (95% CI)	OR (95% CI)	OR (95% CI)	OR (95% CI)	OR (95% CI)	OR (95% CI)
I. Low-lower-middle-income countries						
AOO 4–12 (Spline)	1.01 (0.9–1.2)	0.99 (0.8–1.2)	0.96 (0.7–1.3)	1.05 (0.8–1.4)	0.99 (0.8–1.3)	0.85 (0.6–1.2)
AOO 13–29+ (Spline)	0.94* (0.9–1.0)	0.91* (0.9–1.0)	0.92 (0.8–1.0)	1.01 (0.9–1.1)	1.08 (1.0–1.2)	1.20* (1.1–1.3)
AAI – AOO (Linear)	0.99 (1.0–1.0)	1.01 (1.0–1.0)	0.96 (0.9–1.0)	0.98 (0.9–1.0)	1.00 (1.0–1.0)	1.04 (1.0–1.1)
II. Upper-middle-income countries						
AOO 13–19 (Spline)	0.92 (0.8–1.0)	0.87 (0.7–1.0)	0.86 (0.6–1.1)	0.93 (0.7–1.2)	0.94 (0.8–1.2)	0.98 (0.7–1.3)
AOO 20–29+ (Spline)	1.02 (1.0–1.1)	1.04 (0.9–1.1)	1.06 (0.8–1.4)	0.97 (0.8–1.2)	1.27 (1.0–1.7)	1.49* (1.0–2.1)
AAI-AOO (Linear)	–	1.01 (1.0–1.0)	0.92* (0.9–1.0)	0.92* (0.9–1.0)	0.97 (0.9–1.0)	1.07 (1.0–1.2)
AAI-AOO 0–5 (Spline)	1.40* (1.2–1.6)	–	–	–	–	–
AAI-AAO 6–10+ (Spline)	0.83* (0.8–0.9)	–	–	–	–	–
III. High-income countries						
AOO 4–19+ (Spline)	0.94* (0.9–1.0)	0.87* (0.8–0.9)	1.01 (1.0–1.1)	0.97 (0.9–1.0)	1.01 (1.0–1.1)	1.04 (1.0–1.1)
AAI-AOO (Linear)	0.99* (1.0–1.0)	1.02* (1.0–1.0)	0.96* (0.9–1.0)	0.95* (0.9–1.0)	0.98* (1.0–1.0)	1.02 (1.0–1.0)
Age at interview 18–25	0.92* (0.9–1.0)	1.04 (1.0–1.2)	0.01* (0.0–0.0)	0.71 (0.4–1.1)	1.01 (0.7–1.4)	1.14 (0.8–1.6)
Age at interview 25–54	0.99* (1.0–1.0)	1.00 (1.0–1.0)	0.98 (0.9–1.0)	1.00 (1.0–1.0)	0.99 (1.0–1.0)	0.99 (1.0–1.0)
Age at interview 55–64+	0.96 (1.0–1.0)	0.94* (0.9–1.0)	0.99 (1.0–1.0)	1.00 (1.0–1.0)	1.02 (1.0–1.1)	1.05* (1.0–1.1)

AOO, age-of-onset.

AAI, age at interview.

* Significant at the 0.05 level, two-sided test.

– Not included due to small cell size.

[a] A discrete-time survival model estimated among respondents with a lifetime history of suicide ideation and an AOO more than one year before interview. Person–year is the unit of analysis. The outcome is number of years since most recent occurrence of ideation. See the text for a more detailed description of the model.

[b] A logistic regression model estimated among respondents with a lifetime history of suicide ideation and an AOO two or more years before interview. The outcome is a dichotomy for recency more than two years (coded 1) vs. 0–2 years (coded 0) after AOO.

[c] A logistic regression model estimated among respondents with a lifetime history of suicide ideation, an AOO fifteen or more years before interview, and recency more than two years after AOO. The outcome is a dichotomy for recency within ten years of interview (coded 1) vs. 11+ years earlier than interview (coded 0).

[d] A logistic regression model estimated among respondents with a lifetime history of suicide ideation, an AOO ten or more years before interview, and recency more than two years after AOO. The outcome is a dichotomy for recency within five years of interview (coded 1) vs. 6+ years earlier than interview (coded 0).

[e] A logistic regression model estimated among respondents with a lifetime history of suicide ideation, an AOO ten or more years before interview, and recency more than two years after AOO. The outcome is a dichotomy for recency within the year of interview (coded 1) vs. 1+ years earlier than interview (coded 0).

[f] A logistic regression model estimated among respondents with a lifetime history of suicide ideation, an AOO ten or more years before interview, and recency within five years of interview. The outcome is a dichotomy for recency within the year of interview (coded 1) vs. 1+ years earlier than interview (coded 0).

Appendix Table 5.5. Joint associations of age-of-onset, age at interview, and time between age-of-onset and interview with persistence of suicide plans in the overall backward recency model and logistic regression models for components of recency

| | Backward recency model[a] | Logistic regression models | | | | |
	OR (95% CI)	M1[b] OR (95% CI)	M2[c] OR (95% CI)	M3[d] OR (95% CI)	M4[e] OR (95% CI)	M5[f] OR (95% CI)
I. Low/lower-middle-income countries						
AOO 4–12 (spline)	0.72* (0.6–0.9)	0.59* (0.4–1.0)	18.64* (6.0–58.2)	0.98 (0.6–1.6)	1.05 (0.5–2.0)	1.03 (0.5–2.0)
AOO 13–39+ (spline)	0.97 (0.9–1.0)	0.95 (0.9–1.0)	1.21 (0.9–1.7)	1.04 (0.9–1.2)	1.05 (0.9–1.2)	1.03 (0.9–1.2)
AAI – AOO (linear)	0.98 (0.9–1.0)	1.00 (1.0–1.1)	1.07 (1.0–1.2)	1.05 (1.0–1.1)	1.08 (1.0–1.2)	1.08 (1.0–1.2)
II. Upper-middle-income countries						
AOO 3–12 (spline)	0.81* (0.7–1.0)	0.64 (0.4–1.1)	1.21 (0.8–1.8)	1.15 (0.7–1.8)	1.08 (0.8–1.5)	0.89 (0.5–1.6)
AOO 13–39+ (spline)	0.96 (0.9–1.0)	0.89 (0.7–1.1)	1.15 (0.5–2.5)	0.80 (0.6–1.1)	44.53* (30.6–64.7)	11.01* (7.6–15.9)
AAI-AOO (linear)	0.98 (1.0–1.0)	0.98 (0.9–1.0)	1.04 (0.9–1.2)	0.95 (0.9–1.1)	1.05 (0.9–1.2)	1.10 (1.0–1.3)
III. High-income countries						
AOO 4–19+ (spline)	0.86* (0.8–0.9)	0.80* (0.7–0.9)	1.11 (1.0–1.3)	1.08 (0.9–1.2)	1.11 (1.0–1.3)	1.08 (0.9–1.3)
AAI-AOO (linear)	0.98* (1.0–1.0)	1.02 (1.0–1.0)	0.94* (0.9–1.0)	0.94* (0.9–1.0)	0.98 (0.9–1.0)	1.02 (1.0–1.1)
Age at interview 18–64+ (spline)	0.99 (1.0–1.0)	1.00 (1.0–1.0)	1.00 (0.9–1.0)	1.01 (1.0–1.0)	1.00 (1.0–1.0)	1.00 (1.0–1.0)

AOO, age-of-onset.
AAI, age at interview.
* Significant at the 0.05 level, two-sided test.
[a] A discrete-time survival model estimated among respondents with a lifetime history of suicide plans and an AOO more than one year before interview. Person–year is the unit of analysis. The outcome is number of years since most recent occurrence of a plan. See the text for a more detailed description of the model.
[b] A logistic regression model estimated among respondents with a lifetime history of suicide plans and an AOO five or more years before interview. The outcome is a dichotomy for recency more than two years (coded 1) vs. 0–2 years (coded 0) after AOO.
[c] A logistic regression model estimated among respondents with a lifetime history of suicide plans, an AOO fifteen or more years before interview, and recency more than two years after AOO. The outcome is a dichotomy for recency within ten years of interview (coded 1) vs. 11+ years earlier than interview (coded 0).
[d] A logistic regression model estimated among respondents with a lifetime history of suicide plans, an AOO ten or more years before interview, and recency more than two years after AOO. The outcome is a dichotomy for recency within five years of interview (coded 1) vs. 6+ years earlier than interview (coded 0).
[e] A logistic regression model estimated among respondents with a lifetime history of suicide plans, an AOO ten or more years before interview, and recency more than two years after AOO. The outcome is a dichotomy for recency within the year of interview (coded 1) vs. 1+ years earlier than interview (coded 0).
[f] A logistic regression model estimated among respondents with a lifetime history of suicide plans, an AOO ten or more years before interview, and recency within five years of interview. The outcome is a dichotomy for recency within the year of interview (coded 1) vs. 1+ years earlier than interview (coded 0).

Appendix Table 5.6. Joint associations of age-of-onset, age at interview, and time between age-of-onset and interview with persistence of suicide attempts in the overall backward recency model and logistic regression models for components of recency

| | Backward recency model[a] | Logistic regression models | | | | |
	OR (95% CI)	M1[b] OR (95% CI)	M2[c] OR (95% CI)	M3[d] OR (95% CI)	M4[e] OR (95% CI)	M5[f] OR (95% CI)
I. Low/lower-middle-income countries						
AOO 4–19 (spline)	1.00 (0.9–1.1)	1.00 (0.9–1.1)	0.99 (0.7–1.3)	0.99 (0.8–1.3)	1.00 (0.8–1.3)	1.03 (0.6–1.7)
AOO 30–39+ (spline)	0.93 (0.8–1.1)	0.89 (0.7–1.1)	13.84* (7.7–24.9)	14.98* (9.0–24.8)	17.86* (11.7–27.3)	6.77* (4.4–10.4)
AAI – AOO (linear)	–	1.06* (1.0–1.1)	1.03 (1.0–1.1)	1.04 (1.0–1.1)	1.03 (1.0–1.1)	1.00 (0.8–1.2)
AAI-AOO 0–5 (spline)	1.40* (1.1–1.7)	–	–	–	–	–
AAI-AOO 6–10 (spline)	0.73* (0.6–0.9)	–	–	–	–	–
AAI-AOO 11–15+ (spline)	1.08* (1.0–1.1)	–	–	–	–	–
II. Upper-middle-income countries						
AOO (linear)	0.97 (0.9–1.0)	0.99 (0.9–1.0)	0.94 (0.8–1.1)	1.05 (0.9–1.2)	1.12 (0.9–1.4)	48.56* (33.0–71.4)
AAI-AOO (linear)	0.98 (0.9–1.0)	0.99 (1.0–1.0)	1.11 (0.9–1.4)	1.03 (0.9–1.2)	1.15 (1.0–1.4)	365.92 (185.4–722.0)
III. High-income countries						
AOO 4–29 (spline)	0.90* (0.9–0.9)	0.90* (0.9–0.9)	0.95 (0.9–1.0)	0.96 (0.9–1.0)	1.00 (0.9–1.1)	1.07 (1.0–1.2)
AOO 30–39 (spline)	1.13* (1.1–1.2)	1.09* (1.0–1.2)	1.21 (0.9–1.6)	0.97 (0.8–1.2)	0.95 (0.7–1.2)	0.88 (0.6–1.3)
AOO 4064+ (spline)	0.90* (0.8–1.0)	0.91* (0.8–1.0)	1.26 (0.6–2.7)	1.47* (1.1–2.0)	0.96 (0.6–1.6)	0.74 (0.3–1.7)
AAI-AOO (linear)	1.02 (1.0–1.0)	0.96* (0.9–1.0)	0.94* (0.9–1.0)	0.93* (0.9–1.0)	0.96 (0.9–1.0)	1.04 (1.0–1.1)

AOO, age-of-onset.

AAI, age at interview.

* Significant at the 0.05 level, two-sided test.

– Not included due to small cell size.

[a] A discrete-time survival model estimated among respondents with a lifetime history of suicide attempts and an AOO more than one year before interview. Person-year is the unit of analysis. The outcome is number of years since most recent attempt. See the text for a more detailed description of the model.

[b] A logistic regression model estimated among respondents with a lifetime history of suicide attempts and an AOO five or more years before interview. The outcome is a dichotomy for recency more than two years (coded 1) vs. 0–2 years (coded 0) after AOO.

[c] A logistic regression model estimated among respondents with a lifetime history of suicide attempts, an AOO fifteen or more years before interview, and recency more than two years after AOO. The outcome is a dichotomy for recency within ten years of interview (coded 1) vs. 11+ years earlier than interview (coded 0).

[d] A logistic regression model estimated among respondents with a lifetime history of suicide attempts, an AOO ten or more years before interview, and recency more than two years after AOO. The outcome is a dichotomy for recency within five years of interview (coded 1) vs. 6+ years earlier than interview (coded 0).

[e] A logistic regression model estimated among respondents with a lifetime history of suicide attempts, an AOO ten or more years before interview, and recency more than two years after AOO. The outcome is a dichotomy for recency within the year of interview (coded 1) vs. 1+ years earlier than interview (coded 0).

[f] A logistic regression model estimated among respondents with a lifetime history of suicide attempts, an AOO ten or more years before interview, and recency within five years of interview. The outcome is a dichotomy for recency within the year of interview (coded 1) vs. 1+ years earlier than interview (coded 0).

Appendix Table 6.1. Sociodemographic risk factors for suicidal behavior[a] (high-income countries)

Demographics	Among total sample		Among ideators		
	Ideation	Attempt	Plan	Planned attempt	Unplanned attempt
	OR (95% CI)	OR (95% CI)	OR (95% CI)	OR (95% CI)	OR (95% CI)
Gender					
Female	1.3* (1.2–1.4)	1.8* (1.6–2.1)	1.1 (0.9–1.3)	1.1 (0.8–1.5)	1.7* (1.3–2.3)
Male					
χ^2 (p-value)	53.8 (<0.001)*	71.4 (<0.001)*	0.9 (0.33)	0.6 (0.45)	13.5 (<0.001)*
Age group (years)					
18–34	9.1* (7.7–10.7)	13.2* (9.6–18.1)	0.8 (0.5–1.2)	0.9 (0.5–1.9)	1.4 (0.7–3.0)
35–49	4.7* (4.0–5.5)	6.8* (5.0–9.2)	0.9 (0.6–1.3)	1.2 (0.6–2.4)	1.5 (0.7–3.0)
50–64	2.8* (2.4–3.2)	4.0* (2.9–5.5)	0.9 (0.6–1.4)	1.4 (0.7–2.8)	1.4 (0.7–2.9)
65+					
χ^2 (p-value)	819.1 (<0.001)*	299.9 (<0.001)*	2.5 (0.48)	4.0 (0.26)	1.2 (0.75)
5-Category education					
Currently a student	1.2 (1.0–1.4)	1.4* (1.0–1.9)	1.4* (1.0–2.0)	1.8* (1.1–3.2)	1.4 (0.7–2.6)
Low	1.5* (1.3–1.8)	2.7* (2.1–3.5)	1.2 (0.9–1.5)	2.4* (1.5–3.9)	3.2* (1.9–5.3)
Low-average	1.0 (0.9–1.2)	1.5* (1.1–1.9)	1.2 (1.0–1.6)	1.6* (1.0–2.5)	2.1* (1.2–3.7)
High-average	1.1 (0.9–1.3)	1.3* (1.0–1.8)	1.0 (0.8–1.4)	1.1 (0.7–1.7)	1.3 (0.8–2.3)
High					
χ^2 (p-value)	43.3 (<0.001)*	81.7 (<0.001)*	5.9 (0.21)	18.0 (0.001)*	31.5 (<0.001)*
Marital status					
Never married	1.4* (1.2–1.6)	2.0* (1.6–2.5)	1.2 (0.9–1.5)	1.6* (1.1–2.3)	1.1 (0.8–1.7)
Previously married	1.8* (1.5–2.3)	2.8* (2.0–3.8)	1.1 (0.8–1.6)	2.2* (1.3–3.8)	1.8* (1.0–3.0)
History of marriage, current marital status unknown	2.4* (2.1–2.8)	3.1* (2.4–4.0)	2.0* (1.5–2.7)	2.4* (1.5–3.8)	1.8* (1.1–2.9)
Currently in first marriage					
χ^2 (p-value)	139.4 (<0.001)*	92.7 (<0.001)*	25.0 (<0.001)*	18.4 (<0.001)*	8.4 (0.04)*

* Significant at the 0.05 level, two-sided test.
[a] Each column is a separate multivariate model in survival framework, with all rows as predictors controlling for person–years and countries. Outcome variable indicated in each column header.

Appendix Table 6.2. Sociodemographic risk factors for suicidal behavior[a] (middle-income countries)

Demographics	Among total sample		Among ideators		
	Ideation	Attempt	Plan	Planned attempt	Unplanned attempt
	OR (95% CI)	OR (95% CI)	OR (95% CI)	OR (95% CI)	OR (95% CI)
Gender					
Female	1.6* (1.4–1.9)	2.3* (1.7–3.0)	1.2 (0.8–1.6)	2.0* (1.2–3.5)	1.6 (1.0–2.6)
Male					
χ^2 (p-value)	31.7 (<0.001)*	34.2 (<0.001)*	0.7 (0.40)	6.6 (0.01)*	3.4 (0.06)
Age group (years)					
18–34	9.4* (6.4–13.9)	7.5* (4.2–13.2)	2.3* (1.0–5.4)	0.5 (0.2–1.7)	2.9 (0.9–9.1)
35–49	3.3* (2.2–4.8)	2.4* (1.3–4.4)	1.5 (0.7–3.2)	0.5 (0.1–1.7)	1.8 (0.5–6.8)
50–64	1.9* (1.3–2.8)	1.8 (1.0–3.4)	1.4 (0.7–2.8)	1.0 (0.3–3.8)	2.1 (0.6–7.6)
65+					
χ^2 (p-value)	259.3 (<0.001)*	144.1 (<0.001)*	7.3 (0.06)	3.8 (0.29)	5.5 (0.14)
5-Category education					
Currently a student	1.0 (0.7–1.4)	1.1 (0.6–2.0)	0.9 (0.5–1.9)	1.6 (0.6–4.4)	0.5 (0.2–1.4)
Low	1.5* (1.0–2.2)	1.6 (0.9–2.8)	1.6 (0.8–3.2)	2.2 (0.9–5.5)	0.6 (0.3–1.4)
Low-average	1.4 (1.0–1.9)	1.9* (1.1–3.2)	1.4 (0.7–2.8)	3.3* (1.5–7.3)	0.9 (0.3–2.2)
High-average	1.3 (1.0–1.9)	1.6 (1.0–2.8)	1.2 (0.6–2.2)	1.4 (0.7–2.8)	0.6 (0.2–1.4)
High					
χ^2 (p-value)	12.5 (0.01)*	14.5 (0.01)*	3.4 (0.50)	9.6 (0.05)*	3.9 (0.42)
Marital status					
Never married	1.1 (0.9–1.4)	1.3 (1.0–1.8)	1.0 (0.7–1.5)	2.5* (1.2–5.1)	1.6 (0.7–3.2)
Previously married	2.0* (1.6–2.7)	2.4* (1.6–3.8)	1.5 (1.0–2.3)	1.1 (0.6–2.3)	1.3 (0.6–2.8)
Currently in first marriage	27.9 (<0.001)*	15.5 (<0.001)*	3.9 (0.14)	6.8 (0.03)*	1.6 (0.45)
χ^2 (p-value)					

*Significant at the 0.05 level, two-sided test.
[a] Each column is a separate multivariate model in survival framework, with all rows as predictors controlling for person–years and countries. Outcome variable indicated in each column header.

Appendix Table 6.3. Sociodemographic risk factors for suicidal behavior[a] (low-income countries)

	Among total sample		Among ideators		
	Ideation	Attempt	Plan	Planned attempt	Unplanned attempt
Demographics	OR (95% CI)	OR (95% CI)	OR (95% CI)	OR (95% CI)	OR (95% CI)
Gender					
Female	1.3* (1.1–1.5)	1.3* (1.1–1.6)	0.9 (0.7–1.3)	1.6* (1.0–2.5)	1.1 (0.7–1.7)
Male					
χ^2 (p-value)	12.3 (<0.001)*	6.0 (0.01)*	0.1 (0.72)	4.1 (0.04)*	0.1 (0.80)
Age group (years)					
18–34	7.6* (5.1–11.4)	8.5* (4.6–15.5)	2.6* (1.1–5.9)	5.0* (1.7–14.9)	1.4 (0.3–6.2)
35–49	3.7* (2.6–5.4)	4.3* (2.3–7.9)	2.1 (0.9–4.7)	4.0* (1.4–11.6)	2.1 (0.5–8.6)
50–64	2.0* (1.4–2.9)	1.6 (0.8–3.0)	1.3 (0.6–2.9)	1.1 (0.3–4.1)	0.8 (0.1–3.8)
65+					
χ^2 (p-value)	147.7 (<0.001)*	111.5 (<0.001)*	9.9 (0.02)*	21.8 (<0.001)*	6.9 (0.08)
5-Category education					
Currently a student	0.7* (0.5–0.9)	0.5* (0.3–0.9)	1.0 (0.5–1.9)	0.5 (0.2–1.3)	0.6 (0.2–1.9)
Low	1.2 (0.9–1.7)	1.3 (0.8–2.0)	1.7* (1.1–2.8)	1.3 (0.6–2.8)	1.0 (0.4–2.9)
Low-average	1.1 (0.9–1.5)	1.3 (0.8–2.0)	1.4 (0.9–2.3)	1.0 (0.4–2.2)	1.1 (0.5–2.7)
High-average	0.9 (0.7–1.3)	1.1 (0.7–1.9)	1.0 (0.6–1.7)	1.4 (0.6–3.1)	2.2 (0.8–6.0)
High					
χ^2 (p-value)	20.1 (<0.001)*	26.4 (<0.001)*	10.1 (0.04)*	5.6 (0.23)	8.1 (0.09)
Marital status					
Never married	0.9 (0.7–1.2)	0.8 (0.6–1.2)	0.7 (0.5–1.0)	1.4 (0.8–2.5)	0.6 (0.3–1.1)
Previously married	1.7* (1.3–2.3)	2.3* (1.6–3.4)	1.0 (0.7–1.7)	1.1 (0.6–2.1)	1.9 (0.8–4.4)
Currently in first marriage					
χ^2 (p-value)	14.9 (<0.001)*	21.1 (<0.001)*	4.0 (0.13)	1.7 (0.43)	6.7 (0.04)*

* Significant at the 0.05 level, two-sided test.
[a] Each column is a separate multivariate model in survival framework, with all rows as predictors controlling for person–years and countries. Outcome variable indicated in each column header.

Appendix Table 6.4. Interactions between sociodemographic factors and respondent age (4–12, 13–19, 20–29, 30+ years) in the prediction of suicidal behavior[a] (high-income countries)

		Among total sample		Among ideators		
		Ideation	Attempt	Plan	Planned attempt	Unplanned attempt
Interactions		OR (95% CI)	OR (95% CI)	OR (95% CI)	OR (95% CI)	OR (95% CI)
Gender						
Female	13–19	1.2 (0.9–1.6)	1.0 (0.6–1.9)	1.1 (0.5–2.5)	2.9 (0.5–16.1)	0.0* (0.0–0.0)
	20–29	1.1 (0.8–1.5)	1.0 (0.5–1.8)	0.9 (0.4–2.1)	3.9 (0.7–21.8)	0.0* (0.0–0.0)
	30+	0.9 (0.7–1.3)	0.7 (0.4–1.3)	0.8 (0.3–1.7)	2.5 (0.5–13.1)	0.0* (0.0–0.0)
Male	13–19					
	20–29					
	30+					
χ^2 (p-value)		4.5 (0.21)	5.4 (0.15)	3.4 (0.3)	4.7 (0.19)	58.9 (<0.001)*
Age group (years)						
18–34	13–19	0.7 (0.3–1.8)	4.6* (1.8–12.0)	0.8 (0.2–2.8)	0.6 (0.0–9.9)	0.5 (0.1–2.4)
	20–29	0.5 (0.2–1.2)	1.5 (0.7–3.4)	0.4* (0.2–0.9)	0.6 (0.2–2.1)	0.4 (0.1–3.1)
	30+	0.2* (0.1–0.5)	1.5 (0.6–3.6)	–	–	–
35–49	13–19	0.8 (0.3–2.0)	3.3* (1.1–9.6)	2.0 (0.4–9.2)	2.2 (0.1–51.1)	–
	20–29	0.8 (0.3–2.0)	1.9 (0.7–4.7)	0.8 (0.2–2.7)	3.2 (0.5–21.4)	–
	30+	0.6 (0.2–1.4)	1.8 (0.8–4.1)	2.2 (0.8–6.0)	3.8 (0.7–20.5)	–
50–64	13–19	0.6 (0.2–1.5)	2.9 (0.9–9.4)	1.7 (0.3–8.9)	0.1 (0.0–3.3)	–
	20–29	0.9 (0.4–2.3)	4.2* (1.6–10.7)	1.8 (0.5–6.6)	0.4 (0.0–5.6)	–
	30+	0.6 (0.3–1.5)	1.9 (0.9–4.2)	2.0 (0.6–6.2)	0.1 (0.0–1.5)	–
65+	13–19					
	20–29					
	30+					
χ^2 (p-value)		59.9 (<0.001)*	46.0 (<0.001)*	29.7 (<0.001)*	33.9 (<0.001)*	6.0 (0.4)
5-Category education						
Currently a student	13–19	0.6 (0.1–2.9)	3.4 (0.5–22.3)	0.2 (0.0–1.5)	–	18.4* (1.7–201.1)
	20–29	0.4 (0.1–1.9)	1.0 (0.2–7.1)	0.3 (0.0–2.6)	–	–
	30+					
Low	13–19	0.9 (0.1–7.4)	2.0 (0.2–19.1)	0.0* (0.0–0.0)	1.3 (0.4–4.3)	3.9 (0.6–24.1)
	20–29	0.5 (0.1–4.3)	0.5 (0.1–4.8)	0.0* (0.0–0.0)	1.0 (0.4–2.1)	0.7 (0.3–1.8)
	30+	0.4 (0.1–3.1)	0.5 (0.1–4.4)	0.0* (0.0–0.0)	–	–
Low-average	13–19	–	3.0 (0.3–26.2)	0.7 (0.2–2.1)	2.8 (0.8–9.5)	3.5 (0.6–21.8)
	20–29	–	0.8 (0.1–6.8)	1.6 (1.0–2.5)	2.0 (1.0–4.2)	0.5 (0.2–1.6)
	30+	–	0.5 (0.1–4.9)	–	–	–
High-average	13–19	2.2* (1.3–3.8)	3.6* (1.7–7.9)	0.5 (0.2–1.7)	2.2 (0.6–8.4)	–
	20–29	1.6* (1.2–2.2)	1.4 (0.9–2.3)	1.2 (0.7–1.8)	2.3* (1.2–4.5)	0.9 (0.2–5.6)
	30+	–	–	–	–	1.9 (0.3–13.0)
High	13–19					
	20–29					
	30+					
χ^2 (p-value)		172.1 (<0.001)*	32.3 (<0.001)*	435.2 (<0.001)*	104.1 (<0.001)*	18.2* (0.01)

Appendix Table 6.4. (cont.)

Interactions		Among total sample			Among ideators	
		Ideation	Attempt	Plan	Planned attempt	Unplanned attempt
		OR (95% CI)	OR (95% CI)	OR (95% CI)	OR (95% CI)	OR (95% CI)
Marital status						
Never married	13–19	0.5 (0.2–1.0)	1.6 (0.7–3.7)	0.6 (0.1–5.2)	–	1.3 (0.4–4.0)
	20–29	0.3* (0.1–0.7)	1.1 (0.5–2.6)	0.4 (0.1–3.1)	–	2.0 (0.8–5.2)
	30+	0.3* (0.1–0.6)	1.0 (0.4–2.6)	0.3 (0.0–2.1)	–	–
Previously married	13–19	6.1* (1.9–20.0)	–	–	–	–
	20–29	2.0* (1.4–2.9)	2.4* (1.5–3.9)	0.3 (0.0–2.2)	0.0* (0.0–0.0)	0.0* (0.0–0.0)
	30+	–	–	0.2 (0.0–1.1)	0.0* (0.0–0.0)	0.0* (0.0–0.0)
History of marriage, current marital status unknown	13–19	2.0 (0.9–4.5)	4.0* (1.4–11.1)	–	–	–
	20–29	1.3 (0.9–1.7)	1.1 (0.7–1.8)	0.4 (0.1–1.1)	0.4 (0.1–2.1)	–
	30+	–	–	0.2* (0.1–0.7)	0.2 (0.0–1.2)	–
Currently in first marriage	13–19					
	20–29					
	30+					
χ^2 (p-value)		43.4 (<0.001)*	8.5 (0.20)	15.2 (0.03)*	167.6 (<0.001)*	111.9 (<0.001)*

* Significant at the 0.05 level, two-sided test.
– Not included due to small cell size.
0.0* (0.0–0.0) OR is ≤ 0.05 indicating very low risk.
[a] Each column is a separate multivariate model in survival framework; models control for all the demographic predictors in each row, life course intervals (4–12, 13–19, 20–29, 30+ years) and countries. Only the results of interaction terms for life course interval variables by each sociodemographic variable are shown. Outcome variable indicated in each column header.

Appendix Table 6.5. Interactions between sociodemographic factors and respondent age (4–12, 13–19, 20–29, 30+ years) in the prediction of suicidal behavior[a] (middle-income countries)

Interactions		Among total sample			Among ideators	
		Ideation	Attempt	Plan	Planned attempt	Unplanned attempt
		OR (95% CI)	OR (95% CI)	OR (95% CI)	OR (95% CI)	OR (95% CI)
Gender						
Female	13–19	2.0 (0.9–4.6)	1.9 (0.8–4.7)	0.7 (0.1–4.6)	1.6 (0.1–49.2)	–
	20–29	1.6 (0.7–3.9)	1.3 (0.5–3.2)	0.6 (0.1–3.6)	0.8 (0.0–21.5)	1.1 (0.3–4.2)
	30+	1.6 (0.7–3.5)	0.9 (0.4–2.2)	0.5 (0.1–3.0)	0.5 (0.0–13.6)	0.5 (0.2–1.7)
Male	13–19					
	20–29					
	30+					
χ^2 (p-value)		3.7 (0.29)	5.1 (0.16)	1.1 (0.78)	4.3 (0.23)	2.4 (0.29)
Age group (years)						
18–34	13–19	1.3 (0.7–2.6)	2.0 (0.8–4.8)	0.0* (0.0–0.0)	0.4 (0.0–20.2)	0.7 (0.0–10.7)
	20–29	1.2 (0.5–3.3)	3.0 (0.7–13.1)	0.0* (0.0–0.0)	0.3 (0.0–12.7)	0.8 (0.1–5.5)
	30+	2.4* (1.1–5.1)	2.2 (0.9–5.6)	0.0* (0.0–0.0)	1.0 (0.0–33.9)	–

Appendix Table 6.5. (cont.)

Interactions		Among total sample		Among ideators		
		Ideation	Attempt	Plan	Planned attempt	Unplanned attempt
		OR (95% CI)	OR (95% CI)	OR (95% CI)	OR (95% CI)	OR (95% CI)
35–49	13–19	0.6 (0.2–1.3)	1.3 (0.5–3.7)	0.0* (0.0–0.0)	0.1 (0.0–16.2)	0.4 (0.0–22.6)
	20–29	0.5 (0.2–1.7)	1.8 (0.4–7.8)	0.0* (0.0–0.0)	0.0 (0.0–6.3)	0.6 (0.0–31.6)
	30+	0.9 (0.4–2.3)	2.6* (1.1–5.9)	0.0* (0.0–0.0)	0.1 (0.0–12.0)	1.5 (0.1–54.8)
50–64	13–19	1.26 (0.5–3.0)	1.3 (0.5–3.5)	0.0* (0.0–0.0)	1.1 (0.1–18.3)	–
	20–29	0.6 (0.2–1.6)	1.4 (0.3–5.9)	0.0* (0.0–0.0)	0.4 (0.0–5.1)	–
	30+	2.2* (1.2–3.9)	2.3* (1.1–4.6)	0.0* (0.0–0.0)	–	1.6 (0.3–11.8)
65+	13–19					
	20–29					
	30+					
χ^2 (p-value)		23.7 (0.005)*	17.5 (0.04)*	133.1 (<.001)*	3.8 (0.87)	2.8 (0.84)
5-Category education						
Currently a student	13–19	0.4 (0.1–2.0)	–	1.4 (0.1–13.6)	0.0* (0.0–0.0)	0.2 (0.0–1.7)
	20–29	1.5 (0.3–6.5)	2.2 (0.3–16.1)	1.9 (0.2–17.7)	0.6 (0.0–35.1)	0.1 (0.0–1.0)
	30+	1.1 (0.2–8.4)	0.2 (0.0–1.2)	–	–	–
Low	13–19	0.1* (0.0–0.7)	–	–	0.0* (0.0–0.0)	–
	20–29	0.4 (0.1–2.2)	2.5 (0.3–23.7)	–	0.0* (0.0–0.0)	–
	30+	0.4 (0.1–1.9)	3.1 (0.5–20.6)	–	0.0* (0.0–0.0)	–
Low-average	13–19	0.3* (0.1–0.9)	–	0.0* (0.0–0.0)	0.0* (0.0–0.0)	0.0* (0.0–0.0)
	20–29	0.9 (0.4–1.9)	0.7 (0.2–2.3)	0.0* (0.0–0.0)	0.6 (0.1–4.0)	0.0* (0.0–0.0)
	30+	–	–	0.0* (0.0–0.0)	–	0.0* (0.0–0.0)
High-average	13–19	0.5 (0.2–1.2)	–	2.1 (0.6–6.8)	0.0* (0.0–0.0)	–
	20–29	1.1 (0.5–2.1)	0.9 (0.2–3.0)	1.6 (0.6–4.2)	1.2 (0.3–5.8)	–
	30+					
High	13–19					
	20–29					
	30+					
χ^2 (p-value)		16.3 (0.09)	0.7 (0.41)	73.1 (<0.001)*	240.4 (<0.001)*	90.7 (<0.001)*
Marital status						
Never married	13–19	0.5 (0.3–1.1)	1.8 (0.7–4.6)	0.4 (0.0–4.4)	1.3 (0.0–38.9)	2.2 (0.3–13.5)
	20–29	0.6 (0.3–1.1)	1.2 (0.5–2.8)	0.2 (0.0–2.8)	2.5 (0.1–73.3)	2.1 (0.4–13.0)
	30+	0.4* (0.2–0.9)	1.0 (0.3–3.1)	0.2 (0.0–2.7)	2.3 (0.06–88.45)	–
Previously married	13–19	–	7.4 (0.45–116.9)	–	1.4 (0.0–46.6)	–
	20–29	–	3.9 (0.3–52.1)	0.0* (0.0–0.0)	1.2 (0.3–5.1)	–
	30+	–	2.7 (0.2–35.8)	0.0* (0.0–0.0)	–	0.4 (0.1–1.6)
Currently in first marriage	13–19					
	20–29					
	30+					
χ^2 (p-value)		18.5 (0.005)*	6.3 (0.40)	214.7 (<0.001)*	1.2 (0.94)	2.2 (0.53)

* Significant at the 0.05 level, two-sided test.
– Not included due to small cell size.
0.0* (0.0–0.0) OR is ≤ 0.05 indicating very low risk.
[a] Each column is a separate multivariate model in survival framework; models control for all the demographic predictors in each row, life course intervals (4–12, 13–19, 20–29, 30+ years) and countries. Only the results of interaction terms for life course interval variables by each sociodemographic variable are shown. Outcome variable indicated in each column header.

Appendix Table 6.6. Interactions between sociodemographic factors and respondent age (4–12, 13–19, 20–29, 30+ years) in the prediction of suicidal behavior[a] (low-income countries)

Interactions		Among total sample		Plan	Among ideators			
		Ideation	Attempt		Planned attempt		Unplanned attempt	
		OR (95% CI)	OR (95% CI)	OR (95% CI)	OR (95% CI)		OR (95% CI)	
Gender								
Female	13–19	1.0 (0.6–1.6)	1.2 (0.4–3.0)	1.3 (0.3–6.4)	2.6 (0.0–145.7)		1.8	(0.4–9.7)
	20–29	1.1 (0.7–1.7)	1.6 (0.7–3.8)	2.4 (0.5–11.3)	4.0 (0.1–203.6)		1.4	(0.3–7.0)
	30+	1.1 (0.7–1.8)	1.3 (0.6–3.0)	1.0 (0.2–4.8)	1.9 (0.0–101.6)		1.5	(0.3–8.0)
Male	13–19							
	20–29							
	30+							
χ^2 (p-value)		0.7 (0.87)	1.7 (0.63)	9.1 (0.03)*	3.1 (0.38)		0.6	(0.90)
Age group (years)								
18–34	13–19	2.1* (1.0–4.1)	0.2 (0.0–1.9)	0.0* (0.0–0.0)	–		2.2	(0.1–45.1)
	20–29	1.6 (0.8–3.2)	5.1 (0.3–86.2)	0.0* (0.0–0.0)	–		1.6	(0.2–10.4)
	30+	1.8* (1.0–3.1)	0.5 (0.1–5.2)	0.0* (0.0–0.0)	–		–	
35–49	13–19	1.3 (0.6–2.7)	0.1 (0.0–1.4)	0.0* (0.0–0.0)	0.0* (0.0–0.0)		7.8	(0.2–283.2)
	20–29	1.2 (0.6–2.6)	2.2 (0.1–38.0)	0.0* (0.0–0.0)	0.0* (0.0–0.0)		1.6	(0.1–21.2)
	30+	2.2* (1.3–3.5)	0.3 (0.0–2.6)	0.0* (0.0–0.0)	0.0* (0.0–0.0)		1.7	(0.2–20.5)
50–64	13–19	1.1 (0.5–2.6)	0.1 (0.0–1.7)	0.0* (0.0–0.0)	–		–	
	20–29	0.8 (0.3–1.2)	3.4 (0.1–82.0)	0.0* (0.0–0.0)	0.9 (0.1–7.4)		–	
	30+	0.9 (0.5–1.7)	0.2 (0.0–2.4)	0.0* (0.0–0.0)	0.4 (0.1–2.2)		1.2	(0.2–8.6)
65+	13–19							
	20–29							
	30+							
χ^2 (p-value)		23.3 (0.01)*	19.9 (0.02)*	572.6 (<0.001)*	110.7 (<0.001)*		5.2	(0.52)
5-Category education								
Currently a student	13–19	0.6 (0.1–3.2)	–	–	–		0.6	(0.1–4.5)
	20–29	0.5 (0.2–1.6)	1.2 (0.1–11.9)	–	–		–	
	30+	–	0.0* (0.0–0.0)	–	–		–	
Low	13–19	0.8 (0.1–4.5)	–	–	–		–	
	20–29	0.7 (0.2–2.5)	0.5 (0.0–5.9)	–	–		8.4	(0.9–80.2)
	30+	1.6 (0.5–5.8)	1.0 (0.1–12.5)	–	–		7.8	(0.6–103.4)
Low-average	13–19	1.2 (0.3–4.8)	–	0.0* (0.0–0.0)	0.0* (0.0–0.0)		–	
	20–29	1.1 (0.6–1.8)	1.0 (0.5–2.0)	0.0* (0.0–0.0)	0.0* (0.0–0.0)		8.5	(0.8–84.4)
	30+	–	–	0.0* (0.0–0.0)	0.0* (0.0–0.0)		16.1*	(1.2–215.4)
High-average	13–19	1.0 (0.2–4.8)	–	0.9 (0.3–3.1)	–		–	
	20–29	0.9 (0.5–1.6)	1.1 (0.4–2.7)	1.8 (0.8–3.8)	1.2 (0.2–7.4)		3.9	(0.3–50.4)
	30+	–	–	–	0.7 (0.1–4.7)		2.9	(0.2–45.4)
High	13–19							
	20–29							
	30+							
χ^2 (p-value)		2.4 (0.49)	228.9 (<0.001)*	144.3 (<0.001)*	47.9 (<0.001)*		7.3	(0.40)

Appendix Table 6.6. (cont.)

		Among total sample		Among ideators		
		Ideation	Attempt	Plan	Planned attempt	Unplanned attempt
Interactions		OR (95% CI)	OR (95% CI)	OR (95% CI)	OR (95% CI)	OR (95% CI)
Marital status						
Never married	13–19	0.3* (0.1–0.8)	0.0* (0.0–0.0)	0.1 (0.0–1.8)	0.0* (0.0–0.0)	–
	20–29	1.0 (0.4–2.5)	0.0* (0.0–0.0)	0.4 (0.0–9.0)	0.0* (0.0–0.0)	0.8 (0.1–7.0)
	30+	0.9 (0.3–2.3)	0.0* (0.0–0.0)	0.4 (0.0–8.4)	0.0* (0.0–0.0)	1.5 (0.1–14.8)
Previously married	13–19	–	0.0* (0.0–0.0)	–	–	–
	20–29	0.0* (0.0–0.0)	1.8 (0.8–4.0)	4.1 (0.4–41.9)	0.0* (0.0–0.0)	–
	30+	0.0* (0.0–0.0)	2.1* (2.1–2.1)	4.6 (0.5–43.1)	0.0* (0.0–0.0)	3.1 (0.6–16.0)
Currently in first marriage	13–19					
	20–29					
	30+					
χ^2 (p-value)		26.3 (<0.001)*	889.6 (<0.001)*	12.2 (0.03)*	138.1 (<0.001)*	2.0 (0.57)

* Significant at the 0.05 level, two-sided test.
– Not included due to small cell size.
0.0* (0.0–0.0) OR is ≤ 0.05 indicating very low risk.
[a] Each column is a separate multivariate model in survival framework; models control for all the demographic predictors in each row, life course intervals (4–12, 13–19, 20–29, 30+ years) and countries. Only the results of interaction terms for life course interval variables by each sociodemographic variable are shown. Outcome variable indicated in each column header.

Appendix Table 6.7. Sociodemographic risk factors for suicidal behavior during childhood (person–years: 4–12)[a] (high-income countries)

	Among total sample			Among ideators	
	Ideation	Attempt	Plan	Planned attempt	Unplanned attempt
Demographics	OR (95% CI)	OR (95% CI)	OR (95% CI)	OR (95% CI)	OR (95% CI)
Gender					
Female	1.2 (0.9–1.7)	2.2* (1.2–4.2)	1.1 (0.5–2.4)	0.5 (0.0–4.6)	7.3* (1.5–35.0)
Male					
χ^2 (p-value)	2.2 (0.14)	5.8 (0.02)*	0.1 (0.73)	0.4 (0.51)	6.1 (0.01)*
Age group (years)					
18–34	19.3* (8.3–44.5)	17.1* (3.8–78.1)	0.0* (0.0–0.0)	0.0* (0.0–0.0)	3.2 (0.2–55.0)
35–49	7.8* (3.3–18.2)	9.7* (2.0–45.7)	0.0* (0.0–0.0)	0.0* (0.0–0.0)	6.1 (0.3–118.5)
50–64	4.5* (1.9–10.7)	2.9 (0.5–15.0)	0.0* (0.0–0.0)	0.4 (0.1–2.7)	0.4 (0.0–12.1)
65+					
χ^2 (p-value)	94.1 (<0.001)*	25.6 (<0.001)*	106.8 (<0.001)*	412.9 (<0.001)*	6.5 (0.09)
5-Category education					
Currently a student	–	–	–	–	–
Low	–	–	–	–	–
Low-average					
High-average					
High	–	–	–	–	–
χ^2 (p-value)	–	–	–	–	–
Marital status					
Never married	–	–	–	–	–
Previously married					
History of marriage, current marital status unknown					
Currently in first marriage	–	–	–	–	–
χ^2 (p-value)	–	–	–	–	–

* Significant at the 0.05 level, two-sided test.
– Not included due to small cell size.
0.0* (0.0–0.0) OR is ≤0.05 indicating very low risk.
[a] Each column is a separate multivariate model in survival framework, with all rows as predictors controlling for person–years and countries. Outcome variable indicated in each column header.

Appendix Table 6.8. Sociodemographic risk factors for suicidal behavior during adolescence (person–years: 13–19)[a] (high-income countries)

	Among total sample			Among ideators	
	Ideation	Attempt	Plan	Planned attempt	Unplanned attempt
Demographics	OR (95% CI)	OR (95% CI)	OR (95% CI)	OR (95% CI)	OR (95% CI)
Gender					
Female	1.4* (1.3–1.6)	1.9* (1.5–2.5)	1.3 (0.9–1.7)	1.1 (0.7–1.8)	1.9* (1.2–3.0)
Male					
χ^2 (p-value)	30.9 (<0.001)*	29.3 (<0.001)*	2.6 (0.11)	0.1 (0.73)	8.6 (0.003)*
Age group (years)					
18–34	13.4* (9.2–19.3)	21.1* (9.8–45.3)	1.1 (0.4–3.4)	0.8 (0.0–13.1)	1.8 (0.6–5.3)
35–49	5.9* (4.1–8.5)	8.7* (4.1–18.4)	1.4 (0.5–4.1)	0.8 (0.0–13.8)	1.4 (0.5–4.6)
50–64	2.6* (1.8–3.9)	3.5* (1.5–8.0)	1.0 (0.3–3.3)	0.6 (0.0–11.1)	0.9 (0.3–2.9)
65+	–	–	–	–	–
χ^2 (p-value)	442.5 (<0.001)*	156.7 (<0.001)*	3.2 (0.37)	0.5 (0.93)	5.0 (0.17)
5-Category education					
Currently a student	1.0 (0.7–1.3)	1.2 (0.2–5.7)	1.8 (0.9–3.4)	3.0* (1.1–8.2)	5.2* (1.8–14.7)
Low	1.4 (1.0–2.0)	2.5 (0.5–12.1)	1.2 (0.6–2.5)	2.4 (0.8–7.5)	10.2* (3.4–31.0)
Low-average	1.1 (0.8–1.7)	1.5 (0.3–7.5)	1.3 (0.7–2.7)	2.5 (0.7–8.5)	6.5* (2.1–20.0)
High-average	–	1.1 (0.2–5.5)	–	–	–
High					
χ^2 (p-value)	11.0 (0.01)*	18.6 (<0.001)*	5.7 (0.13)	5.0 (0.18)	18.6 (<0.001)*
Marital status					
Never married	1.5 (0.9–2.4)	0.9 (0.5–1.7)	1.6 (0.6–4.1)	0.3 (0.0–1.9)	0.7 (0.2–2.3)
Previously married	5.2* (1.6–16.8)	–	3.4 (0.4–30.1)	–	–
History of marriage, current marital status unknown	2.9* (1.2–6.8)	2.8* (1.0–7.9)	5.1* (1.4–18.6)	1.1 (0.1–13.9)	2.7 (0.2–41.8)
Currently in first marriage					
χ^2 (p-value)	12.3 (0.01)*	6.5 (0.09)	7.0 (0.07)	143.0 (<0.001)*	133.4 (<0.001)*

* Significant at the 0.05 level, two-sided test.
– Not included due to small cell size.
[a] Each column is a separate multivariate model in survival framework, with all rows as predictors controlling for person–years and countries. Outcome variable indicated in each column header.

Appendix Table 6.9. Sociodemographic risk factors for suicidal behavior during young adulthood (person–years: 20–29)[a] (high-income countries)

Demographics	Among total sample		Plan	Among ideators	
	Ideation	Attempt		Planned attempt	Unplanned attempt
	OR (95% CI)	OR (95% CI)	OR (95% CI)	OR (95% CI)	OR (95% CI)
Gender					
Female	1.3* (1.1–1.5)	1.9* (1.4–2.4)	1.1 (0.8–1.5)	1.4 (1.0–2.2)	1.5 (0.9–2.4)
Male					
X^2 (p-value)	14.5 (<0.001)*	22.7 (<0.001)*	0.5 (0.47)	3.1 (0.08)	2.4 (0.12)
Age group (years)					
18–34	9.5* (6.8–13.2)	9.7* (5.0–18.9)	0.6 (0.4–1.1)	1.2 (0.4–3.5)	1.5 (0.3–8.2)
35–49	6.3* (4.5–8.7)	6.9* (3.6–13.3)	0.6 (0.3–1.1)	1.8 (0.6–5.0)	1.7 (0.3–9.0)
50–64	4.2* (3.0–5.8)	7.0* (3.6–13.4)	1.1 (0.6–1.9)	4.2* (1.4–12.5)	2.9 (0.5–16.2)
65+					
X^2 (p-value)	188.7 (<0.001)*	46.1 (<0.001)*	11.0 (0.01)*	13.5 (0.004)*	5.2 (0.15)
5-Category education					
Currently a student	1.3 (0.9–1.9)	1.4 (0.8–2.6)	1.7 (1.0–3.1)	2.2 (0.9–5.5)	0.6 (0.1–2.5)
Low	1.7* (1.3–2.1)	2.5* (1.6–3.9)	1.2 (0.8–1.9)	2.3* (1.1–4.8)	2.4* (1.2–5.2)
Low-average	1.1 (0.9–1.5)	1.7* (1.1–2.6)	1.8* (1.2–2.6)	2.4* (1.3–4.4)	1.4 (0.6–3.8)
High-average	1.4* (1.1–1.8)	1.7* (1.1–2.5)	1.2 (0.8–1.8)	1.9* (1.0–3.5)	1.2 (0.5–2.6)
High					
X^2 (p-value)	24.2 (<0.001)*	19.4 (<0.001)*	10.9 (0.03)*	9.2 (0.06)	12.8 (0.01)*
Marital status					
Never married	1.4* (1.1–1.7)	2.0* (1.5–2.8)	1.2 (0.9–1.7)	1.8* (1.0–3.0)	1.5 (0.8–2.8)
Previously married	3.2* (2.2–4.6)	5.0* (2.8–8.8)	1.6 (0.9–2.8)	3.0* (1.3–7.1)	1.8 (0.8–4.3)
History of marriage, current marital status unknown	2.3* (1.7–3.1)	2.4* (1.6–3.7)	2.0* (1.3–3.2)	2.9* (1.4–6.3)	1.7 (0.7–4.0)
Currently in first marriage					
X^2 (p-value)	65.0 (<0.001)*	43.8 (<0.001)*	10.3 (0.02)*	11.9 (0.01)*	3.9 (0.27)

* Significant at the 0.05 level, two-sided test.
[a] Each column is a separate multivariate model in survival framework, with all rows as predictors controlling for person–years and countries. Outcome variable indicated in each column header.

Appendix Table 6.10. Sociodemographic risk factors for suicidal behavior during later adulthood (person-years: 30+)[a] (high-income countries)

	Among total sample			Among ideators	
	Ideation	Attempt	Plan	Planned attempt	Unplanned attempt
Demographics	OR (95% CI)	OR (95% CI)	OR (95% CI)	OR (95% CI)	OR (95% CI)
Gender					
Female	1.2* (1.0–1.3)	1.4* (1.1–1.8)	0.9 (0.7–1.2)	0.9 (0.6–1.4)	1.4 (0.9–2.1)
Male					2.4 (0.12)
X^2 (p-value)	4.9 (0.03)*	7.5 (0.01)*	0.5 (0.49)	0.1 (0.71)	
Age group (years)					
18–34	3.7* (2.4–5.6)	9.1* (4.6–17.8)	1.6 (0.8–3.2)	1.8 (0.6–5.1)	2.9 (0.9–9.9)
35–49	4.3* (3.5–5.3)	6.5* (4.4–9.8)	1.6* (1.1–2.5)	1.9* (1.0–3.7)	2.2* (1.1–4.2)
50–64	2.7* (2.2–3.2)	3.1* (2.1–4.6)	1.2 (0.8–1.8)	1.3 (0.7–2.3)	1.5 (0.8–2.8)
65+					
X^2 (p-value)	194.2 (<0.001)*	89.8 (<0.001)*	7.7 (0.05)	5.2 (0.16)	6.6 (0.09)
4-Category education					
Low	1.2 (1.0–1.5)	2.1* (1.4–3.2)	1.1 (0.8–1.6)	2.2* (1.2–3.8)	3.6* (1.7–7.6)
Low-average	0.8* (0.7–1.0)	1.0 (0.7–1.5)	1.0 (0.7–1.4)	1.0 (0.6–1.9)	2.9* (1.3–6.4)
High-average	0.9 (0.8–1.1)	1.1 (0.8–1.7)	1.1 (0.8–1.5)	0.8 (0.4–1.4)	2.4* (1.2–5.1)
High					
X^2 (p-value)	16.5 (<0.001)*	19.8 (<0.001)*	0.5 (0.92)	12.6 (0.01)*	11.4 (0.01)*
Marital status					
Never married	1.4* (1.1–1.8)	2.8* (1.9–4.3)	1.1 (0.7–1.6)	2.6* (1.4–4.9)	1.1 (0.5–2.2)
Previously married	1.8* (1.4–2.3)	3.0* (2.1–4.3)	0.9 (0.5–1.4)	1.9 (0.8–4.2)	1.6 (0.8–3.4)
History of marriage, current marital status unknown	2.4* (1.9–2.9)	3.5* (2.4–5.1)	2.0* (1.4–2.8)	2.3* (1.3–4.1)	1.8 (0.9–3.6)
Currently in first marriage					
X^2 (p-value)	87.5 (<0.001)*	65.8 (<0.001)*	16.5 (<0.001)*	12.9 (0.01)*	5.3 (0.15)

* Significant at the 0.05 level, two-sided test.
[a] Each column is a separate multivariate model in survival framework, with all rows as predictors controlling for person-years and countries. Outcome variable indicated in each column header.

Appendix Table 6.11. Sociodemographic risk factors for suicidal behavior during childhood (person–years: 4–12)[a] (middle-income countries)

	Among total sample			Among ideators	
	Ideation	Attempt	Plan	Planned attempt	Unplanned attempt
Demographics	OR (95% CI)	OR (95% CI)	OR (95% CI)	OR (95% CI)	OR (95% CI)
Gender					
Female	1.0 (0.4–2.2)	2.5 (0.8–7.9)	2.1 (0.3–16.0)	–	0.0* (0.0–0.0)
Male					
X² (p-value)	0.0 (0.93)	2.3 (0.13)	0.5 (0.46)	–	469.1 (<0.001)*
Age group (years)					
18–34	39.0* (5.2–289.0)	–	–	1.1 (0.0–33.9)	–
35–49	28.8* (3.4–244.8)	–	–	5.2 (0.0–542.2)	–
50–64	3.8 (0.4–33.3)	–	–	–	–
65+					
X² (p-value)	32.5 (<0.001)*	–	–	0.9 (0.63)	–
5-Category education					
Currently a student	0.4 (0.1–1.6)	0.2* (0.0–0.7)	0.0* (0.0–0.0)	0.6 (0.0–27.4)	0.0* (0.0–0.0)
Low	3.2 (0.7–14.1)	0.3 (0.0–2.3)	0.0* (0.0–0.0)	–	0.0* (0.0–0.0)
Low-average					
High-average					
High					
X² (p-value)	24.1 (<0.001)*	5.7 (0.06)	36.9 (<0.001)*	107.2 (<0.001)*	540.1 (<0.001)*
Marital status					
Never married	–	–	–	–	–
Previously married	–	–	–	–	–
Currently in first marriage					
X² (p-value)	–	–	–	–	–

* Significant at the 0.05 level, two-sided test.
– Not included due to small cell size.
0.0* (0.0–0.0) OR is ≤0.05 indicating very low risk.
[a] Each column is a separate multivariate model in survival framework, with all rows as predictors controlling for person–years and countries. Outcome variable indicated in each column header.

Appendix Table 6.12. Sociodemographic risk factors for suicidal behavior during adolescence (person–years: 13–19)[a] (middle-income countries)

Demographics	Among total sample				Among ideators		
	Ideation	Attempt	Plan		Planned attempt	Unplanned attempt	
	OR (95% CI)	OR (95% CI)	OR (95% CI)		OR (95% CI)	OR (95% CI)	
Gender							
Female	1.9* (1.4–2.5)	3.1* (2.0–4.9)	1.3 (0.6–2.9)		4.1* (1.4–11.7)	2.9* (1.1–7.7)	
Male							
X^2 (p-value)	18.9 (<0.001)*	24.8 (<0.001)*	0.5 (0.48)		6.9 (0.01)*	4.5 (0.03)*	
Age group (years)							
18–34	5.3* (2.9–9.9)	3.8* (1.8–8.2)	0.4 (0.1–2.4)		0.3 (0.0–2.8)	0.0* (0.0–0.0)	
35–49	1.9 (1.0–3.6)	1.3 (0.6–2.9)	0.2 (0.0–1.5)		0.5 (0.0–5.5)	0.0* (0.0–0.0)	
50–64	1.3 (0.6–2.6)	1.1 (0.4–2.6)	0.6 (0.1–4.0)		0.8 (0.1–10.2)	0.0* (0.0–0.0)	
65+							
X^2 (p-value)	94.9 (<0.001)*	43.3 (<0.001)*	4.4 (0.22)		1.7 (0.63)	280.3 (<0.001)*	
5-Category education							
Currently a student	0.4 (0.2–1.0)	0.1* (0.0–0.3)	0.3 (0.0–2.7)		0.0* (0.0–0.0)	0.0* (0.0–0.0)	
Low	0.5 (0.2–1.3)	0.1* (0.0–0.4)	0.3 (0.0–2.3)		0.0* (0.0–0.0)	0.0* (0.0–0.0)	
Low-average	0.5 (0.2–1.3)	0.2* (0.1–0.5)	0.3 (0.0–2.3)		0.0* (0.0–0.0)	0.0* (0.0–0.0)	
High-average	0.6 (0.3–1.6)	0.2* (0.1–0.6)	0.4 (0.0–3.6)		0.0* (0.0–0.0)	0.0* (0.0–0.0)	
High							
X^2 (p-value)	8.5 (0.07)	21.1 (<0.001)*	2.1 (0.71)		246.2 (<0.001)*	195.3 (<0.001)*	
Marital status							
Never married	1.0 (0.6–1.5)	1.1 (0.6–1.9)	2.2 (1.0–4.9)		2.1 (0.4–10.7)	2.0 (0.4–9.8)	
Previously married	4.4* (1.1–17.5)	2.8 (0.6–12.7)	–		1.9 (0.1–24.1)	2.9 (0.3–28.4)	
Currently in first marriage							
X^2 (p-value)	5.1 (0.08)	1.9 (0.40)	188.5 (<0.001)*		0.9 (0.64)	1.1 (0.58)	

* Significant at the 0.05 level, two-sided test.
0.0* (0.0–0.0) OR is ≤0.05 indicating very low risk.
[a] Each column is a separate multivariate model in survival framework, with all rows as predictors controlling for person–years and countries. Outcome variable indicated in each column header.

Appendix Table 6.13. Sociodemographic risk factors for suicidal behavior during young adulthood (person–years: 20–29)[a] (middle-income countries)

Demographics	Among total sample		Among ideators		
	Ideation	Attempt	Plan	Planned attempt	Unplanned attempt
	OR (95% CI)	OR (95% CI)	OR (95% CI)	OR (95% CI)	OR (95% CI)
Gender					
Female	1.6* (1.2–2.1)	2.2* (1.4–3.4)	1.1 (0.7–1.7)	2.2* (1.1–4.3)	2.1 (0.8–5.8)
Male					
χ² (p-value)	8.6 (0.003)*	11.4 (<0.001)*	0.1 (0.75)	5.3 (0.02)*	2.2 (0.14)
Age group (years)					
18–34	5.6* (2.3–13.5)	6.9* (1.6–31.1)	2.9 (0.7–12.5)	0.4 (0.1–2.6)	7.7 (0.7–89.6)
35–49	1.8 (0.8–4.3)	2.0 (0.4–8.8)	1.7 (0.4–7.0)	0.3 (0.0–2.2)	3.2 (0.3–38.6)
50–64	0.6 (0.2–1.5)	1.2 (0.3–5.7)	2.0 (0.4–10.1)	0.5 (0.0–5.1)	6.6 (0.5–93.9)
65+					
χ² (p-value)	119.9 (<0.001)*	64.0 (<0.001)*	5.5 (0.14)	1.6 (0.66)	5.5 (0.14)
5-Category education					
Currently a student	1.4 (0.7–2.6)	1.4 (0.6–3.4)	1.9 (0.5–7.2)	6.5* (1.9–22.5)	0.2* (0.0–0.8)
Low	1.7 (0.9–3.4)	1.8 (0.8–4.3)	2.1 (0.6–7.1)	4.5* (1.4–14.6)	0.5 (0.2–1.5)
Low-average	1.4 (0.8–2.5)	1.9 (0.9–4.3)	2.1 (0.7–6.8)	4.3* (1.4–13.1)	0.3 (0.1–1.5)
High-average	1.4 (0.8–2.6)	1.7 (0.8–3.7)	1.7 (0.5–5.4)	2.0 (0.8–4.9)	0.5 (0.1–1.7)
High					
χ² (p-value)	2.6 (0.62)	3.8 (0.44)	2.2 (0.70)	11.5 (0.02)*	5.6 (0.23)
Marital status					
Never married	1.3 (0.9–1.8)	1.3 (0.8–2.0)	1.1 (0.6–1.8)	2.3 (1.0–5.3)	1.4 (0.6–3.6)
Previously married	2.8* (1.7–4.5)	3.2* (1.5–6.7)	1.6 (0.7–3.6)	1.3 (0.4–4.4)	1.8 (0.4–7.1)
Currently in first marriage					
χ² (p-value)	16.9 (<0.001)*	9.9 (0.01)*	1.6 (0.44)	3.9 (0.14)	0.9 (0.62)

* Significant at the 0.05 level, two-sided test.

[a] Each column is a separate multivariate model in survival framework, with all rows as predictors controlling for person-years and countries. Outcome variable indicated in each column header.

Appendix Table 6.14. Sociodemographic risk factors for suicidal behavior during later adulthood (person–years: 30+)[a] (middle-income countries)

	Among total sample			Among ideators	
	Ideation	Attempt	Plan	Planned attempt	Unplanned attempt
Demographics	OR (95% CI)	OR (95% CI)	OR (95% CI)	OR (95% CI)	OR (95% CI)
Gender					
Female	1.5* (1.2–1.9)	1.5* (1.0–2.3)	1.0 (0.6–1.5)	1.7 (0.8–3.4)	1.0 (0.5–2.1)
Male					
χ^2 (p-value)	10.2 (0.001)*	3.9 (0.05)*	0.0 (0.88)	2.1 (0.15)	0.0 (0.96)
Age group (years)					
18–34	12.9* (6.8–24.2)	7.9* (3.3–18.9)	4.5* (1.4–14.3)	2.6 (0.3–23.0)	2.4 (0.4–15.2)
35–49	4.2* (2.9–6.2)	4.2* (2.0–9.2)	2.6* (1.2–5.6)	1.5 (0.2–11.0)	3.1 (0.7–14.4)
50–64	2.7* (1.8–3.9)	2.7* (1.3–5.5)	1.2 (0.5–2.7)	1.6 (0.2–10.7)	2.2 (0.6–9.1)
65+					
χ^2 (p-value)	82.7 (<0.001)*	26.0 (<0.001)*	16.0 (0.001)*	1.0 (0.81)	2.1 (0.55)
4-Category education					
Low	1.9* (1.2–2.9)	3.0* (1.2–7.7)	1.7 (0.7–4.0)	3.1 (0.6–15.8)	1.5 (0.5–4.3)
Low-average	1.6* (1.0–2.5)	3.3* (1.2–9.1)	1.5 (0.7–3.2)	8.4* (1.7–41.7)	1.7 (0.5–6.6)
High-average	1.3 (0.8–2.0)	2.0 (0.7–5.9)	0.9 (0.4–1.9)	1.8 (0.4–7.2)	0.7 (0.2–2.7)
High					
χ^2 (p-value)	9.6 (0.02)*	9.1 (0.03)*	4.1 (0.25)	13.8 (0.003)*	3.5 (0.32)
Marital status					
Never married	0.8 (0.5–1.3)	1.1 (0.5–2.4)	0.8 (0.3–2.1)	2.8 (0.6–12.2)	0.8 (0.1–5.3)
Previously married	1.9* (1.3–2.6)	2.3* (1.2–4.3)	1.1 (0.6–1.9)	1.1 (0.4–3.1)	1.3 (0.5–3.1)
Currently in first marriage					
χ^2 (p-value)	17.2 (<0.001)*	6.4 (0.04)*	0.4 (0.83)	1.9 (0.38)	0.4 (0.82)

* Significant at the 0.05 level, two-sided test.
[a] Each column is a separate multivariate model in survival framework, with all rows as predictors controlling for person–years and countries. Outcome variable indicated in each column header.

Appendix Table 6.15. Sociodemographic risk factors for suicidal behavior during childhood (person–years: 4–12)[a] (low-income countries)

Demographics	Among total sample				Among ideators	
	Ideation	Attempt	Plan		Planned attempt	Unplanned attempt
	OR (95% CI)	OR (95% CI)	OR (95% CI)		OR (95% CI)	OR (95% CI)
Gender						
Female	1.4 (0.9–2.3)	1.0 (0.5–2.1)	0.8 (0.1–4.9)		0.0* (0.0–0.0)	1.0 (0.2–4.7)
Male						
X^2 (p-value)	2.0 (0.16)	0.0 (0.94)	0.0 (0.84)		331.0 (<0.001)*	0.0 (0.95)
Age group (years)						
18–34	50.5* (6.5–390.8)	7.6 (1.0–60.6)	9.2 (0.1–850.7)		0.0* (0.0–0.0)	0.0* (0.0–0.0)
35–49	27.2* (3.5–212.3)	7.6 (0.8–68.5)	26.1 (0.2–3220.3)		–	0.0* (0.0–0.0)
50–64	25.5* (3.1–213.1)	3.3 (0.3–37.9)	0.3 (0.0–34.0)		–	0.0* (0.0–0.0)
65+						
X^2 (p-value)	18.2 (<0.001)*	4.1 (0.25)	5.8 (0.12)		361.6 (<0.001)*	66.6 (<0.001)*
5-Category education						
Currently a student	2.5 (0.3–20.2)	0.6 (0.1–5.0)	0.0* (0.0–0.0)		0.0* (0.0–0.0)	–
Low	2.6 (0.3–26.6)	1.5 (0.1–16.4)	0.0* (0.0–0.0)		0.0* (0.0–0.0)	–
Low-average						
High-average						
High						
X^2 (p-value)	0.8 (0.67)	1.5 (0.47)	56.1 (<0.001)*		443.3 (<0.001)*	276.9 (<0.001)*
Marital status						
Never married	–	–	–		–	–
Previously married	–	–	–		–	–
Currently in first marriage						
X^2 (p-value)	–	–	–		–	–

* Significant at the 0.05 level, two-sided test.
– Not included due to small cell size.
0.0* (0.0–0.0) OR is ≤0.05 indicating very low risk.
[a] Each column is a separate multivariate model in survival framework, with all rows as predictors controlling for person–years and countries. Outcome variable indicated in each column header.

Appendix Table 6.16. Sociodemographic risk factors for suicidal behavior during adolescence (person–years: 13–19)^a (low-income countries)

Demographics	Among total sample			Among ideators	
	Ideation	Attempt	Plan	Planned attempt	Unplanned attempt
	OR (95% CI)	OR (95% CI)	OR (95% CI)	OR (95% CI)	OR (95% CI)
Gender					
Female	1.2 (0.9–1.7)	1.1 (0.8–1.6)	0.9 (0.5–1.7)	2.6 (0.9–7.9)	1.6 (0.7–4.0)
Male					
χ^2 (p-value)	1.5 (0.22)	0.2 (0.63)	0.1 (0.75)	3.1 (0.08)	1.1 (0.29)
Age group (years)					
18–34	8.5* (3.6–19.8)	2.7* (1.1–7.0)	0.0* (0.0–0.0)	1.3 (0.1–11.6)	0.1 (0.0–1.4)
35–49	2.9* (1.2–6.8)	1.6 (0.6–4.2)	0.0* (0.0–0.0)	0.6 (0.1–7.5)	0.3 (0.0–5.1)
50–64	2.1 (0.8–5.2)	0.5 (0.1–1.5)	0.0* (0.0–0.0)	0.4 (0.0–4.7)	0.0* (0.0–0.2)
65+					
χ^2 (p-value)	60.4 (<0.001)*	22.8 (<0.001)*	194.8 (<0.001)*	2.3 (0.51)	10.8 (0.01)*
5-Category education					
Currently a student	0.9 (0.2–3.7)	0.1* (0.0–0.6)	0.5 (0.0–7.1)	1.2 (0.1–18.1)	0.0* (0.0–0.3)
Low	1.2 (0.3–4.8)	0.2 (0.0–1.0)	0.9 (0.1–12.5)	1.6 (0.1–29.5)	0.0* (0.0–0.2)
Low-average	1.4 (0.3–6.2)	0.3 (0.1–1.5)	0.6 (0.0–8.6)	4.4 (0.2–94.2)	0.0* (0.0–0.3)
High-average	1.2 (0.2–6.1)	0.3 (0.1–1.8)	0.4 (0.0–6.0)	3.1 (0.1–78.0)	0.1 (0.0–1.4)
High					
χ^2 (p-value)	5.5 (0.24)	17.3 (0.002)*	3.2 (0.52)	3.3 (0.51)	10.1 (0.04)*
Marital status					
Never married	0.4* (0.2–0.7)	0.4* (0.2–0.7)	0.2* (0.1–0.5)	1.8 (0.4–8.8)	0.7 (0.1–5.4)
Previously married	–	7.9* (1.4–45.9)	0.3 (0.0–2.5)	–	–
Currently in first marriage					
χ^2 (p-value)	0.6 (0.44)	19.3 (<0.001)*	14.1 (<0.001)*	95.3 (<0.001)*	0.1 (0.72)

*Significant at the 0.05 level, two-sided test.
– Not included due to small cell size.
0.0* (0.0–0.0) OR is ≤0.05 indicating very low risk.
^{a}Each column is a separate multivariate model in survival framework, with all rows as predictors controlling for person–years and countries. Outcome variable indicated in each column header.

Appendix Table 6.17. Sociodemographic risk factors for suicidal behavior during young adulthood (person-years: 20–29)[a] (low-income countries)

	Among total sample				Among ideators		
	Ideation	Attempt	Plan		Planned attempt	Unplanned attempt	
Demographics	OR (95% CI)	OR (95% CI)	OR (95% CI)		OR (95% CI)	OR (95% CI)	
Gender							
Female	1.3* (1.0–1.7)	1.6* (1.0–2.4)	2.0* (1.2–3.3)		2.2* (1.1–4.3)	0.9 (0.4–2.1)	
Male							
X^2 (p-value)	5.1 (0.02)*	4.3 (0.04)*	6.3 (0.01)*		5.3 (0.021)*	0.1 (0.82)	
Age group[b] (years)							
18–34	4.2* (2.0–8.5)	–	2.1 (0.5–9.2)		0.7 (0.2–2.9)	11.3 (1.0–130.0)	
35–49	2.1* (1.0–4.4)	35.3* (4.8–261.9)	1.8 (0.4–7.4)		0.6 (0.1–2.3)	11.4 (0.9–138.0)	
50–64	1.3 (0.6–2.7)	22.5* (2.9–173.2)	1.0 (0.2–5.7)			4.6 (0.3–63.0)	
65+							
X^2 (p-value)	42.6 (<0.001)*	63.6 (<0.001)*	3.0 (0.39)		0.8 (0.64)	6.5 (0.09)	
5-Category education							
Currently a student	0.6 (0.4–1.1)	1.0 (0.5–2.2)	1.5 (0.5–4.5)		6.5 (1.9–22.4)	0.8 (0.1–5.2)	
Low	0.7 (0.5–1.2)	1.2 (0.7–2.1)	0.8 (0.3–1.8)		4.4 (1.4–13.9)	1.8 (0.5–6.8)	
Low-average	1.2 (0.8–1.8)	1.6 (0.9–2.6)	1.7 (0.8–3.6)		4.3 (1.4–13.2)	1.7 (0.7–4.5)	
High-average	0.9 (0.6–1.4)	1.3 (0.7–2.4)	1.3 (0.6–2.7)		2.1 (0.9–4.9)	3.3 (1.0–11.5)	
High							
X^2 (p-value)	11.5 (0.02)*	3.8 (0.43)	6.4 (0.17)		11.6 (0.021)*	4.9 (0.30)	
Marital status							
Never married	1.2 (0.9–1.5)	1.1 (0.7–1.6)	0.9 (0.5–1.6)		2.3 (1.0–5.4)	0.4 (0.2–1.1)	
Previously married	2.2* (1.3–3.8)	1.8 (0.9–3.8)	1.3 (0.5–2.9)		1.3 (0.4–4.4)	0.7 (0.2–2.7)	
Currently in first marriage							
X^2 (p-value)	9.3 (0.01)*	2.8 (0.24)	0.6 (0.73)		3.9 (0.14)	2.9 (0.23)	

* Significant at the 0.05 level, two-sided test.
[a] Each column is a separate multivariate model in survival framework, with all rows as predictors controlling for person-years and countries. Outcome variable indicated in each column header.
[b] For the planned attempt model, the reference level was changed to 50 or older due to having too few cases that are 65+ years.

Appendix Table 6.18. Sociodemographic risk factors for suicidal behavior during later adulthood (person-years: 30+)[a] (low-income countries)

	Among total sample			Among ideators	
	Ideation	Attempt	Plan	Planned attempt	Unplanned attempt
Demographics	OR (95% CI)	OR (95% CI)	OR (95% CI)	OR (95% CI)	OR (95% CI)
Gender					
Female	1.4* (1.1–1.8)	1.3 (0.9–1.9)	0.6* (0.4–1.0)	1.3 (0.7–2.4)	1.0 (0.4–2.6)
Male					
χ^2 (p-value)	7.8 (0.01)*	2.6 (0.11)	4.8 (0.03)*	0.7 (0.41)	0.0 (0.97)
Age group (years)					
18–34	6.8* (4.1–11.4)	9.5* (4.0–22.2)	4.2* (1.6–11.1)	6.0* (1.4–25.6)	2.8 (0.3–27.3)
35–49	4.6* (3.0–7.0)	4.8* (2.4–9.3)	2.7* (1.2–6.1)	2.7 (0.9–8.0)	3.6 (0.5–25.3)
50–64	1.8* (1.2–2.7)	1.3 (0.6–2.8)	1.2 (0.5–2.7)	0.7 (0.2–2.3)	1.5 (0.2–12.1)
65+					
χ^2 (p-value)	89.7 (<0.001)*	63.0 (<0.001)*	19.3 (<0.001)*	23.1 (<0.001)*	4.9 (0.18)
4-Category education					
Low	1.9* (1.2–2.8)	2.4* (1.3–4.5)	2.3* (1.1–4.9)	1.3 (0.5–3.7)	1.7 (0.4–7.3)
Low-average	1.0 (0.7–1.5)	1.6 (0.9–3.0)	1.8 (0.9–3.7)	0.7 (0.2–1.9)	2.9 (0.8–10.6)
High-average	0.9 (0.6–1.4)	1.1 (0.5–2.2)	1.1 (0.5–2.4)	0.9 (0.3–3.0)	2.1 (0.5–9.1)
High					
χ^2 (p-value)	25.2 (<0.001)*	12.6 (0.01)*	8.9 (0.03)*	4.3 (0.23)	2.7 (0.43)
Marital status					
Never married	1.5* (1.0–2.2)	1.4 (0.9–2.4)	0.9 (0.5–1.5)	1.5 (0.6–3.9)	1.3 (0.3–5.1)
Previously married	2.0* (1.5–2.6)	3.1* (2.0–4.9)	1.1 (0.6–1.8)	0.9 (0.4–1.8)	2.5 (0.9–6.9)
Currently in first marriage					
χ^2 (p-value)	23.2 (<0.001)*	25.0 (<0.001)*	0.4 (0.81)	1.0 (0.61)	3.2 (0.20)

* Significant at the 0.05 level, two-sided test.
[a] Each column is a separate multivariate model in survival framework, with all rows as predictors controlling for person-years and countries. Outcome variable indicated in each column header.

Appendix Table 6.19. Associations between sociodemographic factors and persistence of suicidal behavior[a] (high-income countries)

Demographics	Ideation OR (95% CI)	Plan OR (95% CI)	Attempt OR (95% CI)
Gender			
Female	0.9 (0.8–1.0)	0.9 (0.8–1.2)	1.0 (0.7–1.3)
Male			
χ^2 (p-value)	1.6 (0.20)	0.3 (0.60)	0.1 (0.78)
Education as of the age of each outcome			
Currently a student	1.0 (0.8–1.2)	1.2 (0.7–2.0)	1.2 (0.6–2.3)
Low	1.2 (1.0–1.5)	1.3 (0.8–2.0)	1.7 (0.9–3.3)
Low-average	1.0 (0.8–1.3)	1.1 (0.7–1.7)	1.2 (0.6–2.3)
High-average	1.0 (0.8–1.2)	1.3 (0.9–2.0)	1.4 (0.7–2.7)
High			
χ^2 (p-value)	7.1 (0.13)	2.2 (0.70)	7.5 (0.11)
Marital status as of the age of each outcome			
Never married	1.0 (0.8–1.2)	0.9 (0.6–1.4)	1.0 (0.7–1.6)
Previously married	0.6* (0.4–0.9)	0.8 (0.5–1.3)	0.6 (0.3–1.3)
History of marriage, current marital status unknown	0.9 (0.7–1.2)	1.0 (0.6–1.5)	0.6 (0.3–1.1)
Currently in first marriage			
χ^2 (p-value)	7.7 (0.05)	0.9 (0.82)	4.3 (0.23)

* Significant at the 0.05 level, two-sided test.
[a] Results are based on multivariate discrete time survival models with countries and age-related variables as a control.

Appendix Table 6.20. Associations between sociodemographic factors and persistence of suicidal behavior[a] (middle-income countries)

Demographics	Ideation OR (95% CI)	Plan OR (95% CI)	Attempt OR (95% CI)
Gender			
Female	1.6* (1.2–2.2)	1.2 (0.7–1.9)	1.4 (0.7–2.6)
Male			
χ^2 (p-value)	10.9* (0.001)	0.3 (0.56)	1.0 (0.33)
Education as of the age of each outcome			
Currently a student	1.1 (0.5–2.5)	1.0 (0.4–2.5)	1.2 (0.3–4.7)
Low	1.1 (0.5–2.3)	0.6 (0.2–1.4)	1.5 (0.4–5.6)
Low-average	1.3 (0.6–2.5)	0.8 (0.3–2.1)	2.5 (0.6–10.0)
High-average	1.4 (0.7–2.6)	0.8 (0.3–2.1)	2.6 (0.7–10.1)
High			
χ^2 (p-value)	2.2 (0.70)	3.7 (0.45)	6.2 (0.18)
Marital status as of the age of each outcome			
Never married	1.0 (0.7–1.5)	1.3 (0.8–2.3)	1.5 (0.8–2.6)
Previously married	1.3 (0.8–2.2)	1.2 (0.5–2.5)	1.4 (0.5–3.8)
Currently in first marriage			
χ^2 (p-value)	1.5 (0.48)	1.0 (0.60)	1.6 (0.45)

* Significant at the 0.05 level, two-sided test.
[a] Results are based on multivariate discrete time survival models with countries and age-related variables as a control.

Appendix Table 6.21. Associations between sociodemographic factors and persistence of suicidal behavior[a] (low-income countries)

Demographics	Ideation OR (95% CI)	Plan OR (95% CI)	Attempt OR (95% CI)
Gender			
Female	1.0 (0.8–1.3)	0.6* (0.4–0.9)	0.8 (0.4–1.4)
Male			
χ^2 (p-value)	0.0 (0.93)	4.9* (0.03)	0.7 (0.41)
Education as of the age of each outcome			
Currently a student	1.3 (0.6–2.7)	3.8* (1.4–10.3)	0.5 (0.1–2.4)
Low	1.3 (0.8–2.3)	4.2* (1.8–9.9)	0.8 (0.2–2.9)
Low-average	1.5 (0.8–2.7)	2.6* (1.1–6.0)	0.8 (0.2–2.8)
High-average	1.0 (0.5–1.8)	2.2 (0.8–5.8)	0.8 (0.2–4.3)
High			
χ^2 (p-value)	3.6 (0.47)	15.1* (0.01)	1.2 (0.88)
Marital status as of the age of each outcome			
Never married	0.8 (0.5–1.2)	0.9 (0.5–1.5)	1.5 (0.8–2.8)
Previously married	1.0 (0.6–1.7)	2.1* (1.1–3.7)	1.2 (0.5–3.1)
Currently in first marriage			
χ^2 (p-value)	1.6 (0.45)	7.5* (0.02)	1.4 (0.50)

* Significant at the 0.05 level, two-sided test.
0.0* (0.0–0.0) OR is ≤0.05 indicating very low risk.
[a] Results are based on multivariate discrete time survival models with countries and age-related variables as a control.

Appendix Table 6.22. Control model[a] (all countries)

	Among total sample		Among ideators		
	Ideation	Attempt	Plan	Planned attempt	Unplanned attempt
Main effects	Female	Female	Female	Female	Female
	18–34	18–34	18–34	18–34	18–34
	35–49	35–49	35–49	35–49	35–49
	50–64	50–64	50–64	50–64	50–64
	Currently a student	Currently a student	Currently a student	Currently a student	Currently a student
	Low	Low	Low	Low	Low
	Low-average	Low-average	Low-average	Low-average	Low-average
	High-average	High-average	High-average	High-average	High-average
	Never married	Never married	Never married	Never married	Never married
	Previously married	Previously married	Previously married	Previously married	Previously married
	History of marriage, current marital status unknown	History of marriage, current marital status unknown	History of marriage, current marital status unknown	History of marriage, current marital status unknown	History of marriage, current marital status unknown

Appendix Table 6.22. (cont.)

	Among total sample			Among ideators	
	Ideation	**Attempt**	**Plan**	**Planned attempt**	**Unplanned attempt**
Interaction effects	Education	Gender	Age	Age	Age
	Marital status	Age	Education	Education	Marital status
	–	Education	–	–	–
	–	Marital status	–	–	–

[a] All main effects are included as controls, in addition with interactions that were significant.

Appendix Table 6.23. Control model[a] (high-income countries)

	Among total sample			Among ideators	
	Ideation	**Attempt**	**Plan**	**Planned attempt**	**Unplanned attempt**
Main effects	Female	Female	Female	Female	Female
	18–34	18–34	18–34	18–34	18–34
	35–49	35–49	35–49	35–49	35–49
	50–64	50–64	50–64	50–64	50–64
	Currently a student	Currently a student	Currently a student	Currently a student	Currently a student
	Low	Low	Low	Low	Low
	Low-average	Low-average	Low-average	Low-average	Low-average
	High-average	High-average	High-average	High-average	High-average
	Never married	Never married	Never married	Never married	Never married
	Previously married	Previously married	Previously married	Previously married	Previously married
	History of marriage, current marital status unknown	History of marriage, current marital status unknown	History of marriage, current marital status unknown	History of marriage, current marital status unknown	History of marriage, current marital status unknown
Interaction effects	Age	Age	Age	Age	Gender
	Education	Education	Education	Education	Education
	Marital status	Marital status	Marital status	Marital status	Marital status
	–	–	–	–	–

[a] All main effects are included as controls, in addition with interactions that were significant.

Appendix Table 6.24. Control model[a] (middle-income countries)

	Among total sample			Among ideators	
	Ideation	Attempt	Plan	Planned attempt	Unplanned attempt
Main effects	Female	Female	Female	Female	Female
	18–34	18–34	18–34	18–34	18–34
	35–49	35–49	35–49	35–49	35–49
	50–64	50–64	50–64	50–64	50–64
	Currently a student	Currently a student	Currently a student	Currently a student	Currently a student
	Low	Low	Low	Low	Low
	Low-average	Low-average	Low-average	Low-average	Low-average
	High-average	High-average	High-average	High-average	High-average
	Never married	Never married	Never married	Never married	Never married
	Previously married	Previously married	Previously married	Previously married	Previously married
Interaction effects	Age	Age	Age	Education	Age
	Marital status	–	Education	–	Education
	–	–	Marital status	–	–
	–	–	–	–	–

[a] All main effects are included as controls, in addition with interactions that were significant.

Appendix Table 6.25. Control model[a] (low-income countries)

	Among total sample			Among ideators	
	Ideation	Attempt	Plan	Planned attempt	Unplanned attempt
Main effects	Female	Female	Female	Female	Female
	18–34	18–34	18–34	18–34	18–34
	35–49	35–49	35–49	35–49	35–49
	50–64	50–64	50–64	50–64	50–64
	Currently a student	Currently a student	Currently a student	Currently a student	Currently a student
	Low	Low	Low	Low	Low
	Low-average	Low-average	Low-average	Low-average	Low-average
	High-average	High-average	High-average	High-average	High-average
	Never married	Never married	Never married	Never married	Never married
	Previously married	Previously married	Previously married	Previously married	Previously married
Interaction effects	Age	Age	Gender	Age	–
	–	Education	Age	Education	–
	–	Marital status	Education	Marital status	–
	–	–	Marital status	–	–

[a] All main effects are included as controls, in addition with interactions that were significant.

Appendix Table 7.1. Prevalence of parental psychopathology among those with each type of suicidal behavior (high-income countries)

Parental disorder	Among total sample %ª (SE) with parental disorder				Among ideators %ª (SE) with parental disorder					
	Ideation	No ideation	Attempt	No attempt	Plan	No plan	Planned attempt	No planned attempt	Unplanned attempt	No unplanned attempt
Type of parental disorder										
Depression	7.6 (0.7)	1.9 (0.2)	10.8 (1.4)	2.1 (0.2)	10.4 (1.1)	5.2 (0.7)	10.7 (1.5)	12.7 (1.7)	11.5 (2.7)	4.2 (0.6)
Panic disorder	11.1 (0.8)	3.8 (0.2)	15.6 (1.7)	4.1 (0.2)	12.6 (1.2)	10.6 (1.1)	13.8 (1.9)	12.0 (2.0)	19.8 (3.2)	8.4 (1.1)
Generalized anxiety disorder	8.1 (0.8)	2.0 (0.2)	10.9 (1.4)	2.2 (0.2)	11.0 (1.1)	5.5 (0.7)	11.2 (1.4)	13.9 (2.1)	11.1 (2.7)	4.9 (0.7)
Substance abuse	11.0 (0.8)	3.4 (0.2)	15.8 (1.8)	3.7 (0.2)	15.1 (1.8)	9.4 (1.1)	15.6 (2.2)	12.4 (2.3)	16.9 (3.1)	8.0 (1.0)
Antisocial personality disorder	6.8 (0.7)	1.5 (0.2)	11.8 (1.4)	1.7 (0.2)	10.2 (1.5)	4.8 (0.6)	11.8 (1.7)	8.0 (1.8)	12.7 (2.8)	3.8 (0.5)
Suicidal behavior	0.3 (0.1)	0.1 (0.0)	0.4 (0.2)	0.1 (0.0)	0.3 (0.2)	0.3 (0.2)	0.4 (0.3)	0.3 (0.3)	0.4 (0.4)	0.4 (0.2)
Number of parental disorders [b]										
1	13.7 (0.8)	5.8 (0.3)	16.3 (1.5)	6.1 (0.3)	14.3 (1.5)	13.6 (1.2)	14.9 (2.0)	14.9 (2.3)	19.4 (2.8)	12.4 (1.3)
2	5.9 (0.6)	1.7 (0.2)	7.9 (1.2)	1.8 (0.2)	8.0 (1.3)	5.1 (0.8)	7.7 (1.4)	7.8 (1.7)	17.7 (3.2)	7.0 (0.9)
3	3.4 (0.5)	0.7 (0.1)	3.4 (0.8)	0.8 (0.1)	4.3 (0.6)	2.2 (0.4)	3.1 (0.7)	6.3 (1.2)		
4+	2.1 (0.3)	0.4 (0.1)	5.2 (1.1)	0.4 (0.1)	3.8 (0.6)	1.2 (0.4)	5.5 (1.0)	2.3 (0.8)		
N[c]	(2762)	(65,360)	(859)	(67,676)	(978)	(3332)	(533)	(733)	(295)	(2610)

[a] % represents the percentage of people with the parental disorder among the cases with the outcome variable indicated in the column header. Prevalence estimates are from person–year data. For example, the first cell is the % of those with parental depression among those with attempts.

[b] For number of parental disorders, the last OR represents the odds for that number of parental disorders or more. For example, for unplanned attempt, 2 represents ≥ 2 (that is, 2+).

[c] Number of cases with the outcome variable; N represents the number of person–years.

Appendix Table 7.2. Prevalence of parental psychopathology among those with each type of suicidal behavior (middle-income countries)

Parental disorder	Among total sample %[a] (SE) with parental disorder						Among ideators %[a] (SE) with parental disorder			
	Ideation	No ideation	Attempt	No attempt	Plan	No plan	Planned attempt	No planned attempt	Unplanned attempt	No unplanned attempt
Type of parental disorder										
Depression	5.3 (0.6)	1.8 (0.2)	6.9 (1.0)	1.9 (0.2)	6.2 (1.1)	5.7 (1.3)	6.9 (1.5)	5.1 (1.7)	7.2 (2.0)	5.3 (1.4)
Panic disorder	11.4 (1.0)	4.8 (0.3)	17.1 (1.9)	4.9 (0.3)	16.8 (1.9)	8.0 (1.5)	18.7 (2.5)	12.0 (3.0)	11.4 (2.7)	6.0 (1.2)
Generalized anxiety disorder	6.7 (0.8)	1.9 (0.2)	9.4 (1.3)	1.9 (0.2)	8.3 (1.4)	6.0 (1.2)	7.8 (1.4)	10.8 (4.2)	11.7 (3.1)	4.2 (1.0)
Substance abuse	9.5 (0.8)	4.5 (0.3)	11.7 (1.5)	4.6 (0.3)	9.4 (1.4)	10.2 (1.6)	10.6 (1.9)	10.2 (2.4)	15.1 (2.8)	8.2 (1.3)
Antisocial personality disorder	7.5 (0.9)	2.2 (0.2)	9.3 (1.4)	2.3 (0.2)	7.3 (0.8)	8.5 (1.7)	7.8 (1.2)	6.0 (1.7)	13.8 (3.6)	6.7 (1.5)
Suicidal behavior	1.6 (0.4)	0.5 (0.1)	1.4 (0.6)	0.5 (0.1)	1.2 (0.6)	2.3 (1.5)	1.5 (0.9)	1.5 (1.5)	1.2 (0.7)	3.5 (1.9)
Number of parental disorders[b]										
1	15.1 (1.0)	7.4 (0.3)	19.3 (1.8)	7.5 (0.3)	16.5 (2.0)	15.6 (2.2)	17.5 (2.2)	19.3 (5.0)	21.9 (3.9)	15.8 (2.6)
2	6.4 (0.7)	2.1 (0.2)	8.8 (1.3)	2.2 (0.2)	8.0 (1.1)	6.3 (1.3)	8.8 (1.8)	5.1 (1.6)	13.6 (2.9)	6.9 (1.4)
3	2.2 (0.4)	0.9 (0.1)	5.1 (0.8)	1.2 (0.1)	4.7 (0.9)	3.3 (0.8)	5.1 (1.2)	4.7 (1.8)		
4+	1.7 (0.4)	0.3 (0.0)								
N[c]	(1687)	(57,216)	(635)	(57,623)	(721)	(1234)	(411)	(320)	(194)	(911)

[a] % represents the percentage of people with the parental disorder among the cases with the outcome variable indicated in the column header. Prevalence estimates are from person–year data. For example, the first cell is the % of those with parental depression among those with attempts.
[b] For number of parental disorders, the last OR represents the odds for that number of parental disorders or more. For example, for unplanned attempt, 2 represents ≥ 2 (that is, 2+).
[c] Number of cases with the outcome variable; N represents the number of person–years.

Appendix Table 7.3. Prevalence of parental psychopathology among those with each type of suicidal behavior (low-income countries)

Parental disorder	Among total sample %[a] (SE) with parental disorder						Among ideators %[a] (SE) with parental disorder			
	Ideation	No ideation	Attempt	No attempt	Plan	No plan	Planned attempt	No planned attempt	Unplanned attempt	No unplanned attempt
Type of parental disorder										
Depression	4.5 (0.7)	1.3 (0.1)	4.6 (1.3)	1.3 (0.1)	5.7 (1.3)	4.4 (1.1)	3.5 (1.0)	4.7 (1.5)	2.4 (1.0)	3.9 (1.3)
Panic disorder	11.9 (1.1)	4.9 (0.3)	14.0 (2.0)	5.0 (0.3)	13.3 (1.8)	12.5 (2.0)	12.2 (2.5)	7.6 (2.0)	11.5 (2.8)	12.9 (2.4)
Generalized anxiety disorder	4.2 (0.8)	0.9 (0.1)	4.6 (1.3)	1.0 (0.1)	6.1 (1.6)	3.6 (1.0)	3.6 (1.0)	11.1 (5.8)	3.9 (1.8)	2.9 (1.0)
Substance abuse	10.3 (0.9)	2.9 (0.3)	9.8 (1.3)	3.1 (0.3)	11.6 (1.2)	9.2 (1.7)	10.7 (1.7)	8.6 (2.1)	7.1 (1.6)	12.0 (2.5)
Antisocial personality disorder	3.5 (0.6)	1.1 (0.2)	4.7 (0.9)	1.1 (0.2)	3.8 (0.7)	2.3 (0.7)	5.1 (1.3)	2.3 (0.9)	4.4 (1.6)	3.2 (1.2)
Suicidal behavior	0.5 (0.2)	0.2 (0.1)	0.8 (0.4)	0.2 (0.1)	1.0 (0.4)	0.5 (0.3)	1.0 (0.6)	0.7 (0.5)	0.1 (0.1)	0.4 (0.4)
Number of parental disorders[b]										
1	16.0 (1.3)	6.4 (0.3)	16.4 (1.8)	6.6 (0.3)	17.7 (1.8)	14.8 (2.2)	16.6 (2.6)	17.2 (5.8)	14.3 (2.5)	16.5 (2.8)
2	4.6 (0.6)	1.5 (0.2)	9.0 (1.5)	2.2 (0.2)	10.0 (1.7)	7.0 (1.3)	8.0 (1.5)	7.7 (2.1)	6.4 (2.0)	7.2 (1.8)
3+	2.9 (0.6)	0.6 (0.1)								
N[c]	(1639)	(40,936)	(583)	(39,548)	(717)	(1292)	(353)	(384)	(192)	(843)

[a] % represents the percentage of people with the parental disorder among the cases with the outcome variable indicated in the column header. Prevalence estimates are from person-year data. For example, the first cell is the % of those with parental depression among those with attempts.

[b] For number of parental disorders, the last OR represents the odd for that number of parental disorders or more. For example, for unplanned attempt, 2 represents ≥ 2 (that is, 2+).

[c] Number of cases with the outcome variable; N represents the number of person-years.

Appendix Table 7.4. Final multivariate models for associations between parental psychopathology and lifetime suicidal behavior[a] (high-income countries)

Parental disorder	Among total sample			Among ideators	
	Ideation	Attempt	Plan	Planned attempt	Unplanned attempt
	OR (95% CI)	OR (95% CI)	OR (95% CI)	OR (95% CI)	OR (95% CI)
Type of parental disorder					
Depression	2.3* (1.7–3.2)	2.1* (1.3–3.4)	1.0 (0.6–1.6)	0.7 (0.3–1.5)	1.9 (0.8–4.5)
Panic disorder	2.0* (1.7–2.3)	2.4* (1.8–3.1)	0.8 (0.6–1.1)	1.2 (0.7–2.1)	1.9* (1.2–3.1)
Generalized anxiety disorder	2.7* (2.1–3.4)	2.1* (1.4–3.0)	0.9 (0.6–1.6)	0.6 (0.3–1.1)	1.2 (0.5–2.9)
Substance abuse	2.1* (1.7–2.6)	1.9* (1.4–2.5)	1.0 (0.7–1.4)	0.8 (0.5–1.3)	1.1 (0.6–2.1)
Antisocial personality disorder	2.5* (1.9–3.2)	3.1* (2.2–4.5)	0.9 (0.5–1.7)	1.2 (0.6–2.4)	1.9 (1.0–3.4)
Suicidal behavior	1.0 (0.5–2.0)	0.8 (0.3–2.0)	1.4 (0.4–5.8)	0.9 (0.1–5.2)	1.1 (0.1–12.5)
6 df χ^2 for 6 types	149.2 (<.001)*	80.6 (<.001)*	2.3 (0.90)	5.5 (0.48)	11.4 (0.08)
5 df χ^2 for difference between types	11.5 (0.04)*	12.3 (0.03)*	2.6 (0.76)	6.3 (0.28)	5.5 (0.36)
Number of parental disorders[b]					
2	0.5* (0.4–0.7)	0.6* (0.4–0.9)	1.8 (1.0–3.1)	1.1 (0.5–2.3)	0.6 (0.2–1.4)
3	0.3* (0.2–0.6)	0.3* (0.1–0.6)	1.7 (0.6–4.8)	0.7 (0.2–2.7)	
4+	0.1* (0.1–0.2)	0.3* (0.1–0.7)	3.0 (0.8–11.9)	3.0 (0.5–16.6)	
χ^2 (p-value)	38.6 (<0.001)*	10.0 (0.02)*	4.0 (0.27)	7.6 (0.06)	1.4 (0.24)

*Significant at the 0.05 level, two-sided test.
[a] Assessed in the Part 2 sample due to having Part 2 controls. Models control for person–years, country, and significant variables from the chapter on sociodemographics.
[b] For number of parental disorders, the last OR represents the odds for that number of parental disorders or more. For example, for unplanned attempt, 2 represents ≥2 (that is, 2+).

Appendix Table 7.5. Final multivariate models for associations between parental psychopathology and lifetime suicidal behavior[a] (middle-income countries)

| | Among total sample | | | Among ideators | |
| | Ideation | Attempt | Plan | Planned attempt | Unplanned attempt |
Parental disorder	OR (95% CI)	OR (95% CI)	OR (95% CI)	OR (95% CI)	OR (95% CI)
Type of parental disorder					
Depression	1.9* (1.3–3.0)	1.8* (1.1–3.0)	0.6 (0.3–1.3)	1.3 (0.4–4.8)	0.6 (0.2–1.9)
Panic disorder	1.8* (1.5–2.3)	2.9* (2.0–4.1)	2.2* (1.4–3.6)	1.6 (0.7–3.9)	1.3 (0.6–2.8)
Generalized anxiety disorder	2.4* (1.7–3.5)	3.2* (2.0–5.2)	1.0 (0.4–2.1)	0.4 (0.1–1.4)	2.8 (1.0–8.1)
Substance abuse	1.2 (1.0–1.6)	1.5* (1.0–2.2)	0.7 (0.4–1.3)	0.9 (0.4–1.9)	1.5 (0.7–3.5)
Antisocial personality disorder	2.7* (2.0–3.8)	3.1* (1.9–5.0)	0.5* (0.3–0.9)	1.1 (0.4–2.9)	1.7 (0.7–4.4)
Suicidal behavior	3.1* (1.7–5.6)	2.2 (0.8–5.9)	0.3 (0.1–1.0)	0.6 (0.1–3.2)	0.6 (0.1–3.1)
6 df χ^2 for 6 types	73.1 (<0.001)*	72.0 (<0.001)*	27.9 (<0.001)*	4.9 (0.56)	6.9 (0.33)
5 df χ^2 for difference between types	22.5 (<0.001)*	21.1 (<0.001)*	24.4 (<0.001)*	4.9 (0.43)	3.8 (0.58)
Number of parental disorders[b]					
2	0.7 (0.4–1.0)	0.6 (0.4–1.0)	1.4 (0.6–3.7)	1.6 (0.5–5.0)	0.8 (0.2–3.0)
3	0.3* (0.2–0.5)	0.2* (0.1–0.4)	1.8 (0.3–9.5)	1.1 (0.2–8.0)	
4+	0.2* (0.1–0.5)				
χ^2 (p-value)	24.2 (<0.001)*	18.4 (<0.001)*	0.6 (0.73)	0.8 (0.68)	0.1 (0.77)

* Significant at the 0.05 level, two-sided test.
[a] Assessed in the Part 2 sample due to having Part 2 controls. Models control for person–years, country, and significant variables from the chapter on sociodemographics.
[b] For number of parental disorders, the last OR represents the odds for that number of parental disorders or more. For example, for unplanned attempt, 2 represents ≥2 (that is, 2+).

Appendix Table 7.6. Final multivariate models for associations between parental psychopathology and lifetime suicidal behavior[a] (low-income countries)

	Among total sample			Among ideators	
	Ideation	Attempt	Plan	Planned attempt	Unplanned attempt
Parental disorder	OR (95% CI)	OR (95% CI)	OR (95% CI)	OR (95% CI)	OR (95% CI)
Type of parental disorder					
Depression	2.6* (1.5–4.4)	1.9 (1.0–3.6)	1.1 (0.5–2.5)	2.3 (0.5–10.5)	0.8 (0.1–4.2)
Panic disorder	2.3* (1.8–3.1)	2.4* (1.5–3.8)	1.0 (0.5–1.7)	3.2* (1.1–9.3)	0.8 (0.4–1.7)
Generalized anxiety disorder	2.9* (1.4–5.9)	1.7* (1.0–3.1)	1.5 (0.6–3.7)	0.2* (0.0–0.8)	3.2 (0.8–12.8)
Substance abuse	2.4* (1.8–3.2)	1.6* (1.0–2.4)	0.8 (0.4–1.3)	0.8 (0.3–1.7)	0.5 (0.2–1.1)
Antisocial personality disorder	1.5 (0.9–2.6)	1.4 (0.7–2.7)	1.5 (0.6–4.0)	2.5 (0.6–10.1)	2.4 (0.5–11.2)
Suicidal behavior	3.5* (1.2–10.4)	5.7* (1.9–17.2)	2.5 (0.5–11.9)	1.2 (0.0–33.6)	0.7 (0.0–10.2)
6 df χ^2 for 6 types	85.0 (<0.001)*	36.4 (<0.001)*	4.1 (0.67)	11.5 (0.07)	8.0 (0.23)
5 df χ^2 for difference between types	5.9 (0.31)	7.0 (0.22)	6.1 (0.30)	10.2 (0.07)	8.1 (0.15)
Number of parental disorders[b]					
2	0.6* (0.3–1.0)	0.8 (0.4–1.6)	1.1 (0.4–3.1)	0.5 (0.1–3.2)	0.3 (0.1–1.6)
3+	0.2* (0.1–0.7)				
χ^2 (p-value)	6.2 (0.05)*	0.6 (0.45)	0.0 (0.85)	0.5 (0.49)	1.9 (0.16)

*Significant at the 0.05 level, two-sided test.
[a] Assessed in the Part 2 sample due to having Part 2 controls. Models control for person–years, country, and significant variables from the chapter on sociodemographics.
[b] For number of parental disorders, the last OR represents the odds for that number of parental disorders or more. For example, for unplanned attempt, 2 represents ≥2 (that is, 2+).

Appendix Table 7.7. Interactions between parental psychopathology and respondent age in the prediction of suicidal behavior[a] (high-income countries)

Interactions		Among total sample			Among ideators	
		Ideation	Attempt	Plan	Planned attempt	Unplanned attempt
		OR (95% CI)	OR (95% CI)	OR (95% CI)	OR (95% CI)	OR (95% CI)
Type of parental disorder						
Depression	13–19	1.6 (0.6–4.1)	2.1 (0.5–8.9)	0.2 (0.0–5.0)	3.5 (0.1–222.3)	1.2 (0.3–4.9)
	20–29	1.9 (0.7–4.8)	1.7 (0.3–8.8)	0.5 (0.0–7.6)	1.8 (0.0–88.0)	–
	30+	1.6 (0.6–4.5)	1.4 (0.2–8.6)	0.3 (0.0–5.1)	3.6 (0.1–188.0)	–
χ^2 (p-value)		1.8 (0.62)	1.3 (0.74)	1.5 (0.69)	1.1 (0.77)	0.0 (0.84)
Panic	13–19	0.9 (0.4–2.0)	2.3 (0.6–8.0)	0.5 (0.1–2.5)	0.3 (0.0–2.2)	1.7 (0.6–4.5)
disorder	20–29	1.0 (0.4–2.1)	1.8 (0.5–6.4)	0.8 (0.2–3.9)	0.2 (0.0–1.9)	–
	30+	0.8 (0.4–1.6)	2.0 (0.6–7.0)	1.0 (0.2–5.8)	0.3 (0.0–2.1)	–
χ^2 (p-value)		1.6 (0.67)	1.7 (0.63)	3.3 (0.35)	1.9 (0.60)	1.2 (0.28)
Generalized	13–19	2.5 (0.9–7.2)	2.4 (0.7–9.1)	0.9 (0.1–8.9)	–	0.9 (0.2–4.3)
anxiety	20–29	1.2 (0.4–3.1)	2.7 (0.6–12.3)	0.3 (0.0–4.2)	–	–
disorder	30+	1.9 (0.6–5.7)	1.9 (0.5–7.3)	0.4 (0.1–2.9)	–	–
χ^2 (p-value)		5.9 (0.11)	2.1 (0.56)	3.4 (0.33)	–	0.0 (0.93)
Substance	13–19	1.0 (0.5–1.9)	0.9 (0.3–3.4)	2.4 (0.3–16.3)	1.1 (0.0–84.9)	0.9 (0.3–3.0)
abuse	20–29	1.0 (0.5–1.7)	0.9 (0.2–2.9)	1.8 (0.3–11.3)	0.7 (0.0–46.1)	–
	30+	1.0 (0.5–1.8)	0.7 (0.2–2.6)	1.5 (0.3–8.8)	0.7 (0.0–55.3)	–
χ^2 (p-value)		0.1 (1.00)	0.9 (0.83)	1.4 (0.72)	0.9 (0.82)	0.0 (0.91)
Antisocial	13–19	1.3 (0.5–2.9)	1.9 (0.5–8.4)	5.7 (0.8–40.2)	0.8 (0.1–4.5)	1.6 (0.3–8.0)
personality	20–29	1.1 (0.4–2.5)	1.9 (0.5–7.2)	5.8 (0.6–56.0)	1.4 (0.3–6.6)	–
disorder	30+	0.9 (0.4–2.0)	1.9 (0.5–7.7)	4.5 (0.5–43.6)	–	–
χ^2 (p-value)		1.1 (0.78)	1.0 (0.80)	3.2 (0.36)	0.9 (0.63)	0.3 (0.60)
Suicidal	13–19	0.1* (0.0–0.8)	–	–	–	–
behavior	20–29	0.2 (0.0–1.2)	–	–	–	–
	30+	0.1* (0.0–0.6)	–	–	–	–
χ^2 (p-value)		7.6 (0.06)	–	–	–	–
18 df χ^2 test for all parental disorders		30.6 (0.03)*	7.0 (0.96)	22.1 (0.11)	6.4 (0.84)	1.2 (0.94)
30 df χ^2 test for all parental disorders and dummies for number of disorders		45.7 (0.01)*	38.9 (0.03)*	30.2 (0.09)	10.3 (0.89)	1.3 (0.97)
Number of parental disorders[b]						
2	13–19	0.5 (0.2–1.6)	0.3 (0.0–2.2)	0.7 (0.1–8.4)	1.0 (0.0–102.8)	0.8 (0.2–3.6)
	20–29	0.5 (0.2–1.6)	0.2 (0.0–1.8)	0.4 (0.0–4.6)	1.3 (0.0–112.9)	–
	30+	0.8 (0.3–2.3)	0.5 (0.1–4.3)	0.6 (0.1–7.4)	1.7 (0.0–146.4)	–
3	13–19	0.5 (0.1–2.8)	0.0* (0.0–0.8)	0.6 (0.0–65.2)	0.2 (0.0–260.5)	
	20–29	0.5 (0.1–2.7)	0.0* (0.0–0.9)	0.6 (0.0–66.4)	0.5 (0.0–424.4)	
	30+	0.6 (0.1–3.1)	0.2 (0.0–3.8)	1.4 (0.0–121.8)	0.5 (0.0–347.0)	
4+	13–19	0.1 (0.0–1.9)	0.1 (0.0–8.6)	3.9 (0.69)	1.7 (0.95)	0.1 (0.74)
	20–29	0.1 (0.0–1.9)	0.1 (0.0–8.8)			
	30+	0.2 (0.0–3.1)	0.1 (0.0–16.4)			
χ^2 (p-value)		5.4 (0.80)	14.4 (0.11)			

*Significant at the 0.05 level, two-sided test.
– Not included due to small cell size.
[a] Assessed in the Part 2 sample due to having Part 2 controls. Models control for life course intervals (4–12, 13–19, 20–29, 30+ years), country, and the significant interaction terms from the chapter on sociodemographics, and the interaction of the life course intervals (4–12, 13–19, 20–29, 30+ years) and all controls. Only the interactions for parental psychopathology and life course intervals are shown.
[b] For number of parental disorders, the last OR represents the odds for that number of parental disorders or more. For example, for unplanned attempt, 2 represents ≥2 (that is, 2+).

Appendix Table 7.8. Interactions between parental psychopathology and respondent age in the prediction of suicidal behavior[a] (middle-income countries)

Interactions		Among total sample		Among ideators		
		Ideation	Attempt	Plan	Planned attempt	Unplanned attempt
		OR (95% CI)	OR (95% CI)	OR (95% CI)	OR (95% CI)	OR (95% CI)
Type of parental disorder						
Depression	13–19	5.8* (1.5–23.3)	4.4 (0.6–32.2)	1.6 (0.1–29.0)	12.1 (0.3–464.9)	–
	20–29	2.1 (0.5–9.0)	3.2 (0.4–22.8)	1.5 (0.1–18.7)	4.1 (0.2–92.7)	–
	30+	2.2 (0.5–9.3)	1.4 (0.2–12.3)	1.9 (0.1–28.2)	–	–
χ^2 (p-value)		9.8 (0.02)*	4.2 (0.24)	0.3 (0.97)	1.9 (0.38)	–
Panic	13–19	7.6* (1.6–35.4)	2.6 (0.8–8.8)	0.0* (0.0–0.0)	0.0 (0.0–2.0)	5.2 (0.8–33.3)
disorder	20–29	4.4 (1.0–19.6)	2.4 (0.7–7.5)	0.0* (0.0–0.0)	0.0 (0.0–8.5)	–
	30+	5.3* (1.1–25.7)	1.9 (0.7–5.8)	0.0* (0.0–0.0)	0.1 (0.0–11.3)	–
χ^2 (p-value)		8.2 (0.04)*	2.6 (0.46)	16.6 (<0.001)	6.9 (0.08)	3.1 (0.08)
Generalized	13–19	0.6 (0.2–2.2)	0.3 (0.1–1.9)	0.0* (0.0–0.0)	1.2 (0.1–28.1)	–
anxiety	20–29	0.6 (0.2–2.2)	0.3 (0.1–1.9)	0.0* (0.0–0.0)	2.2 (0.5–9.2)	–
disorder	30+	0.3 (0.1–1.4)	0.1* (0.0–0.8)	0.0* (0.0–0.0)	–	–
χ^2 (p-value)		2.3 (0.50)	5.1 (0.16)	50.7 (<0.001)*	1.2 (0.55)	–
Substance	13–19	1.4 (0.5–4.2)	2.2 (0.5–9.8)	2.6 (0.1–58.3)	–	–
abuse	20–29	1.5 (0.5–4.1)	2.9 (0.6–13.9)	2.1 (0.1–53.0)	–	5.6 (0.9–34.4)
	30+	1.0 (0.3–3.0)	1.9 (0.4–9.1)	2.4 (0.1–62.5)	–	1.8 (0.2–13.8)
χ^2 (p-value)		2.7 (0.43)	1.9 (0.60)	0.4 (0.94)	–	4.3 (0.12)
Antisocial	13–19	1.7 (0.4–6.8)	1.3 (0.4–4.3)	0.0* (0.0–0.0)	2.8 (0.1–100.5)	–
personality	20–29	1.2 (0.3–4.8)	0.9 (0.3–3.3)	0.0* (0.0–0.0)	1.6 (0.2–15.2)	–
disorder	30+	1.6 (0.4–6.7)	1.5 (0.3–8.0)	0.0* (0.0–0.0)	–	–
χ^2 (p-value)		1.3 (0.73)	0.7 (0.86)	58.8 (<0.001)*	0.4 (0.83)	–
Suicidal	13–19	0.5 (0.1–3.3)	0.5 (0.0–13.4)	–	–	–
behavior	20–29	0.9 (0.1–8.3)	1.6 (0.1–20.7)	–	–	–
	30+	0.0* (0.0–0.0)	0.0* (0.0–0.0)	–	–	–
χ^2 (p-value)		857.5 (<0.001)*	471.2 (<0.001)*	–	–	–
18 df χ^2 test for all parental disorders		1091.6 (<0.001)*	776.5 (<0.001)*	145.3 (<0.001)*	11.5 (0.24)	7.3 (0.06)
27 df χ^2 test for all parental disorders and dummies for number of disorders		1169.4 (<0.001)*	996.1 (<0.001)*	149.7 (<0.001)*	28.8 (0.004)*	10.6 (0.10)
Number of parental disorders[b]						
	13–19	0.4 (0.1–2.5)	0.4 (0.0–3.4)	387.4* (5.0–30186.1)	1.2 (0.0–234.8)	1.0 (0.0–21.8)
2	20–29	0.4 (0.1–2.9)	0.4 (0.0–3.6)	338.2* (4.9–23357.9)	1.2 (0.0–128.5)	0.3 (0.0–5.8)
	30+	1.0 (0.2–6.2)	1.0 (0.1–10.0)	281.0* (3.7–21098.3)	0.3 (0.0–26.5)	0.6 (0.0–16.5)
	13–19	0.1 (0.0–1.3)	0.2 (0.0–5.8)			
3	20–29	0.4 (0.0–4.9)	0.1 (0.0–3.9)			
	30+	0.4 (0.0–6.3)	0.4 (0.0–16.8)			
	13–19	0.0 (0.0–1.3)				
4+	20–29	0.1 (0.0–2.4)				
	30+	0.1 (0.0–3.8)				
χ^2 (p-value)		11.3 (0.26)	2.5 (0.87)	7.6 (0.05)	1.0 (0.81)	1.8 (0.60)

*Significant at the 0.05 level, two-sided test.
– Not included due to small cell size.
0.0* (0.0–0.0) OR is ≤ 0.05 indicating very low risk.
[a] Assessed in the Part 2 sample due to having Part 2 controls. Models control for life course intervals (4–12, 13–19, 20–29, 30+ years), country, and significant interaction terms from the chapter on sociodemographics, and the interaction of the life course intervals (4–12, 13–19, 20–29, 30+ years) and all controls. Only the interactions for parental psychopathology and life course intervals are shown.
[b] For number of parental disorders, the last OR represents the odds for that number of parental disorders or more. For example, for unplanned attempt, 2 represents ≥2 (that is, 2+).

Appendix Table 7.9. Interactions between parental psychopathology and respondent age in the prediction of suicidal behavior[a] (low-income countries)

		Among total sample		Among ideators		
		Ideation	Attempt	Plan	Planned attempt	Unplanned attempt
Interactions		OR (95% CI)	OR (95% CI)	OR (95% CI)	OR (95% CI)	OR (95% CI)
Type of parental disorder						
	13–19	3.5* (1.2–10.2)	–	–	–	–
Depression	20–29	2.0 (0.6–7.2)	–	–	–	–
	30+	6.9* (2.1–23.1)	–	0.6 (0.1–2.8)	–	–
χ^2 (p-value)		10.5 (0.02)*	–	0.4 (0.55)	–	–
	13–19	1.3 (0.4–4.5)	2.2 (0.5–10.4)	0.2 (0.0–2.5)	0.4 (0.1–2.6)	0.1 (0.0–1.2)
Panic disorder	20–29	1.3 (0.4–4.0)	2.7 (0.8–8.9)	0.2 (0.0–1.9)	0.2 (0.0–1.2)	0.3 (0.0–3.1)
	30+	0.9 (0.3–2.8)	1.9 (0.6–6.0)	0.4 (0.0–5.3)	–	–
χ^2 (p-value)		1.6 (0.66)	2.7 (0.44)	4.6 (0.20)	3.7 (0.16)	12.0 (0.06)
Generalized	13–19	2.2 (0.5–10.4)	2.5 (0.2–29.2)	3.6 (0.6–22.8)	–	–
anxiety	20–29	0.5 (0.1–3.5)	1.4 (0.2–9.3)	–	–	–
disorder	30+	0.4 (0.1–2.8)	0.9 (0.1–9.6)	0.5 (0.1–3.2)	–	–
χ^2 (p-value)		7.7 (0.05)	2.0 (0.58)	5.2 (0.07)	–	–
	13–19	1.2 (0.4–4.3)	2.5 (0.7–9.6)	8.4 (0.7–95.8)	1.0 (0.1–8.1)	–
Substance	20–29	1.1 (0.3–3.5)	2.2 (0.6–7.9)	3.0 (0.3–34.2)	1.0 (0.2–4.8)	–
abuse						
	30+	0.8 (0.2–2.6)	1.2 (0.3–5.4)	2.9 (0.3–30.7)	–	–
χ^2 (p-value)		2.1 (0.54)	3.0 (0.39)	6.5 (0.09)	0.0 (1.00)	–
Antisocial	13–19	3.6 (0.6–21.2)	4.3 (0.2–103.4)	–	–	–
personality	20–29	6.0* (1.1–33.3)	7.3 (0.4–139.5)	–	–	–
disorder	30+	2.4 (0.4–16.3)	8.3 (0.4–183.5)	0.4 (0.1–2.5)	–	–
χ^2 (p-value)		5.0 (0.17)	2.4 (0.48)	1.1 (0.30)	–	–
	13–19	0.3 (0.0–3.0)	–	–	–	–
Suicidal	20–29	0.1 (0.0–1.0)	–	–	–	–
behavior						
	30+	0.2 (0.0–1.2)	–	–	–	–
χ^2 (p-value)		4.5 (0.22)	–	–	–	–
18 df χ^2 test for all parental disorders		32.3 (0.02)*	8.3 (0.76)	19.2 (0.04)*	3.9 (0.42)	–
24 df χ^2 test for all parental disorders and dummies for number of disorders		46.9 (0.003)*	10.2 (0.81)	25.2 (0.02)*	12.0 (0.06)	–
Number of parental disorders[b]						
	13–19	0.3 (0.0–1.6)	0.2 (0.0–2.7)	1.0 (0.0–29.2)	0.1 (0.0–1.2)	–
2	20–29	0.4 (0.1–2.2)	0.2 (0.0–1.3)	3.4 (0.1–90.7)	0.3 (0.0–3.1)	–
	30+	0.5 (0.1–3.4)	0.5 (0.1–4.3)	8.1 (0.2–275.7)	–	–

Appendix Table 7.9. (cont.)

Interactions		Among total sample		Among ideators		
		Ideation	Attempt	Plan	Planned attempt	Unplanned attempt
		OR (95% CI)	OR (95% CI)	OR (95% CI)	OR (95% CI)	OR (95% CI)
	13–19	0.1 (0.0–1.7)				
3+	20–29	0.2 (0.0–4.0)				
	30+	0.2 (0.0–6.6)				
χ^2 (p-value)		3.3 (0.77)	3.3 (0.34)	5.6 (0.13)	3.7 (0.16)	–

*Significant at the 0.05 level, two-sided test.
– Not included due to small cell size.
[a] Assessed in the Part 2 sample due to having Part 2 controls. Models control for life course intervals (4–12, 13–19, 20–29, 30+ years), country, and significant interaction terms from the chapter on sociodemographics, and the interaction of the life course intervals (4–12, 13–19, 20–29, 30+ years) and all controls. Only the interactions for parental psychopathology and life course intervals are shown.
[b] For number of parental disorders, the last OR represents the odds for that number of parental disorders or more. For example, for planned attempt, 2 represents ≥2 (that is, 2+).

Appendix Table 7.10. Parental psychopathology and risk of persistence of suicidal behavior in the respondent[a] (high-income countries)

Parental disorder	Ideation	Plan	Attempt
	OR (95% CI)	OR (95% CI)	OR (95% CI)
Type of parental disorder			
Depression	1.0 (0.8–1.4)	1.1 (0.6–2.0)	0.8 (0.4–1.6)
Panic disorder	1.1 (0.9–1.5)	1.1 (0.8–1.6)	1.3 (0.7–2.3)
Generalized anxiety disorder	1.3 (1.0–1.8)	1.0 (0.6–1.7)	0.8 (0.4–1.4)
Substance abuse	0.9 (0.7–1.2)	0.7 (0.4–1.2)	1.0 (0.6–1.6)
Antisocial personality disorder	0.9 (0.6–1.3)	0.8 (0.5–1.4)	0.8 (0.4–1.6)
Suicidal behavior	1.4 (0.7–3.2)	1.0 (0.3–3.4)	2.1 (0.2–18.0)
χ^2_6 (p-value)	6.9 (0.33)	4.7 (0.59)	4.1 (0.67)
χ^2_5 (p-value)	6.0 (0.30)	7.9 (0.17)	4.3 (0.51)
Number of parental disorders			
2	1.0 (0.7–1.5)	1.1 (0.6–2.3)	1.4 (0.6–3.1)
3	1.0 (0.5–1.8)	1.1 (0.4–3.3)	1.2 (0.3–4.5)
4+	1.0 (0.5–2.4)	1.9 (0.4–9.0)	2.0 (0.4–10.1)
χ^2 (p-value)	0.2 (0.98)	1.3 (0.73)	1.3 (0.73)

*Significant at the 0.05 level, two-sided test.
– Not included due to small cell size.
[a] Results are based on multivariate discrete time survival models. Models control for country, age-related variables, and significant variables from the chapter on sociodemographics.

Appendix Table 7.11. Parental psychopathology and risk of persistence of suicidal behavior in the respondent[a] (middle-income countries)

Parental disorder	Ideation OR (95% CI)	Plan OR (95% CI)	Attempt OR (95% CI)
Type of parental disorder			
Depression	1.8* (1.1–3.2)	1.9 (0.6–6.5)	2.5 (0.5–14.2)
Panic disorder	1.6* (1.1–2.4)	1.6 (0.9–3.0)	2.5* (1.4–4.8)
Generalized anxiety disorder	0.7 (0.3–1.5)	0.9 (0.3–2.6)	1.4 (0.5–4.3)
Substance abuse	1.3 (0.8–2.2)	1.5 (0.6–3.6)	1.2 (0.5–2.7)
Antisocial personality disorder	1.3 (0.8–2.3)	0.8 (0.2–2.6)	1.0 (0.5–2.2)
Suicidal behavior	1.0 (0.3–3.1)	0.0* (0.0–0.0)	6.4* (1.0–39.4)
χ^2_6 (p-value)	13.7 (0.03)*	210.0 (<0.001)*	16.8 (0.01)*
χ^2_5 (p-value)	5.0 (0.42)	200.3 (<0.001)*	9.0 (0.11)
Number of parental disorders[b]			
2	1.1 (0.5–2.4)	0.7 (0.2–3.1)	0.8 (0.2–2.9)
3	0.8 (0.2–2.4)	0.3 (0.0–2.7)	0.1 (0.0–1.0)
4+	0.5 (0.1–2.7)		
χ^2 (p-value)	1.9 (0.60)	1.5 (0.47)	6.1 (0.05)*

* Significant at the 0.05 level, two-sided test.
0.0* (0.0–0.0) OR is ≤0.05 indicating very low risk.
[a] Results are based on multivariate discrete time survival models. Models control for country, age-related variables, and significant variables from the chapter on sociodemographics.
[b] For number of parental disorders, the last OR represents the odds of that number of parental disorders or more. For example, for attempt, 3 represents ≥3 (that is, 3+).

Appendix Table 7.12. Parental psychopathology and risk of persistence of suicidal behavior in the respondent[a] (low-income countries)

Parental disorder	Ideation OR (95% CI)	Plan OR (95% CI)	Attempt OR (95% CI)
Type of parental disorder			
Depression	2.5* (1.2–5.3)	3.2* (1.0–10.0)	2.3 (0.4–12.1)
Panic disorder	0.9 (0.6–1.4)	1.2 (0.6–2.2)	1.8 (0.8–4.0)
Generalized anxiety disorder	0.9 (0.4–2.3)	0.6 (0.1–2.6)	1.7 (0.2–16.6)
Substance abuse	1.0 (0.6–1.7)	1.4 (0.8–2.5)	1.1 (0.4–2.9)
Antisocial personality disorder	1.4 (0.6–3.1)	2.7 (0.6–12.1)	1.4 (0.3–6.7)
Suicidal behavior	1.2 (0.5–3.3)	2.5 (0.6–9.5)	2.0 (0.2–16.7)
χ^2_6 (p-value)	7.1 (0.31)	8.9 (0.18)	3.3 (0.78)
χ^2_5 (p-value)	7.4 (0.19)	6.5 (0.26)	1.8 (0.88)
Number of parental disorders[b]			
2	1.5 (0.7–3.1)	0.6 (0.1–2.8)	0.9 (0.1–7.4)
3+	0.8 (0.2–2.8)	0.5 (0.50)	0.0 (0.90)
χ^2 (p-value)	2.8 (0.25)		

* Significant at 0.05 level, two-sided test.
0.0* (0.0–0.0) OR is ≤0.05 indicating very low risk.
[a] Results are based on multivariate discrete time survival models. Models control for country, age-related variables, and significant variables from the chapter on sociodemographics.
[b] For number of parental disorders, the last OR represents the odds of that number of parental disorders or more. For example, for attempt, 2 represents ≥2 (that is, 2+).

Appendix Table 8.1. Prevalence of childhood adversities in high-, middle-, and low-income countries (all countries combined)

Type of childhood adversity	High-income countries	Middle-income countries	Low-income countries
Physical abuse	8.6	13.1	12.6
Sexual abuse	5.0	0.9	1.2
Neglect	2.5	5.0	5.1
Parental death	8.4	12.8	15.2
Parental divorce	6.7	5.3	4.5
Other parental loss	3.4	4.7	10.7
Family violence	9.3	8.6	6.8
Physical illness	4.4	2.8	1.4
Financial adversity	4.9	2.4	3.8

Appendix Table 8.2. Prevalence of childhood adversities among those with each type of suicidal behavior (high-income countries)

Childhood adversity	Among total sample						Among ideators			
	%[a] (SE) with adversities						%[a] (SE) with adversities			
	Ideation	No ideation	Attempt	No attempt	Plan	No plan	Planned attempt	No planned attempt	Unplanned attempt	No unplanned attempt
Type of adversity										
Physical abuse	17.9 (0.7)	4.8 (0.2)	28.2 (1.6)	5.2 (0.2)	24.1 (1.3)	16.5 (1.0)	30.5 (2.1)	19.4 (2.3)	23.2 (2.2)	14.4 (1.0)
Sexual abuse	12.4 (0.5)	2.4 (0.1)	21.5 (1.2)	2.7 (0.1)	18.4 (1.1)	11.0 (0.7)	23.1 (1.6)	15.0 (1.6)	17.9 (1.7)	8.9 (0.8)
Neglect	13.2 (0.6)	5.1 (0.2)	21.0 (1.3)	5.3 (0.2)	18.5 (1.1)	12.1 (1.0)	23.0 (1.7)	12.8 (1.5)	16.4 (2.2)	10.5 (1.0)
Parental death	12.5 (0.5)	13.4 (0.3)	15.0 (1.1)	13.3 (0.3)	13.3 (1.0)	14.7 (1.0)	15.1 (1.4)	13.8 (1.9)	15.6 (2.1)	14.5 (1.1)
Parental divorce	13.7 (0.7)	6.1 (0.2)	19.2 (1.5)	6.3 (0.2)	14.2 (1.0)	11.9 (0.8)	17.2 (1.7)	10.6 (1.6)	22.5 (2.5)	10.5 (0.9)
Other parental loss	7.9 (0.4)	4.4 (0.2)	12.4 (1.0)	4.5 (0.2)	8.6 (0.9)	8.4 (0.8)	10.6 (1.2)	5.7 (1.2)	15.4 (1.7)	7.1 (1.0)
Family violence	19.8 (0.7)	6.3 (0.2)	28.8 (1.5)	6.8 (0.2)	25.2 (1.3)	17.8 (0.9)	29.0 (1.9)	20.4 (2.0)	26.9 (2.6)	16.2 (1.1)
Physical illness	8.0 (0.5)	4.1 (0.2)	11.8 (1.0)	4.2 (0.2)	10.5 (0.9)	8.3 (0.7)	13.1 (1.4)	9.2 (1.7)	10.5 (1.9)	7.0 (0.7)
Financial adversity	5.8 (0.3)	3.7 (0.2)	8.4 (0.7)	3.8 (0.2)	5.5 (0.5)	6.2 (0.6)	6.8 (0.9)	3.8 (0.8)	11.2 (1.4)	5.3 (0.7)
Number of adversities[b]										
1	29.5 (0.9)	23.6 (0.4)	27.9 (1.4)	23.8 (0.4)	29.4 (1.4)	31.4 (1.3)	26.6 (1.8)	30.3 (2.3)	29.2 (2.5)	32.1 (1.4)
2	15.8 (0.7)	8.2 (0.3)	19.0 (1.2)	8.5 (0.2)	19.1 (1.3)	15.1 (0.9)	19.7 (1.6)	20.2 (2.2)	18.3 (1.9)	14.3 (1.1)
3	8.6 (0.6)	2.2 (0.1)	14.0 (1.2)	2.4 (0.1)	10.9 (0.8)	8.0 (0.8)	14.4 (1.4)	7.6 (1.2)	13.3 (2.4)	7.3 (0.8)
4	3.3 (0.3)	0.6 (0.1)	6.8 (0.8)	0.6 (0.1)	5.0 (0.6)	3.0 (0.4)	6.8 (0.9)	3.4 (0.8)	6.1 (1.4)	1.9 (0.3)
5	1.5 (0.2)	0.2 (0.0)	3.9 (0.6)	0.2 (0.0)	3.4 (0.6)	1.8 (0.3)	5.9 (1.1)	0.8 (0.3)	5.4 (0.9)	0.8 (0.2)
6+	0.6 (0.1)	0.1 (0.0)	1.9 (0.3)	0.1 (0.0)						
N[c]	(5056)	(112,028)	(1613)	(116,041)	(1885)	(5646)	(1002)	(1330)	(551)	(4338)

[a] % represents the percentage of people with the adversity among the cases with the outcome variable indicated in the column header. For example, the first cell is the % of those with physical abuse among those with ideation.

[b] For number of adversities, the last OR represents the odds for that number of adversities or more. For example, for unplanned attempt, 5 represents ≥5 (that is, 5+).

[c] N represents the number of person-years.

Appendix Table 8.3. Prevalence of childhood adversities among those with each type of suicidal behavior (middle-income countries)

Childhood adversity	Among total sample %[a] (SE) with adversities						Among ideators %[a] (SE) with adversities			
	Ideation	No ideation	Attempt	No attempt	Plan	No plan	Planned attempt	No planned attempt	Unplanned attempt	No unplanned attempt
Type of adversity										
Physical abuse	25.7 (1.3)	9.9 (0.3)	31.0 (2.3)	10.2 (0.3)	29.8 (2.1)	28.4 (2.9)	30.8 (2.7)	27.5 (4.4)	31.4 (3.9)	26.5 (3.3)
Sexual abuse	2.1 (0.3)	0.4 (0.1)	4.0 (0.8)	0.4 (0.1)	3.6 (0.7)	1.6 (0.4)	4.6 (1.1)	2.2 (0.9)	2.0 (0.8)	1.3 (0.4)
Neglect	15.0 (1.1)	5.3 (0.3)	19.3 (1.7)	5.5 (0.3)	18.9 (1.6)	16.3 (2.2)	21.5 (2.3)	17.3 (3.7)	15.5 (2.9)	14.4 (2.8)
Parental death	16.2 (1.2)	12.7 (0.4)	15.8 (1.7)	12.7 (0.4)	14.7 (1.4)	16.3 (2.1)	14.8 (1.8)	13.9 (3.6)	16.9 (3.9)	17.6 (2.4)
Parental divorce	8.9 (0.9)	4.2 (0.2)	12.7 (2.0)	4.2 (0.2)	10.3 (1.4)	8.1 (1.6)	14.4 (2.4)	8.3 (2.4)	10.5 (3.1)	7.5 (1.7)
Other parental loss	7.6 (1.0)	3.9 (0.3)	8.7 (1.6)	4.0 (0.2)	8.8 (1.5)	8.4 (1.6)	8.9 (1.8)	7.6 (2.0)	9.4 (2.5)	7.8 (1.6)
Family violence	15.5 (1.1)	6.1 (0.3)	19.2 (1.7)	6.3 (0.3)	18.6 (1.8)	15.9 (2.2)	18.1 (2.0)	15.3 (3.0)	21.3 (3.4)	12.9 (2.2)
Physical illness	3.3 (0.5)	1.9 (0.2)	3.9 (1.0)	2.0 (0.2)	3.6 (0.9)	3.9 (1.1)	4.0 (1.4)	3.2 (1.4)	3.9 (1.7)	3.9 (1.1)
Financial adversity	3.7 (0.5)	2.8 (0.2)	3.7 (0.9)	2.8 (0.2)	4.6 (1.0)	3.7 (1.0)	4.7 (1.4)	1.6 (0.8)	2.0 (1.0)	3.6 (1.1)
Number of adversities[b]										
1	32.0 (1.6)	22.2 (0.5)	30.9 (2.5)	22.4 (0.5)	30.0 (2.0)	34.2 (3.8)	29.6 (2.8)	30.9 (4.7)	34.2 (4.3)	36.7 (4.2)
2	15.9 (1.1)	7.5 (0.3)	19.0 (1.9)	7.6 (0.3)	17.9 (1.7)	16.0 (2.2)	19.3 (2.4)	12.8 (2.7)	30.2 (3.9)	23.2 (3.1)
3	6.6 (0.9)	2.4 (0.2)	9.0 (1.2)	2.5 (0.2)	9.2 (1.5)	6.7 (1.2)	9.4 (1.5)	7.9 (3.1)		
4+	3.3 (0.4)	0.7 (0.1)	5.1 (0.8)	0.7 (0.1)	4.4 (0.7)	3.8 (1.0)	5.8 (1.0)	3.9 (1.6)		
N[c]	(1687)	(57,216)	(635)	(57,623)	(721)	(1234)	(411)	(320)	(194)	(911)

[a] % represents the percentage of people with the adversity among the cases with the outcome variable indicated in the column header. For example, the first cell is the % of those with physical abuse among those with ideation.

[b] For number of adversities, the last OR represents the odds for that number of adversities or more. For example, for unplanned attempt, 2 represents ≥2 (that is, 2+).

[c] N represents the number of person–years.

Appendix Table 8.4. Prevalence of childhood adversities among those with each type of suicidal behavior (low-income countries)

Childhood adversity	Among total sample						Among ideators			
	%ᵃ (SE) with adversities						%ᵃ (SE) with adversities			
	Ideation	No ideation	Attempt	No attempt	Plan	No plan	Planned attempt	No planned attempt	Unplanned attempt	No unplanned attempt
Type of adversity										
Physical abuse	23.5 (1.5)	9.8 (0.4)	30.5 (2.7)	10.1 (0.4)	23.8 (1.9)	29.2 (2.9)	25.2 (3.0)	22.0 (4.6)	33.1 (4.3)	28.6 (3.4)
Sexual abuse	3.5 (0.6)	0.8 (0.1)	6.6 (1.4)	0.8 (0.1)	4.4 (1.2)	3.4 (0.8)	6.0 (2.1)	1.6 (0.6)	6.7 (2.2)	2.0 (0.7)
Neglect	10.3 (1.0)	4.4 (0.3)	13.7 (1.9)	4.5 (0.3)	12.2 (1.9)	11.1 (1.6)	11.7 (2.0)	16.9 (5.7)	11.8 (2.9)	9.7 (1.7)
Parental death	17.2 (1.4)	16.3 (0.5)	20.3 (2.1)	16.2 (0.5)	20.6 (2.1)	17.5 (2.4)	24.9 (2.9)	26.2 (5.6)	14.4 (3.9)	17.4 (2.6)
Parental divorce	8.9 (1.1)	4.0 (0.3)	7.8 (1.5)	4.2 (0.3)	6.7 (1.1)	7.4 (1.4)	6.2 (1.5)	7.1 (2.2)	10.9 (3.4)	8.2 (1.7)
Other parental loss	10.8 (1.1)	9.3 (0.4)	11.0 (1.4)	9.4 (0.4)	10.1 (1.2)	11.5 (1.6)	11.4 (2.0)	8.1 (2.3)	9.3 (2.3)	11.7 (2.0)
Family violence	12.7 (1.1)	4.7 (0.2)	19.8 (2.4)	4.9 (0.2)	13.3 (1.9)	14.5 (1.9)	11.7 (1.9)	16.3 (5.8)	25.7 (4.1)	12.5 (2.0)
Physical illness	5.8 (0.8)	3.4 (0.3)	5.5 (1.4)	3.4 (0.2)	5.3 (1.2)	6.3 (1.3)	4.0 (1.1)	7.9 (2.9)	5.8 (1.7)	6.7 (1.5)
Financial adversity	2.5 (0.6)	1.4 (0.2)	1.7 (0.6)	1.5 (0.2)	2.4 (0.7)	2.8 (1.3)	2.2 (1.0)	3.3 (1.6)	1.3 (0.6)	2.9 (1.4)
Number of adversitiesᵇ										
1	29.0 (1.5)	26.5 (0.7)	26.6 (2.4)	26.4 (0.7)	27.3 (2.1)	30.2 (2.7)	27.0 (3.0)	27.5 (4.1)	27.4 (4.1)	31.2 (3.3)
2	14.5 (1.1)	8.2 (0.3)	17.9 (1.9)	8.4 (0.3)	14.7 (1.6)	14.7 (2.0)	17.5 (2.5)	14.0 (3.5)	33.3 (4.4)	26.8 (3.2)
3	7.2 (0.9)	2.7 (0.2)	8.0 (1.4)	2.8 (0.3)	7.5 (1.4)	9.1 (1.9)	11.8 (2.3)	16.5 (5.9)		
4+	3.7 (0.8)	0.8 (0.1)	7.1 (2.3)	0.8 (0.1)	4.6 (1.2)	3.9 (1.2)				
Nᶜ	(1639)	(40,936)	(583)	(39,548)	(717)	(1292)	(353)	(384)	(192)	(843)

ᵃ % represents the percentage of people with the adversity among the cases with the outcome variable indicated in the column header. For example, the first cell is the % of those with physical abuse among those with ideation.

ᵇ For number of adversities, the last OR represents the odds for that number of adversities or more. For example, for no unplanned attempt, 2 represents ≥2 (that is, 2+).

ᶜ N represents the number of person–years.

Appendix Table 8.5. Multivariate associations between number of childhood adversities and subsequent onset of suicidal behavior[a] (high-income countries)

Number of childhood adversities[b]	Among total sample			Among ideators	
	Ideation	Attempt	Plan	Planned attempt	Unplanned attempt
	OR (95% CI)	OR (95% CI)	OR (95% CI)	OR (95% CI)	OR (95% CI)
1	1.9* (1.7–2.1)	2.7* (2.3–3.2)	1.2 (0.9–1.4)	1.3 (0.9–1.9)	1.3 (0.9–1.8)
2	2.5* (2.2–2.8)	4.3* (3.5–5.2)	1.4* (1.1–1.8)	1.2 (0.8–1.8)	1.6* (1.1–2.4)
3	4.5* (3.8–5.4)	9.6* (7.5–12.2)	1.4* (1.0–1.9)	2.4* (1.5–4.0)	1.9* (1.2–3.0)
4	5.8* (4.4–7.5)	15.4* (11.7–20.4)	1.5* (1.1–2.2)	2.5* (1.2–4.9)	2.7* (1.4–5.4)
5	6.1* (4.2–9.0)	18.9* (12.2–29.3)	1.2 (0.7–2.0)	8.4* (3.4–20.6)	2.9* (1.5–5.6)
6+	5.5* (3.6–8.3)	23.2* (15.7–34.2)			
χ^2 (p-value)	574.6 (<0.001)*	622.0 (<0.001)*	11.1 (0.05)	34.3 (<0.001)*	16.8 (0.01)*

* Significant at the 0.05 level, two-sided test.
[a] Assessed in the Part 2 sample due to having Part 2 controls. Models control for person–years, country, and significant variables from the chapters on sociodemographics and parental psychopathology.
[b] For number of adversities, the last OR represents the odds for that number of adversities or more. For example, for unplanned attempt, 5 represents ≥5 (that is, 5+).

Appendix Table 8.6. Multivariate associations between number of childhood adversities and subsequent onset of suicidal behavior[a] (middle-income countries)

Number of childhood adversities[b]	Among total sample			Among ideators	
	Ideation	Attempt	Plan	Planned attempt	Unplanned attempt
	OR (95% CI)	OR (95% CI)	OR (95% CI)	OR (95% CI)	OR (95% CI)
1	1.8* (1.5–2.1)	1.9* (1.4–2.5)	0.8 (0.6–1.1)	1.0 (0.6–1.9)	1.2 (0.7–2.0)
2	2.3* (1.9–2.7)	2.9* (2.2–4.0)	1.1 (0.7–1.7)	1.9 (0.9–4.0)	1.4 (0.8–2.5)
3	2.6* (1.8–3.6)	3.5* (2.3–5.2)	1.4 (0.9–2.3)	1.5 (0.6–3.9)	
4+	4.2* (2.9–6.0)	6.2* (3.9–9.9)	1.1 (0.6–2.2)	1.7 (0.7–3.8)	
χ^2 (p-value)	156.4 (<0.001)*	107.6 (<0.001)*	7.9 (0.09)	4.8 (0.31)	1.5 (0.47)

* Significant at the 0.05 level, two-sided test.
[a] Assessed in the Part 2 sample due to having Part 2 controls. Models control for person–years, country, and significant variables from the chapters on sociodemographics and parental psychopathology.
[b] For number of adversities, the last OR represents the odds for that number of adversities or more. For example, for unplanned attempt, 2 represents ≥2 (that is, 2+).

Appendix Table 8.7. Multivariate associations between number of childhood adversities and subsequent onset of suicidal behavior[a] (low-income countries)

Number of childhood adversities[b]	Among total sample		Among ideators		
	Ideation	Attempt	Plan	Planned attempt	Unplanned attempt
	OR (95% CI)	OR (95% CI)	OR (95% CI)	OR (95% CI)	OR (95% CI)
1	1.6* (1.4–2.0)	1.6* (1.2–2.1)	0.9 (0.7–1.4)	1.0 (0.6–1.7)	0.8 (0.5–1.5)
2	2.5* (2.0–3.0)	2.9* (2.1–3.9)	1.1 (0.7–1.8)	1.1 (0.5–2.3)	1.0 (0.5–1.7)
3	2.8* (2.0–3.9)	2.6* (1.5–4.3)	0.8 (0.4–1.4)	0.6 (0.2–1.3)	
4+	5.3* (3.1–9.0)	7.6* (3.7–15.5)	1.0 (0.5–1.9)		
χ^2 (p-value)	89.9 (<0.001)*	61.6 (<0.001)*	1.4 (0.85)	2.1 (0.55)	0.4 (0.81)

* Significant at the 0.05 level, two-sided test.
[a] Assessed in the Part 2 sample due to having Part 2 controls. Models control for person–years, country, and significant variables from the chapters on sociodemographics and parental psychopathology.
[b] For number of adversities, the last OR represents the odds for that number of adversities or more. For example, for unplanned attempt, 2 represents ≥2 (that is, 2+).

Appendix Table 8.8. Multivariate interactive associations between type and number of childhood adversities and subsequent onset of suicidal behavior[a] (high-income countries)

Childhood adversity	Among total sample		Among ideators		
	Ideation	Attempt	Plan	Planned attempt	Unplanned attempt
	OR (95% CI)	OR (95% CI)	OR (95% CI)	OR (95% CI)	OR (95% CI)
Type of adversity					
Physical abuse	3.0* (2.5–3.5)	4.3* (3.2–5.7)	1.2 (0.9–1.6)	1.3 (0.8–2.2)	1.0 (0.6–1.7)
Sexual abuse	3.4* (2.9–4.0)	4.8* (3.7–6.2)	1.2 (0.9–1.6)	1.3 (0.8–2.0)	1.0 (0.6–1.7)
Neglect	2.5* (2.1–3.0)	3.7* (2.9–4.9)	1.5* (1.1–2.0)	1.9* (1.2–3.0)	1.2 (0.7–2.1)
Parental death	1.3* (1.2–1.6)	1.9* (1.5–2.4)	1.1 (0.8–1.5)	1.5 (0.9–2.5)	1.3 (0.8–2.1)
Parental divorce	1.7* (1.5–2.0)	2.4* (1.9–3.0)	0.9 (0.7–1.2)	1.4 (0.9–2.4)	1.5 (1.0–2.4)
Other parental loss	1.8* (1.5–2.2)	2.5* (1.9–3.3)	0.9 (0.6–1.3)	1.2 (0.6–2.2)	1.6 (0.9–2.8)
Family violence	1.8* (1.5–2.1)	2.1* (1.6–2.8)	1.2 (0.9–1.6)	1.1 (0.7–1.8)	1.1 (0.7–1.7)
Physical illness	2.2* (1.8–2.5)	3.1* (2.4–4.0)	1.2 (0.9–1.7)	1.2 (0.6–2.3)	1.6 (0.9–2.8)
Financial adversity	1.3 (1.0–1.6)	1.5* (1.1–1.9)	0.6* (0.4–0.9)	0.9 (0.4–1.9)	1.3 (0.7–2.7)
9 df χ^2 test for 9 types	410.0 (<0.001)*	239.3 (<0.001)*	30.1 (<0.001)*	10.3 (0.33)	9.4 (0.40)
8 df χ^2 test for difference between types	194.4 (<0.001)*	113.1 (<0.001)*	28.7 (<0.001)*	6.6 (0.58)	6.4 (0.60)
Number of adversities[b]					
2	0.7* (0.5–0.8)	0.6* (0.4–0.8)	1.1 (0.8–1.6)	0.7 (0.4–1.3)	1.1 (0.6–2.0)
3	0.6* (0.4–0.8)	0.4* (0.3–0.7)	1.0 (0.6–1.7)	1.0 (0.4–2.8)	1.0 (0.4–2.6)
4	0.3* (0.2–0.5)	0.2* (0.1–0.4)	1.0 (0.5–2.1)	0.8 (0.2–2.8)	1.1 (0.3–4.2)
5	0.2* (0.1–0.3)	0.1* (0.0–0.2)	0.7 (0.3–2.2)	2.1 (0.3–14.9)	1.0 (0.2–5.9)
6+	0.1* (0.0–0.1)	0.0* (0.0–0.1)			
χ^2 (p-value)	68.7 (<0.001)*	55.1 (<0.001)*	2.1 (0.71)	8.3 (0.08)	0.2 (0.99)

* Significant at the 0.05 level, two-sided test.
[a] Assessed in the Part 2 sample due to having Part 2 controls. Models control for person–years, country, and significant variables from the chapters on sociodemographics and parental psychopathology.
[b] For number of adversities, the last OR represents the odds for that number of adversities or more. For example, for unplanned attempt, 5 represents ≥5 (that is, 5+).

Appendix Table 8.9. Multivariate interactive associations between type and number of childhood adversities and subsequent onset of suicidal behavior[a] (middle-income countries)

	Among total sample			Among ideators	
	Ideation	Attempt	Plan	Planned attempt	Unplanned attempt
Childhood adversity	OR (95% CI)	OR (95% CI)	OR (95% CI)	OR (95% CI)	OR (95% CI)
Type of adversity					
Physical abuse	2.4* (1.9–3.0)	2.4* (1.8–3.4)	0.8 (0.5–1.4)	1.0 (0.5–2.2)	0.9 (0.5–1.8)
Sexual abuse	2.6* (1.5–4.3)	4.0* (2.2–7.5)	1.6 (0.7–3.5)	1.1 (0.3–3.7)	0.7 (0.2–2.1)
Neglect	2.3* (1.7–3.1)	2.5* (1.6–3.8)	1.1 (0.7–1.8)	1.1 (0.5–2.5)	1.2 (0.6–2.5)
Parental death	1.5* (1.2–1.8)	1.4 (1.0–1.9)	0.7 (0.5–1.1)	1.0 (0.5–2.3)	1.0 (0.6–2.0)
Parental divorce	1.6* (1.2–2.1)	2.2* (1.4–3.5)	0.8 (0.4–1.5)	2.0 (0.7–5.2)	1.4 (0.5–3.7)
Other parental loss	1.6* (1.1–2.2)	1.4 (0.8–2.6)	0.9 (0.5–1.6)	1.1 (0.4–2.9)	1.1 (0.4–2.8)
Family violence	1.6* (1.2–2.1)	1.5 (1.0–2.2)	0.8 (0.4–1.3)	0.9 (0.4–2.3)	1.4 (0.7–2.7)
Physical illness	1.7* (1.1–2.5)	1.6 (0.8–3.2)	0.5* (0.2–0.9)	0.5 (0.2–1.4)	0.9 (0.3–2.6)
Financial adversity	1.6* (1.1–2.4)	1.4 (0.7–2.7)	1.0 (0.4–2.2)	2.4 (0.5–10.2)	0.6 (0.1–2.8)
9 df χ^2 test for 9 types	85.5 (<0.001)*	59.8 (<0.001)*	10.3 (0.32)	8.6 (0.47)	2.4 (0.98)
8 df χ^2 test for difference between types	35.5 (<0.001)*	32.0 (<0.001)*	8.8 (0.36)	8.2 (0.41)	1.9 (0.98)
Number of adversities[b]					
2	0.7* (0.5–0.9)	0.8 (0.5–1.4)	1.5 (0.8–2.8)	1.5 (0.6–3.9)	1.1 (0.4–2.8)
3	0.4* (0.2–0.7)	0.5 (0.2–1.1)	2.3 (0.9–5.7)	1.1 (0.2–5.5)	
4+	0.3* (0.1–0.6)	0.3 (0.1–1.1)	2.1 (0.5–8.2)	1.0 (0.1–10.4)	
χ^2 (p-value)	16.0 (0.001)*	5.2 (0.16)	4.1 (0.25)	1.6 (0.65)	0.0 (0.91)

* Significant at the 0.05 level, two-sided test.
[a] Assessed in the Part 2 sample due to having Part 2 controls. Models control for person–years, country, and significant variables from the chapters on sociodemographics and parental psychopathology.
[b] For number of adversities, the last OR represents the odds for that number of adversities or more. For example, for unplanned attempt, 2 represents ≥2 (that is, 2+).

Appendix Table 8.10. Multivariate interactive associations between type and number of childhood adversities and subsequent onset of suicidal behavior[a] (low-income countries)

Childhood adversity	Among total sample		Among ideators		
	Ideation	Attempt	Plan	Planned attempt	Unplanned attempt
	OR (95% CI)	OR (95% CI)	OR (95% CI)	OR (95% CI)	OR (95% CI)
Type of adversity					
Physical abuse	2.4* (1.8–3.2)	2.5* (1.7–3.8)	0.7 (0.4–1.1)	1.5 (0.6–3.4)	0.8 (0.4–1.5)
Sexual abuse	2.7* (1.5–5.0)	4.8* (2.2–10.4)	1.3 (0.7–2.3)	3.8 (0.8–18.5)	4.0* (1.5–11.0)
Neglect	1.5* (1.0–2.2)	1.4 (0.8–2.4)	1.1 (0.6–2.1)	0.9 (0.3–2.4)	0.7 (0.3–1.5)
Parental death	1.3 (1.0–1.6)	1.4* (1.0–1.9)	1.2 (0.7–1.8)	1.3 (0.7–2.4)	0.6 (0.3–1.3)
Parental divorce	1.8* (1.3–2.5)	1.1 (0.7–1.8)	0.9 (0.5–1.7)	1.1 (0.4–3.2)	0.8 (0.3–2.0)
Other parental loss	1.4* (1.0–1.9)	1.3 (0.8–2.1)	1.0 (0.6–1.5)	1.6 (0.7–3.7)	0.9 (0.4–2.0)
Family violence	1.4 (1.0–1.9)	1.6 (1.0–2.6)	0.9 (0.5–1.6)	0.5 (0.2–1.3)	1.5 (0.7–3.0)
Physical illness	1.9* (1.3–2.8)	1.3 (0.7–2.4)	0.7 (0.3–1.4)	0.5 (0.1–1.4)	0.7 (0.3–1.7)
Financial adversity	1.3 (0.7–2.4)	0.7 (0.3–1.7)	1.1 (0.4–3.3)	0.6 (0.1–4.5)	0.4 (0.1–1.7)
9 df χ^2 test for 9 types	51.6 (<0.001)*	38.1 (<0.001)*	8.3 (0.51)	12.0 (0.21)	17.8 (0.04)*
8 df χ^2 test for difference between types	37.6 (<0.001)*	36.5 (<0.001)*	8.3 (0.40)	11.4 (0.18)	16.2 (0.04)*
Number of adversities[b]					
2 s	0.9 (0.6–1.3)	1.1 (0.6–1.9)	1.4 (0.7–2.8)	1.2 (0.4–3.8)	1.3 (0.5–3.3)
3	0.6 (0.3–1.0)	0.6 (0.2–1.5)	1.1 (0.4–3.4)	0.5 (0.1–3.7)	
4+	0.5 (0.2–1.5)	0.8 (0.2–4.2)	1.5 (0.3–7.3)		
χ^2 (p-value)	5.1 (0.16)	5.0 (0.17)	1.6 (0.66)	1.8 (0.40)	0.3 (0.61)

* Significant at the 0.05 level, two-sided test.
[a] Assessed in the Part 2 sample due to having Part 2 controls. Models control for person–years, country, and significant variables from the chapters on sociodemographics and parental psychopathology.
[b] For number of adversities, the last OR represents the odds for that number of adversities or more. For example, for unplanned attempt, 2 represents ≥2 (that is, 2+).

Appendix Table 8.11. Multivariate interactive associations between type and number of childhood adversities and subsequent onset of suicidal behavior after adjustment for respondents' lifetime mental disorders[a] (high-income countries)

Childhood adversity	Among total sample			Among ideators	
	Ideation	Attempt	Plan	Planned attempt	Unplanned attempt
	OR (95% CI)	OR (95% CI)	OR (95% CI)	OR (95% CI)	OR (95% CI)
Type of adversity					
Physical abuse	2.4* (2.1–2.9)	3.2* (2.4–4.2)	1.1 (0.8–1.5)	1.4 (0.8–2.2)	1.0 (0.6–1.6)
Sexual abuse	2.5* (2.1–2.9)	3.3* (2.5–4.2)	1.1 (0.8–1.5)	1.4 (0.9–2.2)	1.0 (0.6–1.6)
Neglect	2.3* (2.0–2.8)	3.3* (2.5–4.3)	1.5* (1.1–2.0)	1.9* (1.2–3.1)	1.3 (0.7–2.2)
Parental death	1.3* (1.2–1.5)	1.9* (1.5–2.3)	1.1 (0.8–1.5)	1.6 (1.0–2.5)	1.2 (0.8–2.0)
Parental divorce	1.7* (1.5–2.0)	2.3* (1.8–3.0)	0.9 (0.7–1.2)	1.5 (0.9–2.4)	1.5 (1.0–2.4)
Other parental loss	1.6* (1.3–2.0)	2.3* (1.8–3.1)	0.8 (0.6–1.2)	1.3 (0.7–2.5)	1.6 (0.9–2.8)
Family violence	1.6* (1.4–1.8)	1.9* (1.4–2.4)	1.2 (0.9–1.5)	1.1 (0.7–1.9)	1.1 (0.7–1.6)
Physical illness	1.9* (1.7–2.3)	2.6* (2.0–3.4)	1.2 (0.9–1.7)	1.2 (0.6–2.2)	1.6 (1.0–2.8)
Financial adversity	1.2 (0.9–1.5)	1.3 (0.9–1.7)	0.6* (0.4–0.9)	0.9 (0.4–1.8)	1.4 (0.7–2.6)
9 df χ² test for 9 types	287.9 (<0.001)*	159.7 (<0.001)*	29.3 (<0.001)*	10.1 (0.34)	11.5 (0.24)
8 df χ² test for difference between types	113.8 (<0.001)*	69.8 (<0.001)*	27.5 (<0.001)*	6.0 (0.65)	10.2 (0.25)
Number of adversities[b]					
2	0.7* (0.6–0.9)	0.6* (0.5–0.9)	1.1 (0.8–1.6)	0.7 (0.4–1.3)	1.1 (0.6–2.0)
3	0.6* (0.4–0.8)	0.5* (0.3–0.7)	1.0 (0.6–1.8)	0.9 (0.3–2.5)	1.0 (0.4–2.6)
4	0.4* (0.2–0.5)	0.3* (0.1–0.5)	1.0 (0.5–2.1)	0.7 (0.2–2.5)	1.1 (0.3–4.1)
5	0.2* (0.1–0.3)	0.1* (0.0–0.3)	0.8 (0.3–2.3)	2.1 (0.3–14.8)	0.9 (0.2–5.2)
6+	0.1* (0.0–0.2)	0.0* (0.0–0.1)			
χ² (p-value)	50.2 (<0.001)*	37.1 (<0.001)*	2.0 (0.73)	10.3 (0.04)*	0.4 (0.98)

* Significant at the 0.05 level, two-sided test.
[a] Assessed in the Part 2 sample due to having Part 2 controls. Models control for person–years, country, and significant variables from the chapters on sociodemographics and parental psychopathology.
[b] For number of adversities, the last OR represents the odds for that number of adversities or more. For example, for unplanned attempt, 5 represents ≥5 (that is, 5+).

Appendix Table 8.12. Multivariate interactive associations between type and number of childhood adversities and subsequent onset of suicidal behavior after adjustment for respondents' lifetime mental disorders[a] (middle-income countries)

Childhood adversity	Among total sample			Among ideators	
	Ideation	Attempt	Plan	Planned attempt	Unplanned attempt
	OR (95% CI)	OR (95% CI)	OR (95% CI)	OR (95% CI)	OR (95% CI)
Type of adversity					
Physical abuse	2.0* (1.6–2.5)	2.0* (1.4–2.8)	0.9 (0.5–1.4)	1.1 (0.5–2.3)	0.9 (0.5–1.8)
Sexual abuse	2.1* (1.3–3.4)	3.1* (1.7–5.5)	1.5 (0.7–3.3)	1.1 (0.3–4.0)	0.7 (0.2–2.1)
Neglect	2.2* (1.7–2.9)	2.3* (1.5–3.5)	1.0 (0.6–1.7)	1.3 (0.6–2.9)	1.2 (0.6–2.5)
Parental death	1.5* (1.2–1.8)	1.3 (0.9–1.9)	0.7 (0.5–1.1)	0.8 (0.4–1.9)	1.0 (0.6–2.0)
Parental divorce	1.5* (1.1–1.9)	2.0* (1.3–3.1)	0.8 (0.4–1.4)	2.0 (0.7–5.4)	1.4 (0.5–3.7)
Other parental loss	1.5* (1.1–2.0)	1.4 (0.8–2.4)	0.9 (0.5–1.5)	1.1 (0.4–2.8)	1.1 (0.4–2.8)

Appendix Table 8.12. (cont.)

Childhood adversity	Among total sample			Among ideators	
	Ideation	Attempt	Plan	Planned attempt	Unplanned attempt
	OR (95% CI)	OR (95% CI)	OR (95% CI)	OR (95% CI)	OR (95% CI)
Family violence	1.4* (1.1–1.9)	1.3 (0.9–1.9)	0.8 (0.4–1.3)	0.9 (0.3–2.4)	1.4 (0.7–2.7)
Physical illness	1.5 (1.0–2.2)	1.4 (0.7–2.5)	0.5* (0.2–0.9)	0.8 (0.3–2.3)	0.9 (0.3–2.6)
Financial adversity	1.5* (1.0–2.1)	1.3 (0.7–2.5)	1.0 (0.4–2.3)	1.8 (0.4–8.0)	0.6 (0.1–2.8)
9 df χ^2 test for 9 types	62.6 (<0.001)*	34.5 (<0.001)*	9.9 (0.36)	6.2 (0.72)	2.4 (0.98)
8 df χ^2 test for difference between types	24.1 (0.002)*	19.5 (0.01)*	7.8 (0.45)	5.9 (0.66)	1.9 (0.98)
Number of adversities[b]					
2	0.7* (0.5–0.9)	0.8 (0.5–1.4)	1.4 (0.7–2.6)	1.6 (0.6–4.5)	1.1 (0.4–2.8)
3	0.4* (0.2–0.7)	0.5 (0.2–1.1)	2.1 (0.9–5.1)	0.9 (0.2–5.1)	
4+	0.3* (0.1–0.6)	0.3 (0.1–1.0)	1.9 (0.5–7.3)	0.8 (0.1–7.8)	
χ^2 (p-value)	15.8 (0.001)*	6.0 (0.11)	3.3 (0.35)	2.8 (0.42)	0.0 (0.91)

* Significant at the 0.05 level, two-sided test.
[a] Assessed in the Part 2 sample due to having Part 2 controls. Models control for person–years, country, and significant variables from the chapters on sociodemographics and parental psychopathology.
[b] For number of adversities, the last OR represents the odds for that number of adversities or more. For example, for unplanned attempt, 2 represents ≥2 (that is, 2+).

Appendix Table 8.13. Multivariate interactive associations between type and number of childhood adversities and subsequent onset of suicidal behavior after adjustment for respondents' lifetime mental disorders[a] (low-income countries)

Childhood adversity	Among total sample			Among ideators	
	Ideation	Attempt	Plan	Planned attempt	Unplanned attempt
	OR (95% CI)	OR (95% CI)	OR (95% CI)	OR (95% CI)	OR (95% CI)
Type of adversity					
Physical abuse	2.1* (1.6–2.9)	2.2* (1.4–3.2)	0.6* (0.4–1.0)	1.4 (0.5–3.4)	0.8 (0.4–1.5)
Sexual abuse	2.5* (1.4–4.5)	3.9* (1.8–8.5)	1.0 (0.6–1.9)	3.9 (0.9–17.1)	4.0* (1.5–11.0)
Neglect	1.4* (1.0–2.1)	1.3 (0.8–2.2)	0.9 (0.5–1.7)	0.7 (0.2–2.3)	0.7 (0.3–1.5)
Parental death	1.2 (1.0–1.5)	1.3* (1.0–1.8)	1.2 (0.7–1.8)	1.5 (0.8–2.8)	0.6 (0.3–1.3)
Parental divorce	1.7* (1.2–2.4)	1.1 (0.7–1.7)	0.8 (0.5–1.5)	1.2 (0.3–4.0)	0.8 (0.3–2.0)
Other parental loss	1.4* (1.0–1.8)	1.2 (0.8–2.0)	0.9 (0.6–1.4)	1.7 (0.7–4.2)	0.9 (0.4–2.0)
Family violence	1.3 (0.9–1.8)	1.5 (0.9–2.3)	0.7 (0.4–1.4)	0.4 (0.1–1.1)	1.5 (0.7–3.0)
Physical illness	1.7* (1.2–2.5)	1.1 (0.6–2.0)	0.6 (0.3–1.2)	0.5 (0.2–1.9)	0.7 (0.3–1.7)
Financial adversity	1.3 (0.7–2.5)	0.7 (0.3–1.6)	0.9 (0.3–3.1)	0.4 (0.0–4.8)	0.4 (0.1–1.7)
9 df χ^2 test for 9 types	37.3 (<0.001)*	29.7 (<0.001)*	10.4 (0.32)	15.5 (0.08)	17.8 (0.04)*
8 df χ^2 test for difference between types	28.2 (<0.001)*	28.7 (<0.001)*	9.6 (0.29)	15.5 (0.05)	16.2 (0.04)*

Appendix Table 8.13. (cont.)

| | Among total sample | | | Among ideators | |
| Childhood adversity | Ideation | Attempt | Plan | Planned attempt | Unplanned attempt |
	OR (95% CI)	OR (95% CI)	OR (95% CI)	OR (95% CI)	OR (95% CI)
Number of adversities[b]					
2	0.9 (0.6–1.3)	1.1 (0.6–1.9)	1.5 (0.7–3.0)	1.1 (0.3–3.8)	1.3 (0.5–3.3)
3	0.6 (0.4–1.1)	0.6 (0.3–1.4)	1.4 (0.5–4.4)	0.6 (0.1–4.6)	
4+	0.6 (0.2–1.6)	0.9 (0.2–4.2)	2.2 (0.4–10.6)		
χ^2 (p-value)	4.2 (0.24)	5.7 (0.13)	1.8 (0.62)	1.0 (0.60)	0.3 (0.61)

* Significant at the 0.05 level, two-sided test.
[a] Assessed in the Part 2 sample due to having Part 2 controls. Models control for person–years, country, and significant variables from the chapters on sociodemographics and parental psychopathology.
[b] For number of adversities, the last OR represents the odds for that number of adversities or more. For example, for unplanned attempt, 2 represents ≥2 (that is, 2+).

Appendix Table 8.14. Multivariate interactive associations between type and number of childhood adversities with subsequent onset of suicide attempt across the lifespan[a] (high-income countries)

| Childhood adversity | Lifetime attempt during childhood (age 4–12 years) | Lifetime attempt during teen years (age 13–19 years) | Lifetime attempt during young adulthood (age 20–29 years) | Lifetime attempt during later adulthood (age 30+ years) |
	OR (95% CI)	OR (95% CI)	OR (95% CI)	OR (95% CI)
Type of adversity				
Physical abuse	6.1* (2.4–15.6)	5.5* (3.6–8.3)	3.1* (1.9–5.2)	3.4* (2.0–5.9)
Sexual abuse	8.8* (2.8–27.1)	6.6* (4.6–9.5)	3.3* (2.1–5.3)	3.3* (1.9–5.5)
Neglect	4.8 (1.0–24.1)	2.9* (2.0–4.1)	3.3* (2.0–5.2)	5.2* (3.3–8.1)
Parental death	1.3 (0.4–4.1)	2.2* (1.5–3.2)	1.4 (0.9–2.2)	1.9* (1.2–2.9)
Parental divorce	2.8* (1.2–6.5)	2.6* (1.8–3.7)	2.0* (1.3–3.1)	2.3* (1.4–3.9)
Other parental loss	5.4* (2.1–14.0)	2.7* (1.7–4.4)	1.9* (1.2–3.1)	2.9* (1.7–5.2)
Family violence	2.8 (0.9–8.3)	2.2* (1.5–3.3)	1.8* (1.1–2.9)	2.4* (1.4–3.9)
Physical illness	3.7* (1.5–9.1)	3.2* (2.1–4.8)	3.2* (2.0–5.1)	2.6* (1.5–4.7)
Financial adversity	1.5 (0.5–4.1)	1.6* (1.0–2.6)	1.2 (0.7–2.1)	1.6 (0.7–3.5)
9 df χ^2 test for 9 types	44.5 (<0.001)*	150.4 (<0.001)*	61.0 (<0.001)*	62.1 (<0.001)*
8 df χ^2 test for difference between types	37.4 (<0.001)*	83.8 (<0.001)*	32.0 (<0.001)*	20.2 (0.01)*
Number of adversities[b]				
2	0.9 (0.2–3.5)	0.5* (0.3–0.8)	0.7 (0.4–1.3)	0.6 (0.3–1.1)
3	0.6 (0.1–4.2)	0.3* (0.1–0.6)	0.7 (0.3–1.6)	0.5 (0.2–1.3)
4	0.2 (0.0–3.9)	0.2* (0.1–0.5)	0.4 (0.1–1.4)	0.2* (0.0–0.5)
5	0.1 (0.0–5.4)	0.2* (0.1–1.0)	0.3 (0.1–1.3)	0.0* (0.0–0.2)
6+	0.0 (0.0–3.1)		0.0* (0.0–0.4)	0.0* (0.0–0.1)
χ^2 (p-value)	12.1 (0.03)*	24.7 (<0.001)*	10.7 (0.06)	38.9 (<0.001)*

* Significant at the 0.05 level, two-sided test.
[a] Assessed in the Part 2 sample due to having Part 2 controls. Models control for person–years, country, and significant variables from the chapters on sociodemographics and parental psychopathology.
[b] For number of adversities, the last OR represents the odds for that number of adversities or more. For example, for lifetime attempt during teen years (ages 13–19 years), 5 represents ≥5 (that is, 5+).

Appendix Table 8.15. Multivariate interactive associations between type and number of childhood adversities with subsequent onset of suicide attempt across the lifespan[a] (middle-income countries)

Childhood adversity	Lifetime attempt during childhood (age 4–12 years) OR (95% CI)	Lifetime attempt during teen years (age 13–19 years) OR (95% CI)	Lifetime attempt during young adulthood (age 20–29 years) OR (95% CI)	Lifetime attempt during later adulthood (age 30+ years) OR (95% CI)
Type of adversity				
Physical abuse	4.8* (1.3–18.1)	3.3* (2.1–5.3)	1.8* (1.0–3.0)	2.0* (1.1–3.8)
Sexual abuse	96.1* (16.4–562.5)	4.2* (1.6–11.2)	1.6 (0.5–5.4)	3.1 (0.8–11.9)
Neglect	6.8* (1.0–45.9)	2.8* (1.3–6.1)	1.7 (0.8–3.4)	2.8* (1.3–5.8)
Parental death	3.9 (0.5–28.6)	1.5 (0.9–2.7)	1.2 (0.7–2.3)	1.2 (0.6–2.6)
Parental divorce	6.5 (0.8–50.2)	2.8* (1.6–4.9)	1.9 (0.9–4.0)	1.4 (0.4–4.7)
Other parental loss	2.8 (0.2–47.2)	2.0 (0.9–4.5)	1.0 (0.4–2.5)	1.1 (0.5–2.1)
Family violence	2.1 (0.5–8.3)	1.7 (0.9–3.5)	1.0 (0.5–1.9)	1.6 (0.8–3.2)
Physical illness	2.5 (0.5–12.1)	2.5 (0.8–7.8)	0.3 (0.0–2.1)	2.8* (1.2–6.6)
Financial adversity	0.0* (0.0–0.0)	1.6 (0.5–5.1)	1.1 (0.4–3.2)	1.2 (0.4–3.8)
9 df χ^2 test for 9 types	758.6 (<0.001)*	40.1 (<0.001)*	16.5 (0.06)	20.7 (0.01)*
8 df χ^2 test for difference between types	700.6 (<0.001)*	16.1 (0.04)*	10.6 (0.22)	14.7 (0.06)
Number of adversities				
2	0.1* (0.0–0.5)	0.5 (0.2–1.3)	1.6 (0.7–3.6)	1.0 (0.4–2.7)
3	0.1 (0.0–1.5)	0.2* (0.1–0.9)	1.7 (0.5–5.8)	0.6 (0.1–2.8)
4+	0.0 (0.0–4.3)	0.1* (0.0–1.0)	0.7 (0.1–4.5)	0.8 (0.1–5.9)
χ^2_2 (p-value)	10.4 (0.02)*	5.1 (0.17)	5.7 (0.13)	1.3 (0.72)

* Significant at the 0.05 level, two-sided test.
0.0* (0.0–0.0) OR is ≤ .05 indicating very low risk.
[a] Assessed in the Part 2 sample due to having Part 2 controls. Models control for person–years, country, and significant variables from the chapters on sociodemographics and parental psychopathology.

Appendix Table 8.16. Multivariate interactive associations between type and number of childhood adversities with subsequent onset of suicide attempt across the lifespan[a] (low-income countries)

Childhood adversity	Lifetime attempt during childhood (age 4–12 years)	Lifetime attempt during teen years (age 13–19 years)	Lifetime attempt during young adulthood (age 20–29 years)	Lifetime attempt during later adulthood (age 30+ years)
	OR (95% CI)	OR (95% CI)	OR (95% CI)	OR (95% CI)
Type of adversity				
Physical abuse	3.9* (1.2–12.9)	1.8 (0.9–3.6)	2.8* (1.6–5.2)	2.6* (1.3–5.5)
Sexual abuse	10.1* (3.7–27.7)	5.0* (1.9–13.2)	2.5 (0.7–9.6)	3.9* (1.3–11.7)
Neglect	2.6 (0.7–9.6)	1.2 (0.5–2.7)	1.0 (0.4–2.5)	2.3* (1.0–5.0)
Parental death	2.2 (0.6–8.2)	0.8 (0.4–1.6)	1.4 (0.8–2.2)	2.0* (1.2–3.3)
Parental divorce	1.2 (0.1–9.2)	0.5 (0.2–1.2)	1.4 (0.7–3.0)	1.5 (0.6–3.6)
Other parental loss	2.2 (0.6–8.5)	1.7 (0.9–3.1)	0.6 (0.2–1.7)	1.4 (0.5–3.7)
Family violence	1.9 (0.7–5.5)	1.2 (0.6–2.6)	1.7 (0.7–3.9)	1.7 (0.7–4.2)
Physical illness	1.3 (0.3–6.1)	2.2 (0.8–6.0)	0.5 (0.2–1.7)	1.3 (0.5–4.0)
Financial adversity	0.0* (0.0–0.0)	0.4 (0.1–2.2)	0.5 (0.1–2.4)	1.5 (0.4–5.3)
9 df χ^2 test for 9 types	1179.8 (<0.001)*	41.1 (<0.001)*	26.5 (0.002)*	16.5 (0.06)
8 df χ^2 test for difference between types	1084.6 (<0.001)*	38.1 (<0.001)*	22.0 (0.01)*	8.3 (0.40)
Number of adversities				
2	1.0 (0.2–3.9)	1.0 (0.4–2.4)	1.6 (0.6–4.1)	0.8 (0.3–2.4)
3	0.7 (0.1–5.2)	0.9 (0.3–3.3)	1.1 (0.3–5.0)	0.2* (0.0–0.8)
4+	0.3 (0.0–8.8)	1.4 (0.2–8.7)	2.4 (0.2–29.8)	0.2 (0.0–2.5)
χ^2_2 (p-value)	0.9 (0.82)	0.5 (0.92)	2.6 (0.46)	9.6 (0.02)*

* Significant at the 0.05 level, two-sided test.
0.0* (0.0–0.0) OR is ≤0.05 indicating very low risk.
[a] Assessed in the Part 2 sample due to having Part 2 controls. Models control for person–years, country, and significant variables from the chapters on sociodemographics and parental psychopathology.

Appendix Table 8.17. Multivariate interactive analyses between type and number of childhood adversities and persistence of suicidal behavior[a] (high-income countries)

Childhood adversity	Ideation OR (95% CI)	Plan OR (95% CI)	Attempt OR (95% CI)
Type of adversity			
Physical abuse	1.3* (1.0–1.6)	1.4 (1.0–2.0)	2.4* (1.4–3.9)
Sexual abuse	1.2 (1.0–1.5)	1.3 (0.9–1.8)	1.7* (1.1–2.8)
Neglect	1.0 (0.8–1.3)	0.9 (0.6–1.3)	1.1 (0.7–1.8)
Parental death	0.9 (0.7–1.1)	1.1 (0.7–1.5)	0.8 (0.4–1.4)
Parental divorce	0.9 (0.7–1.1)	0.8 (0.5–1.2)	0.9 (0.6–1.5)
Other parental loss	1.2 (0.9–1.5)	1.2 (0.8–1.8)	1.0 (0.5–1.8)
Family violence	1.0 (0.8–1.2)	0.9 (0.7–1.3)	1.1 (0.7–1.9)
Physical illness	0.9 (0.7–1.2)	0.8 (0.6–1.2)	1.5 (0.9–2.7)
Economic adversity	1.0 (0.7–1.4)	1.1 (0.6–2.0)	1.2 (0.7–2.2)
9 df χ^2 test for 9 types	18.3 (0.03)*	15.8 (0.07)	53.7 (<0.001)*
8 df χ^2 test for difference between types	18.1 (0.02)*	14.8 (0.06)	48.3 (<0.001)*
Number of adversities[b]			
2	1.0 (0.8–1.4)	1.2 (0.7–1.9)	1.0 (0.5–2.0)
3	1.1 (0.7–1.7)	1.3 (0.6–2.6)	0.7 (0.2–1.9)
4	1.1 (0.5–2.1)	1.3 (0.4–3.5)	0.6 (0.1–2.5)
5	1.1 (0.5–2.6)	1.5 (0.4–5.7)	0.3 (0.0–1.8)
6+	1.1 (0.3–3.4)	0.7 (0.1–7.6)	
χ^2 (p-value)	0.3 (1.00)	0.7 (0.95)	13.2 (0.02)*

* Significant at the 0.05 level, two-sided test.
[a] Results are based on multivariate discrete time survival models. Models control for country, age-related variables, and significant variables from the chapters on sociodemographics and parental psychopathology.
[b] For number of adversities, the last OR represents the odds for that number of adversities or more. For example, for plan, 5 represents ≥5 (that is, 5+).

Appendix Table 8.18. Multivariate interactive analyses between type and number of childhood adversities and persistence of suicidal behavior[a] (middle-income countries)

Childhood adversity	Ideation OR (95% CI)	Plan OR (95% CI)	Attempt OR (95% CI)
Type of adversity			
Physical abuse	1.1 (0.7–1.6)	1.5 (0.8–2.8)	0.7 (0.3–1.5)
Sexual abuse	1.2 (0.6–2.4)	1.9 (0.6–6.1)	1.3 (0.5–3.6)
Neglect	1.0 (0.6–1.5)	1.5 (0.8–3.0)	0.8 (0.4–1.7)
Parental death	1.0 (0.7–1.5)	0.9 (0.4–2.0)	0.4 (0.2–1.1)
Parental divorce	0.8 (0.5–1.2)	0.8 (0.3–2.0)	0.5 (0.2–1.1)
Other parental loss	1.8* (1.1–3.0)	1.9 (0.6–5.5)	0.9 (0.3–2.6)
Family violence	1.0 (0.6–1.5)	1.5 (0.8–3.1)	0.8 (0.3–2.2)
Physical illness	1.2 (0.6–2.3)	1.3 (0.3–6.3)	1.1 (0.3–4.3)
Economic adversity	2.1* (1.0–4.1)	0.9 (0.2–3.6)	0.7 (0.2–2.7)
9 df χ^2 test for 9 types	13.4 (0.14)	7.9 (0.55)	7.4 (0.59)
8 df χ^2 test for difference between types	15.0 (0.06)	8.0 (0.44)	7.1 (0.53)

Appendix Table 8.18. (cont.)

Childhood adversity	Ideation OR (95% CI)	Plan OR (95% CI)	Attempt OR (95% CI)
Number of adversities			
2	1.4 (0.8–2.5)	1.0 (0.4–2.4)	2.5 (0.9–7.3)
3	1.4 (0.6–3.5)	0.4 (0.1–1.9)	2.0 (0.4–10.6)
4+	1.2 (0.3–4.8)	0.2 (0.0–3.7)	3.1 (0.3–37.2)
χ^2 (p-value)	2.6 (0.45)	5.0 (0.17)	4.4 (0.22)

* Significant at the 0.05 level, two-sided test.
[a] Results are based on multivariate discrete time survival models. Models control for country, age-related variables, and significant variables from the chapters on sociodemographics and parental psychopathology.

Appendix Table 8.19. Multivariate interactive analyses between type and number of childhood adversities and persistence of suicidal behavior[a] (low-income countries)

Childhood adversity	Ideation OR (95% CI)	Plan OR (95% CI)	Attempt OR (95% CI)
Type of adversity			
Physical abuse	0.9 (0.6–1.4)	1.1 (0.6–2.2)	1.0 (0.4–2.1)
Sexual abuse	0.9 (0.5–1.5)	1.6 (0.7–3.7)	1.1 (0.3–3.8)
Neglect	1.2 (0.7–2.1)	0.8 (0.3–2.2)	1.2 (0.4–4.0)
Parental death	0.8 (0.5–1.2)	1.3 (0.8–2.1)	0.6 (0.2–1.5)
Parental divorce	0.8 (0.5–1.5)	1.7 (0.8–3.6)	0.5 (0.1–1.9)
Other parental loss	0.9 (0.6–1.4)	1.0 (0.5–1.9)	0.4* (0.1–1.0)
Family violence	0.7 (0.4–1.2)	1.5 (0.7–3.5)	1.1 (0.4–3.5)
Physical illness	0.9 (0.5–1.8)	1.0 (0.3–2.7)	1.0 (0.3–4.1)
Economic adversity	0.3* (0.1–0.9)	0.2* (0.0–0.9)	0.2 (0.0–2.6)
9 df χ^2 test for 9 types	8.9 (0.45)	12.2 (0.20)	11.7 (0.23)
8 df χ^2 test for difference between types	8.3 (0.41)	11.4 (0.18)	9.7 (0.29)
Number of adversities			
2	1.5 (0.8–2.7)	0.8 (0.3–1.9)	0.5 (0.2–1.6)
3	1.2 (0.5–3.3)	0.6 (0.2–2.1)	1.1 (0.2–7.6)
4+	1.7 (0.5–6.3)	0.4 (0.1–3.3)	1.4 (0.1–18.1)
χ^2 (p-value)	2.6 (0.46)	0.8 (0.84)	3.8 (0.28)

* Significant at the 0.05 level, two-sided test.
[a] Results are based on multivariate discrete time survival models. Models control for country, age-related variables, and significant variables from the chapters on sociodemographics and parental psychopathology.

Appendix Table 9.1. Prevalence of traumatic events among those with each type of suicidal behavior (high-income countries)

Traumatic events	Among total sample %^{a} (SE) with adversities				Among ideators %^{a} (SE) with adversities					
	Ideation	No ideation	Attempt	No attempt	Plan	No plan	Planned attempt	No planned attempt	Unplanned attempt	No unplanned attempt
Disasters/accidents										
All man-made disasters	7.3 (0.5)	4.7 (0.2)	8.4 (0.9)	4.8 (0.2)	9.5 (0.9)	9.6 (0.8)	9.1 (1.2)	15.6 (2.0)	7.5 (1.2)	9.2 (0.8)
Natural disaster	7.5 (0.6)	4.8 (0.2)	10.0 (1.2)	4.8 (0.2)	9.7 (0.9)	9.4 (1.0)	10.7 (1.3)	11.8 (1.8)	9.6 (2.0)	8.9 (0.8)
Accident	15.1 (0.7)	8.2 (0.2)	15.3 (1.2)	8.6 (0.2)	17.5 (1.1)	21.5 (1.3)	16.4 (1.7)	26.2 (2.3)	13.8 (1.9)	20.7 (1.3)
War/combat/refugee experiences										
Exposure to war	11.2 (0.6)	18.9 (0.3)	11.7 (1.2)	18.5 (0.3)	12.3 (1.1)	12.2 (0.9)	14.2 (1.6)	13.2 (1.9)	6.1 (1.3)	13.5 (1.0)
Combat	2.1 (0.3)	3.6 (0.2)	1.3 (0.3)	3.4 (0.1)	2.3 (0.4)	3.5 (0.7)	1.6 (0.4)	2.3 (0.8)	0.8 (0.4)	3.7 (0.8)
Refugee	1.1 (0.2)	2.5 (0.1)	0.8 (0.3)	2.4 (0.1)	0.9 (0.3)	1.6 (0.3)	0.9 (0.4)	0.8 (0.3)	0.7 (0.3)	1.7 (0.4)
Sexual/interpersonal violence										
Sexual violence	11.7 (0.6)	3.5 (0.2)	14.8 (1.0)	3.8 (0.2)	13.1 (1.0)	15.2 (1.1)	13.3 (1.2)	16.7 (1.9)	18.3 (2.3)	13.6 (1.0)
Interpersonal violence	16.3 (0.7)	8.2 (0.2)	16.8 (1.1)	8.6 (0.2)	18.0 (1.3)	23.1 (1.1)	15.3 (1.5)	28.1 (2.2)	20.2 (2.1)	22.4 (1.3)
Witness/perpetrator violence										
Witness violence	15.0 (0.6)	12.5 (0.3)	13.4 (1.0)	12.6 (0.3)	16.9 (1.2)	20.4 (1.0)	12.9 (1.3)	23.2 (2.4)	14.5 (1.9)	20.5 (1.1)
Perpetrator violence	2.0 (0.2)	1.1 (0.1)	2.2 (0.4)	1.2 (0.1)	3.6 (0.7)	3.3 (0.4)	2.5 (0.5)	5.5 (1.6)	2.0 (0.7)	3.7 (0.5)
Loss/trauma										
Death of loved one	21.0 (0.8)	14.1 (0.3)	23.2 (1.2)	14.4 (0.3)	22.8 (1.2)	31.5 (1.1)	22.8 (1.6)	35.4 (2.8)	24.7 (2.4)	32.0 (1.3)
Trauma to loved one	9.6 (0.5)	4.8 (0.2)	12.7 (1.1)	5.0 (0.2)	11.8 (0.9)	15.0 (0.8)	13.1 (1.3)	18.4 (1.7)	12.1 (1.7)	13.5 (0.9)
All others	10.6 (0.6)	4.4 (0.1)	13.1 (1.1)	4.8 (0.1)	12.9 (1.1)	16.0 (0.8)	13.2 (1.4)	20.4 (2.4)	12.5 (1.6)	14.8 (0.9)

Number of traumatic events[b]

1	27.4 (0.8)	25.7 (0.3)	28.1 (1.5)	25.5 (0.3)	28.0 (1.4)	25.9 (1.0)	28.4 (1.8)	25.8 (2.4)	26.0 (2.5)	25.8 (1.1)
2	17.5 (0.6)	11.9 (0.2)	18.4 (1.3)	12.0 (0.2)	18.8 (1.1)	20.1 (0.9)	19.1 (1.8)	22.1 (1.9)	18.0 (2.2)	21.1 (1.0)
3	10.0 (0.6)	6.0 (0.2)	9.7 (0.8)	6.1 (0.2)	11.1 (0.9)	12.7 (0.8)	9.3 (1.1)	16.4 (1.4)	9.9 (1.5)	12.7 (0.9)
4	4.5 (0.4)	2.7 (0.1)	5.6 (0.7)	2.9 (0.1)	5.9 (0.8)	9.0 (0.6)	6.2 (1.0)	10.2 (1.4)	5.0 (1.0)	8.9 (0.7)
5	2.0 (0.2)	1.3 (0.1)	2.3 (0.4)	1.4 (0.1)	2.7 (0.4)	4.1 (0.4)	2.4 (0.5)	5.3 (0.9)	2.5 (0.8)	3.1 (0.4)
6	1.0 (0.1)	0.6 (0.0)	1.8 (0.4)	0.6 (0.0)	1.5 (0.3)	2.3 (0.4)	1.7 (0.4)	2.3 (0.6)	3.0 (1.3)	3.2 (0.4)
7	0.4 (0.1)	0.2 (0.0)	0.7 (0.2)	0.4 (0.0)	0.9 (0.3)	1.0 (0.2)	0.6 (0.3)	2.3 (0.9)		
8+	0.2 (0.1)	0.1 (0.0)								
N[c]	(5056)	(112,028)	(1613)	(116,041)	(1885)	(5646)	(1002)	(1330)	(551)	(4338)

[a] % represents the percentage of people with the adversity among the cases with the outcome variable indicated in the column header. For example, the first cell is the % of those who experienced a man-made disaster among those with suicide ideation.

[b] For number of traumatic events, the last OR represents the odds for that number of traumatic events or more. For example, for unplanned attempt, 7 represents ≥ 7 (that is, 7+).

[c] Number of cases with the outcome variable; N represents the number of person–years.

Appendix Table 9.2. Prevalence of traumatic events among those with each type of suicidal behavior (middle-income countries)

Traumatic events	Among total sample %^{a} (SE) with adversities						Among ideators %^{a} (SE) with adversities			
	Ideation	No ideation	Attempt	No attempt	Plan	No plan	Planned attempt	No planned attempt	Unplanned attempt	No unplanned attempt
Disasters/accidents										
All man-made disasters	5.1 (0.9)	1.8 (0.1)	5.0 (1.3)	1.9 (0.1)	5.4 (1.4)	10.2 (2.3)	4.5 (1.5)	9.2 (2.9)	6.8 (2.1)	9.1 (2.0)
Natural disaster	2.7 (0.5)	2.1 (0.2)	2.3 (0.6)	2.1 (0.1)	2.1 (0.5)	4.2 (1.1)	2.0 (0.5)	2.2 (0.9)	3.0 (1.5)	4.4 (1.3)
Accident	14.2 (1.2)	5.8 (0.2)	15.4 (1.9)	5.9 (0.2)	15.6 (2.0)	21.1 (2.6)	14.4 (2.3)	24.1 (4.9)	17.7 (3.9)	20.5 (3.0)
War/combat/refugee experiences										
Exposure to war	4.4 (0.7)	3.8 (0.2)	4.8 (1.1)	3.7 (0.2)	5.7 (1.0)	5.6 (1.5)	5.4 (1.4)	3.1 1.9)	4.1 (1.5)	6.0 (1.9)
Combat	1.8 (0.6)	0.9 (0.1)	0.5 (0.2)	0.9 (0.1)	1.6 (0.7)	3.2 (1.8)	0.2 (0.2)	0.1 (0.1)	1.1 (0.7)	4.1 (1.8)
Refugee	1.9 (0.5)	1.7 (0.2)	2.8 (0.8)	1.7 (0.2)	2.4 (0.7)	1.2 (0.3)	3.6 (1.1)	0.5 (0.5)	1.6 (0.8)	1.1 (0.6)
Sexual/interpersonal violence										
Sexual violence	5.9 (0.7)	1.0 (0.1)	9.8 (1.4)	1.1 (0.1)	7.4 (1.1)	8.4 (1.5)	9.6 (1.8)	6.5 2.1)	10.3 (2.2)	6.3 (1.4)
Interpersonal violence	16.9 (1.5)	6.5 (0.2)	16.5 (1.8)	6.7 (0.2)	17.4 (2.2)	17.6 (1.7)	17.4 (2.4)	25.0 (5.1)	15.2 (3.1)	18.1 (1.9)
Witness/perpetrator violence										
Witness violence	17.0 (1.5)	7.4 (0.2)	17.8 (1.9)	7.7 (0.2)	18.6 (2.1)	23.0 (2.6)	19.7 (2.4)	23.6 (5.3)	15.7 (3.4)	25.0 (3.1)
Perpetrator violence	2.8 (0.6)	0.5 (0.1)	3.6 (0.9)	0.6 (0.1)	2.3 (0.7)	3.3 (0.9)	3.6 (0.9)	3.5 (1.9)	4.3 (1.7)	3.1 (1.4)
Loss/trauma										
Death of loved one	19.7 (1.4)	8.0 (0.2)	18.2 (1.7)	8.2 (0.3)	23.3 (2.0)	25.3 (2.8)	21.2 (2.3)	24.2 (4.0)	13.6 (2.7)	25.8 (3.1)
Trauma to loved one	6.2 (0.7)	3.0 (0.2)	8.5 (1.5)	3.2 (0.1)	7.9 (1.4)	11.2 (1.7)	8.6 (1.6)	8.4 (2.9)	7.2 (2.4)	12.1 (2.1)
All others	4.8 (0.7)	1.7 (0.1)	6.3 (1.6)	1.8 (0.1)	6.5 (1.4)	7.8 (1.3)	6.6 (2.1)	8.8 (2.7)	6.3 (2.4)	6.7 (1.3)

Number of traumatic events[b]

1	26.0 (1.5)	14.5 (0.3)	28.8 (2.5)	14.7 (0.3)	26.8 (2.3)	26.0 (2.2)	28.6 (3.2)	27.7 (4.9)	28.5 (4.4)	27.1 (2.6)
2	15.9 (1.2)	6.6 (0.2)	17.2 (1.7)	6.6 (0.2)	18.0 (1.8)	19.8 (2.0)	17.7 (2.1)	22.8 (3.8)	16.2 (3.3)	17.3 (2.0)
3	6.7 (0.7)	2.6 (0.1)	7.6 (1.2)	2.8 (0.1)	7.0 (1.2)	7.7 (1.1)	8.1 (1.8)	9.0 (2.4)	7.4 (2.3)	9.1 (1.4)
4	2.4 (0.5)	1.1 (0.1)	2.6 (0.7)	1.2 (0.1)	3.0 (0.8)	6.5 (1.8)	2.9 (0.9)	4.7 (1.8)	4.8 (1.8)	11.6 (2.4)
5	1.8 (0.4)	0.5 (0.0)	2.6 (0.8)	0.8 (0.1)	3.5 (1.2)	5.0 (1.3)	3.0 (1.1)	3.3 (1.9)		
6+	1.0 (0.3)	0.3 (0.0)								
N[c]	(1687)	(57,216)	(635)	(57,623)	(721)	(1234)	(411)	(320)	(194)	(911)

[a] % represents the percentage of people with the adversity among the cases with the outcome variable indicated in the column header. For example, the first cell is the % of those who experienced a man-made disaster among those with suicide ideation.

[b] For number of traumatic events, the last OR represents the odds for that number of traumatic events or more. For example, for unplanned attempt, 4 represents ≥4 (that is, 4+).

[c] Number of cases with the outcome variable; N represents the number of person–years.

Appendix Table 9.3. Prevalence of traumatic events among those with each type of suicidal behavior (low-income countries)

Traumatic events	Among total sample %^{a} (SE) with adversities						Among ideators %^{a} (SE) with adversities			
	Ideation	No ideation	Attempt	No attempt	Plan	No plan	Planned attempt	No planned attempt	Unplanned attempt	No unplanned attempt
Disasters/accidents										
All man-made disasters	4.6 (0.7)	3.1 (0.3)	5.3 (1.2)	3.0 (0.2)	7.3 (1.5)	7.0 (1.5)	6.2 (1.7)	10.0 (2.4)	4.8 (2.0)	7.6 (1.7)
Natural disaster	5.6 (0.8)	4.6 (0.3)	7.4 (1.3)	4.6 (0.3)	7.1 (1.3)	7.6 (1.4)	6.8 (1.6)	12.2 (3.5)	8.8 (2.4)	6.4 (1.3)
Accident	13.0 (1.3)	7.0 (0.3)	13.5 (2.0)	7.1 (0.3)	16.0 (2.0)	19.6 (2.3)	12.4 (2.1)	23.4 (4.6)	14.7 (4.0)	16.7 (2.6)
War/combat/refugee experiences										
Exposure to war	6.3 (0.8)	6.5 (0.5)	7.2 (1.4)	6.0 (0.4)	6.8 (1.3)	8.2 (1.2)	9.2 (2.2)	11.6 (3.8)	4.3 (1.5)	8.4 (1.6)
Combat	1.8 (0.4)	1.6 (0.2)	2.1 (0.6)	1.4 (0.1)	3.1 (0.8)	2.9 (1.0)	2.8 (1.0)	2.6 (1.4)	0.9 (0.4)	3.0 (1.3)
Refugee	0.9 (0.3)	1.6 (0.2)	1.1 (0.4)	1.4 (0.2)	1.2 (0.4)	2.1 (1.2)	0.9 (0.5)	2.0 (1.0)	0.9 (0.7)	2.6 (1.3)
Sexual/interpersonal violence										
Sexual violence	7.3 (0.8)	1.5 (0.1)	9.3 (1.4)	1.7 (0.1)	9.1 (1.7)	8.0 (1.1)	9.6 (1.9)	13.9 (4.0)	9.4 (2.6)	7.6 (1.3)
Interpersonal violence	14.7 (1.5)	6.8 (0.3)	12.2 (1.7)	6.7 (0.3)	15.9 (2.0)	13.1 (1.9)	14.5 (2.3)	26.1 (6.8)	9.6 (2.5)	13.2 (2.1)
Witness/perpetrator violence										
Witness violence	13.7 (1.4)	8.5 (0.3)	14.8 (1.9)	8.7 (0.3)	13.4 (1.7)	16.0 (1.9)	14.6 (2.2)	14.5 (3.1)	16.2 (4.0)	18.0 (2.8)
Perpetrator violence	1.5 (0.4)	0.5 (0.1)	2.1 (0.7)	0.5 (0.1)	2.8 (0.7)	1.6 (0.5)	2.1 (0.8)	6.7 (2.9)	2.6 (1.4)	0.8 (0.4)
Loss/trauma										
Death of loved one	17.1 (1.4)	9.9 (0.3)	16.8 (2.2)	9.9 (0.3)	18.1 (2.0)	24.8 (2.6)	17.7 (2.2)	19.6 (3.6)	16.8 (4.2)	26.0 (2.9)
Trauma to loved one	8.0 (1.1)	3.8 (0.2)	8.1 (1.6)	3.7 (0.2)	6.6 (1.1)	12.7 (1.8)	6.6 (1.5)	8.5 (1.9)	10.0 (3.7)	14.3 (2.1)
All others	5.5 (0.7)	2.1 (0.2)	8.0 (1.5)	2.1 (0.1)	8.8 (1.5)	7.1 (1.4)	9.1 (2.0)	7.2 (2.5)	6.6 (2.4)	7.1 (1.5)

Number of traumatic events[b]

1	20.5 (1.4)	16.8 (0.4)	22.1 (2.0)	17.2 (0.4)	21.2 (1.8)	24.7 (2.5)	20.7 (2.2)	19.8 (3.2)	22.0 (4.3)	22.6 (2.9)
2	12.5 (1.3)	8.0 (0.3)	12.0 (1.6)	7.8 (0.3)	11.6 (1.5)	14.4 (1.7)	11.3 (2.1)	11.1 (1.9)	14.5 (3.3)	15.9 (2.4)
3	6.3 (0.9)	3.7 (0.2)	7.8 (1.5)	3.8 (0.2)	7.5 (1.4)	11.5 (1.3)	7.2 (1.5)	17.2 (2.8)	9.6 (3.6)	9.9 (1.5)
4	4.6 (0.8)	1.8 (0.1)	3.8 (1.0)	1.6 (0.1)	4.3 (1.1)	3.1 (0.6)	4.1 (1.5)	10.8 (2.5)	5.6 (2.0)	9.3 (1.7)
5	1.5 (0.3)	0.8 (0.1)	2.8 (0.8)	0.7 (0.1)	3.8 (1.2)	2.5 (0.5)	5.6 (1.4)	3.8 (1.4)		
6+	1.5 (0.5)	0.4 (0.1)	1.4 (0.6)	0.4 (0.1)	1.9 (0.6)	2.7 (0.8)				
N[c]	(1383)	(34,170)	(530)	(32,878)	(645)	(1071)	(330)	(323)	(162)	(683)

[a] % represents the percentage of people with the adversity among the cases with the outcome variable indicated in the column header. For example, the first cell is the % of those who experienced a man-made disaster among those with suicide ideation. Because Shenzhen did not assess traumatic events, it was excluded from these prevalence estimates.
[b] For number of traumatic events, the last OR represents the odds for that number of traumatic events or more. For example, for unplanned attempt, 4 represents ≥4 (that is, 4+).
[c] Number of cases with the outcome variable; N represents the number of person–years.

Appendix Table 9.4. Final multivariate models for associations between traumatic events and suicidal behavior[a] (high-income countries)

	Among total sample			Among ideators	
	Ideation	Attempt	Plan	Planned attempt	Unplanned attempt
Traumatic events	OR (95% CI)	OR (95% CI)	OR (95% CI)	OR (95% CI)	OR (95% CI)
Disasters/accidents					
All man-made disasters	1.3* (1.1–1.6)	1.3 (1.0–1.8)	1.5* (1.0–2.1)	0.7 (0.4–1.2)	0.9 (0.5–1.6)
Natural disaster	1.1 (0.9–1.3)	1.4 (1.0–1.9)	1.4* (1.0–2.0)	1.0 (0.6–1.7)	0.9 (0.5–1.6)
Accident	1.4* (1.2–1.7)	1.2 (0.9–1.7)	1.1 (0.8–1.5)	0.6 (0.4–1.0)	0.6 (0.4–1.0)
War/combat/refugee experiences					
Exposure to war	1.0 (0.9–1.3)	1.6* (1.1–2.2)	1.2 (0.8–1.7)	1.2 (0.7–2.4)	0.7 (0.3–1.4)
Combat	1.1 (0.8–1.5)	0.8 (0.5–1.4)	1.4 (0.7–2.4)	0.9 (0.3–3.3)	0.5 (0.2–1.7)
Refugee	1.1 (0.7–1.5)	0.9 (0.4–1.9)	1.0 (0.5–2.0)	1.0 (0.3–3.5)	1.6 (0.4–5.6)
Sexual/interpersonal violence					
Sexual violence	2.2* (1.9–2.6)	2.5* (2.0–3.3)	1.0 (0.7–1.4)	0.9 (0.6–1.4)	1.4 (0.9–2.3)
Interpersonal violence	1.7* (1.4–2.0)	1.8* (1.4–2.3)	1.0 (0.8–1.4)	0.6* (0.4–0.9)	1.1 (0.7–1.7)
Witness/perpetrator violence					
Witness violence	1.3* (1.1–1.6)	1.3 (1.0–1.6)	1.4* (1.0–1.9)	0.7 (0.4–1.2)	1.1 (0.7–1.7)
Perpetrator violence	1.4* (1.1–1.8)	1.0 (0.6–1.6)	1.3 (0.8–2.1)	0.4* (0.2–1.0)	0.6 (0.2–1.3)
Loss/trauma					
Death of loved one	1.1 (1.0–1.3)	1.1 (0.9–1.4)	0.9 (0.7–1.2)	0.6* (0.4–1.0)	0.7 (0.4–1.1)
Trauma to loved one	1.3* (1.1–1.6)	1.3 (0.9–1.7)	0.9 (0.7–1.3)	0.7 (0.4–1.1)	0.8 (0.5–1.3)
All others	1.7* (1.4–2.0)	1.6* (1.2–2.0)	1.0 (0.7–1.3)	0.7 (0.4–1.1)	0.8 (0.5–1.4)
13 df χ^2 test for 13 types	139.1 (<0.001)*	87.5 (<0.001)*	25.2 (0.02)*	17.1 (0.20)	19.3 (0.12)
12 df χ^2 test for difference between types	109.6 (<0.001)*	62.8 (<0.001)*	24.2 (0.02)*	13.0 (0.37)	19.4 (0.08)
Number of traumatic events[b]					
2	1.0 (0.8–1.2)	0.9 (0.7–1.3)	1.0 (0.7–1.5)	1.2 (0.7–2.1)	1.1 (0.6–2.1)
3	0.8 (0.6–1.1)	0.7 (0.4–1.1)	0.8 (0.5–1.5)	1.2 (0.5–2.9)	1.2 (0.5–2.8)
4	0.6* (0.4–0.9)	0.6 (0.3–1.2)	0.6 (0.3–1.3)	2.2 (0.6–7.4)	1.3 (0.4–4.6)
5	0.5* (0.3–0.8)	0.5 (0.2–1.3)	0.7 (0.3–1.7)	3.4 (0.6–17.7)	2.2 (0.5–10.7)
6	0.4* (0.2–0.8)	0.6 (0.2–1.8)	0.6 (0.2–2.3)	4.0 (0.5–29.6)	5.2 (0.6–43.2)
7	0.3* (0.1–0.7)	0.3 (0.1–1.1)	0.6 (0.1–3.1)	3.4 (0.3–41.3)	
8+	0.2* (0.1–0.6)				
χ^2 (p-value)	29.9 (<0.001)*	8.7 (0.19)	5.5 (0.48)	6.6 (0.36)	6.2 (0.29)

* Significant at the 0.05 level, two-sided test.
[a] Assessed in the Part 2 sample due to having Part 2 controls. Models control for person–years, country, and significant variables from the chapters on sociodemographics, parental psychopathology, and childhood adversities.
[b] For number of traumatic events, the last OR represents the odds for that number of traumatic events or more. For example, for unplanned attempt, 6 represents ≥6 (that is, 6+).

Appendix Table 9.5. Final multivariate models for associations between traumatic events and suicidal behavior[a] (middle-income countries)

| | Among total sample | | | Among ideators | |
| | Ideation | Attempt | Plan | Planned attempt | Unplanned attempt |
Traumatic events	OR (95% CI)	OR (95% CI)	OR (95% CI)	OR (95% CI)	OR (95% CI)
Disasters/accidents					
All man-made disasters	1.8* (1.2–2.9)	1.8* (1.0–3.4)	0.6 (0.3–1.2)	0.4 (0.1–1.7)	1.2 (0.5–3.0)
Natural disaster	1.1 (0.7–1.7)	1.0 (0.6–1.8)	0.6 (0.3–1.3)	0.6 (0.2–1.9)	2.0 (0.6–7.1)
Accident	1.9* (1.4–2.5)	2.2* (1.4–3.6)	1.0 (0.6–1.6)	0.5 (0.2–1.1)	1.4 (0.6–3.1)
War/combat/refugee experiences					
Exposure to war	1.2 (0.8–1.9)	1.1 (0.6–2.1)	1.1 (0.6–2.1)	0.7 (0.3–2.0)	0.3 (0.1–1.1)
Combat	3.3* (1.6–6.8)	0.7 (0.3–1.8)	0.7 (0.3–1.7)	20.5 (0.2–1828.1)	0.7 (0.1–4.2)
Refugee	1.4 (0.7–2.9)	1.6 (0.6–4.3)	1.2 (0.4–3.4)	5.0 (0.3–78.1)	0.5 (0.1–2.6)
Sexual/interpersonal violence					
Sexual violence	2.8* (2.0–3.8)	3.9* (2.3–6.4)	0.8 (0.5–1.4)	0.9 (0.3–2.3)	2.1 (0.9–4.6)
Interpersonal violence	2.0* (1.6–2.5)	2.5* (1.8–3.5)	1.2 (0.8–1.9)	0.6 (0.2–1.2)	1.0 (0.5–1.9)
Witness/perpetrator violence					
Witness violence	1.5* (1.1–2.0)	1.9* (1.2–3.0)	1.2 (0.7–2.0)	0.8 (0.3–2.2)	1.0 (0.4–2.4)
Perpetrator violence	2.3* (1.4–3.6)	3.1* (1.7–5.4)	1.0 (0.4–2.4)	1.6 (0.4–6.8)	2.4 (0.6–10.5)
Loss/trauma					
Death of loved one	1.6* (1.2–2.0)	1.5* (1.0–2.1)	1.2 (0.8–1.9)	1.0 (0.5–1.9)	0.6 (0.3–1.1)
Trauma to loved one	1.2 (0.8–1.7)	1.6 (1.0–2.6)	1.0 (0.6–1.8)	1.3 (0.4–3.6)	0.5 (0.2–1.5)
All others	1.6* (1.1–2.3)	2.0* (1.0–3.8)	1.0 (0.5–1.9)	0.5 (0.2–1.1)	0.8 (0.3–2.0)
13 df χ^2 test for 13 types	91.7 (<0.001)*	67.3 (<0.001)*	14.6 (0.33)	13.3 (0.43)	20.7 (0.08)
12 df χ^2 test for difference between types	37.5 (<0.001)*	41.9 (<0.001)*	12.4 (0.41)	9.8 (0.63)	18.5 (0.10)
Number of traumatic events[b]					
2	0.8 (0.6–1.1)	0.7 (0.4–1.1)	0.8 (0.5–1.4)	1.8 (0.7–5.0)	0.7 (0.3–1.7)
3	0.5* (0.3–0.9)	0.4* (0.2–0.9)	0.7 (0.3–1.8)	1.7 (0.3–9.0)	0.8 (0.2–3.3)
4	0.3* (0.1–0.7)	0.2* (0.1–0.7)	0.5 (0.1–1.8)	2.8 (0.3–24.9)	0.8 (0.1–7.0)
5	0.4* (0.2–0.9)	0.1* (0.0–0.7)	1.2 (0.2–7.3)	5.8 (0.4–77.2)	
6+	0.2* (0.1–0.7)				
χ^2 (p-value)	12.8 (0.03)*	9.4 (0.05)	3.6 (0.46)	2.5 (0.65)	1.0 (0.79)

* Significant at the 0.05 level, two-sided test.
[a] Assessed in the Part 2 sample due to having Part 2 controls. Models control for person–years, country, and significant variables from the chapters on sociodemographics, parental psychopathology, and childhood adversities.
[b] For number of traumatic events, the last OR represents the odds for that number of traumatic events or more. For example, for unplanned attempt, 4 represents ≥4 (that is, 4+).

Appendix Table 9.6. Final multivariate models for associations between traumatic events and suicidal behavior[a] (low-income countries)

Traumatic events	Among total sample		Among ideators		
	Ideation	Attempt	Plan	Planned attempt	Unplanned attempt
	OR (95% CI)	OR (95% CI)	OR (95% CI)	OR (95% CI)	OR (95% CI)
Disasters/accidents					
All man-made disasters	0.9 (0.6–1.3)	1.1 (0.6–2.1)	1.5 (0.7–2.9)	0.7 (0.2–1.9)	0.5 (0.1–1.6)
Natural disaster	1.2 (0.8–1.7)	1.8* (1.0–3.1)	1.7 (0.8–3.3)	0.4 (0.2–1.2)	1.8 (0.7–4.5)
Accident	1.4* (1.0–1.9)	1.7 (1.0–3.0)	1.0 (0.6–1.7)	0.8 (0.3–2.1)	0.7 (0.3–1.7)
War/combat/refugee experiences					
Exposure to war	1.2 (0.9–1.7)	1.8* (1.0–3.2)	1.2 (0.6–2.3)	1.9 (0.7–5.2)	0.8 (0.2–2.9)
Combat	1.3 (0.7–2.5)	1.9 (0.8–4.2)	1.9 (0.7–5.8)	0.7 (0.2–3.0)	0.7 (0.1–3.7)
Refugee	1.1 (0.6–2.0)	1.9 (0.8–4.5)	1.5 (0.3–8.2)	0.7 (0.1–6.7)	2.2 (0.3–18.1)
Sexual/interpersonal violence					
Sexual violence	2.2* (1.6–3.2)	2.9* (1.7–4.9)	1.2 (0.7–2.3)	0.8 (0.3–1.9)	1.3 (0.5–3.8)
Interpersonal violence	2.1* (1.5–2.9)	2.0* (1.1–3.5)	1.9* (1.1–3.2)	0.8 (0.3–1.9)	0.5 (0.2–1.1)
Witness/perpetrator violence					
Witness violence	1.3 (0.9–2.0)	1.7* (1.1–2.6)	1.0 (0.6–1.9)	1.5 (0.7–3.4)	1.2 (0.4–4.2)
Perpetrator violence	1.4 (0.7–2.7)	2.1 (0.9–4.8)	1.4 (0.6–3.0)	0.2* (0.0–0.8)	1.9 (0.2–21.2)
Loss/trauma					
Death of loved one	1.2 (0.9–1.6)	1.2 (0.8–1.9)	0.9 (0.5–1.4)	1.1 (0.5–2.7)	0.7 (0.3–1.8)
Trauma to loved one	1.4 (0.9–2.1)	1.5 (0.8–2.7)	0.5 (0.3–1.0)	1.1 (0.5–2.6)	0.8 (0.3–2.5)
All others	1.4 (0.9–2.2)	2.4* (1.2–4.6)	1.8 (0.9–3.4)	1.4 (0.5–4.5)	0.7 (0.2–2.3)
13 df χ^2 test for 13 types	45.5 (<0.001)*	30.2 (0.004)*	19.5 (0.11)	16.1 (0.24)	11.8 (0.54)
12 df χ^2 test for difference between types	29.7 (0.003)*	16.3 (0.18)	17.7 (0.13)	15.7 (0.21)	15.2 (0.23)
Number of traumatic events[b]					
2	0.8 (0.6–1.3)	0.7 (0.4–1.2)	0.8 (0.4–1.7)	1.6 (0.5–5.1)	1.6 (0.5–5.4)
3	0.6 (0.3–1.2)	0.5 (0.2–1.2)	0.7 (0.3–1.9)	0.8 (0.2–4.0)	3.1 (0.5–17.9)
4	0.7 (0.3–1.6)	0.3* (0.1–1.0)	1.5 (0.4–6.5)	0.9 (0.1–6.7)	3.3 (0.1–81.6)
5	0.4 (0.1–1.4)	0.5 (0.1–2.4)	1.2 (0.2–6.6)	7.2 (0.4–132.6)	
6+	0.5 (0.1–2.4)	0.1* (0.0–1.0)	0.3 (0.0–2.8)		
χ^2 (p-value)	3.4 (0.63)	7.2 (0.20)	7.8 (0.17)	9.5 (0.05)*	2.0 (0.57)

* Significant at the 0.05 level, two-sided test.
[a] Assessed in the Part 2 sample due to having Part 2 controls. Models control for person–years, country, and significant variables from the chapters on sociodemographics, parental psychopathology, and childhood adversities.
[b] For number of traumatic events, the last OR represents the odds for that number of traumatic events or more. For example, for unplanned attempt, 4 represents ≥4 (that is, 4+).

Appendix Table 9.7. Interactions between traumatic events and suicidal behavior over the life course[a] (high-income countries)

		Among total sample						Among ideators			
		Ideation		Attempt		Plan		Planned attempt		Unplanned attempt	
Interactions		OR (95% CI)	χ² (p-value)	OR (95% CI)	χ² (p-value)	OR (95% CI)	χ² (p-value)	OR (95% CI)	χ² (p-value)	OR (95% CI)	χ² (p-value)
Disasters/accidents											
All man-made disasters	13–19	0.6 (0.3–1.5)	1.1 (0.78)	0.5 (0.1–2.0)	9.6 (0.02)*	0.1 (0.0–1.1)	7.2 (0.07)	0.1 (0.0–2.5)	6.0 (0.11)	—	—
	20–29	0.7 (0.3–1.5)		0.2* (0.0–0.9)		0.1* (0.0–0.8)		0.1 (0.0–1.8)		—	
	30+	0.7 (0.3–1.5)		0.7 (0.2–2.9)		0.2 (0.0–1.7)		0.2 (0.0–6.1)		—	
Natural disaster	13–19	1.2 (0.6–2.5)	1.2 (0.74)	1.3 (0.4–3.9)	2.2 (0.53)	0.6 (0.1–6.7)	8.0 (0.05)*	8.3 (0.5–135.3)	3.1 (0.38)	—	—
	20–29	1.0 (0.5–2.0)		1.0 (0.3–3.2)		0.2 (0.0–2.4)		9.0 (0.6–132.1)		—	
	30+	1.1 (0.5–2.2)		1.6 (0.5–4.9)		0.3 (0.0–3.0)		9.9 (0.7–131.2)		—	
Accident	13–19	0.8 (0.4–1.6)	3.0 (0.39)	0.6 (0.2–1.8)	1.3 (0.74)	0.4 (0.1–3.0)	0.7 (0.86)	3.6 (0.2–51.6)	0.9 (0.82)	—	—
	20–29	1.1 (0.6–2.0)		0.8 (0.3–2.2)		0.4 (0.1–3.3)		3.6 (0.2–53.0)		—	
	30+	0.8 (0.4–1.5)		0.7 (0.3–1.7)		0.5 (0.1–3.3)		3.5 (0.2–50.0)		—	
War/combat/refugee experiences											
Exposure to war	13–19	0.4 (0.1–1.6)	2.8 (0.43)	1.7 (0.5–6.3)	1.3 (0.73)	0.0* (0.0–0.0)	54.0 (<0.001)*	1.1 (0.2–5.4)	0.0 (0.98)	0.0* (0.0–0.0)	11.6 (<0.001)*
	20–29	0.5 (0.1–2.2)		1.9 (0.6–6.3)		0.0* (0.0–0.0)		1.0 (0.3–3.9)		0.0* (0.0–0.0)	
	30+	0.5 (0.1–2.0)		1.9 (0.6–5.7)		0.0* (0.0–0.0)		—		0.0* (0.0–0.0)	
Combat	13–19	—	184.2 (<0.001)*	0.2 (0.0–10.3)	1.2 (0.76)	0.1* (0.0–0.5)	8.0 (0.02)*	1.7 (0.1–38.0)	0.2 (0.89)	0.0* (0.0–0.0)	19.3 (<0.001)*
	20–29	817.2* (275.7–2422.1)		0.4 (0.1–2.6)		0.3 (0.1–1.0)		0.8 (0.1–6.5)		0.5 (0.0–6.8)	
	30+	—		0.5 (0.1–2.9)		—		—		—	
Refugee	13–19	—	253.8 (<0.001)*	3.3* (1.2–9.5)	6.9 (0.07)	5.3 (0.6–44.2)	2.5 (0.29)	4.3 (0.6–863.8)	3.1 (0.21)	0.0* (0.0–0.0)	34.5 (<0.001)*
	20–29	187.8* (53.6–658.3)		1.2 (0.3–4.7)		1.9 (0.3–11.4)		46.8 (0.6–3484.6)		—	
	30+	478.6* (216.6–1057.8)		0.8 (0.3–2.2)		—		—		—	
Sexual/interpersonal violence											
Sexual violence	13–19	0.5 (0.3–1.1)	4.9 (0.18)	0.4 (0.2–1.0)	3.8 (0.28)	0.5 (0.1–4.2)	1.2 (0.75)	1.9 (0.1–25.0)	0.7 (0.88)	—	—
	20–29	0.5 (0.2–1.0)		0.5 (0.2–1.3)		0.4 (0.0–3.4)		2.5 (0.2–31.4)		—	
	30+	0.5* (0.2–0.9)		0.5 (0.2–1.3)		0.5 (0.1–4.1)		2.4 (0.2–26.9)		—	
Interpersonal violence	13–19	0.4 (0.1–1.5)	12.7 (0.01)*	0.6 (0.2–1.6)	6.9 (0.08)	1.3 (0.0–35.5)	5.4 (0.14)	0.1 (0.0–14.2)	2.9 (0.41)	2.0 (0.0–482.4)	4.5 (0.21)
	20–29	0.2* (0.1–0.8)		0.4 (0.1–1.1)		1.1 (0.0–30.6)		0.0 (0.0–11.0)		0.8 (0.0–186.8)	
	30+	0.3 (0.1–1.0)		0.8 (0.3–2.0)		2.3 (0.1–59.5)		0.1 (0.0–21.7)		1.9 (0.0–446.9)	
Witness/perpetrator violence											
Witness violence	13–19	0.3* (0.1–0.6)	11.3 (0.01)*	0.4 (0.1–1.1)	3.5 (0.32)	0.5 (0.1–3.8)	5.7 (0.12)	0.0* (0.0–0.0)	74.1 (<0.001)*	—	—
	20–29	0.3* (0.2–0.7)		0.4 (0.1–1.1)		0.2 (0.0–1.6)		0.0* (0.0–0.0)		—	
	30+	0.4* (0.2–0.7)		0.4 (0.1–1.1)		0.3 (0.0–2.3)		0.0* (0.0–0.0)		—	
Perpetrator violence	13–19	0.3 (0.1–1.3)	4.0 (0.27)	0.6 (0.0–12.0)	4.3 (0.23)	0.0* (0.0–0.0)	77.6 (<0.001)*	0.0 (0.0–8.5)	4.6 (0.20)	0.6 (0.1–6.8)	0.2 (0.90)
	20–29	0.3 (0.1–1.1)		0.4 (0.0–8.6)		0.0* (0.0–0.0)		0.0 (0.0–8.4)		0.9 (0.1–11.2)	
	30+	0.3* (0.1–1.0)		1.3 (0.1–25.0)		0.0* (0.0–0.0)		0.0 (0.0–34.6)		—	
Loss/trauma											
Death of loved one	13–19	0.5* (0.2–0.9)	5.7 (0.13)	0.4 (0.1–1.4)	2.2 (0.54)	0.8 (0.2–4.1)	0.4 (0.93)	0.1 (0.0–4.9)	1.4 (0.70)	4.6 (0.0–5512.2)	0.3 (0.96)
	20–29	0.5 (0.3–1.1)		0.4 (0.1–1.5)		0.8 (0.2–3.7)		0.2 (0.0–5.6)		4.9 (0.0–6318.1)	
	30+	0.5* (0.2–0.9)		0.4 (0.1–1.4)		0.7 (0.1–3.3)		0.1 (0.0–4.3)		4.2 (0.0–5486.9)	

Appendix Table 9.7. (cont.)

		Among total sample						Among ideators			
		Ideation		Attempt		Plan		Planned attempt		Unplanned attempt	
Interactions		OR (95% CI)	χ² (p-value)	OR (95% CI)	χ² (p-value)	OR (95% CI)	χ² (p-value)	OR (95% CI)	χ² (p-value)	OR (95% CI)	χ² (p-value)
Trauma to loved one	13–19	0.7 (0.3–1.5)	6.1 (0.11)	0.4 (0.2–1.0)	6.6 (0.09)	0.4 (0.0–5.6)	3.3 (0.35)	1.0 (0.0–25.7)	2.1 (0.55)	0.0* (0.0–0.0)	44.9 (<0.001)*
	20–29	0.6 (0.3–1.2)		0.3* (0.1–0.8)		0.2 (0.0–3.0)		0.5 (0.0–15.3)		0.0* (0.0–0.0)	
	30+	0.5* (0.2–1.0)		0.5 (0.2–1.1)		0.3 (0.0–3.9)		1.1 (0.0–28.9)		0.0* (0.0–0.0)	
All others	13–19	0.8 (0.3–1.7)	1.9 (0.59)	0.5 (0.2–1.3)	5.2 (0.16)	0.6 (0.1–4.0)	1.3 (0.73)	0.6 (0.0–20.3)	1.2 (0.74)	0.0* (0.0–0.0)	110.1 (<0.001)*
	20–29	0.8 (0.4–1.8)		0.3* (0.1–0.9)		0.4 (0.1–2.9)		0.5 (0.0–20.8)		0.0* (0.0–0.0)	
	30+	0.7 (0.3–1.4)		0.5 (0.2–1.4)		0.5 (0.1–3.2)		0.9 (0.0–34.9)		0.0* (0.0–0.0)	
39 df χ² test for all trauma			552.7 (<0.001)*		52.2 (0.08)		229.4 (<0.001)*		192.9 (<0.001)*		480.2 (<0.001)*
χ² test for all trauma and dummies for number of traumas			1651.9 (<0.001)*		76.8 (0.04)*		630.1 (<0.001)*		396.5 (<0.001)*		–
Number of traumatic events[b]											
2	13–19	1.4 (0.6–3.2)	401.2 (<0.001)*	5.0* (1.5–16.1)	24.9 (0.13)	2.9 (0.2–37.3)	49.3 (<0.001)*	–	29.7 (0.01)*	–	179.1 (<0.001)*
	20–29	1.3 (0.5–3.3)		4.6* (1.4–15.8)		4.6 (0.3–62.2)		–		–	
	30+	1.4 (0.6–3.2)		4.2* (1.3–13.4)		3.0 (0.3–36.5)		–		–	
3	13–19	2.8 (0.6–11.9)		2.7 (0.3–22.0)		2.6 (0.1–70.7)		5.4 (0.1–534.8)		–	
	20–29	3.6 (0.9–15.4)		2.9 (0.4–22.6)		7.8 (0.3–191.1)		3.4 (0.0–353.9)		–	
	30+	3.3 (0.8–13.6)		1.5 (0.2–11.8)		3.6 (0.1–89.7)		–		–	
4	13–19	3.0 (0.4–21.2)		7.8 (0.4–152.0)		0.0* (0.0–0.1)		0.0 (0.0–27.6)		–	
	20–29	3.1 (0.4–23.2)		8.7 (0.5–152.8)		0.0* (0.0–0.7)		0.0 (0.0–2.5)		–	
	30+	3.7 (0.5–25.9)		3.7 (0.2–70.1)		0.0* (0.0–0.2)		0.0* (0.0–0.7)		–	
5	13–19	–		36.8 (0.4–3244.4)		0.8 (0.1–10.5)		1.8 (0.0–315.5)		0.0* (0.0–0.0)	
	20–29	–		–		1.9 (0.2–19.5)		2.3 (0.0–149.4)		0.9 (0.0–44.5)	
	30+	–		–		–		–		–	
6	13–19	64.4* (2.0–2123.2)		22.7 (0.4–1378.5)		2.1 (0.1–56.8)		2.1 (0.0–374.9)		1.5 (0.0–222.5)	
	20–29	–		88.7* (1.4–5448.5)		4.2 (0.2–72.9)		2.6 (0.0–379.0)		–	
	30+	–		16.5 (0.3–992.8)		–		–		–	
7	13–19	0.0* (0.0–0.0)		0.8 (0.0–341784.8)		0.0* (0.0–0.0)		0.0* (0.0–0.0)		–	
	20–29	1.3 (0.2–8.9)		–		16.4 (0.5–521.9)		4.8 (0.0–3199.6)		–	
	30+	–		–		–		–		–	
8+	13–19	0.0* (0.0–0.0)		4.5 (0.0–463.9)		–		–		–	
	20–29	2.4 (0.1–61.8)		–		–		–		–	
	30+	–		–		–		–		–	

* Significant at the 0.05 level, two-sided test.

0.0* (0.0–0.0) OR is ≤0.05 indicating very low risk.

– Not included due to small cell size.

[a] Assessed in the Part 2 sample. Models control for person-years, country, significant variables from the chapters on sociodemographics, parental psychopathology, childhood adversities, and interaction terms between life course intervals (4–12, 13–19, 20–29, 30+ years) and each control. Only the interaction terms between the life course intervals and PTSD variables are shown in table.

[b] For number of traumatic events, the last OR represents the odds for that number of traumatic events or more. For example, for unplanned attempt, 6 represents ≥6 (that is, 6+).

Appendix Table 9.8. Interactions between traumatic events and suicidal behavior over the life course[a] (middle-income countries)

Interactions		Among total sample						Among ideators			
		Ideation		Attempt		Plan		Planned attempt		Unplanned attempt	
		OR (95% CI)	χ² (p-value)	OR (95% CI)	χ² (p-value)	OR (95% CI)	χ² (p-value)	OR (95% CI)	χ² (p-value)	OR (95% CI)	χ² (p-value)
Disasters/accidents											
All man-made disasters	13–19	0.6 (0.1–3.0)	7.4 (0.06)	—	—	—	—	205.3* (6.1–6965.7)	9.6 (0.01)*	0.2 (0.0–1.8)	3.4 (0.18)
	20–29	0.6 (0.2–2.0)		—		—		1.0 (0.1–17.6)		0.1 (0.0–2.3)	
	30+	0.3* (0.1–0.8)		—		—		—		—	
Natural disaster	13–19	1.0 (0.2–6.3)	0.1 (0.99)	0.3 (0.0–5.9)	0.7 (0.88)	—	—	0.5 (0.0–11.7)	50.0 (<0.001)*	—	—
	20–29	1.1 (0.2–6.6)		0.4 (0.0–6.1)		—		0.0* (0.0–0.0)		—	
	30+	1.2 (0.2–6.5)		0.3 (0.0–5.1)		—		0.0* (0.0–0.0)		—	
Accident	13–19	1.3 (0.3–6.1)	6.1 (0.11)	—	—	—	—	—	—	0.6 (0.1–5.1)	1.4 (0.50)
	20–29	0.6 (0.1–2.7)		—		—		—		0.3 (0.0–2.2)	
	30+	0.5 (0.1–2.3)		—		—		—		—	
War/combat/refugee experience											
Exposure to war	13–19	4.1 (0.4–37.8)	17.0 (<0.001)*	0.5 (0.1–44)	4.4 (0.22)	—	—	—	—	0.0* (0.0–0.0)	70.2 (<0.001)*
	20–29	0.6 (0.1–6.3)		0.3 (0.0–2.7)		—		—		0.0* (0.0–0.0)	
	30+	1.1 (0.1–11.4)		0.1 (0.0–1.5)		—		—		0.0* (0.0–0.0)	
Combat	13–19	0.2 (0.0–1.8)	11.9 (0.003)*	4.2 (0.4–40.0)	2.0 (0.38)	0.0 (0.0–3.3)	3.0 (0.22)	—	—	—	—
	20–29	6.3* (1.3–29.0)		1.6 (0.1–22.7)		2.5 (0.2–30.5)		—		—	
	30+	—		—		—		—		—	
Refugee	13–19	96.8* (11.6–806.6)	27.5 (<.001)*	31.3* (5.0–195.9)	26.9 (<0.001)*	6.0 (0.3–105.3)	2.6 (0.27)	0.0* (0.0–0.1)	25.8 (<0.001)*	0.0* (0.0–0.0)	45.9 (<0.001)*
	20–29	—		65.7* (10.3–418.1)		5.1 (0.5–52.9)		0.0* (0.0–0.0)		0.2 (0.0–6.2)	
	30+	92.5* (12.4–691.5)		84.1* (11.8–597.3)		—		—		—	
Sexual/interpersonal violence											
Sexual violence	13–19	1.4 (0.4–5.2)	2.4 (0.50)	—	—	0.0* (0.0–0.0)	1.2 (0.56)	—	—	3.2 (0.4–27.9)	2.4 (0.30)
	20–29	0.8 (0.2–2.9)		—		0.0* (0.0–0.0)		—		0.5 (0.1–3.2)	
	30+	1.0 (0.3–3.8)		—		0.0* (0.0–0.0)		—		—	
Interpersonal violence	13–19	0.8 (0.1–6.8)	0.1 (1.00)	—	—	—	—	16.7* (1.2–238.9)	4.4 (0.11)	—	—
	20–29	0.9 (0.1–7.0)		—		—		1.0 (0.2–5.3)		—	
	30+	0.9 (0.1–6.9)		—		—		—		—	
Witness/perpetrator violence											
Witness violence	13–19	0.5 (0.1–2.1)	1.9 (0.59)	0.4 (0.1–1.4)	6.7 (0.08)	0.6 (0.2–2.3)	4.1 (0.13)	8.3 (0.7–93.5)	7.2 (0.03)*	0.0* (0.0–0.0)	2.5 (0.28)
	20–29	0.5 (0.1–1.9)		0.3* (0.1–0.8)		2.6 (0.9–8.0)		5.4* (1.4–21.3)		0.0* (0.0–0.0)	
	30+	0.7 (0.2–2.6)		0.2* (0.1–0.8)		—		—		0.0* (0.0–0.0)	
Perpetrator violence	13–19	—	—	—	—	1.1 (0.1–14.3)	0.1 (0.97)	9.5 (0.3–270.9)	39.2 (<0.001)*	14.8 (0.9–242.1)	4.7 (0.10)
	20–29	—		—		0.8 (0.1–7.1)		—		—	
	30+	—		—		—		—		—	
Loss/trauma											
Death of loved one	13–19	1.0 (0.2–4.8)	1.5 (0.69)	1.1 (0.3–4.0)	0.4 (0.93)	1.1 (0.1–19.5)	1.5 (0.69)	0.0* (0.0–0.0)	52.9 (<0.001)*	0.5 (0.1–4.0)	0.6 (0.73)
	20–29	0.7 (0.2–3.5)		1.0 (0.2–3.7)		2.1 (0.1–37.0)		0.0* (0.0–0.0)		0.6 (0.1–4.1)	
	30+	0.7 (0.1–3.2)		0.9 (0.2–3.2)		1.7 (0.1–28.7)		0.0* (0.0–0.0)		—	

Appendix Table 9.8. (cont.)

Interactions	Among total sample						Among ideators			
	Ideation		Attempt		Plan		Planned attempt		Unplanned attempt	
	OR (95% CI)	χ² (p-value)	OR (95% CI)	χ² (p-value)	OR (95% CI)	χ² (p-value)	OR (95% CI)	χ² (p-value)	OR (95% CI)	χ² (p-value)
Trauma to loved one 13–19	0.2 (0.0–1.7)	2.9 (0.41)	—	—	3.2 (0.7–14.8)	5.1 (0.08)	0.4 (0.0–9.2)	1.9 (0.40)	0.3 (0.0–2.3)	1.5 (0.46)
20–29	0.4 (0.0–2.9)		—		4.7* (1.2–18.8)		2.7 (0.3–23.5)		0.7 (0.1–5.2)	
30+	0.3 (0.0–2.2)		—		—		—		—	
All others 13–19	0.6 (0.1–7.7)		—	—	0.9 (0.1–5.2)	0.2 (0.90)	0.1 (0.0–5.7)	5.1 (0.08)	0.6 (0.1–15.4)	0.2 (0.91)
20–29	0.9 (0.2–5.0)		—		0.7 (0.2–3.2)		2.7 (0.2–36.2)		0.6 (0.1–6.5)	
30+	—		—		—		—		—	
39 df χ² test for all trauma		1419.9 (<0.001)*		856.5 (<0.001)*		455.9 (<0.001)*		738.0 (<0.001)*		881.4 (<0.001)*
χ² test for all trauma and dummies for number of traumas		1697.6 (<0.001)*		1678.1 (<0.001)*		771.2 (<0.001)*		1160.4 (<0.001)*		1128.1 (<0.001)*
Number of traumatic events[b] 2, 13–19	1.2 (0.2–7.8)	94.6 (<0.001)*	234.6* (51.4–1071.8)	155.5 (<0.001)*	0.0* (0.0–0.0)	6.9 (0.55)	1.6 (0.1–31.5)	109.3 (<0.001)*		13.6 (0.034)*
20–29	1.8 (0.2–12.7)		251.2* (52.7–1197.5)		0.0* (0.0–0.0)		3.7 (0.4–35.3)			
30+	1.7 (0.3–11.5)		220.8* (39.7–1226.3)		0.0* (0.0–0.0)		—			
3, 13–19	—		14.6* (1.1–190.6)		1.2 (0.1–18.0)		0.6 (0.0–48.2)			
20–29	—		15.6* (1.3–191.9)		0.3 (0.0–2.4)		3.4 (0.1–84.6)			
30+	—		11.3 (0.8–152.2)		—		—			
4, 13–19	0.6 (0.1–7.7)		0.1 (0.0–3.2)		0.2 (0.0–15.3)		0.0* (0.0–0.8)			
20–29	0.9 (0.2–5.0)		0.5 (0.0–8.0)		0.1 (0.0–1.5)		0.1 (0.0–3.0)			
30+	—		0.4 (0.0–9.1)		—		—			
5, 13–19	0.4 (0.0–92.6)		0.1 (0.0–7.5)		0.2 (0.0–38.2)		0.0* (0.0–0.0)			
20–29	2.2 (0.0–254.5)		0.1 (0.0–6.4)		0.2 (0.0–9.4)		0.2 (0.0–15.0)			
30+	9.9 (0.1–968.4)		0.6 (0.0–46.5)		—		—			
6+, 13–19	0.5 (0.0–15.9)		—		—		0.0 (0.0–2.3)			
20–29	0.2 (0.0–3.9)		—		—		—			
30+	—		—		—		—			

* Significant at the 0.05 level, two-sided test.

0.0* (0.0–0.0) OR is ≤0.05 indicating very low risk.

— Not included due to small cell size.

[a] Assessed in the Part 2 sample. Models control for person–years, country, significant variables from the chapters on sociodemographics, parental psychopathology, childhood adversities, and interaction terms between life course intervals (4–12, 13–19, 20–29, 30+ years) and each control. Only the interaction terms between the life course intervals and PTSD variables are shown in table.

[b] For number of traumatic events, the last OR represents the odds for that number of traumatic events or more. For example, for unplanned attempt, 4 represents ≥4 (that is, 4+).

Appendix Table 9.9. Interactions between traumatic events and suicidal behavior over the life course[a] (low-income countries)

Interactions		Among total sample						Among ideators			
		Ideation		Attempt		Plan		Planned attempt		Unplanned attempt	
		OR (95% CI)	χ² (p-value)	OR (95% CI)	χ² (p-value)	OR (95% CI)	χ² (p-value)	OR (95% CI)	χ² (p-value)	OR (95% CI)	χ² (p-value)
Disasters/accidents											
All man-made disasters	13–19	0.3 (0.0–2.7)	2.5 (0.48)	44.1* (3.4–572.2)	106.5 (<0.001)*	0.0* (0.0–0.0)	131.9 (<0.001)*	—	—	—	—
	20–29	0.4 (0.0–3.8)		—		0.0* (0.0–0.0)		—		—	
	30+	0.2 (0.0–2.1)		—		0.0* (0.0–0.0)		—		—	
Natural disaster	13–19	0.4 (0.0–3.5)	5.4 (0.15)	0.1 (0.0–1.1)	5.5 (0.14)	5.8 (0.6–57.8)	3.1 (0.22)	0.1* (0.0–1.0)	51.0 (<0.001)*	0.0* (0.0–0.0)	145.0 (<0.001)*
	20–29	0.3 (0.0–3.0)		0.1* (0.0–0.6)		0.8 (0.2–3.0)		—		0.0* (0.0–0.0)	
	30+	0.2 (0.0–1.5)		0.1 (0.0–1.0)		—		—		0.0* (0.0–0.0)	
Accident	13–19	9.3 (0.9–100.9)	7.1 (0.07)	—	—	0.0* (0.0–0.0)	168.0 (<0.001)*	0.9 (0.0–22.3)	0.8 (0.66)	—	—
	20–29	7.1 (0.7–76.1)		—		0.0* (0.0–0.0)		2.3 (0.3–15.1)		—	
	30+	4.1 (0.4–44.6)		—		0.0* (0.0–0.0)		—		—	
War/combat/refugee experiences											
Exposure to war	13–19	1.2 (0.2–9.2)	4.5 (0.21)	—	86.5 (<0.001)*	—	—	—	—	0.0* (0.0–0.0)	114.7 (<0.001)*
	20–29	0.9 (0.1–7.4)		—		—		—		0.0* (0.0–0.9)	
	30+	0.4 (0.1–2.5)		—		—		—		0.0 (0.0–2.2)	
Combat	13–19	—	—	79.6* (15.5–408.3)	8.9 (0.01)*	52.8* (2.4–1155.1)	6.4 (0.04)*	3.3 (0.0–25275.1)	0.6 (0.73)	—	2.2 (0.14)
	20–29	—		—		1.1 (0.1–11.4)		4.0 (0.1–149.0)		0.1 (0.0–2.6)	
	30+	—		—		—		—		—	
Refugee	13–19	0.6 (0.1–3.5)	25.1 (<0.001)*	—	57.9 (<0.001)*	0.0* (0.0–0.2)	11.0 (0.004)*	—	—	0.0 (0.0–2.3)	2.6 (0.11)
	20–29	0.1* (0.0–0.6)		—		0.3 (0.0–3.3)		—		—	
	30+	0.1* (0.0–0.7)		—		—		—		—	
Sexual/interpersonal violence											
Sexual violence	13–19	—	1.5 (0.69)	0.5 (0.0–6.1)	0.3 (0.95)	0.0* (0.0–0.0)	3.4 (0.18)	0.3 (0.0–2.0)	2.0 (0.36)	0.8 (0.1–9.7)	6.6 (0.04)*
	20–29	—		0.6 (0.1–6.2)		0.0* (0.0–0.0)		1.2 (0.1–10.9)		0.1* (0.0–0.6)	
	30+	—		0.6 (0.1–5.0)		0.0* (0.0–0.0)		—		—	
Interpersonal violence	13–19	—	—	0.0* (0.0–0.3)	10.7 (0.01)*	—	—	1.1 (0.0–37.4)	0.1 (0.94)	0.0* (0.0–0.0)	30.9 (<0.001)*
	20–29	—		0.0* (0.0–0.2)		—		0.8 (0.2–3.5)		0.0* (0.0–0.0)	
	30+	—		0.0* (0.0–0.2)		—		—		0.0* (0.0–0.0)	
Witness/perpetrator violence											
Witness violence	13–19	0.0* (0.0–0.2)	31.0 (<0.001)*	0.2 (0.0–1.1)	8.5 (0.04)*	0.0* (0.0–0.0)	93.6 (<0.001)*	0.0* (0.0–0.0)	13.4 (0.001)*	—	—
	20–29	0.1* (0.0–0.2)		0.1* (0.0–0.7)		0.0* (0.0–0.0)		0.0* (0.0–0.0)		—	
	30+	0.1* (0.0–0.2)		0.3 (0.0–2.1)		0.0* (0.0–0.0)		0.0* (0.0–0.0)		—	
Perpetrator violence	13–19	0.2 (0.0–2.6)	9.8 (0.02)*	0.0* (0.0–0.3)	199.6 (<0.001)*	0.0* (0.0–0.0)	108.6 (<0.001)*	0.0* (0.0–0.0)	82.2 (<0.001)*	0.0* (0.0–0.0)	31.1 (<0.001)*
	20–29	0.1* (0.0–0.7)		—		0.0* (0.0–0.0)		0.2 (0.0–2.2)		0.0* (0.0–0.4)	
	30+	0.0* (0.0–0.4)		—		0.0* (0.0–0.0)		—		—	
Loss/trauma											
Death of loved one	13–19	2.9 (0.8–10.6)	7.4 (0.06)	6.1 (0.4–94.9)	8.8 (0.03)*	0.0* (0.0–0.0)	10.9 (0.004)*	0.1* (0.0–1.0)	7.1 (0.03)*	—	—
	20–29	1.9 (0.5–6.9)		1.4 (0.1–19.8)		0.0* (0.0–0.0)		0.1* (0.0–0.5)		—	
	30+	1.2 (0.3–4.0)		2.1 (0.1–30.1)		0.0* (0.0–0.0)		—		—	

Appendix Table 9.9. (cont.)

		Among total sample						Among ideators			
		Ideation		Attempt		Plan		Planned attempt		Unplanned attempt	
		OR (95% CI)	χ^2 (p-value)	OR (95% CI)	χ^2 (p-value)	OR (95% CI)	χ^2 (p-value)	OR (95% CI)	χ^2 (p-value)	OR (95% CI)	χ^2 (p-value)
Interactions											
Trauma to loved one	13–19	–	–	–	–	7.7 (0.6–95.6)	4.1 (0.13)	0.5 (0.0–16.4)	3.6 (0.16)	0.0* (0.0–0.0)	28.3 (<0.001)*
	20–29	–		–		0.5 (0.1–2.1)		0.1 (0.0–1.1)		1.5 (0.1–18.2)	
	30+	–		–		–		–		–	
All others											
	13–19	66.1* (3.1–1423.1)	10.9 (0.012)*	–	–	1.3 (0.2–7.3)	5.7 (0.06)	–	–	0.0* (0.0–0.0)	91.3 (<0.001)*
	20–29	34.6* (1.5–792.4)		–		0.2* (0.0–0.8)		–		0.2 (0.0–3.9)	
	30+	18.3 (0.9–370.6)		–		–		–		–	
39 df χ^2 test for all trauma			705.2 (<0.001)*		2022.5 (<0.001)*		1304.9 (<0.001)*		1046.7 (<0.001)*		1967.1 (<0.001)*
χ^2 test for all trauma and dummies for number of traumas			1497.6 (<0.001)*		4152.7 (<0.001)*		2245.8 (<0.001)*		1508.0 (<0.001)*		2304.1 (<0.001)*
Number of traumatic events[b]											
2	13–19	0.6 (0.1–5.3)	271.4 (<0.001)*	2.1 (0.1–84.4)	144.2 (<0.001)*	–	35.3 (<0.001)*	54.4 (0.4–6823.6)	222.4 (<0.001)*	0.5 (0.0–75.8)	261.1 (<0.001)*
	20–29	0.8 (0.1–7.2)		6.5 (0.2–274.0)		–		–		6.6 (0.6–78.8)	
	30+	1.0 (0.1–7.8)		2.8 (0.1–106.0)		–		–		–	
3	13–19	0.2 (0.0–4.5)		1.7 (0.0–64.1)		0.1 (0.0–1.9)		0.0* (0.0–0.0)		–	
	20–29	0.2 (0.0–5.5)		4.5 (0.2–114.7)		7.9 (0.9–67.2)		7.1 (0.2–222.6)		–	
	30+	0.6 (0.0–12.7)		1.7 (0.1–44.3)		–		–		–	
4	13–19	–		0.1 (0.0–7.0)		4.2 (0.0–628.0)		0.0* (0.0–0.0)		–	
	20–29	0.6 (0.0–40.0)		0.6 (0.0–40.0)		3.8 (0.1–120.8)		30.5 (0.4–2538.0)		–	
	30+	0.2 (0.0–13.3)		0.2 (0.0–13.3)		–		–		–	
5	13–19	0.0* (0.0–0.6)		0.0* (0.0–0.0)		0.0* (0.0–0.8)		–		–	
	20–29	0.5 (0.0–8.7)		17.8 (0.6–520.5)		–		–		–	
	30+	–		–		–		–		–	
6+	13–19	0.0* (0.0–0.0)		0.0* (0.0–0.0)		6.0 (0.0–1254.8)		–		–	
	20–29	0.0 (0.0–2.0)		0.4 (0.0–57.0)		–		–		–	
	30+	–		–		–		–		–	

* Significant at the 0.05 level, two-sided test.

0.0* (0.0–0.0) OR is ≤0.05 indicating very low risk.

– Not included due to small cell size.

[a] Assessed in the Part 2 sample. Models control for person–years, country, significant variables from the chapters on sociodemographics, parental psychopathology, childhood adversities, and interaction terms between life course intervals (4–12, 13–19, 20–29, 30+ years) and each control. Only the interaction terms between the life course intervals and PTSD variables are shown in table.

[b] For number of traumatic events, the last OR represents the odds for that number of traumatic events or more. For example, for unplanned attempt, 3 represents ≥3 (that is, 3+).

Appendix Table 9.10. Associations between traumatic events and the persistence of suicidal behavior[a] (high-income countries)

Traumatic events	Ideation OR (95% CI)	Plan OR (95% CI)	Attempt OR (95% CI)
Disasters/accidents			
All man-made disasters	1.1 (0.9–1.5)	0.9 (0.6–1.5)	1.5 (0.9–2.5)
Natural disaster	1.0 (0.7–1.2)	0.9 (0.6–1.4)	0.8 (0.4–1.5)
Accident	1.2 (0.9–1.5)	1.2 (0.8–1.8)	1.0 (0.6–1.6)
War/combat/refugee experiences			
Exposure to war	1.1 (0.8–1.5)	0.9 (0.6–1.6)	1.4 (0.7–2.6)
Combat	1.0 (0.6–1.7)	0.3* (0.1–0.9)	1.6 (0.4–5.5)
Refugee	1.3 (0.7–2.4)	0.8 (0.2–2.6)	0.8 (0.2–2.8)
Sexual/interpersonal violence			
Sexual violence	1.3* (1.0–1.7)	0.9 (0.6–1.4)	1.1 (0.7–1.8)
Interpersonal violence	1.1 (0.9–1.4)	0.5* (0.3–0.8)	0.6 (0.3–1.1)
Witness/perpetrator violence			
Witness violence	0.9 (0.7–1.2)	1.0 (0.7–1.5)	1.1 (0.7–1.9)
Perpetrator violence	1.0 (0.7–1.5)	1.6 (0.9–3.0)	1.2 (0.6–2.6)
Loss/trauma			
Death of loved one	1.1 (0.9–1.4)	1.1 (0.8–1.5)	1.2 (0.8–1.9)
Trauma to loved one	1.1 (0.9–1.4)	0.8 (0.6–1.2)	1.0 (0.6–1.6)
All others	1.2 (0.9–1.5)	1.1 (0.8–1.6)	1.1 (0.7–1.7)
13 df χ^2 group significance test for 13 types	10.9 (0.62)	22.5 (0.05)*	12.2 (0.51)
12 df χ^2 significance test for difference between types	9.3 (0.68)	23.6 (0.02)*	11.9 (0.45)
Number of traumatic events			
1			
2	0.8 (0.6–1.1)	1.0 (0.6–1.7)	1.1 (0.6–2.0)
3	0.8 (0.5–1.2)	1.1 (0.6–2.3)	0.8 (0.4–2.0)
4	0.5* (0.3–0.9)	0.6 (0.2–1.6)	0.9 (0.3–3.1)
5	0.7 (0.3–1.6)	1.2 (0.3–4.4)	0.7 (0.1–3.5)
6+	0.4 (0.2–1.2)	2.1 (0.5–9.4)	0.9 (0.1–6.5)
χ^2 (p-value)	7.6 (0.18)	6.6 (0.25)	1.8 (0.87)

* Significant at the 0.05 level, two-sided test.

[a] Results are based on multivariate discrete time survival models. Models control for country, age-related variables, and significant variables from the chapters on sociodemographics, parental psychopathology, and childhood adversities.

Appendix Table 9.11. Associations between traumatic events and the persistence of suicidal behavior[a] (middle-income countries)

Traumatic events	Ideation OR (95% CI)	Plan OR (95% CI)	Attempt OR (95% CI)
Disasters/accidents			
All man-made disasters	2.0 (0.8–4.6)	5.4 (1.8–16.6)	2.6 (0.5–14.6)
Natural disaster	2.5* (1.3–4.9)	1.1 (0.4–3.1)	1.2 (0.3–4.5)
Accident	1.6 (0.9–2.9)	1.8 (0.7–4.6)	1.4 (0.4–5.2)
War/combat/refugee experiences			
Exposure to war	1.4 (0.7–3.1)	7.5* (2.2–25.5)	1.8 (0.5–7.2)
Combat	2.2 (0.4–11.3)	0.1 (0.0–1.4)	1.0 (0.0–41.6)
Refugee	5.8* (2.2–15.8)	1.6 (0.1–20.0)	5.6* (1.1–27.4)
Sexual/interpersonal violence			
Sexual violence	1.4 (0.8–2.4)	4.0* (2.0–8.0)	2.6* (1.1–6.0)
Interpersonal violence	1.5 (0.9–2.3)	1.7 (0.8–3.8)	1.7 (0.6–5.1)
Witness/perpetrator violence			
Witness violence	1.6 (1.0–2.5)	1.1 (0.5–2.7)	1.1 (0.4–2.8)
Perpetrator violence	0.9 (0.4–2.3)	4.4 (1.0–19.5)	1.5 (0.3–6.5)
Loss/trauma			
Death of loved one	1.0 (0.6–1.7)	1.7 (0.8–3.7)	1.7 (0.8–3.7)
Trauma to loved one	0.8 (0.4–1.7)	1.9 (0.7–5.3)	2.3 (0.7–7.0)
All others	1.4 (0.8–2.5)	2.1 (0.8–5.5)	0.8 (0.2–2.7)
13 df χ^2 test for 13 types	33.1 (0.002)*	37.4 (<0.001)*	19.4 (0.11)
12 df χ^2 test for difference between types	28.7 (0.004)*	24.1 (0.02)*	14.9 (0.25)
Number of traumatic events[b]			
1			
2	0.4* (0.2–0.8)	0.3* (0.1–0.8)	0.4 (0.1–1.3)
3	0.5 (0.2–1.6)	0.5 (0.1–1.9)	0.7 (0.1–5.1)
4	0.1 (0.0–1.1)	0.0* (0.0–0.3)	0.1 (0.0–1.1)
5+	0.1* (0.0–0.8)		
χ^2 (p-value)	9.6 (0.05)*	10.5 (0.01)*	9.1 (0.03)*

* Significant at the 0.05 level, two-sided test.
[a] Results are based on multivariate discrete time survival models. Models control for country, age-related variables, and significant variables from the chapters on sociodemographics, parental psychopathology, and childhood adversities.
[b] For number of traumatic events, the last OR represents the odds for that number of traumatic events or more. For example, for attempt, 4 represents ≥4 (that is, 4+).

Appendix Table 9.12. Associations between traumatic events and the persistence of suicidal behavior[a] (low-income countries)

Traumatic events	Ideation	Plan	Attempt
	OR (95% CI)	OR (95% CI)	OR (95% CI)
Disasters/accidents			
All man-made disasters	0.6 (0.2–1.4)	0.5 (0.1–2.2)	0.1 (0.0–2.1)
Natural disaster	1.1 (0.5–2.2)	0.4 (0.1–2.0)	1.5 (0.3–8.1)
Accident	1.4 (0.8–2.4)	1.2 (0.5–2.6)	10.0*(2.3–43.9)
War/combat/refugee experiences			
Exposure to war	1.1 (0.5–2.5)	1.4 (0.5–4.0)	2.6 (0.8–8.9)
Combat	1.4 (0.5–4.0)	2.7 (0.7–10.5)	0.8 (0.1–7.5)
Refugee	0.8 (0.2–3.2)	1.1 (0.1–9.6)	4.9 (0.2–109.4)
Sexual/interpersonal violence			
Sexual violence	1.2 (0.6–2.3)	0.8 (0.3–2.2)	1.4 (0.4–4.8)
Interpersonal violence	1.3 (0.8–1.9)	0.7 (0.3–1.5)	1.9 (0.8–4.1)
Witness/perpetrator violence			
Witness violence	1.5 (0.8–2.8)	0.8 (0.4–1.8)	1.7 (0.5–5.5)
Perpetrator violence	1.0 (0.4–2.6)	0.1 (0.1–1.9)	0.5 (0.0–6.0)
Loss/trauma			
Death of loved one	1.5 (0.9–2.6)	1.3 (0.6–2.7)	4.4*(1.5–12.5)
Trauma to loved one	0.9 (0.5–1.8)	0.5 (0.1–2.0)	3.9*(1.1–13.8)
All others	1.6 (0.8–3.5)	4.5*(1.6–12.6)	7.8*(1.5–39.3)
13 df χ^2 test for 13 types	11.1 (0.60)	24.3 (0.03)*	41.0 (<0.001)*
12 df χ^2 test for difference between types	8.9 (0.72)	21.9 (0.04)*	23.3 (0.03)*
Number of traumatic events[b]			
1			
2	0.6 (0.3–1.2)	0.5 (0.2–1.7)	0.1*(0.0–0.4)
3	0.5 (0.2–1.3)	0.9 (0.2–3.9)	0.1 (0.0–1.5)
4	0.7 (0.2–3.3)	0.7 (0.1–6.2)	0.0*(0.0–0.5)
5+	0.3 (0.0–2.4)	0.0 (0.0–1.1)	
χ^2 (p-value)	4.0 (0.40)	5.5 (0.24)	11.8 (0.01)*

* Significant at the 0.05 level, two-sided test.
[a] Results are based on multivariate discrete time survival models. Models control for country, age-related variables, and significant variables from the chapters on sociodemographics, parental psychopathology, and childhood adversities.
[b] For number of traumatic events, the last OR represents the odds for that number of traumatic events or more. For example, for attempt, 4 represents ≥4 (that is, 4+).

Appendix Table 9.13. Interactions between the occurrence of traumatic events and DSM-IV posttraumatic stress disorder in the prediction of suicidal behavior[a] (high-income countries)

Traumatic events	Among total sample			Among ideators	
	Ideation	Attempt	Plan	Planned attempt	Unplanned attempt
	OR (95% CI)	OR (95% CI)	OR (95% CI)	OR (95% CI)	OR (95% CI)
Disasters/accidents					
All man-made disasters	1.0 (0.5–1.7)	0.4* (0.2–0.9)	0.5 (0.3–1.1)	1.2 (0.4–3.8)	0.1* (0.0–0.6)
Natural disaster	1.2 (0.6–2.2)	1.0 (0.4–2.1)	0.9 (0.4–1.8)	1.6 (0.6–4.1)	0.5 (0.1–2.6)
Accident	1.2 (0.8–1.8)	0.9 (0.5–1.5)	1.4 (0.8–2.4)	0.8 (0.4–1.5)	0.7 (0.2–2.4)
War/combat/refugee experiences					
Exposure to war	2.5* (1.3–5.1)	2.1 (0.8–5.3)	1.8 (0.7–4.6)	0.8 (0.2–2.7)	2.6 (0.4–18.8)
Combat	1.0 (0.5–2.4)	1.0 (0.3–3.3)	0.9 (0.2–3.8)	0.6 (0.1–6.4)	0.0* (0.0–0.0)
Refugee	0.3 (0.1–1.0)	0.6 (0.1–3.3)	0.3 (0.1–1.8)	0.0* (0.0–0.6)	7.6 (0.4–139.4)
Sexual/interpersonal violence					
Sexual violence	0.8 (0.6–1.1)	0.8 (0.5–1.3)	0.6 (0.3–1.0)	0.7 (0.3–1.9)	0.6 (0.2–1.4)
Interpersonal violence	0.8 (0.5–1.1)	1.0 (0.6–1.7)	1.3 (0.7–2.3)	1.1 (0.5–2.8)	0.8 (0.3–2.2)
Witness/perpetrator violence					
Witness violence	1.2 (0.8–1.8)	1.2 (0.7–2.3)	0.8 (0.5–1.6)	2.1 (1.0–4.7)	1.2 (0.4–3.8)
Perpetrator violence	0.5 (0.2–1.1)	1.5 (0.7–3.3)	1.1 (0.4–2.6)	1.2 (0.3–4.6)	5.4 (0.8–36.5)
Loss/trauma					
Death of loved one	0.8 (0.6–1.1)	1.1 (0.7–1.7)	0.7 (0.5–1.1)	1.1 (0.6–2.1)	0.9 (0.4–2.4)
Trauma to loved one	0.8 (0.5–1.2)	0.7 (0.4–1.2)	0.8 (0.5–1.4)	0.8 (0.4–1.9)	1.6 (0.5–4.6)
All others	0.6* (0.4–0.8)	0.8 (0.5–1.3)	0.9 (0.5–1.6)	1.6 (0.7–3.6)	0.6 (0.2–1.5)
13 df group χ^2 test	133.9 (<0.001)*	70.1 (<0.001)*	22.3 (0.05)	17.1 (0.20)	20.7 (0.08)
13 df group interaction test	30.5 (0.004)*	18.2 (0.15)	16.3 (0.23)	13.7 (0.40)	123.1 (<0.001)*

* Significant at the 0.05 level, two-sided test.
0.0* (0.0–0.0) OR is ≤0.05 indicating very low risk.
[a] Assessed in the Part 2 sample due to having Part 2 controls. Models included interaction terms between DSM-IV posttraumatic stress disorder (PTSD) and each trauma event. Only interaction terms are shown in the table; however, the main effects are still controlled for. Models control for person–years, country, and significant variables from the chapters on sociodemographics, parental psychopathology, and childhood adversities.

Appendix Table 9.14. Interactions between the occurrence of traumatic events and DSM-IV posttraumatic stress disorder in the prediction of suicidal behavior[a] (middle-income countries)

Traumatic events	Among total sample		Among ideators		
	Ideation	Attempt	Plan	Planned attempt	Unplanned attempt
	OR (95% CI)	OR (95% CI)	OR (95% CI)	OR (95% CI)	OR (95% CI)
Disasters/accidents					
All man-made disasters	1.0 (0.4–2.9)	0.5 (0.0–24.6)	0.6 (0.0–6.7)	0.0* (0.0–0.0)	0.9 (0.0–155.0)
Natural disaster	0.4 (0.1–1.7)	0.8 (0.2–3.6)	17.8* (1.8–172.4)	4.3 (0.0–19677.5)	0.0* (0.0–0.0)
Accident	0.8 (0.3–2.2)	0.5 (0.0–5.2)	1.8 (0.3–12.7)	0.4 (0.1–2.4)	0.0* (0.0–0.0)
War/combat/refugee experiences					
Exposure to war	0.1 (0.0–1.2)	0.8 (0.2–3.5)	0.0* (0.0–0.0)	–	0.0* (0.0–0.4)
Combat	10.6 (0.8–141.8)	0.8 (0.1–5.7)	0.2 (0.0–7.5)	–	0.1 (0.0–6946.0)
Refugee	6.6* (1.1–40.7)	1.2 (0.0–118.0)	–	0.2 (0.0–889.3)	–
Sexual/interpersonal violence					
Sexual violence	1.3 (0.5–3.4)	–	1.0 (0.1–7.9)	0.2 (0.0–2.0)	–
Interpersonal violence	1.0 (0.4–2.2)	1.7 (0.4–7.9)	3.0 (0.6–14.3)	0.0 (0.0–3.3)	40.2* (1.1–1421.0)
Witness/perpetrator violence					
Witness violence	0.9 (0.3–2.4)	1.2 (0.4–4.1)	0.9 (0.2–4.7)	0.1 (0.0–6.5)	0.0 (0.0–23.1)
Perpetrator violence	0.9 (0.2–3.7)	1.7 (0.4–6.4)	–	0.0* (0.0–0.6)	–
Loss/trauma					
Death of loved one	0.9 (0.4–2.0)	0.8 (0.2–2.9)	0.9 (0.1–6.8)	0.0* (0.0–0.3)	0.1 (0.0–16.4)
Trauma to loved one	0.9 (0.3–2.5)	0.7 (0.2–3.0)	0.3 (0.0–1.8)	0.8 (0.0–19.5)	12.7 (0.4–441.9)
All others	0.6 (0.2–1.9)	1.0 (0.2–6.0)	0.8 (0.1–4.3)	0.1 (0.0–3.5)	0.0 (0.0–3.3)
13 df group χ^2 test	73.8 (<0.001)*	62.7 (<0.001)*	14.5 (0.34)	13.0 (0.44)	28.7 (0.007)*
13 df group interaction test	9.5 (0.73)	7.4 (0.88)	87.0 (<0.001)*	179.9 (<0.001)*	669.6 (<0.001)*

*Significant at the 0.05 level, two-sided test.
0.0* (0.0–0.0) OR is ≤0.05 indicating very low risk.
– Not included due to small cell size.
[a] Assessed in the Part 2 sample due to having Part 2 controls. Models included interaction terms between DSM-IV posttraumatic stress disorder (PTSD) and each trauma event. Only interaction terms are shown in the table; however, the main effects are still controlled for. Models control for person–years, country, and significant variables from the chapters on sociodemographics, parental psychopathology, and childhood adversities.

Appendix Table 9.15. Interactions between the occurrence of traumatic events and DSM-IV posttraumatic stress disorder in the prediction of suicidal behavior[a] (low-income countries)

Traumatic events	Among total sample		Among ideators		
	Ideation	Attempt	Plan	Planned attempt	Unplanned attempt
	OR (95% CI)	OR (95% CI)	OR (95% CI)	OR (95% CI)	OR (95% CI)
Disasters/accidents					
All man-made disasters	1.5 (0.2–14.5)	8.7 (0.3–264.1)	6.3 (0.2–176.6)	–	–
Natural disaster	–	–	2.5 (0.0–140.9)	3.5 (0.1–82.8)	–
Accident	2.9 (0.2–54.1)	1.2 (0.0–28.9)	0.9 (0.1–7.8)	0.0 (0.0–1.1)	0.0* (0.0–0.1)
War/combat/refugee experiences					
Exposure to war	0.5 (0.0–16.4)	1.6 (0.1–21.0)	1.7 (0.0–171.5)	0.7 (0.1–6.4)	0.0* (0.0–0.0)
Combat	2.1 (0.0–180.2)	–	0.0* (0.0–0.5)	0.0* (0.0–0.0)	–
Refugee	1.2 (0.0–28.2)	0.9 (0.1–14.7)	–	0.0* (0.0–0.0)	–
Sexual/interpersonal violence					
Sexual violence	–	–	0.0* (0.0–0.5)	0.0 (0.0–1.7)	0.0* (0.0–0.0)
Interpersonal violence	2.7 (0.2–47.6)	2.6 (0.1–66.6)	0.2 (0.0–2.0)	4.4 (0.4–47.6)	–
Witness/perpetrator violence					
Witness violence	1.3 (0.1–23.5)	0.2 (0.0–188.2)	–	–	0.0* (0.0–0.0)
Perpetrator violence	0.0 (0.0–2.2)	0.2 (0.0–7.0)	0.0* (0.0–0.0)	–	–
Loss/trauma					
Death of loved one	1.3 (0.2–8.4)	2.1 (0.1–32.9)	0.6 (0.1–4.4)	–	0.2 (0.0–9.0)
Trauma to loved one	3.7 (0.1–184.1)	1.5 (0.0–438.4)	0.2 (0.0–2.2)	–	0.0* (0.0–0.4)
All others	2.8 (0.0–211.7)	2.9 (0.1–168.9)	–	–	0.0* (0.0–0.0)
13 df group χ² test	40.2 (<0.001)*	29.5 (<0.001)*	19.2 (0.12)	16.6 (0.22)	11.8 (0.55)
13 df group interaction test	41.6 (<0.001)*	18.5 (0.14)	201.9 (<0.001)*	142.5 (<0.001)*	1163.5 (<0.001)*

* Significant at the 0.05 level, two-sided test.
0.0* (0.0–0.0) OR is ≤0.05 indicating very low risk.
– Not included due to small cell size.
[a] Assessed in the Part 2 sample due to having Part 2 controls. Models included interaction terms between DSM-IV posttraumatic stress disorder (PTSD) and each trauma event. Only interaction terms are shown in the table; however, the main effects are still controlled for. Models control for person–years, country, and significant variables from the chapters on sociodemographics, parental psychopathology, and childhood adversities.

Appendix Table 10.1. Prevalence of DSM-IV mental disorders among those with each type of suicidal behavior[a] (high-income countries)

Mental disorders	Among total sample						Among ideators			
	%[b] (SE) with disorder						%[b] (SE) with disorder			
	Ideation	No ideation	Attempt	No attempt	Plan	No plan	Planned attempt	No planned attempt	Unplanned attempt	No unplanned attempt
Anxiety disorders										
Panic disorder	3.8 (0.3)	0.8 (0.0)	7.2 (0.7)	0.9 (0.0)	6.1 (0.6)	4.7 (0.4)	7.9 (1.0)	5.9 (1.2)	6.1 (1.1)	3.9 (0.5)
Generalized anxiety disorder	7.9 (0.4)	1.5 (0.1)	12.5 (1.0)	1.8 (0.1)	11.1 (0.9)	13.1 (0.8)	13.6 (1.4)	18.0 (2.2)	10.7 (1.5)	11.9 (0.8)
Specific phobia	17.5 (0.6)	5.5 (0.2)	23.6 (1.3)	5.9 (0.2)	21.7 (1.1)	16.3 (0.8)	25.3 (1.7)	20.5 (1.9)	20.6 (2.1)	14.3 (1.0)
Social phobia	15.7 (0.7)	3.1 (0.1)	20.8 (1.3)	3.6 (0.1)	21.5 (1.3)	15.9 (1.0)	24.1 (1.7)	21.3 (2.1)	16.1 (2.2)	15.1 (1.1)
Posttraumatic stress	7.7 (0.4)	1.4 (0.1)	13.8 (1.0)	1.7 (0.1)	11.7 (0.8)	9.7 (0.7)	14.9 (1.3)	15.7 (1.7)	12.0 (1.5)	8.1 (0.6)
Separation anxiety disorder	4.4 (0.5)	0.9 (0.1)	6.8 (0.7)	1.1 (0.1)	6.3 (0.9)	5.3 (0.6)	7.3 (0.9)	6.7 (1.4)	5.7 (1.2)	4.8 (0.7)
Agoraphobia	1.9 (0.2)	0.4 (0.0)	2.7 (0.4)	0.5 (0.0)	2.7 (0.4)	2.0 (0.3)	3.5 (0.6)	2.6 (0.6)	1.0 (0.4)	1.9 (0.3)
Mood disorders										
Major depressive disorder	18.9 (0.6)	3.8 (0.1)	27.6 (1.4)	4.6 (0.1)	27.8 (1.4)	30.6 (1.1)	32.0 (2.0)	42.3 (2.5)	21.0 (1.9)	29.0 (1.2)
Dysthymic disorder	4.4 (0.3)	0.6 (0.0)	6.9 (0.8)	0.8 (0.0)	7.5 (0.8)	7.2 (0.5)	8.3 (1.2)	12.3 (1.8)	4.5 (1.1)	6.1 (0.5)
Bipolar disorder	3.1 (0.3)	0.4 (0.0)	6.4 (0.8)	0.5 (0.0)	4.6 (0.5)	4.7 (0.5)	7.0 (1.0)	4.3 (0.8)	6.1 (1.4)	4.1 (0.5)
Impulse-control disorders										
Oppositional defiant disorder	3.9 (0.4)	0.4 (0.0)	6.9 (0.7)	0.5 (0.1)	6.1 (0.9)	2.6 (0.3)	6.9 (1.0)	3.7 (0.8)	6.9 (1.2)	1.9 (0.3)
Conduct disorder	3.6 (0.5)	0.4 (0.0)	5.9 (0.7)	0.5 (0.0)	4.7 (0.8)	2.3 (0.4)	5.2 (1.0)	3.4 (0.7)	6.8 (1.2)	1.6 (0.3)
Attention deficit hyperactivity disorder	3.8 (0.4)	0.6 (0.0)	6.3 (0.7)	0.6 (0.0)	5.9 (0.9)	2.0 (0.3)	6.9 (0.9)	3.4 (0.9)	5.4 (1.3)	1.5 (0.3)
Intermittent explosive disorder	3.9 (0.3)	0.7 (0.1)	5.4 (0.6)	0.8 (0.1)	5.1 (0.6)	4.6 (0.5)	6.0 (0.9)	5.8 (0.9)	4.4 (0.9)	4.3 (0.6)

Appendix Table 10.1. (cont.)

Mental disorders	Among total sample %^b (SE) with disorder				Among ideators %^b (SE) with disorder					
	Ideation	No ideation	Attempt	No attempt	Plan	No plan	Planned attempt	No planned attempt	Unplanned attempt	No unplanned attempt
Substance use disorders										
Alcohol abuse or dependence	9.6 (0.5)	2.8 (0.1)	15.2 (1.0)	3.2 (0.1)	14.7 (1.1)	14.5 (0.8)	15.9 (1.4)	17.7 (1.7)	14.0 (1.7)	12.5 (0.8)
Drug abuse or dependence	5.0 (0.4)	0.8 (0.0)	8.6 (0.9)	1.0 (0.0)	9.1 (0.8)	6.5 (0.5)	10.0 (1.1)	9.9 (1.1)	6.3 (1.2)	5.7 (0.5)
Number of mental disorders^c										
1	22.0 (0.8)	10.1 (0.2)	21.7 (1.3)	10.5 (0.2)	21.7 (1.3)	23.3 (0.9)	21.4 (1.6)	22.5 (2.2)	22.2 (2.1)	23.2 (1.1)
2	12.2 (0.5)	3.1 (0.1)	15.1 (1.1)	3.5 (0.1)	14.8 (1.0)	14.2 (0.7)	15.5 (1.4)	17.7 (1.9)	14.9 (1.8)	14.4 (0.8)
3	7.6 (0.4)	1.1 (0.0)	12.1 (1.0)	1.4 (0.0)	9.8 (0.9)	8.2 (0.6)	13.1 (1.4)	12.2 (1.6)	10.5 (1.6)	8.3 (0.7)
4	4.3 (0.4)	0.5 (0.0)	6.7 (0.8)	0.6 (0.0)	7.3 (0.9)	6.2 (0.5)	7.0 (0.9)	6.2 (0.9)	6.0 (1.4)	4.7 (0.5)
5	2.4 (0.2)	0.2 (0.0)	3.6 (0.5)	0.3 (0.0)	3.1 (0.4)	2.7 (0.3)	4.0 (0.6)	4.6 (1.0)	3.0 (0.7)	2.0 (0.2)
6	1.4 (0.2)	0.1 (0.0)	2.5 (0.5)	0.2 (0.0)	3.0 (0.5)	2.0 (0.2)	3.3 (0.7)	3.3 (0.7)	1.2 (0.5)	1.5 (0.2)
7	0.5 (0.1)	0.0 (0.0)	0.8 (0.3)	0.1 (0.0)	1.3 (0.4)	1.2 (0.2)	0.6 (0.3)	1.6 (0.5)	2.3 (0.7)	1.6 (0.3)
8	0.2 (0.1)	0.0 (0.0)	0.8 (0.2)	0.0 (0.0)	0.5 (0.2)	0.6 (0.2)	1.0 (0.4)	1.6 (0.6)		
9	0.2 (0.1)	0.0 (0.0)	1.7 (0.5)	0.0 (0.0)	1.0 (0.3)	0.3 (0.1)	2.3 (0.7)	0.7 (0.3)		
10+	0.1 (0.1)	0.0 (0.0)								
N^d	(5056)	(112,028)	(1613)	(116,041)	(1885)	(5646)	(1002)	(1330)	(551)	(4338)

^a As all subsequent models are based on the Part 2 sample, the percentages are also all based on the Part 2 sample despite some being Part 1 disorders.
^b % represents the percentage of people with the disorder among the cases with the disorder among the cases with the outcome variable indicated in the column header. For example: the first cell is the % of those with panic disorder among those with suicide ideation.
^c For number of mental disorders, the last OR represents the odds for that number of disorders or more. For example, for unplanned attempt, 7 represents ≥7 (that is, 7+).
^d Number of cases with the outcome variable; N represents the number of person–years.

Appendix Table 10.2. Prevalence of DSM-IV mental disorders among those with each type of suicidal behavior[a] (middle-income countries)

Mental disorders	Among total sample %[b] (SE) with disorder						Among ideators %[b] (SE) with disorder			
	Ideation	No ideation	Attempt	No attempt	Plan	No plan	Planned attempt	No planned attempt	Unplanned attempt	No unplanned attempt
Anxiety disorders										
Panic disorder	2.8 (0.4)	0.5 (0.0)	4.1 (0.9)	0.5 (0.0)	4.3 (0.9)	2.6 (0.7)	5.7 (1.2)	4.4 (1.7)	1.4 (1.2)	3.1 (1.0)
Generalized anxiety disorder	5.2 (0.9)	0.8 (0.1)	7.0 (1.3)	1.0 (0.1)	6.7 (1.2)	8.9 (2.4)	7.2 (1.6)	16.1 (5.4)	7.2 (2.2)	9.2 (2.5)
Specific phobia	13.3 (1.0)	4.4 (0.2)	17.6 (1.9)	4.7 (0.2)	16.0 (1.9)	14.6 (2.2)	19.4 (2.4)	22.3 (4.5)	15.0 (2.6)	14.9 (2.5)
Social phobia	8.1 (0.7)	1.4 (0.1)	10.6 (1.5)	1.5 (0.1)	10.1 (1.6)	8.2 (1.4)	11.0 (2.2)	19.3 (3.8)	10.8 (2.6)	7.0 (1.3)
Posttraumatic stress	4.2 (0.7)	0.6 (0.0)	8.2 (1.3)	0.7 (0.1)	6.3 (1.0)	6.5 (2.1)	9.3 (1.7)	4.7 (2.0)	5.6 (2.2)	5.6 (2.0)
Separation anxiety disorder	6.5 (0.7)	1.4 (0.1)	8.5 (1.3)	1.5 (0.1)	6.4 (0.7)	8.2 (1.6)	6.7 (1.3)	7.2 (2.1)	12.0 (3.2)	9.0 (2.0)
Agoraphobia	5.3 (0.6)	1.5 (0.1)	6.3 (1.1)	1.6 (0.1)	7.2 (1.5)	6.1 (1.1)	5.9 (1.3)	12.4 (4.2)	5.6 (1.8)	5.7 (1.1)
Mood disorders										
Major depressive disorder	14.5 (1.0)	2.7 (0.1)	18.7 (1.9)	3.0 (0.1)	19.0 (1.9)	21.2 (2.1)	21.2 (2.4)	31.5 (4.5)	14.3 (3.0)	22.2 (2.6)
Dysthymic disorder	2.5 (0.4)	0.3 (0.0)	3.9 (1.1)	0.4 (0.0)	2.7 (0.6)	4.1 (0.9)	4.3 (1.2)	8.1 (2.9)	3.8 (2.0)	4.4 (1.0)
Bipolar disorder	1.8 (0.5)	0.3 (0.0)	2.4 (0.5)	0.3 (0.0)	3.3 (0.8)	0.9 (0.3)	3.6 (0.9)	5.9 (1.6)	0.2 (0.2)	0.9 (0.3)
Impulse-control disorders										
Oppositional defiant disorder	2.6 (0.5)	0.2 (0.0)	4.4 (1.1)	0.3 (0.0)	4.9 (1.1)	0.7 (0.3)	5.4 (1.5)	5.7 (2.1)	2.8 (1.3)	0.9 (0.3)
Conduct disorder	2.6 (0.6)	0.2 (0.0)	4.8 (1.3)	0.3 (0.0)	3.8 (1.1)	1.4 (0.4)	5.9 (1.8)	2.6 (1.2)	3.4 (1.4)	1.5 (0.5)
Attention deficit hyperactivity disorder	2.5 (0.4)	0.4 (0.0)	3.9 (0.9)	0.4 (0.0)	3.0 (0.7)	1.8 (0.6)	3.1 (0.8)	1.7 (0.9)	4.4 (1.9)	1.3 (0.5)
Intermittent explosive disorder	6.5 (0.9)	0.9 (0.1)	7.7 (1.4)	1.0 (0.1)	8.6 (1.5)	5.8 (1.3)	9.0 (1.9)	7.7 (3.7)	5.2 (1.8)	6.5 (1.4)
Substance use disorders										
Alcohol abuse or dependence	10.4 (1.1)	2.6 (0.1)	13.0 (1.7)	2.8 (0.2)	14.0 (2.1)	14.1 (3.0)	15.0 (2.3)	23.9 (5.4)	10.7 (2.9)	13.2 (3.3)
Drug abuse or dependence	4.1 (0.6)	0.6 (0.1)	6.5 (1.1)	0.7 (0.1)	6.4 (1.3)	2.5 (0.6)	7.7 (1.5)	16.5 (5.8)	4.1 (1.8)	1.7 (0.5)

Appendix Table 10.2. (cont.)

Mental disorders	Among total sample %[b] (SE) with disorder						Among ideators %[b] (SE) with disorder			
	Ideation	No ideation	Attempt	No attempt	Plan	No plan	Planned attempt	No planned attempt	Unplanned attempt	No unplanned attempt
Number of mental disorders[c]										
1	25.1 (1.3)	9.7 (0.3)	25.8 (2.0)	9.9 (0.3)	26.7 (2.0)	22.5 (1.8)	27.4 (2.7)	20.6 (3.0)	22.0 (3.7)	25.3 (2.2)
2	12.1 (1.1)	2.5 (0.1)	15.3 (2.2)	2.7 (0.1)	16.8 (1.9)	11.9 (1.7)	20.0 (3.0)	18.1 (3.8)	7.4 (2.2)	12.0 (1.9)
3	5.7 (0.8)	0.8 (0.1)	7.4 (1.5)	1.0 (0.1)	5.7 (1.2)	8.8 (2.2)	6.5 (1.8)	11.3 (3.7)	18.5 (3.1)	15.2 (2.5)
4	2.3 (0.4)	0.3 (0.0)	4.4 (1.0)	0.3 (0.0)	3.7 (0.8)	4.1 (1.2)	4.3 (1.0)	8.4 (2.6)		
5	1.9 (0.4)	0.1 (0.0)	2.8 (0.6)	0.1 (0.0)	3.7 (0.9)	1.8 (0.7)	3.9 (0.9)	5.0 (2.2)		
6+	1.2 (0.3)	0.1 (0.0)	2.6 (0.7)	0.1 (0.0)	1.9 (0.6)	1.5 (0.5)	2.5 (0.8)	6.1 (2.3)		
N[d]	(1687)	(57,216)	(635)	(57,623)	(721)	(1234)	(411)	(320)	(194)	(911)

[a] As all subsequent models are based on the Part 2 sample, the percentages are also all based on the Part 2 sample despite some being Part 1 disorders.

[b] % represents the percentage of people with the disorder among those with the disorder among the cases with the outcome variable indicated in the column header. For example: the first cell is the % of those with panic disorder among those with suicide ideation.

[c] For number of mental disorders, the last OR represents the odds for that number of disorders or more. For example, for unplanned attempt, 3 represents ≥ 3 (that is, 3+).

[d] Number of cases with the outcome variable; N represents the number of person–years.

Appendix Table 10.3. Prevalence of DSM-IV mental disorders among those with each type of suicidal behavior[a] (low-income countries)

Mental disorders	Among total sample %[b] (SE) with disorder						Among ideators %[b] (SE) with disorder			
	Ideation	No ideation	Attempt	No attempt	Plan	No plan	Planned attempt	No planned attempt	Unplanned attempt	No unplanned attempt
Anxiety disorders										
Panic disorder	1.6 (0.3)	0.5 (0.1)	2.1 (0.6)	0.5 (0.1)	2.0 (0.5)	2.0 (0.6)	2.5 (0.8)	1.1 (0.5)	1.8 (1.1)	3.3 (0.8)
Generalized anxiety disorder	2.1 (0.4)	0.5 (0.0)	2.9 (0.8)	0.6 (0.0)	3.3 (0.8)	3.7 (0.8)	4.2 (1.3)	3.3 (1.4)	1.4 (0.7)	3.7 (0.9)
Specific phobia	13.8 (1.2)	4.4 (0.2)	19.6 (2.1)	4.8 (0.2)	20.4 (2.3)	14.2 (2.1)	20.5 (2.8)	14.4 (3.2)	13.7 (3.4)	12.6 (2.2)
Social phobia	4.8 (0.7)	1.1 (0.1)	6.7 (1.6)	1.2 (0.1)	6.5 (1.2)	5.0 (1.3)	8.1 (2.1)	7.7 (2.6)	5.1 (2.3)	5.6 (1.6)
Posttraumatic stress	2.0 (0.5)	0.4 (0.1)	2.2 (0.6)	0.4 (0.1)	3.2 (0.8)	1.8 (0.6)	3.0 (1.1)	4.1 (1.8)	1.4 (0.7)	2.1 (0.8)
Separation anxiety disorder	4.3 (0.6)	0.9 (0.1)	6.2 (1.2)	0.9 (0.1)	6.1 (1.4)	4.0 (0.9)	5.6 (1.4)	2.6 (0.8)	6.8 (1.7)	3.7 (1.0)
Agoraphobia	1.2 (0.3)	0.4 (0.1)	2.3 (0.8)	0.4 (0.1)	1.7 (0.6)	1.0 (0.5)	2.1 (0.9)	2.4 (1.4)	2.4 (1.5)	1.2 (0.8)
Mood disorders										
Major depressive disorder	11.5 (0.8)	2.8 (0.2)	16.9 (1.9)	3.0 (0.1)	21.3 (1.7)	14.6 (1.5)	22.0 (2.7)	40.6 (4.9)	9.0 (2.2)	15.8 (2.2)
Dysthymic disorder	2.8 (0.4)	0.7 (0.1)	5.2 (1.2)	0.7 (0.1)	5.0 (1.0)	2.9 (0.7)	5.5 (1.6)	8.6 (3.2)	3.6 (1.6)	2.6 (0.8)
Bipolar disorder	1.4 (0.4)	0.2 (0.0)	2.1 (0.7)	0.3 (0.0)	2.7 (1.0)	1.2 (0.4)	2.4 (1.0)	3.7 (1.7)	0.8 (0.6)	1.2 (0.6)
Impulse-control disorders										
Oppositional defiant disorder	2.0 (0.5)	0.2 (0.0)	3.8 (1.1)	0.3 (0.0)	2.0 (0.6)	1.6 (0.7)	2.3 (0.9)	0.4 (0.4)	4.7 (2.0)	1.5 (0.8)
Conduct disorder	2.5 (0.4)	0.3 (0.0)	4.9 (1.0)	0.3 (0.1)	4.2 (0.8)	2.3 (0.8)	5.0 (1.5)	2.7 (1.4)	3.8 (1.5)	2.7 (1.1)
Attention deficit hyperactivity disorder	1.2 (0.3)	0.2 (0.0)	2.4 (0.9)	0.2 (0.0)	1.8 (0.7)	0.8 (0.4)	2.2 (1.1)	0.8 (0.5)	2.0 (1.3)	0.5 (0.3)
Intermittent explosive disorder	7.1 (0.7)	1.3 (0.1)	9.5 (1.4)	1.5 (0.1)	11.0 (1.3)	8.2 (1.3)	10.0 (1.8)	10.0 (2.3)	8.1 (2.2)	6.6 (1.1)
Substance use disorders										
Alcohol abuse or dependence	5.2 (0.8)	2.2 (0.1)	7.8 (1.7)	2.4 (0.1)	8.7 (1.4)	7.6 (1.4)	7.6 (1.8)	14.1 (3.4)	8.1 (3.5)	7.1 (1.7)
Drug abuse or dependence	1.3 (0.3)	0.2 (0.0)	1.9 (0.5)	0.3 (0.0)	2.4 (0.7)	2.3 (0.8)	2.7 (0.9)	4.7 (1.7)	0.4 (0.4)	2.4 (0.9)

Appendix Table 10.3. (cont.)

Mental disorders	Among total sample %^b (SE) with disorder						Among ideators %^b (SE) with disorder			
	Ideation	No ideation	Attempt	No attempt	Plan	No plan	Planned attempt	No planned attempt	Unplanned attempt	No unplanned attempt
Number of mental disorders[a]										
1	22.9 (1.4)	9.2 (0.3)	26.2 (2.6)	9.6 (0.3)	25.7 (1.8)	25.2 (2.2)	27.7 (2.8)	30.4 (3.8)	23.1 (4.1)	25.6 (2.7)
2	9.2 (0.9)	2.0 (0.1)	11.3 (1.7)	2.2 (0.1)	14.9 (1.8)	11.8 (1.7)	12.1 (2.1)	19.5 (3.8)	17.4 (3.0)	16.7 (2.4)
3	3.7 (0.6)	0.6 (0.1)	6.6 (1.3)	0.6 (0.1)	7.3 (1.3)	3.0 (0.7)	8.7 (2.2)	7.1 (2.3)		
4	1.5 (0.3)	0.2 (0.0)	5.5 (1.2)	0.4 (0.0)	3.0 (0.8)	1.2 (0.4)	6.0 (1.6)	6.7 (2.3)		
5+	1.0 (0.2)	0.1 (0.0)			2.0 (0.6)	1.7 (0.6)				
N[d]	(1639)	(40,936)	(583)	(39,548)	(717)	(1292)	(353)	(384)	(192)	(843)

[a] As all subsequent models are based on the Part 2 sample, the percentages are also all based on the Part 2 sample despite some being Part 1 disorders.

[b] % represents the percentage of people with the disorder among the cases with the outcome variable indicated in the column header. For example: the first cell is the % of those with panic disorder among those with suicide ideation.

[c] For number of mental disorders, the last OR represents the odds for that number of disorders or more. For example, for unplanned attempt, 2 represents ≥2 (that is, 2+).

[d] Number of cases with the outcome variable; N represents the number of person–years.

Appendix Table 10.4. Associations between number of DSM-IV mental disorders and each type of suicidal behavior[a] (high-income countries)

Number of mental disorders[b]	Among total sample			Among ideators	
	Ideation	Attempt	Plan	Planned attempt	Unplanned attempt
	OR (95% CI)	OR (95% CI)	OR (95% CI)	OR (95% CI)	OR (95% CI)
1	2.3* (2.1–2.6)	2.9* (2.4–3.6)	1.1 (0.9–1.4)	1.1 (0.7–1.6)	1.1 (0.8–1.5)
2	3.3* (2.9–3.8)	4.6* (3.7–5.7)	1.2 (1.0–1.5)	0.9 (0.6–1.4)	1.2 (0.8–1.8)
3	4.6* (4.0–5.4)	7.1* (5.4–9.4)	1.5* (1.2–2.1)	1.2 (0.7–1.9)	0.9 (0.5–1.5)
4	5.1* (4.0–6.6)	7.3* (5.3–10.1)	1.3 (0.9–1.9)	1.5 (0.9–2.5)	0.9 (0.6–1.6)
5	4.9* (3.9–6.2)	6.5* (4.6–9.4)	1.2 (0.8–1.8)	1.3 (0.7–2.5)	0.9 (0.4–2.1)
6	5.7* (4.1–7.9)	7.4* (4.5–12.3)	1.8* (1.1–2.9)	1.1 (0.5–2.4)	0.4 (0.1–1.3)
7	6.0* (3.3–10.7)	3.9* (2.0–7.4)	1.7 (0.7–3.7)	0.7 (0.2–3.0)	1.0 (0.5–2.1)
8	3.8* (2.2–6.4)	9.2* (5.2–16.1)	0.9 (0.3–2.3)	1.1 (0.4–3.0)	
9	5.3* (2.4–11.8)	19.6* (10.5–36.6)	4.4* (1.9–10.6)	5.4* (1.4–21.1)	
10+	3.6* (1.5–8.8)				
χ^2 (p-value)	682.2 (<0.001)*	345.2 (<0.001)*	19.8 (0.02)*	13.1 (0.16)	3.5 (0.84)

* Significant at the 0.05 level, two-sided test.
[a] Assessed in the Part 2 sample due to having Part 2 controls. Models control for person–years, country, and significant variables from the chapters on sociodemographics, parental psychopathology, childhood adversities, and traumatic events.
[b] For number of mental disorders, the last OR represents the odds for that number of disorders or more. For example, for unplanned attempt, 7 represents ≥7 (that is, 7+).

Appendix Table 10.5. Associations between number of DSM-IV mental disorder and each type of suicidal behavior[a] (middle-income countries)

Number of mental disorders[b]	Among total sample			Among ideators	
	Ideation	Attempt	Plan	Planned attempt	Unplanned attempt
	OR (95% CI)	OR (95% CI)	OR (95% CI)	OR (95% CI)	OR (95% CI)
1	2.6* (2.2–3.0)	2.3* (1.8–3.0)	1.6* (1.2–2.3)	1.3 (0.8–2.3)	1.1 (0.6–1.9)
2	3.5* (2.8–4.4)	4.6* (3.3–6.3)	1.7* (1.1–2.6)	1.0 (0.5–2.2)	0.4 (0.2–1.0)
3	4.8* (3.5–6.7)	4.0* (2.4–6.7)	1.0 (0.5–1.9)	0.5 (0.2–1.3)	1.1 (0.6–2.2)
4	5.1* (3.1–8.2)	6.8* (3.1–14.8)	1.6 (0.7–3.4)	0.5 (0.2–1.7)	
5	–	6.7* (1.1–39.5)	3.2* (1.3–7.8)	1.2 (0.3–4.2)	
6+	–	0.0* (0.0–0.0)	1.8 (0.7–4.6)	0.6 (0.2–1.7)	
χ^2 (p-value)	304.8 (<0.001)*	264.7 (<0.001)*	15.5 (0.02)*	9.4 (0.15)	5.1 (0.17)

* Significant at the 0.05 level, two-sided test.
0.0* (0.0–0.0) OR is ≤ 0.05 indicating very low risk.
– Not included due to small cell size.
[a] Assessed in the Part 2 sample due to having Part 2 controls. Models control for person–years, country, and significant variables from the chapters on sociodemographics, parental psychopathology, childhood adversities, and traumatic events.
[b] For number of mental disorders, the last OR represents the odds for that number of disorders or more. For example, for unplanned attempt, 3 represents ≥3 (that is, 3+).

Appendix Table 10.6. Associations between number of DSM-IV mental disorders and each type of suicidal behavior[a] (low-income countries)

Number of mental disorders[b]	Among total sample			Among ideators	
	Ideation	Attempt	Plan	Planned attempt	Unplanned attempt
	OR (95% CI)	OR (95% CI)	OR (95% CI)	OR (95% CI)	OR (95% CI)
1	2.1* (1.8–2.4)	2.6* (2.0–3.4)	1.2 (0.9–1.7)	0.5* (0.3–0.9)	0.8 (0.5–1.5)
2	3.3* (2.6–4.2)	3.6* (2.4–5.5)	1.7* (1.2–2.5)	0.4* (0.2–0.8)	1.1 (0.5–2.3)
3	2.5* (1.7–3.8)	5.6* (2.8–11.3)	3.5* (1.9–6.6)	0.9 (0.4–2.0)	
4	4.3* (2.5–7.3)	3.3* (1.1–9.7)	4.7* (1.7–12.9)	0.7 (0.3–1.7)	
5+	3.4* (1.6–7.3)		1.8 (0.8–4.2)		
χ^2 (p-value)	154.7 (<0.001)*	81.2 (<0.001)*	28.4 (<0.001)*	11.4 (0.02)*	0.9 (0.63)

* Significant at the 0.05 level, two-sided test.
[a] Assessed in the Part 2 sample due to having Part 2 controls. Models control for person–years, country, and significant variables from the chapters on sociodemographics, parental psychopathology, childhood adversities, and traumatic events.
[b] For number of mental disorders, the last OR represents the odds for that number of disorders or more. For example, for unplanned attempt, 2 represents ≥2 (that is, 2+).

Appendix Table 10.7. Final multivariate models for associations between DSM-IV mental disorders and each type of suicidal behavior[a] (high-income countries)

Mental disorders	Among total sample			Among ideators	
	Ideation	Attempt	Plan	Planned attempt	Unplanned attempt
	OR (95% CI)	OR (95% CI)	OR (95% CI)	OR (95% CI)	OR (95% CI)
Anxiety disorders					
Panic disorder	2.2* (1.7–2.7)	2.8* (1.9–4.1)	1.3 (0.9–1.9)	1.6 (0.8–3.2)	1.2 (0.6–2.5)
Generalized anxiety disorder	2.9* (2.3–3.5)	3.2* (2.3–4.4)	0.9 (0.7–1.3)	1.2 (0.7–2.0)	1.5 (0.9–2.5)
Specific phobia	1.9* (1.6–2.1)	2.0* (1.6–2.6)	1.1 (0.9–1.5)	1.3 (0.8–2.0)	1.3 (0.8–2.2)
Social phobia	2.4* (2.1–2.9)	2.2* (1.7–2.9)	1.2 (0.9–1.7)	1.2 (0.7–1.9)	0.9 (0.5–1.4)
Posttraumatic stress	2.0* (1.6–2.4)	2.4* (1.8–3.2)	1.1 (0.8–1.6)	1.1 (0.6–1.9)	1.6 (0.9–3.0)
Separation anxiety disorder	1.9* (1.4–2.7)	1.8* (1.3–2.5)	1.4 (0.9–2.2)	1.3 (0.6–2.6)	1.1 (0.6–1.8)
Agoraphobia	2.2* (1.7–2.9)	2.5* (1.6–3.9)	1.5 (0.9–2.6)	2.3 (1.0–5.2)	0.4 (0.1–1.5)
Mood disorders					
Major depressive disorder	3.6* (3.1–4.2)	3.9* (2.9–5.1)	0.9 (0.7–1.2)	0.9 (0.5–1.4)	0.8 (0.5–1.2)
Dysthymic disorder	2.0* (1.6–2.5)	1.5 (1.0–2.2)	1.1 (0.7–1.7)	0.6 (0.3–1.2)	0.7 (0.4–1.6)
Bipolar disorder	2.5* (1.9–3.3)	3.1* (2.1–4.8)	0.8 (0.5–1.3)	2.2* (1.2–4.2)	1.4 (0.7–2.8)

Appendix Table 10.7. (cont.)

Mental disorders	Among total sample			Among ideators		
	Ideation	Attempt	Plan	Planned attempt	Unplanned attempt
	OR (95% CI)	OR (95% CI)	OR (95% CI)	OR (95% CI)	OR (95% CI)
Impulse-control disorders					
Oppositional defiant disorder	2.7* (2.0–3.5)	3.1* (2.2–4.3)	1.3 (0.7–2.2)	1.4 (0.7–2.9)	1.5 (0.8–2.7)
Conduct disorder	2.3* (1.8–3.0)	1.9* (1.3–2.8)	1.0 (0.6–1.7)	1.0 (0.5–2.0)	1.3 (0.7–2.5)
Attention deficit hyperactivity disorder	1.9* (1.4–2.5)	2.2* (1.4–3.4)	1.4 (0.9–2.0)	1.4 (0.6–2.9)	1.4 (0.6–3.2)
Intermittent explosive disorder	2.3* (1.9–2.9)	2.2* (1.5–3.2)	1.1 (0.7–1.7)	0.8 (0.4–1.7)	0.8 (0.4–1.6)
Substance use disorders					
Alcohol abuse or dependence	2.0* (1.7–2.4)	3.0* (2.2–4.0)	1.4 (1.0–2.0)	1.2 (0.7–2.1)	1.6 (0.9–2.7)
Drug abuse or dependence	2.5* (1.9–3.3)	2.3* (1.6–3.4)	1.4 (1.0–2.0)	1.0 (0.5–2.2)	0.8 (0.4–1.7)
13 df χ^2 test for 13 types	366.2 (<0.001)*	142.4 (<0.001)*	27.1 (0.04)*	31.5 (0.01)*	24.6 (0.08)
12 df χ^2 test for difference between types	96.0 (<0.001)*	88.1 (<0.001)*	26.6 (0.03)*	28.5 (0.02)*	27.5 (0.03)*
Number of mental disorders[b]					
2	0.6* (0.5–0.7)	0.7* (0.5–1.0)	1.0 (0.6–1.5)	0.8 (0.4–1.5)	1.0 (0.5–1.7)
3	0.3* (0.2–0.5)	0.4* (0.2–0.7)	1.1 (0.6–2.0)	1.0 (0.3–2.8)	0.6 (0.2–1.6)
4	0.2* (0.1–0.2)	0.2* (0.1–0.3)	0.8 (0.3–1.8)	0.9 (0.2–4.1)	0.7 (0.2–2.2)
5	0.1* (0.0–0.1)	0.1* (0.0–0.2)	0.6 (0.2–1.7)	0.8 (0.1–5.6)	0.5 (0.1–2.8)
6	0.0* (0.0–0.1)	0.0* (0.0–0.1)	0.8 (0.2–3.2)	0.6 (0.1–5.6)	0.2 (0.0–2.1)
7	0.0* (0.0–0.0)	0.0* (0.0–0.0)	0.6 (0.1–3.0)	0.3 (0.0–6.3)	0.4 (0.0–5.0)
8	0.0* (0.0–0.0)	0.0* (0.0–0.0)	0.3 (0.0–2.6)	0.3 (0.0–7.0)	
9	0.0* (0.0–0.0)	0.0* (0.0–0.0)	1.0 (0.1–10.6)	1.6 (0.0–71.0)	
10+	0.0* (0.0–0.0)				
χ^2 (p-value)	191.9 (<0.001)*	109.5 (<0.001)*	8.7 (0.36)	10.9 (0.21)	3.2 (0.78)

* Significant at the 0.05 level, two-sided test.
0.0* (0.0–0.0) OR is ≤ 0.05 indicating very low risk.
[a] Assessed in the Part 2 sample due to having Part 2 controls. Models control for person–years, country, and significant variables from the chapters on sociodemographics, parental psychopathology, childhood adversities, and traumatic events.
[b] For number of mental disorders, the last OR represents the odds for that number of disorders or more. For example, for unplanned attempt, 7 represents ≥7 (that is, 7+).

Appendix Table 10.8. Final multivariate models for associations between DSM-IV mental disorders and each type of suicidal behavior[a] (middle-income countries)

Mental disorders	Among total sample		Among ideators		
	Ideation	Attempt	Plan	Planned attempt	Unplanned attempt
	OR (95% CI)	OR (95% CI)	OR (95% CI)	OR (95% CI)	OR (95% CI)
Anxiety disorders					
Panic disorder	3.4* (2.3–5.1)	–	2.5* (1.1–6.1)	2.5 (0.7–8.8)	–
Generalized anxiety disorder	3.3* (2.1–5.1)	2.5* (1.3–4.5)	1.4 (0.8–2.6)	0.7 (0.3–2.0)	2.1 (0.5–9.3)
Specific phobia	2.3* (1.9–2.9)	2.2* (1.6–3.0)	1.8 (1.0–3.1)	1.5 (0.7–3.6)	0.7 (0.3–1.6)
Social phobia	2.8* (2.1–3.8)	2.1* (1.3–3.4)	1.5 (0.9–2.6)	0.8 (0.4–1.8)	1.5 (0.6–3.7)
Posttraumatic stress	2.8* (1.8–4.6)	–	2.5* (1.2–4.9)	3.8* (1.6–9.4)	2.7 (0.7–9.5)
Separation anxiety disorder	2.0* (1.5–2.8)	1.7* (1.0–2.6)	1.1 (0.6–2.1)	1.9 (0.7–5.4)	2.4 (0.7–7.9)
Agoraphobia	1.6* (1.2–2.2)	1.3 (0.8–2.1)	1.1 (0.5–2.1)	0.6 (0.2–1.7)	2.2 (0.6–7.9)
Mood disorders					
Major depressive disorder	2.7* (2.0–3.5)	2.7* (1.9–3.9)	1.4 (0.9–2.1)	1.0 (0.5–2.0)	0.5 (0.2–1.2)
Dysthymic disorder	3.3* (1.9–5.7)	–	1.3 (0.6–2.8)	1.1 (0.3–3.5)	0.8 (0.2–3.3)
Bipolar disorder	1.6 (0.9–2.9)	–	4.3* (1.3–14.5)	2.3 (0.6–8.8)	–
Impulse-control disorders					
Oppositional defiant disorder	–	–	5.0* (1.8–14.2)	1.0 (0.2–4.2)	
Conduct disorder	–	–	1.5 (0.7–3.5)	3.8 (0.7–21.7)	
Attention deficit hyperactivity disorder	2.0* (1.2–3.2)	–	1.6 (0.8–3.5)	3.5 (0.7–18.2)	
Intermittent explosive disorder	3.9* (2.8–5.4)	–	2.1* (1.1–4.0)	4.0* (1.5–10.8)	0.9 (0.3–2.5)
Substance use disorders					
Alcohol abuse or dependence	2.9* (2.2–3.8)	3.7* (2.5–5.4)	1.5 (0.9–2.6)	1.0 (0.5–2.0)	2.0 (0.8–5.0)
Drug abuse or dependence	2.3* (1.5–3.5)	–	3.0* (1.3–6.8)	1.2 (0.3–4.1)	–
13 df χ^2 test for 13 types	186.8 (<0.001)*	70.2 (<0.001)*	30.1 (0.02)*	32.9 (0.01)*	13.7 (0.19)
12 df χ^2 test for difference between types	47.8 (<0.001)*	19.4 (0.004)*	23.9 (0.07)	31.9 (0.01)*	14.9 (0.13)

Appendix Table 10.8. (cont.)

Mental disorders	Among total sample			Among ideators	
	Ideation	Attempt	Plan	Planned attempt	Unplanned attempt
	OR (95% CI)	OR (95% CI)	OR (95% CI)	OR (95% CI)	OR (95% CI)
Number of mental disorders[b]					
2	0.5* (0.4–0.8)	0.9 (0.6–1.6)	0.6 (0.3–1.2)	0.7 (0.3–2.1)	0.3 (0.1–1.1)
3	0.3* (0.2–0.5)	0.4* (0.2–0.8)	0.2* (0.1–0.6)	0.2 (0.0–1.2)	0.6 (0.1–4.0)
4	0.1* (0.1–0.2)	0.3* (0.1–0.9)	0.2* (0.1–0.9)	0.2 (0.0–1.9)	4.2 (0.12)
5	0.1* (0.0–0.3)	0.1 (0.0–1.6)	0.3 (0.1–1.5)	0.3 (0.0–7.3)	
6+	0.0* (0.0–0.1)	0.0* (0.0–0.0)	0.0* (0.0–0.4)	0.0 (0.0–1.8)	
χ^2 (p-value)	66.4 (<0.001)*	138.8 (<0.001)*	15.8 (0.01)*	7.6 (0.18)	

* Significant at the 0.05 level, two-sided test.
0.0* (0.0–0.0) OR is ≤ 0.05 indicating very low risk.
– Condition not included in model due to small cell size. Small cell size determined by calculating the expected number of cases of the condition based on the % of people with the outcome and the total number of people with the condition. If the expected value was less than 5, the condition was dropped from the model.
[a] Assessed in the Part 2 sample due to having Part 2 controls. Models control for person–years, country, and significant variables from the chapters on sociodemographics, parental psychopathology, childhood adversities, and traumatic events.
[b] For number of mental disorders, the last OR represents the odds for that number of disorders or more. For example, for unplanned attempt, 3 represents ≥3 (that is, 3+).

Appendix Table 10.9. Final multivariate models for associations between DSM-IV mental disorders and each type of suicidal behavior[a] (low-income countries)

Mental disorders	Among total sample			Among ideators	
	Ideation	Attempt	Plan	Planned attempt	Unplanned attempt
	OR (95% CI)	OR (95% CI)	OR (95% CI)	OR (95% CI)	OR (95% CI)
Anxiety disorders					
Panic disorder	1.6 (1.0–2.5)	–	0.8 (0.3–1.8)	1.8 (0.3–9.6)	0.4 (0.1–2.2)
Generalized anxiety disorder	2.2* (1.4–3.4)	–	0.6 (0.3–1.5)	4.1 (1.0–17.0)	0.5 (0.1–2.2)
Specific phobia	1.9* (1.5–2.4)	2.2* (1.6–3.1)	1.2 (0.7–1.8)	0.9 (0.4–1.8)	1.1 (0.4–2.7)
Social phobia	2.1* (1.4–3.0)	2.4* (1.5–4.0)	1.0 (0.5–2.1)	0.7 (0.2–1.9)	0.5 (0.2–1.5)
Posttraumatic stress	2.9* (1.4–5.7)	–	2.5* (1.1–5.7)	0.8 (0.2–2.7)	–
Separation anxiety disorder	2.0* (1.3–3.0)	–	1.3 (0.7–2.3)	0.9 (0.3–2.9)	1.1 (0.4–3.2)
Agoraphobia	1.7 (0.9–3.1)	–	1.1 (0.3–4.6)	1.2 (0.2–6.4)	–
Mood disorders					
Major depressive disorder	2.4* (1.9–3.1)	3.8* (2.7–5.3)	1.4 (0.9–2.1)	0.3* (0.1–0.5)	0.3* (0.2–0.7)
Dysthymic disorder	2.8* (1.8–4.2)	–	1.2 (0.5–2.9)	1.7 (0.5–5.5)	2.2 (0.4–13.1)
Bipolar disorder	2.1* (1.1–4.0)	–	1.5 (0.5–5.1)	0.8 (0.2–2.8)	–

Appendix Table 10.9. (cont.)

	Among total sample		Among ideators		
	Ideation	Attempt	Plan	Planned attempt	Unplanned attempt
Mental disorders	OR (95% CI)	OR (95% CI)	OR (95% CI)	OR (95% CI)	OR (95% CI)
Impulse-control disorders					
Oppositional defiant disorder	–	–	0.7 (0.2–2.4)	–	–
Conduct disorder	–	–	1.3 (0.6–2.9)	2.0 (0.3–14.2)	–
Attention deficit hyperactivity disorder	–	–	1.8 (0.4–8.3)	0.9 (0.2–4.0)	–
Intermittent explosive disorder	2.6* (1.9–3.5)	3.1* (2.0–4.6)	1.0 (0.6–1.7)	0.8 (0.3–2.0)	1.4 (0.6–3.3)
Substance use disorders					
Alcohol abuse or dependence	1.5 (1.0–2.3)	2.2* (1.2–3.9)	1.2 (0.7–2.2)	0.6 (0.3–1.6)	1.2 (0.4–3.5)
Drug abuse or dependence	–	–	0.7 (0.3–2.0)	0.4 (0.1–1.1)	–
13 df χ^2 test for 13 types	98.7 (<0.001)*	83.2 (<0.001)*	14.2 (0.58)	30.2 (0.01)*	12.6 (0.18)
12 df χ^2 test for difference between types	16.1 (0.10)	148.9 (<0.001)*	12.1 (0.67)	27.9 (0.02)*	9.4 (0.31)
Number of mental disorders[b]					
2	0.7 (0.5–1.1)	0.5* (0.3–0.9)	1.3 (0.7–2.3)	1.1 (0.4–2.9)	2.4 (0.9–6.0)
3	0.3* (0.2–0.6)	0.3* (0.1–0.7)	2.4 (0.9–6.1)	3.8* (1.0–14.4)	3.2 (0.07)
4	0.1* (0.1–0.3)	0.1* (0.0–0.2)	2.9 (0.8–11.1)	1.5 (0.1–15.7)	
5	0.1* (0.0–0.2)		0.6 (0.1–4.9)	8.6 (0.04)*	
χ^2 (p-value)	37.0 (<0.001)*	16.8 (<0.001)*	14.7 (0.01)*		

* Significant at the 0.05 level, two-sided test.
– Condition not included in model due to small cell size. Small cell size determined by calculating the expected number of cases of the condition based on the % of people with the outcome and the total number of people with the condition. If the expected value was less than 5, the condition was dropped from the model.
[a] Assessed in the Part 2 sample due to having Part 2 controls. Models control for person–years, country, and significant variables from the chapters on sociodemographics, parental psychopathology, childhood adversities, and traumatic events.
[b] For number of mental disorders, the last OR represents the odds for that number of disorders or more. For example, for unplanned attempt, 2 represents ≥2 (that is, 2+).

Appendix Table 10.10. Interactions between DSM-IV mental disorders and life course intervals[a] (high-income countries)

Interactions		Attempts among total sample	
		OR (95% CI)	χ² (p-value)
Anxiety disorders			
Panic disorder	middle 33%	–	0.0 (0.98)
	upper 33%	1.0 (0.6–1.8)	
Generalized anxiety disorder	middle 33%	–	0.1 (0.75)
	upper 33%	1.1 (0.7–1.7)	
Specific phobia	middle 33%	0.8 (0.6–1.2)	1.8 (0.41)
	upper 33%	0.8 (0.5–1.2)	
Social phobia	middle 33%	0.9 (0.6–1.4)	1.3 (0.51)
	upper 33%	0.8 (0.5–1.2)	
Posttraumatic stress	middle 33%	–	1.1 (0.28)
	upper 33%	1.3 (0.8–1.9)	
Separation anxiety disorder	middle 33%	–	0.7 (0.40)
	upper 33%	1.3 (0.7–2.7)	
Agoraphobia	middle 33%	–	–
	upper 33%	–	
Mood disorders			
Major depressive disorder	middle 33%	1.0 (0.6–1.6)	2.7 (0.26)
	upper 33%	0.7 (0.5–1.2)	
Dysthymic disorder	middle 33%	–	0.8 (0.36)
	upper 33%	1.4 (0.7–2.7)	
Bipolar disorder	middle 33%	–	0.0 (1.00)
	upper 33%	1.0 (0.5–2.0)	
Impulse-control disorders			
Oppositional defiant disorder	middle 33%	–	–
	upper 33%	–	
Conduct disorder	middle 33%	–	–
	upper 33%	–	
Attention deficit hyperactivity disorder	middle 33%	–	–
	upper 33%	–	
Intermittent explosive disorder	middle 33%	–	0.4 (0.55)
	upper 33%	0.8 (0.4–1.5)	
Substance use disorders			
Alcohol abuse or dependence	middle 33%	0.9 (0.5–1.8)	0.0 (0.99)
	upper 33%	1.0 (0.5–1.9)	
Drug abuse or dependence	middle 33%	–	0.1 (0.73)
	upper 33%	1.1 (0.6–2.1)	
26 df χ² test for all chronic conditions			9.8 (0.88)
25 df χ² test for all conditions and dummies for number of conditions			18.2 (0.58)
Number of mental disorders			
2	middle 33%	0.6 (0.4–1.0)	6.9 (0.14)
	upper 33%	0.8 (0.5–1.3)	
3	middle 33%	–	
	upper 33%	1.0 (0.6–1.5)	

Appendix Table 10.10. (cont.)

Interactions		Attempts among total sample	
		OR (95% CI)	χ² (p-value)
4	middle 33%	–	
	upper 33%	0.6 (0.3–1.1)	
5	middle 33%	–	
	upper 33%	–	
6	middle 33%	–	
	upper 33%	–	
7	middle 33%	–	
	upper 33%	–	
8	middle 33%	–	
	upper 33%	–	
9+	middle 33%	–	
	upper 33%	–	

– Condition not included in model due to small cell size. Small cell size determined by calculating the expected number of cases of the condition based on the % of people with the outcome and the total number of people with the condition. If the expected value was less than 5, the condition was dropped from the model.
[a] Assessed in the Part 2 sample. Models control for person–years, country, and significant variables from the chapters on sociodemographics, parental psychopathology, childhood adversities, and traumatic events. Models also included all controls and interaction terms between life course intervals (intervals determined by the 33.3% percentiles of the age-of-onset for the outcome) and each control. Only the interaction terms between the life course intervals and mental disorder variables are shown in table.

Appendix Table 10.11. Interactions between DSM-IV mental disorders and life course intervals[a] (middle-income countries)

Interactions		Attempts among total sample	
		OR (95% CI)	χ² (p-value)
Anxiety disorders			
Panic disorder	middle 33%	–	–
	upper 33%	–	
Generalized anxiety disorder	middle 33%	–	–
	upper 33%	–	
Specific phobia	middle 33%	1.5 (0.7–3.1)	2.3 (0.31)
	upper 33%	0.8 (0.4–1.6)	
Social phobia	middle 33%	–	–
	upper 33%	–	
Posttraumatic stress	middle 33%	–	–
	upper 33%	–	
Separation anxiety disorder	middle 33%	–	–
	upper 33%	–	
Agoraphobia	middle 33%	–	–
	upper 33%	–	
Mood disorders			
Major depressive disorder	middle 33%	–	2.0 (0.16)
	upper 33%	0.6 (0.3–1.2)	
Dysthymic disorder	middle 33%	–	–
	upper 33%	–	
Bipolar disorder	middle 33%	–	–
	upper 33%	–	

Appendix Table 10.11. (cont.)

Interactions		Attempts among total sample	
		OR (95% CI)	χ^2 (p-value)
Impulse-control disorders			
Oppositional defiant disorder	middle 33%	–	–
	upper 33%	–	
Conduct disorder	middle 33%	–	–
	upper 33%	–	
Attention deficit hyperactivity disorder	middle 33%	–	–
	upper 33%	–	
Intermittent explosive disorder	middle 33%	–	–
	upper 33%	–	
Substance use disorders			
Alcohol abuse or dependence	middle 33%	–	8.0 (0.01)*
	upper 33%	0.3* (0.1–0.7)	
Drug abuse or dependence	middle 33%	–	–
	upper 33%	–	
26 df χ^2 test for all chronic conditions			16.4 (0.003)*
25 df χ^2 test for all conditions and dummies for number of conditions			16.7 (0.01)*
Number of mental disorders			
2	middle 33%	–	0.0 (0.83)
	upper 33%	0.9 (0.4–2.0)	
3	middle 33%	–	
	upper 33%	–	
4	middle 33%	–	
	upper 33%	–	
5	middle 33%	–	
	upper 33%	–	
6+	middle 33%	–	
	upper 33%	–	

* Significant at the 0.05 level, two-sided test.
– Condition not included in model due to small cell size. Small cell size determined by calculating the expected number of cases of the condition based on the % of people with the outcome and the total number of people with the condition. If the expected value was less than 5, the condition was dropped from the model.
[a] Assessed in the Part 2 sample. Models control for person–years, country, and significant variables from the chapters on sociodemographics, parental psychopathology, childhood adversities, and traumatic events. Models also included all controls and interaction terms between life course intervals (intervals determined by the 33.3% percentiles of the age-of-onset for the outcome) and each control. Only the interaction terms between the life course intervals and mental disorder variables are shown in table.

Appendix Table 10.12. Interactions between DSM-IV mental disorders and life course intervals[a] (low-income countries)

Interactions		Attempts among total sample	
		OR (95% CI)	χ^2 (p-value)
Anxiety disorders			
Panic disorder	middle 33%	–	–
	upper 33%	–	
Generalized anxiety disorder	middle 33%	–	–
	upper 33%	–	
Specific phobia	middle 33%	–	0.5 (0.49)
	upper 33%	0.8 (0.5–1.4)	
Social phobia	middle 33%	–	–
	upper 33%	–	
Posttraumatic stress	middle 33%	–	–
	upper 33%	–	
Separation anxiety disorder	middle 33%	–	–
	upper 33%	–	
Agoraphobia	middle 33%	–	–
	upper 33%	–	
Mood disorders			
Major depressive disorder	middle 33%	–	1.2 (0.27)
	upper 33%	0.7 (0.3–1.3)	
Dysthymic disorder	middle 33%	–	–
	upper 33%	–	
Bipolar disorder	middle 33%	–	–
	upper 33%	–	
Impulse-control disorders			
Oppositional defiant disorder	middle 33%	–	–
	upper 33%	–	
Conduct disorder	middle 33%	–	–
	upper 33%	–	
Attention deficit hyperactivity disorder	middle 33%	–	–
	upper 33%	–	
Intermittent explosive disorder	middle 33%	–	–
	upper 33%	–	
Substance use disorders			
Alcohol abuse or dependence	middle 33%	–	2.4 (0.12)
	upper 33%	0.5 (0.2–1.3)	
Drug abuse or dependence	middle 33%	–	–
	upper 33%	–	
26 df χ^2 test for all chronic conditions			3.8 (0.28)
25 df χ^2 test for all conditions and dummies for number of conditions			4.1 (0.40)
Number of mental disorders			
2	middle 33%	–	2.0 (0.15)
	upper 33%	1.7 (0.8–3.8)	
3	middle 33%	–	
	upper 33%	–	
4+	middle 33%	–	
	upper 33%	–	

– Condition not included in model due to small cell size. Small cell size determined by calculating the expected number of cases of the condition based on the % of people with the outcome and the total number of people with the condition. If the expected value was less than 5, the condition was dropped from the model.

[a] Assessed in the Part 2 sample. Models control for person–years, country, and significant variables from the chapters on sociodemographics, parental psychopathology, childhood adversities, and traumatic events. Models also included all controls and interaction terms between life course intervals (intervals determined by the 33.3% percentiles of the age-of-onset for the outcome) and each control. Only the interaction terms between the life course intervals and mental disorder variables are shown in table.

Appendix Table 10.13. Associations between DSM-IV mental disorders and persistence of suicidal behavior[a] (high-income countries)

Mental disorders	Ideation OR (95% CI)	Plan OR (95% CI)	Attempt OR (95% CI)
Anxiety disorders			
Panic disorder	1.7* (1.3–2.3)	1.7* (1.1–2.7)	1.3 (0.8–2.3)
Generalized anxiety disorder	1.3 (1.0–1.7)	1.4 (0.9–2.2)	1.2 (0.8–1.9)
Specific phobia	1.4* (1.1–1.7)	1.5* (1.0–2.1)	1.4 (0.9–2.1)
Social phobia	1.5* (1.2–1.9)	1.8* (1.3–2.5)	1.6* (1.0–2.4)
Posttraumatic stress	1.2 (0.9–1.4)	1.3 (0.9–1.8)	1.3 (0.9–2.1)
Separation anxiety disorder	1.2 (0.9–1.7)	1.3 (0.7–2.3)	1.2 (0.7–2.3)
Agoraphobia	1.6* (1.1–2.2)	1.1 (0.6–2.1)	1.3 (0.6–2.6)
Mood disorders			
Major depressive disorder	1.4* (1.1–1.7)	1.4* (1.1–2.0)	1.0 (0.7–1.5)
Dysthymic disorder	1.1 (0.8–1.4)	1.2 (0.7–2.0)	1.1 (0.6–2.3)
Bipolar disorder	1.3 (0.9–2.0)	1.4 (0.7–2.6)	0.9 (0.5–1.5)
Impulse-control disorders			
Oppositional defiant disorder	1.7* (1.2–2.4)	1.4 (0.8–2.4)	1.2 (0.6–2.4)
Conduct disorder	0.7 (0.5–1.1)	1.2 (0.7–2.1)	1.3 (0.7–2.4)
Attention deficit hyperactivity disorder	1.1 (0.8–1.4)	1.0 (0.7–1.6)	0.7 (0.4–1.3)
Intermittent explosive disorder	1.0 (0.7–1.4)	1.2 (0.8–1.8)	0.8 (0.5–1.4)
Substance use disorders			
Alcohol abuse or dependence	1.2 (0.9–1.5)	1.0 (0.6–1.5)	0.9 (0.6–1.4)
Drug abuse or dependence	1.1 (0.7–1.5)	1.1 (0.6–1.9)	1.1 (0.6–1.9)
16 df χ^2 test for 16 types	65.9 (<0.001)*	31.3 (0.01)*	21.6 (0.16)
15 df χ^2 test for difference between types	41.8 (<0.001)*	21.3 (0.13)	18.8 (0.22)
Number of mental disorders			
2	1.1 (0.8–1.4)	1.1 (0.7–1.6)	1.1 (0.6–1.8)
3	0.8 (0.5–1.3)	0.6 (0.3–1.2)	0.9 (0.4–1.9)
4	0.8 (0.4–1.4)	0.7 (0.3–1.7)	1.0 (0.4–2.7)
5	0.8 (0.4–1.7)	0.5 (0.2–1.8)	0.8 (0.2–3.1)
6	0.7 (0.3–1.6)	0.3 (0.1–1.3)	0.7 (0.1–3.7)
7+	0.3* (0.1–1.0)	0.2 (0.0–1.5)	0.9 (0.1–8.2)
χ^2 (p-value)	14.2 (0.03)*	10.0 (0.13)	1.4 (0.97)

* Significant at the 0.05 level, two-sided test.
– Dropped because the expected value is less than 5.
[a] Results are based on multivariate discrete time survival models. Models control for country, age-related variables, and significant variables from the chapters on sociodemographics, parental psychopathology, childhood adversities, and traumatic events.

Appendix Table 10.14. Associations between DSM-IV mental disorders and persistence of suicidal behavior[a] (middle-income countries)

Mental disorders	Ideation OR (95% CI)	Plan OR (95% CI)	Attempt OR (95% CI)
Anxiety disorders			
Panic disorder	1.3 (0.6–3.0)	3.6* (1.0–12.6)	–
Generalized anxiety disorder	1.1 (0.5–2.4)	1.3 (0.4–3.8)	1.2 (0.4–3.3)
Specific phobia	0.8 (0.5–1.3)	0.9 (0.3–2.4)	1.0 (0.5–2.0)
Social phobia	2.1* (1.2–3.6)	2.5 (0.9–6.9)	3.1* (1.3–7.5)
Posttraumatic stress	1.3 (0.7–2.6)	1.2 (0.4–3.8)	2.4 (0.8–7.2)
Separation anxiety disorder	1.9* (1.0–3.8)	2.1 (0.7–6.4)	1.6 (0.6–4.2)
Agoraphobia	2.3* (1.4–3.8)	4.6* (1.9–10.8)	–
Mood disorders			
Major depressive disorder	1.4 (0.9–2.3)	0.8 (0.4–1.6)	1.8 (0.9–3.8)
Dysthymic disorder	1.0 (0.5–2.2)	4.5* (1.0–19.5)	–
Bipolar disorder	1.1 (0.4–2.9)	–	–
Impulse-control disorders			
Oppositional defiant disorder	3.1* (1.7–6.0)	2.4 (1.0–5.8)	–
Conduct disorder	1.7 (0.6–4.8)	2.8 (0.5–16.8)	–
Attention deficit hyperactivity disorder	0.8 (0.4–1.6)	0.3 (0.1–1.6)	–
Intermittent explosive disorder	1.5 (0.9–2.7)	1.0 (0.4–2.9)	2.1 (0.8–5.0)
Substance use disorders			
Alcohol abuse or dependence	0.9 (0.5–1.6)	1.4 (0.6–3.2)	1.7 (0.7–4.5)
Drug abuse or dependence	0.6 (0.2–1.7)	1.0 (0.2–4.8)	–
16 df χ^2 test for 16 types	45.1 (<0.001)*	25.4 (0.04)*	13.4 (0.10)
15 df χ^2 test for difference between types	37.0 (0.001)*	22.4 (0.07)	8.7 (0.27)
Number of mental disorders[b]			
2	0.8 (0.4–1.7)	1.0 (0.4–2.8)	0.4 (0.2–1.1)
3	0.6 (0.2–1.5)	0.1 (0.0–1.7)	0.2* (0.0–0.8)
4	0.6 (0.2–2.1)	0.2 (0.0–2.7)	
5+	0.5 (0.1–2.4)	0.2 (0.0–2.6)	
χ^2 (p-value)	1.4 (0.84)	7.4 (0.12)	5.5 (0.06)

* Significant at the 0.05 level, two-sided test.
– Dropped because the expected value is less than 5.
[a] Results are based on multivariate discrete time survival models. Models control for country, age-related variables, and significant variables from the chapters on sociodemographics, parental psychopathology, childhood adversities, and traumatic events.
[b] For number of mental disorders, the last OR represents the odds for that number of disorders or more. For example, for attempt, 3 represents ≥3 (that is, 3+).

Appendix Table 10.15. Associations between DSM-IV mental disorders and persistence of suicidal behavior[a] (low-income countries)

Mental disorders	Ideation OR (95% CI)	Plan OR (95% CI)	Attempt OR (95% CI)
Anxiety disorders			
Panic disorder	2.8* (1.3–6.2)	–	–
Generalized anxiety disorder	1.0 (0.4–2.5)	–	–
Specific phobia	2.2* (1.4–3.4)	1.7 (0.9–3.0)	2.5* (1.1–5.9)
Social phobia	1.4 (0.8–2.4)	2.6* (1.1–6.0)	1.4 (0.4–5.1)
Posttraumatic stress	3.1 (0.9–10.1)	–	–
Separation anxiety disorder	1.8 (0.8–3.7)	1.5 (0.5–4.8)	0.9 (0.2–3.4)
Agoraphobia	–	–	–
Mood disorders			
Major depressive disorder	1.5 (1.0–2.3)	1.3 (0.7–2.5)	1.7 (0.7–3.7)
Dysthymic disorder	1.1 (0.5–2.4)	0.4 (0.1–1.9)	0.5 (0.0–4.7)
Bipolar disorder	1.1 (0.4–3.0)	–	–
Impulse-control disorders			
Oppositional defiant disorder	1.0 (0.4–2.3)	–	–
Conduct disorder	3.8* (2.1–7.1)	2.2* (1.0–4.8)	2.2 (0.9–5.6)
Attention deficit hyperactivity disorder	1.5 (0.6–3.8)	–	–
Intermittent explosive disorder	2.1* (1.3–3.2)	1.5 (0.7–3.3)	2.1 (0.6–7.2)
Substance use disorders			
Alcohol abuse or dependence	0.7 (0.4–1.4)	1.7 (0.9–3.3)	1.2 (0.3–4.4)
Drug abuse or dependence	1.3 (0.6–2.9)	–	–
16 df χ^2 test for 16 types	44.9 (<0.001)*	18.7 (0.02)*	9.4 (0.31)
15 df χ^2 test for difference between types	20.2 (0.12)	8.5 (0.29)	2.1 (0.95)
Number of mental disorders[b]			
2	0.6 (0.3–1.1)	1.0 (0.4–2.5)	1.0 (0.3–3.5)
3	0.5 (0.2–1.2)	0.6 (0.1–2.7)	0.8 (0.1–7.0)
4	0.2* (0.1–1.0)		
χ^2 (p-value)	4.0 (0.26)	1.1 (0.56)	0.0 (0.98)

* Significant at the 0.05 level, two-sided test.
– Dropped because the expected value is less than 5.
[a] Results are based on multivariate discrete time survival models. Models control for country, age-related variables, and significant variables from the chapters on sociodemographics, parental psychopathology, childhood adversities, and traumatic events.
[b] For number of mental disorders, the last OR represents the odds for that number of disorders or more. For example, for attempt, 3 represents ≥3 (that is, 3+).

Appendix Table 11.1. Prevalence of physical conditions in those with suicidal behavior (high-income countries)

Physical conditions	Among total sample %[a] (SE) with chronic condition						Among ideators %[a] (SE) with chronic condition			
	Ideation	No ideation	Attempt	No attempt	Plan	No plan	Planned attempt	No planned attempt	Unplanned attempt	No unplanned attempt
Cancer	0.8 (0.1)	0.9 (0.1)	1.0 (0.3)	0.8 (0.1)	1.1 (0.3)	2.1 (0.4)	1.2 (0.4)	3.0 (0.7)	0.9 (0.4)	2.0 (0.4)
Cardiovascular										
Heart disease	2.1 (0.3)	1.7 (0.1)	1.5 (0.4)	1.5 (0.1)	1.8 (0.5)	3.3 (0.4)	1.0 (0.3)	3.7 (0.8)	2.4 (0.9)	3.0 (0.5)
High blood pressure	4.9 (0.4)	5.0 (0.1)	5.3 (0.7)	4.6 (0.1)	5.1 (0.7)	9.4 (0.6)	4.7 (0.9)	9.3 (1.4)	6.4 (1.3)	9.4 (0.7)
Heart attack or stroke	1.2 (0.2)	0.9 (0.1)	1.1 (0.3)	0.7 (0.0)	0.8 (0.2)	2.1 (0.2)	0.9 (0.3)	1.1 (0.3)	1.6 (0.7)	1.8 (0.3)
Diabetes	0.8 (0.1)	1.1 (0.1)	0.7 (0.2)	1.0 (0.1)	0.5 (0.2)	2.1 (0.2)	0.6 (0.2)	2.7 (0.9)	1.0 (0.4)	2.0 (0.3)
Ulcer	3.8 (0.3)	2.7 (0.1)	3.6 (0.5)	2.7 (0.1)	3.8 (0.5)	6.8 (0.6)	3.8 (0.7)	6.5 (1.3)	3.1 (0.8)	6.3 (0.6)
Musculoskeletal										
Arthritis	7.4 (0.4)	6.9 (0.2)	6.4 (0.7)	6.6 (0.1)	7.9 (0.8)	14.9 (0.8)	6.0 (0.9)	16.8 (1.8)	6.6 (1.3)	13.9 (0.9)
Back and neck pain	17.0 (0.7)	11.4 (0.2)	16.2 (1.2)	11.5 (0.2)	17.9 (1.1)	28.8 (1.0)	14.4 (1.2)	32.3 (2.2)	18.6 (2.3)	28.5 (1.1)
Headache	18.8 (0.6)	8.8 (0.2)	20.5 (1.3)	9.2 (0.2)	20.7 (1.2)	26.5 (1.1)	20.5 (1.7)	27.5 (2.2)	20.0 (2.0)	25.5 (1.2)
Other chronic pain	6.1 (0.4)	3.2 (0.1)	7.9 (0.8)	3.3 (0.1)	7.4 (0.8)	10.3 (0.7)	6.5 (0.9)	11.9 (1.6)	9.5 (1.7)	9.0 (0.8)
Respiratory										
Allergies	18.2 (0.7)	11.1 (0.3)	19.1 (1.4)	11.4 (0.3)	19.3 (1.3)	23.9 (1.0)	17.4 (1.6)	27.4 (2.3)	21.8 (2.4)	23.6 (1.1)
Other respiratory	12.4 (0.6)	6.0 (0.2)	14.0 (1.1)	6.2 (0.2)	14.1 (1.1)	13.2 (0.8)	13.1 (1.3)	16.4 (1.9)	15.1 (2.0)	12.5 (0.9)
Epilepsy	0.3 (0.1)	0.1 (0.0)	0.3 (0.2)	0.1 (0.0)	0.2 (0.1)	0.8 (0.3)	0.3 (0.2)	0.5 (0.2)	0.5 (0.3)	0.9 (0.3)
Number of physical conditions										
1	28.1 (0.8)	19.8 (0.2)	27.6 (1.4)	19.9 (0.2)	26.7 (1.2)	27.8 (0.8)	28.7 (1.9)	25.1 (1.7)	25.8 (2.3)	28.7 (1.1)
2	13.2 (0.6)	8.9 (0.1)	14.5 (1.1)	9.0 (0.1)	14.8 (1.1)	18.9 (0.8)	13.3 (1.2)	18.3 (1.6)	17.4 (2.2)	18.8 (0.9)
3	5.5 (0.4)	3.6 (0.1)	6.0 (0.7)	3.6 (0.1)	6.8 (0.7)	10.5 (0.6)	5.4 (0.7)	14.8 (1.5)	6.7 (1.2)	10.9 (0.7)
4	3.0 (0.3)	1.6 (0.1)	2.4 (0.4)	1.5 (0.1)	2.8 (0.4)	5.9 (0.4)	2.4 (0.5)	6.1 (0.8)	2.2 (0.7)	5.5 (0.5)
5+	1.9 (0.2)	0.9 (0.0)	2.5 (0.5)	0.9 (0.0)	2.2 (0.4)	4.2 (0.3)	1.6 (0.4)	5.2 (0.9)	3.3 (1.1)	3.1 (0.4)
N[b]	(5056)	(112,028)	(1613)	(116,041)	(1885)	(5646)	(1002)	(1330)	(551)	(4338)

[a] % represents the percentage of people with the chronic condition among the cases with the outcome variable indicated in the column header. For example, the first cell is the % of those with cancer among those with ideation.

[b] Number of cases with the outcome variable; N represents the number of person–years.

Appendix Table 11.2. Prevalence of physical conditions in those with suicidal behavior (lower income countries)

Physical conditions	Among total sample						Among ideators			
	%ᵃ (SE) with chronic condition						%ᵃ (SE) with chronic condition			
	Ideation	No ideation	Attempt	No attempt	Plan	No plan	Planned attempt	No planned attempt	Unplanned attempt	No unplanned attempt
Cancer	0.3 (0.2)	0.1 (0.0)	0.6 (0.4)	0.0 (0.0)	0.6 (0.3)	0.4 (0.3)	1.2 (0.7)	0.9 (0.7)	0.0 (0.0)	0.2 (0.2)
Cardiovascular										
Heart disease	1.5 (0.4)	1.4 (0.1)	2.2 (0.8)	1.2 (0.1)	1.8 (0.5)	3.8 (1.2)	1.4 (0.6)	1.2 (0.9)	2.7 (1.6)	4.5 (1.5)
High blood pressure	3.2 (0.7)	2.5 (0.2)	3.6 (1.7)	2.0 (0.1)	4.9 (1.5)	6.0 (1.2)	2.5 (1.1)	8.2 (3.4)	5.6 (3.9)	6.4 (1.4)
Heart attack or stroke	1.2 (0.4)	0.9 (0.1)	1.7 (0.7)	0.7 (0.1)	2.5 (0.8)	3.7 (1.1)	2.3 (1.0)	2.3 (1.3)	0.0 (0.0)	2.5 (0.9)
Diabetes	0.6 (0.2)	0.5 (0.1)	0.6 (0.5)	0.4 (0.1)	0.7 (0.5)	0.8 (0.3)	0.2 (0.2)	0.8 (0.4)	1.2 (1.2)	0.7 (0.3)
Ulcer	5.3 (0.9)	2.0 (0.1)	5.8 (1.8)	2.0 (0.1)	8.0 (1.5)	8.4 (1.7)	5.8 (1.7)	13.4 (6.5)	5.5 (3.7)	6.3 (1.2)
Musculoskeletal										
Arthritis	8.8 (1.3)	6.4 (0.2)	10.4 (2.4)	5.4 (0.2)	9.1 (1.8)	9.6 (1.6)	10.5 (2.7)	20.5 (7.3)	11.4 (4.2)	8.6 (1.7)
Back and neck pain	9.3 (1.0)	5.2 (0.2)	6.8 (1.4)	4.9 (0.2)	10.4 (2.2)	15.2 (1.8)	8.8 (2.1)	15.3 (3.9)	3.8 (1.7)	15.4 (2.0)
Headache	15.7 (1.4)	5.6 (0.3)	17.3 (2.6)	5.5 (0.3)	17.4 (2.6)	18.2 (2.0)	18.2 (3.3)	32.9 (6.9)	16.7 (4.4)	17.5 (2.4)
Other chronic pain	4.4 (1.0)	1.5 (0.1)	4.9 (1.7)	1.4 (0.1)	5.7 (1.3)	4.7 (1.2)	4.1 (1.5)	13.2 (7.3)	5.5 (3.8)	5.2 (1.6)
Respiratory										
Allergies	2.9 (0.7)	2.1 (0.2)	4.0 (1.7)	2.1 (0.2)	3.1 (0.9)	3.6 (1.0)	3.9 (1.6)	10.5 (4.2)	4.8 (3.8)	2.4 (0.8)
Other respiratory	3.2 (0.6)	1.6 (0.1)	3.7 (1.1)	1.5 (0.1)	5.5 (1.4)	4.3 (1.0)	3.5 (1.0)	5.9 (2.8)	4.7 (2.4)	3.0 (0.8)
Epilepsy	0.7 (0.4)	0.1 (0.0)	2.2 (1.2)	0.1 (0.0)	1.7 (1.0)	0.3 (0.3)	2.7 (1.9)	0.0 (0.0)	1.8 (1.4)	0.6 (0.4)
Number of physical conditions										
1	23.5 (1.5)	12.5 (0.3)	24.6 (2.5)	12.2 (0.3)	27.3 (2.7)	25.4 (2.5)	26.8 (3.3)	27.3 (4.7)	21.4 (4.3)	25.7 (2.6)
2	7.4 (0.9)	3.9 (0.2)	8.4 (1.7)	3.7 (0.2)	8.6 (1.6)	10.9 (1.3)	10.1 (2.5)	13.3 (3.7)	6.4 (2.4)	11.0 (1.4)
3+	5.3 (0.9)	2.6 (0.2)	5.8 (1.9)	2.0 (0.1)	6.8 (1.7)	8.3 (1.3)	5.0 (1.7)	17.7 (7.1)	7.2 (4.1)	7.3 (1.4)
Nᵇ	(1264)	(31,794)	(459)	(31,351)	(483)	(984)	(269)	(203)	(159)	(683)

ᵃ % represents the percentage of people with the chronic condition among the cases with the outcome variable indicated in the column header. For example, the first cell is the % of those with cancer among those with ideation.

ᵇ Number of cases with the outcome variable; N represents the number of person–years.

Appendix Table 11.3. Final multivariate models for associations between each type of physical condition and suicidal behavior, controlling for other types, and number of physical conditions; unadjusted for mental disorder[a] (high-income countries)

	Among total sample		Among ideators		
	Ideation	Attempt	Plan	Planned attempt	Unplanned attempt
Physical conditions	OR (95% CI)	OR (95% CI)	OR (95% CI)	OR (95% CI)	OR (95% CI)
Cancer	1.1 (0.7–1.7)	1.5 (0.9–2.6)	1.1 (0.6–2.0)	1.3 (0.6–2.9)	0.9 (0.4–2.3)
Cardiovascular					
Heart disease	1.4* (1.0–2.0)	0.9 (0.5–1.5)	1.0 (0.5–1.9)	0.5 (0.2–1.3)	1.3 (0.6–2.9)
High blood pressure	1.4* (1.1–1.7)	1.8* (1.2–2.6)	1.1 (0.7–1.6)	1.5 (0.9–2.7)	1.2 (0.7–2.3)
Heart attack or stroke	1.8* (1.2–2.8)	2.1* (1.1–3.9)	0.7 (0.3–1.3)	1.8 (0.5–6.8)	1.7 (0.7–4.2)
Diabetes	1.2 (0.8–1.8)	1.2 (0.6–2.3)	0.6 (0.3–1.3)	0.7 (0.2–2.3)	1.0 (0.3–2.8)
Ulcer	1.4* (1.1–1.7)	1.1 (0.8–1.6)	0.9 (0.6–1.3)	1.4 (0.8–2.6)	0.8 (0.4–1.5)
Musculoskeletal					
Arthritis	1.4* (1.2–1.7)	1.2 (0.8–1.7)	0.9 (0.7–1.3)	1.0 (0.6–1.8)	0.6 (0.4–1.1)
Back and neck pain	1.5* (1.3–1.7)	1.3 (1.0–1.7)	0.9 (0.7–1.2)	0.7 (0.5–1.2)	0.8 (0.5–1.4)
Headache	1.9* (1.6–2.1)	1.6* (1.2–2.0)	0.9 (0.7–1.1)	1.0 (0.7–1.5)	0.7 (0.4–1.1)
Other chronic pain	1.5* (1.2–1.9)	1.9* (1.4–2.5)	1.0 (0.7–1.3)	1.2 (0.7–2.1)	1.3 (0.8–2.2)
Respiratory					
Allergies	1.1 (1.0–1.3)	1.1 (0.9–1.4)	0.8 (0.6–1.0)	0.8 (0.5–1.2)	0.8 (0.6–1.3)
Other respiratory	1.6* (1.3–1.9)	1.5* (1.2–1.9)	1.1 (0.8–1.4)	1.1 (0.7–1.9)	1.0 (0.6–1.6)
Epilepsy	–	–	0.4 (0.2–1.2)	–	–
13 df group χ^2 for 13 types	110.5 (<0.001)*	48.9 (<0.001)*	11.0 (0.61)	13.4 (0.34)	12.9 (0.38)
12 df χ^2 for difference between types	52.4 (<0.001)*	24.6 (0.01)*	9.7 (0.64)	12.6 (0.32)	12.0 (0.36)
Number of physical conditions					
2	0.7* (0.6–0.9)	0.8 (0.6–1.1)	1.0 (0.7–1.4)	1.0 (0.5–1.7)	1.8 (1.0–3.2)
3	0.5* (0.4–0.7)	0.6* (0.3–0.9)	1.2 (0.7–1.9)	0.7 (0.3–1.6)	1.4 (0.6–3.6)
4	0.5* (0.3–0.8)	0.4* (0.2–0.8)	1.1 (0.6–2.2)	0.7 (0.2–2.3)	1.3 (0.3–5.2)
5+	0.3* (0.2–0.6)	0.4 (0.1–1.1)	1.3 (0.5–3.2)	0.6 (0.1–3.3)	5.2 (0.8–32.0)
χ^2 (p-value)	17.1 (0.002)*	9.0 (0.06)	0.9 (0.92)	1.7 (0.80)	8.2 (0.08)

* Significant at the 0.05 level, two-sided test.
– Condition not included in model due to small cell size. Small cell size determined by calculating the expected number of cases of the condition based on the % of people with the outcome and the total number of people with the condition. If the expected value was less than 5, the condition was dropped from the model.
[a] Assessed in the Part 2 sample due to having Part 2 controls. Israel and ESEMeD countries do not have the instrument questions used for epilepsy, and therefore were coded "no." Models control for person–years, country, and significant variables from the chapters on sociodemographics, parental psychopathology, childhood adversities, and traumatic events.

Appendix Table 11.4. Final multivariate models for associations between each physical condition and suicidal behavior, controlling for other types, and number of physical conditions; unadjusted for mental disorder[a] (lower income countries)

Physical conditions	Among total sample		Among ideators		
	Ideation	Attempt	Plan	Planned attempt	Unplanned attempt
	OR (95% CI)	OR (95% CI)	OR (95% CI)	OR (95% CI)	OR (95% CI)
Cancer	–	–	–	–	–
Cardiovascular					
Heart disease	1.0 (0.4–2.0)	–	0.5 (0.2–1.3)	–	0.5 (0.2–1.3)
High blood pressure	1.0 (0.6–1.8)	1.2 (0.5–2.9)	1.1 (0.4–2.8)	0.3 (0.1–1.3)	1.4 (0.2–10.2)
Heart attack or stroke	1.6 (0.6–4.2)	–	1.0 (0.4–2.6)	16.6* (2.2–127.5)	–
Diabetes	–	–	–	–	–
Ulcer	1.9* (1.1–3.3)	1.9 (0.7–5.6)	1.3 (0.7–2.3)	0.7 (0.1–5.0)	1.7 (0.5–5.9)
Musculoskeletal					
Arthritis	2.3* (1.6–3.3)	3.4* (2.1–5.7)	1.3 (0.6–2.6)	1.4 (0.4–5.7)	2.8* (1.0–7.6)
Back and neck pain	1.3 (0.8–1.9)	0.7 (0.4–1.2)	0.8 (0.4–1.7)	0.7 (0.2–2.2)	0.3* (0.1–0.8)
Headache	1.7* (1.3–2.3)	1.7* (1.0–2.7)*	1.1 (0.7–1.9)	0.7 (0.2–2.2)	1.2 (0.5–2.7)
Other chronic pain	1.6 (0.9–3.0)	1.4 (0.6–3.1)	1.9 (0.8–4.6)	0.5 (0.1–1.8)	0.9 (0.2–3.8)
Respiratory					
Allergies	0.8 (0.4–1.3)	0.8 (0.3–2.2)	0.8 (0.3–1.9)	1.4 (0.3–6.4)	–
Other respiratory	1.5 (0.9–2.3)	1.4 (0.7–2.8)	1.4 (0.7–2.7)	0.7 (0.2–2.6)	3.3 (0.9–11.7)
Epilepsy	–	–	–	–	–
13 df group χ^2 for 13 types	52.0 (<0.001)*	41.2 (<0.001)*	8.8 (0.55)	11.4 (0.25)	17.3 (0.03)*
12 df χ^2 for difference between types	21.6 (0.01)*	33.8 (<0.001)*	8.1 (0.52)	12.0 (0.15)	17.1 (0.02)*
Number of physical conditions					
2	0.7 (0.5–1.1)	0.6 (0.3–1.4)	0.6 (0.3–1.3)	1.5 (0.4–6.0)	0.3 (0.1–1.2)
3+	0.5 (0.2–1.1)	0.7 (0.2–2.2)	1.0 (0.3–3.7)	0.7 (0.1–6.3)	0.8 (0.1–6.7)
χ^2 (p-value)	3.2 (0.20)	1.4 (0.51)	3.2 (0.20)	1.3 (0.52)	4.2 (0.12)

*Significant at the 0.05 level, two-sided test.

– Condition not included in model due to small cell size. Small cell size determined by calculating the expected number of cases of the condition based on the % of people with the outcome and the total number of people with the condition. If the expected value was less than 5, the condition was dropped from the model.

[a] Assessed in the Part 2 sample due to having Part 2 controls. Data from Ukraine, Lebanon, Nigeria, South Africa, China, Bulgaria, Brazil, and India were dropped as they do not have age questions for chronic conditions and cannot have time-varying variables. Models control for person–years, country, and significant variables from the chapters on sociodemographics, parental psychopathology, childhood adversities, and traumatic events.

Appendix Table 11.5. Interactions between physical conditions and life course interval during which the suicide attempt was made[a] (high-income countries)

Interactions		Attempts Among total sample	
		OR (95% CI)	χ^2 (p-value)
Cancer	middle 33%	–	1.5 (0.22)
	upper 33%	0.4 (0.1–1.8)	
Cardiovascular			
Heart disease	middle 33%	–	1.7 (0.20)
	upper 33%	0.5 (0.1–1.5)	
High blood pressure	middle 33%	–	1.6 (0.20)
	upper 33%	0.6 (0.3–1.3)	
Heart attack or stroke	middle 33%	–	0.3 (0.60)
	upper 33%	1.5 (0.3–7.1)	
Diabetes	middle 33%	–	4.3 (0.04)*
	upper 33%	0.1* (0.0–0.9)	
Ulcer	middle 33%	–	0.0 (0.90)
	upper 33%	1.1 (0.5–2.3)	
Musculoskeletal			
Arthritis	middle 33%	0.7 (0.2–2.0)	0.9 (0.63)
	upper 33%	0.6 (0.2–1.6)	
Back and neck pain	middle 33%	1.1 (0.5–2.3)	1.8 (0.41)
	upper 33%	0.7 (0.4–1.5)	
Headache	middle 33%	0.7 (0.4–1.3)	4.8 (0.09)
	upper 33%	0.5* (0.3–0.9)	
Other chronic pain	middle 33%	0.8 (0.4–2.0)	0.4 (0.81)
	upper 33%	1.0 (0.5–2.3)	
Respiratory			
Allergies	middle 33%	0.5* (0.3–0.9)	16.4 (<.001)*
	upper 33%	0.4* (0.2–0.6)	
Other respiratory	middle 33%	1.1 (0.6–2.0)	1.0 (0.59)
	upper 33%	0.8 (0.5–1.5)	
Epilepsy	middle 33%	–	–
	upper 33%	–	
26 df χ^2 test for all chronic conditions			30.7 (0.03)*
25 df χ^2 test for all conditions and dummies for number of conditions			41.1 (0.02)*
Number of physical conditions			
2	middle 33%	1.1 (0.6–2.2)	
	upper 33%	1.5 (0.7–3.2)	
3	middle 33%	0.7 (0.2–2.0)	
	upper 33%	1.5 (0.5–4.5)	
4	middle 33%	–	
	upper 33%	2.8 (0.7–10.6)	
5+	middle 33%	–	
	upper 33%	9.7 (1.0–98.2)	

Appendix Table 11.5. (cont.)

Interactions	Attempts Among total sample	
	OR (95% CI)	χ^2 (p-value)
χ^2 (p-value)		4.5 (0.60)

[*] Significant at the 0.05 level, two-sided test.

[–] Condition not included in model due to small cell size. Small cell size determined by calculating the expected number of cases of the condition based on the % of people with the outcome and the total number of people with the condition. If the expected value was less than 5, the condition was dropped from the model.

[a] Assessed in the the Part 2 sample. Models control for person–years, country, and significant variables from the chapters on sociodemographics, parental psychopathology, childhood adversities, and traumatic events. Models also included all controls and interaction terms between life course intervals (intervals determined by the 33.3% percentiles of the age-of-onset for the outcome) and each control. Only the interaction terms between the life course intervals and physical condition variables are shown in the table. Israel and ESEMeD countries do not have the instrument questions used for epilepsy, and therefore were coded "no."

Appendix Table 11.6. Interactions between physical conditions and life course interval during which the suicide attempt was made[a] (lower income countries)

Interactions		Attempts Among total sample	
		OR (95% CI)	χ2 (p-value)
Cancer	middle 33%	–	–
	upper 33%	–	
Cardiovascular			
Heart disease	middle 33%	–	–
	upper 33%	–	
High blood pressure	middle 33%	–	0.0 (1.00)
	upper 33%	1.0 (0.2–6.4)	
Heart attack or stroke	middle 33%	–	–
	upper 33%	–	
Diabetes	middle 33%	–	–
	upper 33%	–	
Ulcer	middle 33%	–	10.6 (0.001)*
	upper 33%	0.1* (0.0–0.4)	
Musculoskeletal			
Arthritis	middle 33%	–	0.0 (0.87)
	upper 33%	0.9 (0.2–3.7)	
Back and neck pain	middle 33%	–	0.0 (0.99)
	upper 33%	1.0 (0.3–3.0)	
Headache	middle 33%	–	0.1 (0.80)
	upper 33%	0.9 (0.4–2.0)	
Other chronic pain	middle 33%	–	–
	upper 33%	–	
Respiratory			
Allergies	middle 33%	–	–
	upper 33%	–	
Other respiratory	middle 33%	–	–
	upper 33%	–	
Epilepsy	middle 33%	–	–
	upper 33%	–	
26 df χ^2 test for all chronic conditions			11.9 (0.04)*
25 df χ^2 test for all conditions and dummies for number of conditions			12.0 (0.06)
Number of physical conditions			
2	middle 33%	–	
	upper 33%	2.5 (0.7–8.1)	
3+	middle 33%	–	
	upper 33%	–	

Appendix Table 11.6. (cont.)

Interactions	Attempts Among total sample	
	OR (95% CI)	χ2 (p-value)
χ² (p-value)		2.2 (0.14)

[*] Significant at the 0.05 level, two-sided test.
– Condition not included in model due to small cell size. Small cell size determined by calculating the expected number of cases of the condition based on the % of people with the outcome and the total number of people with the condition. If the expected value was less than 5, the condition was dropped from the model.
[a] Assessed in the the Part 2 sample. Models control for person–years, country, and significant variables from the chapters on sociodemographics, parental psychopathology, childhood adversities, and traumatic events. Models also included all controls and interaction terms between life course intervals (intervals determined by the 33.3% percentiles of the age-of-onset for the outcome) and each control. Only the interaction terms between the life course intervals and physical condition variables are shown in the table. Data from Ukraine, Lebanon, Nigeria, South Africa, China, Bulgaria, Brazil, and India were dropped as they do not have age questions for chronic conditions and cannot have time-varying variables.

Appendix Table 11.7. Physical conditions and persistence of suicidal behavior (high-income countries)[a]

Physical conditions	Ideation OR (95% CI)	Plan OR (95% CI)	Attempt OR (95% CI)
Cancer	1.1 (0.5–2.5)	–	–
Cardiovascular			
Heart disease	0.8 (0.5–1.5)	1.3 (0.6–2.8)	–
High blood pressure	1.1 (0.8–1.5)	0.6 (0.3–1.2)	0.5 (0.2–1.1)
Heart attack/stroke	0.8 (0.4–1.7)	–	–
Diabetes	2.7* (1.2–6.1)	–	–
Ulcer	1.0 (0.7–1.5)	1.3 (0.7–2.6)	3.0* (1.3–6.7)
Musculoskeletal			
Arthritis	1.0 (0.7–1.4)	1.1 (0.6–2.1)	0.9 (0.5–1.7)
Back and neck pain	1.2 (1.0–1.4)	1.3 (0.9–1.9)	1.2 (0.7–2.0)
Headache	1.2 (1.0–1.4)	1.2 (0.9–1.6)	1.5* (1.0–2.1)
Other chronic pain	1.0 (0.7–1.3)	1.3 (0.8–2.0)	1.6 (0.9–2.8)
Respiratory			
Allergies	0.9 (0.7–1.1)	1.1 (0.8–1.6)	1.2 (0.8–1.9)
Other respiratory	1.0 (0.8–1.2)	0.9 (0.6–1.3)	1.1 (0.8–1.7)
Epilepsy	0.5 (0.2–1.6)	–	–
13 df χ^2 test for 13 types	18.5 (0.14)	12.4 (0.19)	18.0 (0.02)*
12 df χ^2 test for difference between types	18.9 (0.09)	11.2 (0.19)	14.3 (0.05)*
Number of physical conditions			
2	1.0 (0.7–1.3)	0.7 (0.5–1.2)	0.5* (0.3–0.9)
3	1.0 (0.7–1.6)	1.0 (0.5–2.1)	0.9 (0.4–2.1)
4	1.2 (0.7–2.3)	0.6 (0.2–1.9)	0.6 (0.2–1.9)
5+	1.5 (0.6–3.6)	1.7 (0.4–7.4)	0.3 (0.1–1.5)
χ^2 (p-value)	2.3 (0.68)	7.3 (0.12)	9.9 (0.04)*

* Significant at the 0.05 level, two-sided test.
– Dropped because the expected value is less than 5.
[a] Results are based on multivariate discrete time survival models. Models control for country, age-related variables, and significant variables from the chapters on sociodemographics, parental psychopathology, childhood adversities, traumatic events, and mental disorders.

Appendix Table 11.8. Physical conditions and persistence of suicidal behavior^a (lower income countries)

Physical conditions	Ideation OR (95% CI)	Plan OR (95% CI)	Attempt OR (95% CI)
Cancer	–	–	–
Cardiovascular			
Heart disease	0.9 (0.3–2.4)	–	–
High blood pressure	4.0* (1.4–11.5)	–	–
Heart attack/stroke	–	–	–
Diabetes	–	–	–
Ulcer	2.5* (1.2–5.4)	1.5 (0.4–5.4)	–
Musculoskeletal			
Arthritis	1.2 (0.6–2.3)	0.2 (0.0–1.2)	0.5 (0.1–4.3)
Back and neck pain	2.3* (1.1–5.1)	0.4 (0.1–1.4)	1.2 (0.3–5.5)
Headache	1.6 (0.9–3.0)	2.0 (0.9–4.8)	0.5 (0.2–1.6)
Other chronic pain	0.8 (0.3–2.4)	–	1.4 (0.2–11.9)
Respiratory			
Allergies	3.1* (1.3–7.5)	–	–
Other respiratory	1.3 (0.5–3.2)	1.7 (0.4–7.4)	–
Epilepsy	–	–	–
13 df χ^2 test for 13 types	21.5 (0.01)*	12.3 (0.03)*	2.2 (0.70)
12 df χ^2 test for difference between types	13.6 (0.09)	12.1 (0.02)*	1.4 (0.70)
Number of physical conditions			
2	0.5* (0.2–1.0)	1.9 (0.4–8.4)	0.2 (0.0–3.6)
3+	0.3 (0.1–1.2)	4.2 (0.3–54.0)	0.0* (0.0–0.0)
χ^2 (p-value)	4.1 (0.13)	1.3 (0.52)	18.3 (<0.001)*

* Significant at the 0.05 level, two-sided test.
⁻ Dropped because the expected value is less than 5.
^{a} Results are based on multivariate discrete time survival models. Models control for country, age-related variables, and significant variables from the chapters on sociodemographics, parental psychopathology, childhood adversities, traumatic events, and mental disorders.

Appendix Table 12.1. Population attributable risk proportions of risk factors predicting the subsequent first occurrence of suicide ideation[a] (high-income countries)

	Model				
	1	**2**	**3**	**4**	**5**
Conditions cured	**PARP**	**PARP**	**PARP**	**PARP**	**PARP**
Parental psychopathology	9.92%	4.68%	3.79%	3.66%	2.39%
Childhood adversity	–	27.85%	25.16%	23.40%	17.13%
Trauma	–	–	16.64%	14.58%	8.90%
Chronic conditions	–	–	–	11.76%	7.91%
Mental disorders	–	–	–	–	30.81%
All conditions	–	–	–	–	63.92%

PARP, population attributable risk proportions.
[a] Assessed in the Part 2 sample. All models control for country and person–years.

Appendix Table 12.2. Population attributable risk proportions of risk factors predicting the subsequent first occurrence of suicide ideation[a] (middle-income countries)

	Model				
	1	**2**	**3**	**4**	**5**
Conditions cured	**PARP**	**PARP**	**PARP**	**PARP**	**PARP**
Parental psychopathology	13.01%	7.95%	5.52%	5.43%	3.61%
Childhood adversity	–	28.34%	23.89%	23.62%	18.41%
Trauma	–	–	23.05%	22.78%	14.99%
Chronic conditions	–	–	–	3.17%	2.67%
Mental disorders	–	–	–	–	29.41%
All conditions	–	–	–	–	60.23%

PARP, population attributable risk proportions.
[a] Assessed in the Part 2 sample. All models control for country and person–years.

Appendix Table 12.3. Population attributable risk proportions of risk factors predicting the subsequent first occurrence of suicide ideation[a] (low-income countries)

	Model				
	1	2	3	4	5
Conditions cured	PARP	PARP	PARP	PARP	PARP
Parental psychopathology	18.35%	13.60%	11.54%	11.24%	5.91%
Childhood adversity	–	21.81%	17.03%	16.07%	15.95%
Trauma	–	–	12.60%	11.98%	8.65%
Chronic conditions	–	–	–	4.64%	4.20%
Mental disorders	–	–	–	–	20.59%
All conditions	–	–	–	–	50.32%

PARP, population attributable risk proportions.
[a] Assessed in the Part 2 sample. All models control for country and person–years.

Appendix Table 12.4. Population attributable risk proportions of risk factors predicting the subsequent first occurrence of suicide attempt[a] (high-income countries)

	Model				
	1	2	3	4	5
Conditions cured	PARP	PARP	PARP	PARP	PARP
Parental psychopathology	19.24%	6.51%	5.03%	4.92%	2.58%
Childhood adversity	–	59.62%	57.86%	56.44%	46.32%
Trauma	–	–	19.44%	17.46%	8.20%
Chronic conditions	–	–	–	12.02%	6.89%
Mental disorders	–	–	–	–	52.12%
All conditions	–	–	–	–	83.56%

PARP, population attributable risk proportions.
[a] Assessed in the Part 2 sample. All models control for country and person–years.

Appendix Table 12.5. Population attributable risk proportions of risk factors predicting the subsequent first occurrence of suicide attempt[a] (middle-income countries)

	Model				
	1	2	3	4	5
Conditions cured	PARP	PARP	PARP	PARP	PARP
Parental psychopathology	22.11%	15.79%	12.86%	12.78%	9.52%
Childhood adversity	–	41.59%	38.13%	37.78%	30.34%
Trauma	–	–	29.68%	29.25%	17.14%
Chronic conditions	–	–	–	5.10%	4.21%
Mental disorders	–	–	–	–	42.38%
All conditions	–	–	–	–	74.10%

PARP, population attributable risk proportions.
[a] Assessed in the Part 2 sample. All models control for country and person–years.

Appendix Table 12.6. Population attributable risk proportions of risk factors predicting the subsequent first occurrence of suicide attempt[a] (low-income countries)

	Model				
	1	2	3	4	5
Conditions cured	PARP	PARP	PARP	PARP	PARP
Parental psychopathology	15.73%	10.45%	9.27%	9.04%	5.91%
Childhood adversity	–	35.11%	35.43%	34.98%	29.25%
Trauma	–	–	14.96%	14.57%	11.74%
Chronic conditions	–	–	–	3.03%	1.53%
Mental disorders	–	–	–	–	33.55%
All conditions	–	–	–	–	63.64%

PARP, population attributable risk proportions.
[a] Assessed in the Part 2 sample. All models control for country and person–years.

Appendix Table 12.7. Population attributable risk proportions of sociodemographic factors predicting the subsequent first occurrence of suicide attempt among ideators[a] (high-income countries)

	Model				
	1	2	3	4	5
Conditions cured	PARP	PARP	PARP	PARP	PARP
Parental psychopathology	1.32%	−0.68%	−0.67%	−0.66%	−0.96%
Childhood adversity	–	14.70%	15.23%	15.26%	14.13%
Trauma	–	–	−2.38%	−1.95%	−3.32%
Chronic conditions	–	–	–	−2.05%	−2.17%
Mental disorders	–	–	–	–	3.55%
All conditions	–	–	–	–	11.31%

PARP, population attributable risk proportions.
[a] Assessed in the Part 2 sample. All models control for country and person–years.

Appendix Table 12.8. Population attributable risk proportions of sociodemographic factors predicting the subsequent first occurrence of suicide attempt among ideators[a] (middle-income countries)

	Model				
	1	2	3	4	5
Conditions cured	PARP	PARP	PARP	PARP	PARP
Parental psychopathology	2.20%	1.89%	2.14%	2.25%	1.91%
Childhood adversity	–	4.08%	4.41%	4.27%	3.00%
Trauma	–	–	−0.20%	−0.31%	−1.35%
Chronic conditions	–	–	–	0.66%	0.57%
Mental disorders	–	–	–	–	2.78%
All conditions	–	–	–	–	7.00%

PARP, population attributable risk proportions.
[a] Assessed in the Part 2 sample. All models control for country and person–years.

Appendix Table 12.9. Population attributable risk proportions of sociodemographic factors predicting the subsequent first occurrence of suicide attempt among ideators[a] (low-income countries)

Conditions cured	Model				
	1	2	3	4	5
	PARP	PARP	PARP	PARP	PARP
Parental psychopathology	−0.40%	−0.94%	−0.91%	−1.09%	−1.16%
Childhood adversity	–	2.86%	2.05%	2.03%	1.46%
Trauma	–	–	−0.23%	−0.13%	−0.28%
Chronic conditions	–	–	–	−0.90%	−0.84%
Mental disorders	–	–	–	–	−0.57%
All conditions	–	–	–	–	−1.65%

PARP, population attributable risk proportions.
[a] Assessed in the Part 2 sample. All models control for country and person–years.

Appendix Table 13.1. Bivariate associations of sociodemographic variables with 12-month suicide ideation, plan, and attempt[a] (high-income countries)

Categories	Among total sample		Among ideators	
	Ideation	Plan	Planned attempt	Unplanned attempt
	OR (95% CI)	OR (95% CI)	OR (95% CI)	OR (95% CI)
4-Category age (years)				
Less than 35	4.7 (3.4–6.3)	2.0 (0.8–4.7)	1.5 (0.2–13.8)	4.1 (1.4–11.7)
35–49	3.6 (2.6–4.8)	2.0 (0.9–4.8)	1.1 (0.1–9.7)	3.4 (1.2–9.7)
50–64	2.2 (1.6–3.0)	2.0 (0.8–4.8)	0.5 (0.1–4.6)	1.0 (1.0–1.0)
65 or older	1.0 (1.0–1.0)	1.0 (1.0–1.0)	1.0 (1.0–1.0)	–
χ^2_3 (p-value)	120.8 (<0.001)*	2.7 (0.44)	7.3 (0.06)	7.0 (0.03)*
Dichotomized age (years)				
Less than 50	2.5 (2.1–3.0)	1.2 (0.8–1.7)	2.3 (1.0–5.5)	5.3 (2.0–14.2)
50 or older	1.0 (1.0–1.0)	1.0 (1.0–1.0)	1.0 (1.0–1.0)	1.0 (1.0–1.0)
χ^2_1 (p-value)	104.5 (<0.001)*	0.7 (0.40)	3.8 (0.05)	11.2 (<.001)*
Gender				
Female	1.3 (1.1–1.6)	13.5 (<.001)*	1.3 (0.7–2.3)	0.8 (0.4–1.4)
Male	1.0 (1.0–1.0)	0.8 (0.6–1.2)	1.0 (1.0–1.0)	1.0 (1.0–1.0)
χ^2_1 (p-value)	1.0 (1.0–1.0)	1.2 (0.28)	0.6 (0.45)	0.9 (0.35)
Education				
Low	1.8 (1.4–2.3)	1.6 (0.9–2.8)	0.7 (0.3–2.0)	2.4 (0.8–7.0)
Low-average	1.4 (1.1–1.8)	1.4 (0.8–2.5)	0.8 (0.3–2.2)	2.2 (0.7–6.2)
High-average	1.5 (1.2–1.9)	1.9 (1.1–3.2)	0.8 (0.3–2.4)	1.4 (0.5–4.1)
High	1.0 (1.0–1.0)	1.0 (1.0–1.0)	1.0 (1.0–1.0)	1.0 (1.0–1.0)
χ^2_3 (p-value)	20.8 (<0.001)*	5.4 (0.14)	0.4 (0.95)	3.3 (0.35)
Income level[b]				
Low	3.0 (2.2–4.0)	1.5 (0.8–2.8)	2.4 (0.8–7.3)	1.5 (0.5–4.6)
Low-average	2.2 (1.6–2.8)	1.5 (0.8–2.7)	1.9 (0.6–6.0)	0.9 (0.3–2.9)
High-average	1.5 (1.2–2.1)	1.0 (0.5–1.9)	1.2 (0.4–4.0)	0.7 (0.2–2.5)
High	1.0 (1.0–1.0)	1.0 (1.0–1.0)	1.0 (1.0–1.0)	1.0 (1.0–1.0)
χ^2_3 (p-value)	65.9 (<0.001)*	5.9 (0.12)	4.4 (0.22)	2.8 (0.42)
Marital status				
Married or cohabitating	1.0 (1.0–1.0)	1.0 (1.0–1.0)	1.0 (1.0–1.0)	1.0 (1.0–1.0)
Separated, widowed, or divorced	2.1 (1.8–2.6)	1.1 (0.8–1.7)	1.7 (0.8–3.7)	1.3 (0.6–2.6)
Never married	2.8 (2.4–3.3)	1.1 (0.8–1.6)	1.6 (0.8–3.2)	1.6 (0.9–2.9)
χ^2_2 (p-value)	162.9 (<0.001)*	0.6 (0.75)	2.8 (0.25)	2.2 (0.33)
Employment				
Working	1.0 (1.0–1.0)	1.0 (1.0–1.0)	1.0 (1.0–1.0)	1.0 (1.0–1.0)
Student	1.7 (1.2–2.4)	0.5 (0.3–1.0)	2.5 (0.6–10.0)	0.5 (0.1–2.2)
Homemaker	1.1 (0.8–1.4)	1.5 (0.9–2.5)	0.6 (0.2–1.5)	0.4 (0.1–1.3)
Retired	0.4 (0.3–0.5)	0.9 (0.4–1.8)	0.9 (0.1–5.6)	–

Appendix Table 13.1. (cont.)

| Categories | Among total sample | | Among ideators | |
| | Ideation | Plan | Planned attempt | Unplanned attempt |
	OR (95% CI)	OR (95% CI)	OR (95% CI)	OR (95% CI)
Other	3.2 (2.6–3.9)	2.1 (1.4–3.1)	3.0 (1.3–6.6)	0.9 (0.4–2.0)
χ^2_4 (p-value)	205.8 (<0.001)*	19.6 (<0.001)*	12.2 (0.02)*	3.1 (0.38)
(numerator / denominator N)[c]	(1071 / 52,484)	(328 / 1071)	(110 / 328)	(63 / 743)

* Significant at the 0.05 level, two-sided test.

– Not included due to small cell size.

[a] Based on logistic regression analysis controlling for country.

[b] Family income classified into four categories based on the ratio of income to number of family members: less than or equal to the official Department of Labor federal poverty line (defined in the table as families living in poverty), 1–3, 3–6, and 6+ times the poverty line.

[c] Numerator N refers to the number of cases with each suicide outcome, denominator N refers to the number of cases in the total sample or in the conditional sample among ideators, ideators with a plan and ideators without a plan.

Appendix Table 13.2. Bivariate associations of sociodemographic variables with 12-month suicide ideation, plan, and attempt[a] (middle-income countries)

	Among total sample		Among ideators	
	Ideation	Plan	Planned attempt	Unplanned attempt
Categories	OR (95% CI)	OR (95% CI)	OR (95% CI)	OR (95% CI)
4-Category age (years)				
Less than 35	1.7 (1.1–2.7)	1.0 (0.3–3.2)	2.0 (0.3–15.4)	0.9 (0.2–3.0)
35–49	1.1 (0.7–1.9)	0.9 (0.2–3.0)	0.9 (0.1–6.9)	1.0 (0.3–3.6)
50–64	1.1 (0.6–1.8)	0.7 (0.2–2.3)	1.3 (0.2–9.4)	1.0 (1.0–1.0)
65 or older	1.0 (1.0–1.0)	1.0 (1.0–1.0)	1.0 (1.0–1.0)	–
χ^2_3 (p-value)	20.3 (<0.001)*	1.0 (0.80)	3.2 (0.36)	0.1 (0.96)
Dichotomized age (years)				
Less than 50	1.4 (1.1–1.8)	1.2 (0.7–2.3)	1.3 (0.5–3.5)	1.1 (0.3–3.8)
50 or older	1.0 (1.0–1.0)	1.0 (1.0–1.0)	1.0 (1.0–1.0)	1.0 (1.0–1.0)
χ^2_1 (p-value)	7.7 (0.01)*	0.4 (0.52)	0.3 (0.56)	0.0 (0.85)
Gender				
Female	1.7 (1.3–2.3)	1.0 (0.6–1.6)	1.6 (0.7–3.8)	2.0 (0.9–4.3)
Male	1.0 (1.0–1.0)	1.0 (1.0–1.0)	1.0 (1.0–1.0)	1.0 (1.0–1.0)
χ^2_1 (p-value)	17.6 (<0.001)*	0.0 (0.99)	1.3 (0.26)	3.0 (0.08)
Education				
Low	2.0 (1.3–3.0)	1.1 (0.5–2.4)	2.0 (0.5–7.7)	0.4 (0.1–1.5)
Low-average	1.7 (1.2–2.5)	1.2 (0.6–2.3)	2.1 (0.6–7.5)	0.3 (0.1–1.2)
High-average	1.6 (1.1–2.3)	1.3 (0.7–2.5)	3.6 (1.2–10.6)	0.4 (0.1–1.3)
High	1.0 (1.0–1.0)	1.0 (1.0–1.0)	1.0 (1.0–1.0)	1.0 (1.0–1.0)
χ^2_3 (p-value)	11.1 (0.01)*	0.7 (0.88)	6.1 (0.11)	4.1 (0.25)
Income level[b]				
Low	1.5 (1.1–2.2)	1.2 (0.7–2.2)	1.8 (0.7–4.2)	1.6 (0.3–9.0)
Low-average	1.8 (1.2–2.6)	0.6 (0.3–1.2)	0.8 (0.3–2.3)	0.8 (0.1–5.0)
High-average	1.2 (0.7–1.9)	0.7 (0.3–1.6)	1.0 (0.3–3.3)	3.6 (0.5–25.1)
High	1.0 (1.0–1.0)	1.0 (1.0–1.0)	1.0 (1.0–1.0)	1.0 (1.0–1.0)
χ^2_3 (p-value)	10.5 (0.02)*	7.2 (0.07)	2.9 (0.40)	3.9 (0.27)
Marital status				
Married or cohabitating	1.0 (1.0–1.0)	1.0 (1.0–1.0)	1.0 (1.0–1.0)	1.0 (1.0–1.0)
Separated, widowed, or divorced	1.4 (1.0–1.9)	1.3 (0.7–2.5)	0.5 (0.2–1.9)	0.4 (0.1–1.8)
Never married	1.2 (0.9–1.5)	1.1 (0.7–1.7)	0.8 (0.4–1.9)	1.4 (0.4–4.6)
χ^2_2 (p-value)	5.6 (0.06)	0.7 (0.70)	0.9 (0.65)	2.1 (0.35)
Employment				
Working	1.0 (1.0–1.0)	1.0 (1.0–1.0)	1.0 (1.0–1.0)	1.0 (1.0–1.0)
Student	0.8 (0.4–1.6)	0.8 (0.2–3.5)	4.7 (0.4–50.0)	0.9 (0.0–20.1)
Homemaker	1.6 (1.2–2.1)	1.1 (0.7–1.7)	1.5 (0.7–3.1)	0.6 (0.2–1.7)

Appendix Table 13.2. (cont.)

Categories	Among total sample		Among ideators	
	Ideation	Plan	Planned attempt	Unplanned attempt
	OR (95% CI)	OR (95% CI)	OR (95% CI)	OR (95% CI)
Retired	1.3 (0.8–1.9)	0.6 (0.2–1.7)	0.9 (0.1–5.2)	0.2 (0.0–1.5)
Other	2.3 (1.6–3.2)	1.3 (0.6–2.5)	3.3 (1.3–8.8)	0.6 (0.2–1.6)
χ^2_4 (p-value)	25.8 (<0.001)*	2.0 (0.73)	8.3 (0.08)	3.2 (0.52)
(numerator / denominator N)[c]	(555 / 25666)	(207 / 555)	(93 / 207)	(29 / 348)

* Significant at the 0.05 level, two-sided test.
– Not included due to small cell size.
[a] Based on logistic regression analysis controlling for country.
[b] Family income classified into four categories based on the ratio of income to number of family members: less than or equal to the official Department of Labor federal poverty line (defined in the table as families living in poverty), 1–3, 3–6, and 6+ times the poverty line.
[c] Numerator N refers to the number of cases with each suicide outcome, denominator N refers to the number of cases in the total sample or in the conditional sample among ideators, ideators with a plan and ideators without a plan.

Appendix Table 13.3. Bivariate associations of sociodemographic variables with 12-month suicide ideation, plan, and attempt[a] (low-income countries)

	Among total sample		Among ideators	
	Ideation	Plan	Planned attempt	Unplanned attempt
Categories	OR (95% CI)	OR (95% CI)	OR (95% CI)	OR (95% CI)
4-Category age (years)				
Less than 35	1.0 (0.7–1.4)	1.6 (0.7–3.7)	1.1 (0.2–5.3)	4.9 (0.5–45.0)
35–49	0.8 (0.6–1.1)	1.3 (0.6–3.2)	0.9 (0.2–4.0)	6.0 (0.7–50.9)
50–64	0.6 (0.4–0.9)	1.7 (0.7–4.2)	1.0 (0.2–5.2)	2.6 (0.2–27.0)
65 or older	1.0 (1.0–1.0)	1.0 (1.0–1.0)	1.0 (1.0–1.0)	1.0 (1.0–1.0)
χ^2_3 (p-value)	10.9 (0.01)*	1.7 (0.63)	0.4 (0.93)	3.4 (0.34)
Dichotomized age (years)				
Less than 50	1.2 (1.0–1.5)	1.1 (0.6–1.8)	1.0 (0.4–2.3)	2.6 (0.7–9.9)
50 or older	1.0 (1.0–1.0)	1.0 (1.0–1.0)	1.0 (1.0–1.0)	1.0 (1.0–1.0)
χ^2_1 (p-value)	3.8 (0.05)	0.1 (0.77)	0.0 (0.97)	2.0 (0.15)
Gender				
Female	1.3 (1.1–1.6)	0.8 (0.5–1.2)	0.7 (0.3–1.4)	0.5 (0.2–1.2)
Male	1.0 (1.0–1.0)	1.0 (1.0–1.0)	1.0 (1.0–1.0)	1.0 (1.0–1.0)
χ^2_1 (p-value)	7.5 (0.01)*	1.5 (0.22)	1.0 (0.31)	2.3 (0.13)
Education				
Low	1.3 (1.0–1.8)	1.8 (0.8–4.0)	0.8 (0.2–3.2)	0.4 (0.1–2.5)
Low-average	1.5 (1.1–2.1)	1.5 (0.7–3.3)	1.0 (0.3–3.9)	1.4 (0.3–7.2)
High-average	1.2 (0.8–1.8)	1.7 (0.8–3.5)	0.9 (0.2–4.7)	1.4 (0.2–7.7)
High	1.0 (1.0–1.0)	1.0 (1.0–1.0)	1.0 (1.0–1.0)	1.0 (1.0–1.0)
χ^2_3 (p-value)	6.2 (0.10)	2.4 (0.50)	0.4 (0.94)	3.3 (0.35)
Income level[b]				
Low	1.0 (0.7–1.4)	2.8 (1.4–5.7)	1.0 (0.4–2.7)	0.3 (0.1–1.1)
Low-average	1.3 (0.9–1.8)	1.5 (0.8–2.9)	0.8 (0.3–2.1)	0.3 (0.1–1.3)
High-average	1.1 (0.8–1.6)	0.9 (0.4–1.9)	1.0 (0.3–2.8)	0.2 (0.0–0.6)
High	1.0 (1.0–1.0)	1.0 (1.0–1.0)	1.0 (1.0–1.0)	1.0 (1.0–1.0)
χ^2_3 (p-value)	3.5 (0.32)	15.4 (0.001)*	0.6 (0.89)	7.4 (0.06)
Marital status				
Married or cohabitating	1.0 (1.0–1.0)	1.0 (1.0–1.0)	1.0 (1.0–1.0)	1.0 (1.0–1.0)
Separated, widowed, or divorced	1.4 (1.1–1.9)	1.4 (0.8–2.4)	1.2 (0.5–2.8)	0.9 (0.2–4.6)
Never married	1.1 (0.8–1.4)	1.2 (0.7–1.9)	1.6 (0.7–3.5)	0.5 (0.1–1.8)
χ^2_2 (p-value)	6.8 (0.03)*	1.3 (0.52)	1.4 (0.49)	1.2 (0.55)
Employment				
Working	1.0 (1.0–1.0)	1.0 (1.0–1.0)	1.0 (1.0–1.0)	1.0 (1.0–1.0)
Student	1.4 (0.9–2.3)	1.1 (0.4–2.6)	1.3 (0.3–6.2)	15.5 (3.5–67.7)
Homemaker	1.4 (1.1–1.9)	0.9 (0.5–1.5)	0.9 (0.4–2.0)	0.3 (0.1–1.8)
Retired	1.1 (0.8–1.6)	0.8 (0.4–1.7)	1.3 (0.3–5.1)	1.1 (0.2–7.5)
Other	2.5 (2.0–3.3)	1.1 (0.7–2.0)	2.5 (1.0–6.1)	2.2 (0.8–6.2)
χ^2_4 (p-value)	50.2 (<0.001)*	1.2 (0.88)	5.3 (0.26)	21.2 (<0.001)*

Appendix Table 13.3. (cont.)

Categories	Among total sample		Among ideators	
	Ideation	Plan	Planned attempt	Unplanned attempt
	OR (95% CI)	OR (95% CI)	OR (95% CI)	OR (95% CI)
(numerator / denominator N)[c]	(639 / 31,227)	(207 / 639)	(83 / 207)	(31 / 432)

[*] Significant at the 0.05 level, two-sided test.

[a] Based on logistic regression analysis controlling for country.

[b] Family income classified into four categories based on the ratio of income to number of family members: less than or equal to the official Department of Labor federal poverty line (defined in the table as families living in poverty), 1–3, 3–6, and 6+ times the poverty line.

[c] Numerator N refers to the number of cases with each suicide outcome, denominator N refers to the number of cases in the total sample or in the conditional sample among ideators, ideators with a plan and ideators without a plan.

Appendix Table 13.4. Bivariate associations of parental psychopathology and other childhood adversities with 12-month suicide ideation, plan, and attempt[a] (high-income countries)

Risk factors	Among total sample		Among ideators	
	Ideation	Plan	Planned attempt	Unplanned attempt
	OR (95% CI)	OR (95% CI)	OR (95% CI)	OR (95% CI)
Parental psychopathology				
Parental suicidal behavior	3.7* (2.3–5.8)	0.8 (0.3–1.9)	0.4 (0.1–2.0)	1.1 (0.2–7.5)
Parental depression	3.8* (2.4–5.9)	2.0 (0.9–4.2)	2.3 (0.8–6.9)	0.4 (0.1–2.2)
Parental panic disorder	2.7* (1.8–4.3)	1.0 (0.6–1.9)	2.8 (0.8–9.9)	1.9 (0.4–7.8)
Parental generalized anxiety disorder	4.0* (2.7–6.0)	1.5 (0.7–3.1)	1.5 (0.4–5.2)	1.0 (0.3–3.3)
Parental substance abuse	2.1* (1.4–3.0)	1.3 (0.7–2.6)	0.7 (0.2–2.2)	1.6 (0.6–4.4)
Parental antisocial personality disorder	2.9* (2.0–4.2)	1.1 (0.5–2.4)	2.5 (0.6–9.8)	1.2 (0.5–2.8)
Other childhood adversities				
Parental death	1.1 (0.8–1.5)	1.1 (0.5–2.1)	0.7 (0.2–2.3)	1.4 (0.3–5.7)
Parental divorce	2.0* (1.5–2.8)	0.9 (0.5–1.7)	2.7 (0.9–7.6)	0.8 (0.3–2.2)
Other parental loss	2.4* (1.7–3.5)	1.0 (0.5–2.2)	0.5 (0.1–1.5)	2.1 (0.5–8.3)
Parental criminal behavior	2.4* (1.8–3.2)	1.0 (0.4–2.1)	3.7 (0.7–18.6)	2.1 (0.6–7.6)
Physical abuse	4.7* (3.9–5.8)	1.6* (1.0–2.4)	2.3* (1.2–4.4)	2.5* (1.2–5.2)
Sexual abuse	4.3* (3.4–5.4)	1.6* (1.0–2.6)	2.3* (1.1–4.7)	1.9 (0.7–5.1)
Neglect	3.2* (2.1–4.8)	3.6* (2.0–6.6)	2.0 (0.8–5.1)	4.5* (1.2–17.7)
Physical illness	1.7* (1.2–2.3)	1.1 (0.6–2.0)	1.7 (0.7–4.4)	1.6 (0.7–3.6)
Family violence	2.9* (2.4–3.6)	1.5 (1.0–2.3)	1.8 (0.9–3.8)	3.1* (1.6–6.2)
Economic adversity	1.7* (1.2–2.5)	2.2* (1.2–4.0)	1.6 (0.5–4.6)	2.0 (0.5–8.1)
(numerator / denominator N)[b]	(972 / 28340)	(318 / 972)	(107 / 318)	(60 / 654)

* Significant at the 0.05 level, two-sided test.
[a] Based on logistic regression analysis controlling for country.
[b] Numerator N refers to the number of cases with each suicide outcome, denominator N refers to the number of cases in the total sample or in the conditional sample among ideators, ideators with a plan and ideators without a plan.

Appendix Table 13.5. Bivariate associations of parental psychopathology and other childhood adversities with 12-month suicide ideation, plan, and attempt[a] (middle-income countries)

| | Among total sample | | Among ideators | |
| | Ideation | Plan | Planned attempt | Unplanned attempt |
Risk factors	OR (95% CI)	OR (95% CI)	OR (95% CI)	OR (95% CI)
Parental psychopathology				
Parental suicidal behavior	2.3* (1.4–3.7)	4.0* (1.7–9.7)	1.2 (0.3–4.9)	0.2 (0.0–1.8)
Parental depression	2.4* (1.4–4.1)	1.1 (0.4–3.1)	1.0 (0.3–3.3)	1.7 (0.5–5.5)
Parental panic disorder	2.7* (2.0–3.6)	2.4* (1.3–4.6)	1.8 (0.7–5.0)	0.2 (0.1–1.1)
Parental generalized anxiety disorder	2.7* (1.7–4.2)	1.1 (0.5–2.3)	0.9 (0.2–4.8)	2.0 (0.3–11.2)
Parental substance abuse	2.1* (1.4–3.0)	0.4* (0.2–0.8)	0.8 (0.3–2.3)	0.4 (0.1–1.9)
Parental antisocial personality disorder	2.9* (2.0–4.3)	0.8 (0.3–2.1)	1.1 (0.3–3.6)	0.4 (0.0–3.6)
Other childhood adversities				
Parental death	1.8* (1.3–2.5)	0.6 (0.3–1.1)	1.2 (0.5–2.9)	1.0 (0.3–4.1)
Parental divorce	1.1 (0.7–1.7)	0.8 (0.4–1.6)	1.6 (0.4–5.8)	0.5 (0.0–6.9)
Other parental loss	3.2* (2.3–4.5)	0.8 (0.4–1.4)	1.2 (0.3–4.5)	0.4 (0.1–2.5)
Parental criminal behavior	2.2* (1.5–3.2)	1.1 (0.4–2.8)	1.1 (0.3–3.6)	0.5 (0.1–4.8)
Physical abuse	3.2* (2.4–4.1)	1.3 (0.7–2.3)	1.0 (0.5–2.2)	0.9 (0.5–1.9)
Sexual abuse	5.0* (2.7–9.3)	1.9 (0.6–6.3)	3.4 (0.4–27.0)	2.1 (0.4–12.5)
Neglect	2.4* (1.7–3.3)	1.6 (0.7–3.8)	1.0 (0.3–3.4)	0.7 (0.1–4.4)
Physical illness	1.9* (1.2–3.2)	1.0 (0.4–2.7)	1.7 (0.3–8.8)	0.6 (0.1–4.9)
Family violence	2.5* (1.9–3.2)	1.5 (0.8–2.7)	1.0 (0.5–2.1)	1.0 (0.1–8.7)
Economic adversity	2.0* (1.2–3.2)	0.9 (0.4–2.3)	0.2 (0.0–1.1)	0.5 (0.1–2.7)
(numerator / denominator N)[b]	(508 / 15,240)	(205 / 508)	(92 / 205)	(28 / 303)

* Significant at the 0.05 level, two-sided test.
[a] Based on logistic regression analysis controlling for country.
[b] Numerator N refers to the number of cases with each suicide outcome, denominator N refers to the number of cases in the total sample or in the conditional sample among ideators, ideators with a plan and ideators without a plan.

Appendix Table 13.6. Bivariate associations of parental psychopathology and other childhood adversities with 12-month suicide ideation, plan, and attempt[a] (low-income countries)

Risk factors	Among total sample		Among ideators	
	Ideation	Plan	Planned attempt	Unplanned attempt
	OR (95% CI)	OR (95% CI)	OR (95% CI)	OR (95% CI)
Parental psychopathology				
Parental suicidal behavior	3.9* (2.0–7.8)	1.2 (0.5–3.0)	1.7 (0.5–5.8)	1.2 (0.2–8.9)
Parental depression	4.9* (2.6–9.4)	1.6 (0.6–4.3)	1.0 (0.2–3.8)	5.0 (1.0–25.2)
Parental panic disorder	2.9* (1.9–4.4)	2.1 (1.0–4.3)	1.0 (0.4–2.9)	5.6* (1.4–22.1)
Parental generalized anxiety disorder	6.0* (3.1–11.5)	1.9 (0.7–4.9)	1.4 (0.4–5.0)	8.7* (1.7–43.8)
Parental substance abuse	3.3* (2.3–4.7)	1.6 (0.9–2.9)	0.9 (0.4–2.1)	0.5 (0.1–1.8)
Parental antisocial personality disorder	3.4* (2.2–5.2)	1.0 (0.4–2.5)	0.9 (0.2–4.2)	0.7 (0.1–4.3)
Other childhood adversities				
Parental death	1.0 (0.8–1.4)	1.8* (1.1–3.2)	1.4 (0.6–3.1)	0.1 (0.0–1.2)
Parental divorce	1.3 (0.8–2.1)	1.2 (0.5–3.0)	0.7 (0.1–3.2)	0.2* (0.0–0.9)
Other parental loss	1.0 (0.7–1.5)	1.2 (0.6–2.4)	0.7 (0.2–2.1)	0.1* (0.0–0.9)
Parental criminal behavior	3.3* (2.1–5.2)	0.6 (0.3–1.4)	0.6 (0.1–3.0)	2.4 (0.4–15.0)
Physical abuse	2.6* (1.9–3.7)	1.4 (0.8–2.5)	1.4 (0.6–3.5)	1.0 (0.3–3.4)
Sexual abuse	3.0* (1.6–5.6)	2.1 (0.7–6.3)	0.3 (0.1–1.9)	1.6 (0.3–9.7)
Neglect	2.2* (1.5–3.4)	1.7 (0.8–3.7)	0.5 (0.2–1.3)	1.8 (0.4–7.7)
Physical illness	2.0* (1.2–3.4)	1.2 (0.5–2.9)	1.1 (0.2–5.6)	3.8 (0.6–24.5)
Family violence	1.9* (1.2–3.0)	1.9 (0.9–3.9)	3.6* (1.2–10.5)	1.7 (0.4–7.1)
Economic adversity	1.0 (0.5–2.1)	1.8 (0.4–7.1)	2.1 (0.2–23.2)	0.0* (0.0–0.0)
(numerator / denominator N)[b]	(530 / 11,719)	(207 / 530)	(83 / 207)	(31 / 323)

* Significant at the 0.05 level, two-sided test.
0.0* (0.0–0.0) OR is ≤ 0.05 indicating very low risk.
[a] Based on logistic regression analysis controlling for country.
[b] Numerator N refers to the number of cases with each suicide outcome, denominator N refers to the number of cases in the total sample or in the conditional sample among ideators, ideators with a plan and ideators without a plan.

Appendix Table 13.7. Bivariate associations of 12-month DSM-IV/CIDI disorders with 12-month suicide ideation, plan, and attempt[a] (high-income countries)

12-month DSM-IV disorders[b]	Among total sample		Among ideators	
	Ideation	Plan	Planned attempt	Unplanned attempt
	OR (95% CI)	OR (95% CI)	OR (95% CI)	OR (95% CI)
Anxiety disorders				
Panic disorder	10.8* (8.5–13.7)	2.2* (1.3–3.6)	1.8 (0.9–3.5)	1.3 (0.6–3.0)
Agoraphobia without panic	8.8* (5.8–13.3)	1.2 (0.6–2.5)	1.1 (0.3–3.8)	0.3 (0.0–1.8)
Generalized anxiety disorder	8.6* (6.7–11.1)	1.1 (0.7–1.8)	1.1 (0.5–2.7)	0.5 (0.2–1.4)
Specific phobia	4.2* (3.5–5.0)	1.8* (1.2–2.6)	2.5* (1.3–4.9)	0.9 (0.5–1.9)
Social phobia	7.9* (6.6–9.6)	2.0* (1.3–3.0)	0.8 (0.4–1.7)	1.2 (0.5–2.7)
Posttraumatic stress disorder	8.4* (6.6–10.8)	1.3 (0.8–2.1)	1.6 (0.8–3.2)	1.1 (0.5–2.5)
Adult separation anxiety disorder	13.4* (8.4–21.3)	1.6 (0.8–3.3)	1.2 (0.3–4.7)	1.3 (0.4–4.3)
Any anxiety disorder	8.0* (6.7–9.6)	2.1* (1.5–3.1)	1.8 (0.9–3.6)	1.2 (0.6–2.3)
Mood disorders				
Major depressive disorder	13.0* (11.2–15.2)	2.0* (1.4–2.7)	0.8 (0.5–1.6)	1.6 (0.9–2.7)
Dysthymic disorder	9.9* (7.1–13.8)	2.4* (1.3–4.5)	1.0 (0.3–3.6)	0.3 (0.1–1.5)
Bipolar disorder	8.8* (6.8–11.4)	1.4 (0.9–2.3)	1.5 (0.8–3.0)	0.9 (0.3–2.3)
Any mood disorder	15.4* (13.1–18.1)	2.2* (1.6–3.1)	1.0 (0.6–1.9)	1.5 (0.9–2.5)
Impulse-control disorders				
Attention deficit hyperactivity disorder	4.6* (2.9–7.6)	1.7 (0.8–3.9)	1.3 (0.4–4.8)	0.9 (0.2–4.1)
Oppositional defiant disorder	14.8* (8.4–26.2)	2.2 (0.7–7.0)	1.6 (0.3–7.3)	3.9 (0.7–20.1)
Conduct disorder	3.2* (1.5–7.0)	1.4 (0.2–10.2)	16.3* (1.0–255.6)	6.9 (0.7–72.5)
Intermittent explosive disorder	4.8* (3.2–7.1)	1.9* (1.0–3.6)	1.1 (0.3–4.1)	0.6 (0.1–3.0)
Any impulse-control disorder	4.8* (3.4–6.8)	1.6 (0.9–3.0)	1.3 (0.5–3.6)	0.9 (0.3–2.7)
Substance use disorders				
Alcohol abuse or dependence	6.7* (5.2–8.6)	2.5* (1.6–3.8)	1.3 (0.6–2.6)	0.8 (0.3–2.4)
Illicit drug abuse or dependence	11.4* (7.9–16.4)	2.9* (1.5–5.6)	2.6 (0.9–7.8)	1.9 (0.6–5.7)
Any substance use disorder	8.0* (6.3–10.0)	2.5* (1.6–3.8)	1.9 (0.8–4.5)	1.3 (0.6–3.2)
Number of disorders				
Any	12.0* (9.8–14.7)	2.2* (1.4–3.4)	1.2 (0.5–2.9)	0.9 (0.4–1.9)
1[b]	5.9* (4.6–7.6)	1.2 (0.7–2.1)	0.6 (0.2–1.9)	0.8 (0.3–2.1)
2[b]	18.6* (14.4–24.1)	2.1* (1.2–3.6)	1.7 (0.6–4.7)	0.8 (0.3–2.3)
3+[b]	42.6* (32.5–55.7)	3.9* (2.3–6.6)	1.6 (0.6–4.1)	1.1 (0.5–2.6)
χ^2_2 (p-value)	907.1 (<0.001)*	32.7 (<0.001)*	5.1 (0.17)	0.7 (0.87)
(numerator / denominator N)[c]	(1071 / 52,484)	(328 / 1071)	(110 / 328)	(63 / 743)

* Significant at the 0.05 level, two-sided test.
[a] Based on logistic regression analysis controlling for country.
[b] Rows based on multivariate regression analysis controlling for country (no disorder is the reference category).
[c] Numerator N refers to the number of cases with each suicide outcome, denominator N refers to the number of cases in the total sample or in the conditional sample among ideators, ideators with a plan and ideators without a plan.

Appendix Table 13.8. Bivariate associations of 12-month DSM-IV/CIDI disorders with 12-month suicide ideation, plan, and attempt[a] (middle-income countries)

12-month DSM-IV disorders[b]	Among total sample		Among ideators	
	Ideation	Plan	Planned attempt	Unplanned attempt
	OR (95% CI)	OR (95% CI)	OR (95% CI)	OR (95% CI)
Anxiety disorders				
Panic disorder	8.2* (5.1–13.2)	2.4* (1.0–5.7)	3.0 (0.8–11.3)	0.0* (0.0–0.0)
Agoraphobia without panic	4.0* (2.7–6.0)	1.9 (0.9–3.9)	1.1 (0.4–2.7)	2.1 (0.6–7.3)
Generalized anxiety disorder	4.7* (2.8–7.9)	1.2 (0.4–3.4)	0.3 (0.1–1.1)	0.0* (0.0–0.0)
Specific phobia	3.1* (2.3–4.3)	1.1 (0.6–1.9)	0.9 (0.3–2.4)	1.3 (0.4–4.3)
Social phobia	6.7* (4.8–9.4)	1.2 (0.6–2.7)	0.7 (0.3–2.0)	0.9 (0.3–2.9)
Posttraumatic stress disorder	6.4* (4.2–9.8)	0.5 (0.3–1.1)	1.0 (0.1–9.3)	0.3 (0.1–1.6)
Adult separation anxiety disorder	8.9* (5.5–14.3)	2.6 (0.9–7.8)	1.2 (0.3–4.1)	4.2 (0.8–22.6)
Any anxiety disorder	4.7* (3.7–6.2)	1.2 (0.8–2.0)	1.7 (0.7–4.1)	1.1 (0.4–2.7)
Mood disorders				
Major depressive disorder	9.6* (7.4–12.5)	1.0 (0.7–1.6)	1.0 (0.4–2.3)	2.6 (1.0–7.2)
Dysthymic disorder	8.6* (4.6–16.1)	1.8 (0.7–4.5)	1.0 (0.2–5.7)	1.9 (0.3–10.4)
Bipolar disorder	10.5* (6.7–16.5)	3.6* (1.6–7.9)	0.3* (0.1–1.0)	0.0* (0.0–0.0)
Any mood disorder	9.8* (7.6–12.6)	1.2 (0.8–1.8)	0.9 (0.4–2.2)	2.4 (0.9–6.4)
Impulse-control disorders				
Attention deficit hyperactivity disorder	2.6* (1.1–6.4)	2.9 (0.7–11.9)	0.2 (0.0–1.2)	0.0* (0.0–0.0)
Oppositional defiant disorder	8.3* (3.2–21.6)	1.8 (0.3–10.8)	3.0 (0.3–30.5)	0.0* (0.0–0.0)
Conduct disorder	3.0 (0.9–10.6)	1.2 (0.1–13.2)	–	0.0* (0.0–0.0)
Intermittent explosive disorder	6.1* (3.6–10.4)	1.5 (0.7–3.3)	1.4 (0.4–4.4)	1.5 (0.6–4.2)
Any impulse-control disorder	5.2* (3.3–8.2)	1.2 (0.5–2.5)	1.1 (0.4–3.5)	1.4 (0.5–3.7)
Substance use disorders				
Alcohol abuse or dependence	4.1* (2.6–6.6)	1.6 (0.6–4.1)	2.4 (0.7–8.1)	0.5 (0.1–3.8)
Illicit drug abuse or dependence	8.5* (5.1–14.2)	0.8 (0.3–1.9)	7.7* (1.1–54.1)	0.0* (0.0–0.0)
Any substance use disorder	4.7* (3.2–6.8)	1.5 (0.6–3.5)	3.1* (1.0–9.3)	0.3 (0.0–2.7)
Number of disorders				
Any	6.7* (5.0–8.9)	1.4 (0.8–2.3)	2.8* (1.0–7.6)	2.2 (0.7–6.4)
1[b]	4.2* (3.0–6.0)	1.2 (0.6–2.3)	2.6 (0.9–8.0)	2.9 (0.8–9.9)
2[b]	9.4* (6.1–14.3)	1.5 (0.7–2.9)	5.5* (1.7–18.2)	0.4 (0.1–3.5)
3+[b]	21.3* (14.2–31.8)	1.7 (0.8–3.3)	1.2 (0.4–3.7)	3.0 (0.8–11.5)
χ^2_2 (p-value)	241.8 (<0.001)*	2.8 (0.43)	12.6 (0.01)*	7.5 (0.06)
(numerator / denominator N)[c]	(555 / 25,666)	(207 / 555)	(93 / 207)	(29 / 348)

* Significant at the 0.05 level, two-sided test.
– Not included due to small cell size.
0.0* (0.0–0.0) OR is ≤ 0.05 indicating very low risk.
[a] Based on logistic regression analysis controlling for country.
[b] Rows based on multivariate regression analysis controlling for country (no disorder is the reference category).
[c] Numerator N refers to the number of cases with each suicide outcome, denominator N refers to the number of cases in the total sample or in the conditional sample among ideators, ideators with a plan and ideators without a plan.

Appendix Table 13.9. Bivariate associations of 12-month DSM-IV/CIDI disorders with 12-month suicide ideation, plan, and attempt[a] (low-income countries)

12-month DSM-IV disorders[b]	Among total sample		Among ideators	
	Ideation	Plan	Planned attempt	Unplanned attempt
	OR (95% CI)	OR (95% CI)	OR (95% CI)	OR (95% CI)
Anxiety disorders				
Panic disorder	4.8* (2.8–8.1)	0.9 (0.3–2.2)	9.0* (1.2–67.8)	0.0* (0.0–0.0)
Agoraphobia without panic	4.6* (2.2–9.6)	5.0* (1.2–20.7)	1.1 (0.2–6.7)	0.0* (0.0–0.0)
Generalized anxiety disorder	7.1* (4.7–10.8)	1.4 (0.5–3.9)	0.4 (0.1–1.6)	0.0* (0.0–0.0)
Specific phobia	3.9* (3.0–5.1)	2.0* (1.2–3.2)	0.8 (0.3–1.8)	0.9 (0.2–3.8)
Social phobia	3.1* (2.0–4.9)	2.3 (0.9–5.8)	1.4 (0.3–6.8)	0.6 (0.1–3.1)
Posttraumatic stress disorder	3.1* (1.4–6.8)	4.8 (0.9–27.4)	4.1 (0.8–20.4)	0.0* (0.0–0.0)
Adult separation anxiety disorder	7.8* (3.9–15.4)	1.7 (0.6–4.5)	1.1 (0.2–4.8)	3.8 (0.5–28.5)
Any anxiety disorder	5.1* (3.9–6.5)	1.4 (0.9–2.2)	1.0 (0.5–1.9)	1.2 (0.4–3.5)
Mood disorders				
Major depressive disorder	8.7* (6.8–11.0)	2.1* (1.4–3.2)	1.1 (0.6–2.2)	1.1 (0.3–3.9)
Dysthymic disorder	5.7* (3.2–10.1)	3.0* (1.0–9.1)	1.0 (0.2–5.4)	2.7 (0.4–18.7)
Bipolar disorder	5.8* (3.0–11.0)	3.7* (1.4–9.6)	6.3 (1.0–41.4)	2.1 (0.5–9.7)
Any mood disorder	8.7* (6.9–11.0)	2.4* (1.6–3.6)	1.3 (0.7–2.6)	1.3 (0.4–3.8)
Impulse-control disorders				
Attention deficit hyperactivity disorder	0.6 (0.1–4.7)	0.0* (0.0–0.0)	–	0.0* (0.0–0.0)
Oppositional defiant disorder	0.0* (0.0–0.0)	–	–	–
Conduct disorder	6.3* (2.7–15.0)	5.6 (0.8–40.8)	5.2 (0.6–43.8)	8.0 (0.4–159.3)
Intermittent explosive disorder	5.5* (4.0–7.4)	1.8 (1.0–3.4)	1.3 (0.5–3.0)	2.9 (0.7–12.0)
Any impulse-control disorder	4.5* (3.1–6.4)	1.7 (0.7–3.9)	1.5 (0.6–4.0)	1.9 (0.5–7.3)
Substance use disorders				
Alcohol abuse or dependence	3.0* (2.1–4.2)	1.9* (1.0–3.6)	1.7 (0.6–4.5)	0.3 (0.0–2.4)
Illicit drug abuse or dependence	19.9* (8.6–46.1)	1.4 (0.3–6.3)	6.8* (1.3–35.1)	0.0* (0.0–0.0)
Any substance use disorder	3.8* (2.6–5.4)	1.8 (0.9–3.7)	1.9 (0.7–5.0)	0.2 (0.0–1.7)
Number of disorders				
Any	6.8* (5.3–8.7)	2.1* (1.3–3.3)	1.6 (0.7–3.5)	1.4 (0.5–4.3)
1[b]	4.9* (3.6–6.6)	1.6 (1.0–2.8)	1.6 (0.6–3.8)	1.3 (0.4–4.8)
2[b]	12.3* (8.8–17.4)	2.2* (1.2–3.9)	1.6 (0.6–4.0)	2.2 (0.5–8.9)
3+[b]	14.3* (9.8–20.8)	4.2* (1.9–9.3)	1.6 (0.5–4.9)	0.2 (0.0–2.1)
χ^2_2 (p-value)	313.8 (<.001)*	14.7 (0.002)*	1.3 (0.74)	3.9 (0.28)
(numerator / denominator N)[c]	(639 / 31227)	(207 / 639)	(83 / 207)	(31 / 432)

* Significant at the 0.05 level, two-sided test.
– Not included due to small cell size.
0.0* (0.0–0.0) OR is ≤ 0.05 indicating very low risk.
[a] Based on logistic regression analysis controlling for country.
[b] Rows based on multivariate regression analysis controlling for country (no disorder is the reference category).
[c] Numerator N refers to the number of cases with each suicide outcome, denominator N refers to the number of cases in the total sample or in the conditional sample among ideators, ideators with a plan and ideators without a plan.

Appendix Table 13.10. Multivariate associations between respondent history of suicidal behavior and 12-month suicide ideation, plan, and attempt[a] (high-income countries)

History of suicidal behavior prior to current year	Among total sample		Among ideators	
	Ideation	Plan	Planned attempt	Unplanned attempt
	OR (95% CI)	OR (95% CI)	OR (95% CI)	OR (95% CI)
History of ideation only	30.7* (24.7–38.1)	0.3* (0.1–0.6)	0.1* (0.0–0.6)	0.2* (0.1–0.5)
History of ideation and plan but no attempt	28.8* (20.4–40.6)	1.0 (0.6–1.9)	1.3 (0.5–3.6)	5.7* (2.4–13.7)
History of ideation with unplanned attempt	48.6* (37.0–63.9)	11.0* (6.5–18.5)	0.1* (0.1–0.3)	2.8 (0.9–9.0)
History of ideation with planned attempt	47.9* (36.7–62.6)	7.3* (4.2–12.6)	1.8 (0.8–3.7)	0.8 (0.2–2.7)
X^2_4 (p-value)	1334.4 (<0.001)*	164.2 (<0.001)*	38.5 (<0.001)*	51.3 (<0.001)*
(numerator / denominator N)[b]	(1071 / 52,484)	(328 / 1071)	(110 / 328)	(63 / 743)

* Significant at the 0.05 level, two-sided test.
[a] Based on multivariate logistic regression analysis controlling for countries, age, age squared.
[b] Numerator N refers to the number of cases with each suicide outcome, denominator N refers to the number of cases in the total sample or in the conditional sample among ideators, ideators with a plan and ideators without a plan.

Appendix Table 13.11. Multivariate associations between respondent history of suicidal behavior and 12-month suicide ideation, plan, and attempt[a] (middle-income countries)

History of suicidal behavior prior to current year	Among total sample		Among ideators	
	Ideation	Plan	Planned attempt	Unplanned attempt
	OR (95% CI)	OR (95% CI)	OR (95% CI)	OR (95% CI)
History of ideation only	24.4* (17.9–33.1)	0.2* (0.1–0.5)	0.4 (0.1–1.7)	0.5 (0.2–1.7)
History of ideation and plan but no attempt	24.3* (14.0–42.1)	1.1 (0.5–2.3)	2.1 (0.6–7.4)	3.4* (1.1–10.6)
History of ideation with unplanned attempt	35.3* (23.0–54.2)	4.7* (2.0–11.1)	0.1* (0.0–0.3)	0.0* (0.0–0.0)
History of ideation with planned attempt	34.1* (24.2–48.1)	4.9* (2.5–9.7)	3.5* (1.5–8.3)	0.4 (0.1–1.9)
X^2_4 (p-value)	659.9 (<0.001)*	59.9 (<0.001)*	32.5 (<0.001)*	1311.3 (<0.001)*
(numerator / denominator N)[b]	(555 / 25666)	(207 / 555)	(93 / 207)	(29 / 348)

* Significant at the 0.05 level, two-sided test.
0.0* (0.0–0.0) OR is ≤ 0.05 indicating very low risk.
[a] Based on multivariate logistic regression analysis controlling for countries, age, age squared.
[b] Numerator N refers to the number of cases with each suicide outcome, denominator N refers to the number of cases in the total sample or in the conditional sample among ideators, ideators with a plan and ideators without a plan.

Appendix Table 13.12. Multivariate associations between respondent history of suicidal behavior and 12-month suicide ideation, plan, and attempt[a] (low-income countries)

History of suicidal behavior prior to current year	Among total sample		Among ideators	
	Ideation	Plan	Planned attempt	Unplanned attempt
	OR (95% CI)	OR (95% CI)	OR (95% CI)	OR (95% CI)
History of ideation only	32.6* (25.3–42.0)	0.2* (0.1–0.3)	0.1* (0.0–0.6)	0.7 (0.2–2.7)
History of ideation and plan but no attempt	37.1* (22.2–61.9)	0.4* (0.2–0.9)	5.5* (1.1–28.4)	17.0* (4.9–58.8)
History of ideation with unplanned attempt	51.8* (35.1–76.3)	3.3* (1.8–6.0)	0.2* (0.1–0.7)	1.2 (0.2–9.7)
History of ideation with planned attempt	51.5* (35.3–75.3)	3.6* (2.1–6.1)	0.9 (0.4–2.0)	3.6 (0.5–23.9)
X^2_4 (p-value)	929.0 (<0.001)*	94.6 (<0.001)*	21.7 (<0.001)*	41.3 (<0.001)*
(numerator / denominator N)[b]	(639 / 31,227)	(207 / 639)	(83 / 207)	(31 / 432)

* Significant at the 0.05 level, two-sided test.
[a] Based on multivariate logistic regression analysis controlling for countries, age, age squared.
[b] Numerator N refers to the number of cases with each suicide outcome, denominator N refers to the number of cases in the total sample or in the conditional sample among ideators, ideators with a plan and ideators without a plan.

Appendix Table 13.13. Risk factors included in the summary risk indices

Planned attempt total

Psychiatric disorders: panic disorder, oppositional defiant disorder, conduct disorder, drug abuse and dependence
Adversities: sexual abuse
Prior suicidal behavior: no prior attempt but had prior plan, no prior plan or attempt but had prior ideation
Demographics: employment: other

Unplanned attempt total

Psychiatric disorders: adult separation anxiety, oppositional defiant disorder, conduct disorder
Adversities: NONE
Prior suicidal behavior: no prior attempt but had prior plan, no prior plan or attempt but had prior ideation
Demographics: less than 35 years old

Planned attempt (high-income countries)

Psychiatric disorders: specific phobia, conduct disorder, drug abuse or dependence
Adversities: parental depression, parental panic disorder, parental ASPD, parental divorce, parental criminal behavior, physical abuse, sexual abuse, neglect
Prior suicidal behavior: no prior attempt but had prior plan, no prior plan or attempt but had prior ideation
Demographics: employment: student or other

Unplanned attempt (high-income countries)

Psychiatric disorders: NONE
Adversities: other parental loss, parental criminal behavior, physical abuse, neglect, family violence
Prior suicidal behavior: no prior attempt but had prior plan, no prior plan or attempt but had prior ideation
Demographics: less than 50 years old

Planned attempt (middle-income countries)

Psychiatric disorders: panic disorder, oppositional defiant disorder, conduct disorder, alcohol abuse or dependence, drug abuse or dependence
Adversities: NONE
Prior suicidal behavior: prior attempt, no prior attempt but had prior plan, no prior plan or attempt but had prior ideation
Demographics: less than high education

Unplanned attempt (middle-income countries)

Psychiatric disorders: NONE
Adversities: NONE
Prior suicidal behavior: prior attempt, no prior attempt but had prior plan, no prior plan or attempt but had prior ideation
Demographics: Income: low

Planned attempt (low-income countries)

Psychiatric disorders: panic disorder, post-traumatic stress, bipolar disorder, conduct disorder, drug abuse or dependence
Adversities: family violence, economic adversity
Prior suicidal behavior: no prior attempt but had prior plan, no prior plan or attempt but had prior ideation
Demographics: employment: Other

Unplanned attempt (low-income countries)

Psychiatric disorders: NONE
Adversities: parental depression, parental panic, parental GAD, parental criminal behavior, physical illness
Prior suicidal behavior: no prior attempt but had prior plan, no prior plan or attempt but had prior ideation
Demographics: employment: other

Appendix Table 13.14. Concordance (AUC) between predicted probability of suicide attempt using the risk indices and the actual occurrence of suicide attempts[a]

Country group	Planned attempt AUC	Unplanned attempt AUC
High-income countries		
United States	0.74	0.76
Belgium	0.80	0.83
France	0.88	–
Germany	0.92	0.75
Italy	–	–
Netherlands	0.67	0.77
Spain	0.84	0.79
New Zealand	0.84	0.76
Japan	0.95	0.68
Israel	0.90	0.55
Middle-income countries		
Mexico	0.80	0.61
Lebanon	0.87	0.59
South Africa	0.81	0.70
Brazil	0.86	0.75
Bulgaria	0.55	0.55
Romania	0.86	0.82
Low-income countries		
Colombia	0.77	0.60
Ukraine	0.56	–
Nigeria	0.82	–
China	0.84	0.59
India	0.84	0.70
Shenzhen	0.83	0.76

– Data too scarce for model to converge.
[a] A model was fit for each country where the outcome is the planned/unplanned attempt, and the predictor is the predicted probability of planned/unplanned attempt based on the pooled models. AUC is calculated for each model.

Appendix Table 14.1. Treatment of people with suicidal behavior in any care sector (all countries combined)

Country	Suicide ideation only (n=432)			Suicide plan (n=189)			Unplanned suicide attempt (n=66)			Planned suicide attempt (n=136)			Any suicidal behavior (n=823)		
	%	SE	n	%	SE	n	%	SE	n	%	SE	n	%	SE	n
Colombia	11.9	3.5	16	57.7	12.0	11	68.4	17.2	10	14.2	6.0	4	26.0	4.8	41
Mexico	9.4	4.0	9	18.4	8.1	5	29.9	19.9	3	42.8	7.9	10	18.9	3.4	27
USA	63.1	3.9	95	71.6	7.8	31	81.6	9.5	20	76.3	5.7	21	67.9	2.8	167
Belgium	89.2	7.5	10	83.4	14.6	6	75.3	22.8	2	24.8	18.6	3	64.1	14.4	21
France	52.1	15.9	17	93.9	4.9	11	0.0	0.0	0	100.0	0.0	6	62.2	13.6	34
Germany	39.3	19.2	6	79.5	18.2	6	100.0	0.0	1	0.0	0.0	0	49.6	15.4	13
Italy	56.0	17.1	7	100.0	0.0	2	0.0	0.0	0	0.0	0.0	0	62.7	15.1	9
Netherlands	21.7	12.1	6	100.0	0.0	3	100.0	0.0	1	100.0	0.0	3	34.6	15.3	13
Spain	28.5	7.5	13	67.6	16.1	6	100.0	0.0	1	100.0	0.0	4	39.9	9.3	24
Ukraine	25.3	9.0	10	21.4	9.0	5	42.2	28.9	1	12.3	8.9	2	23.4	5.8	18
Israel	41.5	7.4	20	45.4	12.7	7	48.0	25.5	2	82.9	15.4	6	47.0	6.0	35
Lebanon	17.8	12.4	2	0.0	0.0	0	100.0	0.0	2	27.9	21.4	2	20.8	8.4	6
Nigeria	0.4	0.4	1	5.9	5.9	1	0.0	0.0	0	0.0	0.0	0	1.8	1.6	2
South Africa	19.2	4.3	17	23.5	8.6	7	48.8	19.5	3	47.0	9.9	14	27.2	4.3	41
China	8.1	8.1	1	4.2	4.5	1	0.0	0.0	0	45.8	25.5	2	10.0	6.4	4
Japan	19.2	8.6	8	62.9	21.0	4	48.8	27.7	2	84.0	18.1	3	28.6	9.3	17
New Zealand	57.1	3.8	144	52.0	6.8	56	46.7	13.7	12	64.3	13.0	37	56.2	3.2	249
Romania	9.2	7.5	2	25.6	24.1	1	0.0	0.0	0	69.5	30.0	1	17.8	10.0	4
Bulgaria	11.4	5.8	3	92.7	5.8	6	0.0	0.0	0	0.0	0.0	0	23.0	6.8	9
Brazil	27.2	7.3	25	42.6	8.1	14	51.3	18.9	6	65.7	11.6	13	37.0	6.3	58
India	15.0	4.8	12	8.0	3.7	5	0.0	0.0	0	16.0	8.2	4	12.4	3.1	21
Shenzhen	14.1	6.7	8	3.6	4.0	1	0.0	0.0	0	27.6	24.7	1	13.0	5.9	10

Appendix Table 14.2. Treatment of people with suicidal behavior in any mental healthcare sector (all countries combined)

Country	Suicide ideation only (n=240)			Suicide plan (n=111)			Unplanned suicide attempt (n=47)			Planned suicide attempt (n=90)			Any suicidal behavior (n=488)		
	%	SE	n	%	SE	n	%	SE	n	%	SE	n	%	SE	n
Colombia	7.5	2.5	11	39.7	13.1	9	53.4	17.5	7	12.0	5.6	3	18.8	4.1	30
Mexico	5.5	3.3	4	15.8	8.4	4	15.7	15.5	1	33.5	9.4	5	13.8	3.4	14
USA	40.6	4.5	63	49.6	9.5	21	64.8	12.1	16	58.8	7.7	15	46.6	3.4	115
Belgium	60.5	15.9	7	78.6	18.9	5	75.3	22.8	2	16.3	14.4	2	50.9	13.0	16
France	30.1	12.6	12	66.5	15.2	8	0.0	0.0	0	65.6	24.8	4	38.5	10.5	24
Germany	31.2	18.8	3	18.8	12.0	3	100.0	0.0	1	0.0	0.0	0	26.3	12.8	7
Italy	8.1	7.6	1	53.1	35.2	1	0.0	0.0	0	0.0	0.0	0	15.0	9.5	2
Netherlands	3.1	3.4	1	0.0	0.0	0	100.0	0.0	1	57.8	30.1	2	9.5	4.7	4
Spain	28.5	7.5	13	32.5	12.5	4	100.0	0.0	1	100.0	0.0	4	34.4	7.3	22
Ukraine	1.3	1.4	1	0.0	0.0	0	42.2	28.9	1	0.0	0.0	0	2.9	2.1	2
Israel	22.3	6.1	11	17.0	9.2	3	0.0	0.0	0	34.1	17.8	3	21.0	4.7	17
Lebanon	0.0	0.0	0	0.0	0.0	0	0.0	0.0	0	24.4	21.2	1	5.7	5.6	1
Nigeria	0.0	0.0	0	0.0	0.0	0	0.0	0.0	0	0.0	0.0	0	0.0	0.0	0
South Africa	9.1	3.3	8	1.1	1.1	1	43.1	20.2	2	8.7	4.7	4	8.8	2.5	15
China	0.0	0.0	0	0.0	0.0	0	0.0	0.0	0	28.1	23.6	1	2.3	2.3	1
Japan	15.5	7.8	6	38.0	21.9	2	23.0	21.2	1	44.3	28.6	2	19.7	7.6	11
New Zealand	31.9	3.5	74	36.0	6.3	37	29.4	12.2	8	58.5	12.5	31	35.0	2.8	150
Romania	9.2	7.5	2	25.6	24.1	1	0.0	0.0	0	69.5	30.0	1	17.8	10.0	4
Bulgaria	8.7	5.9	2	7.8	7.9	1	0.0	0.0	0	0.0	0.0	0	8.1	5.7	3
Brazil	20.1	5.9	17	32.8	8.3	10	51.3	18.9	6	49.6	13.3	8	28.8	5.5	41
India	0.9	0.9	1	0.0	0.0	0	0.0	0.0	0	14.6	8.1	3	2.3	1.5	4
Shenzhen	5.6	4.6	3	3.6	4.0	1	0.0	0.0	0	27.6	24.7	1	5.6	4.0	5

Appendix Table 14.3. Treatment of people with suicidal behavior in the general medical healthcare sector (all countries combined)

Country	Suicide ideation only (n=257)			Suicide plan (n=116)			Unplanned suicide attempt (n=36)			Planned suicide attempt (n=70)			Any suicidal behavior (n=479)		
	%	SE	n	%	SE	n	%	SE	n	%	SE	n	%	SE	n
Colombia	4.4	2.6	6	14.9	13.2	1	17.7	9.7	4	6.9	5.1	2	8.0	2.7	13
Mexico	4.6	2.4	6	0.0	0.0	0	14.1	11.4	2	10.6	7.1	4	5.3	2.1	12
USA	32.9	4.1	50	36.0	8.7	16	48.3	11.4	12	39.5	8.5	10	35.7	2.2	88
Belgium	82.3	9.9	9	83.4	14.6	6	36.5	28.6	1	24.8	18.6	3	58.5	13.8	19
France	37.5	14.9	11	77.2	10.8	9	0.0	0.0	0	49.8	28.8	5	45.0	12.8	25
Germany	8.1	5.4	3	67.7	19.5	4	0.0	0.0	0	0.0	0.0	0	25.4	11.6	7
Italy	48.1	15.3	6	100.0	0.0	2	0.0	0.0	0	0.0	0.0	0	56.1	13.8	8
Netherlands	21.7	12.1	6	31.7	26.8	2	100.0	0.0	1	77.8	21.2	2	28.5	12.6	11
Spain	16.3	6.8	7	67.6	16.1	6	100.0	0.0	1	18.1	15.3	2	25.4	6.9	16
Ukraine	20.0	9.7	8	17.8	8.5	4	0.0	0.0	0	5.4	5.5	1	16.5	6.2	13
Israel	19.5	6.0	9	8.6	8.1	1	48.0	25.5	2	37.9	18.7	3	20.5	4.9	15
Lebanon	17.8	12.4	2	0.0	0.0	0	62.7	33.1	1	0.0	0.0	0	12.6	6.7	3
Nigeria	0.4	0.4	1	5.9	5.9	1	0.0	0.0	0	0.0	0.0	0	1.8	1.6	2
South Africa	13.8	4.1	10	16.4	8.3	4	43.1	20.2	2	15.4	7.0	5	15.9	3.7	21
China	8.1	8.1	1	4.2	4.5	1	0.0	0.0	0	45.8	25.5	2	10.0	6.4	4
Japan	3.7	2.9	2	11.5	11.3	1	0.0	0.0	0	0.0	0.0	0	4.2	2.6	3
New Zealand	39.5	4.1	101	37.9	5.4	44	28.8	10.8	8	34.8	9.6	24	38.3	3.1	177
Romania	3.3	3.9	1	0.0	0.0	0	0.0	0.0	0	0.0	0.0	0	2.6	2.9	1
Bulgaria	5.4	3.4	2	92.7	5.8	6	0.0	0.0	0	0.0	0.0	0	18.2	5.7	8
Brazil	8.1	3.9	8	20.2	6.5	5	34.2	20.9	2	18.3	8.6	6	14.1	3.7	21
India	5.3	2.4	6	5.5	3.2	3	0.0	0.0	0	1.3	1.3	1	4.6	1.3	10
Shenzhen	7.3	5.3	2	0.0	0.0	0	0.0	0.0	0	0.0	0.0	0	6.3	4.5	2

Appendix Table 14.4. Treatment of people with suicidal behavior in any non-healthcare sector (all countries combined)

Country	Suicide ideation only (n=114)			Suicide plan (n=45)			Unplanned suicide attempt (n=14)			Planned suicide attempt (n=41)			Any suicidal behavior (n=214)		
	%	SE	n	%	SE	n	%	SE	n	%	SE	n	%	SE	n
Colombia	1.3	0.9	2	3.1	3.1	1	17.7	15.8	1	0.0	0.0	0	3.9	2.8	4
Mexico	0.0	0.0	0	2.5	2.6	1	0.0	0.0	0	4.9	3.8	2	1.5	1.2	3
USA	23.1	3.7	32	16.9	6.5	9	27.3	9.6	7	42.6	9.8	11	24.6	2.9	59
Belgium	8.0	7.7	1	17.4	16.1	1	0.0	0.0	0	0.0	0.0	0	6.8	6.7	2
France	11.6	10.1	2	0.0	0.0	0	0.0	0.0	0	7.9	8.6	1	9.4	7.7	3
Germany	4.9	3.8	2	0.0	0.0	0	0.0	0.0	0	0.0	0.0	0	3.0	2.2	2
Italy	16.2	11.1	2	0.0	0.0	0	0.0	0.0	0	0.0	0.0	0	13.7	9.5	2
Netherlands	3.1	3.4	1	68.3	26.8	1	0.0	0.0	0	0.0	0.0	0	7.2	5.9	2
Spain	0.0	0.0	0	7.0	6.9	1	0.0	0.0	0	0.0	0.0	0	1.1	1.1	1
Ukraine	5.3	3.1	2	7.0	4.7	2	0.0	0.0	0	6.9	6.9	1	5.6	2.5	5
Israel	3.0	2.2	2	19.9	10.3	3	0.0	0.0	0	17.1	15.4	1	8.1	3.3	6
Lebanon	0.0	0.0	0	0.0	0.0	0	37.3	33.1	1	3.5	3.8	1	2.6	2.2	2
Nigeria	0.0	0.0	0	5.9	5.9	1	0.0	0.0	0	0.0	0.0	0	1.6	1.6	1
South Africa	5.1	2.7	5	13.6	7.8	3	5.7	5.8	1	26.6	8.3	7	11.4	3.4	16
China	0.0	0.0	0	0.0	0.0	0	0.0	0.0	0	0.0	0.0	0	0.0	0.0	0
Japan	16.1	7.9	6	13.4	12.9	1	25.8	23.0	1	39.7	26.1	1	17.3	6.9	9
New Zealand	16.6	3.1	43	14.3	5.1	15	4.1	3.5	2	27.4	10.4	11	16.5	2.6	71
Romania	0.0	0.0	0	0.0	0.0	0	0.0	0.0	0	0.0	0.0	0	0.0	0.0	0
Bulgaria	0.0	0.0	0	0.0	0.0	0	0.0	0.0	0	0.0	0.0	0	0.0	0.0	0
Brazil	6.4	4.1	4	9.2	5.4	4	5.9	5.8	1	35.3	15.1	4	10.3	2.9	13
India	10.1	4.8	6	2.6	2.0	2	0.0	0.0	0	0.0	0.0	0	6.2	2.6	8
Shenzhen	5.8	4.2	4	0.0	0.0	0	0.0	0.0	0	27.6	24.7	1	5.5	3.7	5

Appendix Table 14.5. Twelve-month treatment of people with suicidal behavior (high-income countries)

Twelve-month treatment	Suicide ideation only (n=594)			Suicide plan (n=211)			Unplanned suicide attempt (n=60)			Planned suicide attempt (n=107)			Any suicidal behavior (n=972)		
	%	SE	n	%	SE	n	%	SE	n	%	SE	n	%	SE	n
Any healthcare	47.9	2.6	302	56.3	4.4	125	58.6	7.5	37	64.4	6.6	76	51.7	2.1	540
Any mental healthcare	30.7	2.3	191	38.2	4.3	84	44.1	8.0	30	52.4	6.4	63	35.0	1.8	368
Psychiatrist	17.0	1.9	102	26.9	3.8	58	22.5	5.0	18	44.3	6.1	50	21.8	1.6	228
Other mental healthcare	21.8	2.1	134	23.8	3.7	54	38.7	8.0	25	39.7	6.3	44	24.8	1.8	257
General medical healthcare	31.7	2.5	204	37.6	3.8	91	40.2	7.3	25	35.7	5.6	49	33.7	1.8	369
Any non-healthcare	14.8	1.8	91	14.8	3.2	31	14.7	4.8	10	26.8	5.6	25	15.9	1.5	157
Human service	7.2	1.3	46	6.3	2.0	14	7.2	3.5	4	17.1	4.0	18	8.0	1.0	82
CAM	9.5	1.5	56	9.7	2.6	21	7.5	3.1	6	16.6	5.2	13	10.1	1.3	96
Any of the above	51.9	2.7	326	60.9	4.4	132	64.7	7.5	41	70.3	6.6	83	56.1	2.1	582

Appendix Table 14.6. Twelve-month treatment of people with suicidal behavior (middle-income countries)

Twelve-month treatment	Suicide ideation only (n=275)			Suicide plan (n=113)			Unplanned suicide attempt (n=28)			Planned suicide attempt (n=92)			Any suicidal behavior (n=508)		
	%	SE	n	%	SE	n	%	SE	n	%	SE	n	%	SE	n
Any healthcare	17.0	2.5	53	25.8	5.0	27	44.4	12.1	12	34.0	5.7	30	23.0	2.2	122
Any mental healthcare	11.2	2.1	33	14.1	3.8	17	40.9	12.4	9	24.0	5.6	19	15.4	2.0	78
Psychiatrist	8.6	1.9	26	8.6	2.9	12	20.4	9.2	7	22.9	5.6	17	11.6	1.8	62
Other mental healthcare	4.5	1.5	13	7.8	3.2	9	35.9	12.6	6	8.7	4.1	8	7.4	1.5	36
General medical healthcare	9.5	2.1	29	17.4	4.6	15	35.2	12.6	7	13.6	4.3	15	13.1	2.0	66
Any non-healthcare	3.8	1.5	9	9.2	4.0	8	6.0	3.6	3	21.6	5.9	14	8.0	1.7	34
Human service	2.9	1.3	8	6.7	3.8	4	6.0	3.6	3	9.4	4.2	7	4.9	1.6	22
CAM	0.8	0.8	1	5.8	3.4	5	0.0	0.0	0	16.0	5.2	9	4.4	1.2	15
Any of the above	18.5	2.7	58	30.9	5.1	33	47.9	11.9	14	49.1	6.2	40	27.6	2.6	145

Appendix Table 14.7. Twelve-month treatment of people with suicidal behavior (low-income countries)

Twelve-month treatment	Suicide ideation only (n=292)			Suicide plan (n=124)			Unplanned suicide attempt (n=31)			Planned suicide attempt (n=83)			Any suicidal behavior (n=530)		
	%	SE	n	%	SE	n	%	SE	n	%	SE	n	%	SE	n
Any healthcare	9.5	2.0	36	15.6	3.8	20	48.1	12.6	11	13.8	3.9	12	14.2	2.0	79
Any mental healthcare	3.5	1.1	16	6.8	2.6	10	38.4	12.9	8	10.9	3.6	8	7.7	1.5	42
Psychiatrist	2.4	0.9	11	4.6	2.3	6	25.0	11.5	6	7.6	2.8	6	5.2	1.3	29
Other mental healthcare	1.1	0.6	6	2.4	1.4	5	23.8	12.1	5	4.5	2.6	4	3.5	1.2	20
General medical healthcare	7.1	1.9	24	8.8	3.2	10	11.5	6.0	4	6.0	2.7	6	7.6	1.4	44
Any non-healthcare	4.7	1.5	14	3.5	1.4	6	11.5	10.6	1	1.4	1.1	2	4.5	1.3	23
Human service	2.9	1.4	8	2.2	1.2	4	11.5	10.6	1	0.4	0.4	1	3.1	1.2	14
CAM	1.7	0.8	6	1.2	0.9	2	0.0	0.0	0	1.0	1.0	1	1.4	0.6	9
Any of the above	13.6	2.3	48	17.8	3.9	24	48.1	12.6	11	14.8	4.0	13	17.2	2.1	96

Appendix Table 14.8. Multivariate predictors of the treatment of people with suicidal behavior[a] (high-income countries)

Category/ sub-category	Among 12-month respondents with any suicidal behavior (n=972)	Among respondents with any suicidal behavior who received treatment (n=582)		
	Any 12-month treatment	Any mental healthcare	General medical healthcare	Any non-healthcare
	OR (95% CI)	OR (95% CI)	OR (95% CI)	OR (95% CI)
Age				
Continuous (divided by 10)	1.1 (0.9–1.3)	0.8 (0.6–1.1)	1.3 (1.0–1.7)	1.2 (0.9–1.5)
χ^2_1 (p-value)	0.3 (0.60)	2.1 (0.15)	3.2 (0.08)	1.6 (0.21)
Gender				
Female	1.0 (0.7–1.5)	0.9 (0.5–1.4)	1.2 (0.7–2.0)	2.7* (1.6–4.3)
Male				
χ^2_1 (p-value)	0.0 (0.99)	0.3 (0.58)	0.6 (0.44)	15.9 (<0.001)*
Education				
Continuous	1.1 (0.9–1.3)	1.1 (0.9–1.4)	0.8* (0.6–1.0)	1.3* (1.0–1.6)
χ^2_1 (p-value)	0.6 (0.43)	0.7 (0.41)	5.4 (0.02)*	5.1 (0.02)*
Marital status				
Never married	0.5* (0.3–0.8)	1.6 (0.9–3.1)	0.4* (0.2–0.8)	2.2* (1.2–4.1)
Previously married	1.1 (0.6–1.7)	1.1 (0.6–1.8)	1.0 (0.5–1.7)	1.2 (0.6–2.3)
Married/ cohabiting				
χ^2_2 (p-value)	9.1 (0.01)*	2.4 (0.30)	7.8 (0.02)*	6.7 (0.04)*
Income				
Continuous	1.1 (0.9–1.3)	1.2* (1.0–1.5)	0.9 (0.7–1.0)	0.7* (0.5–0.9)
χ^2_1 (p-value)	0.6 (0.44)	5.3 (0.02)*	3.7 (0.06)	5.1 (0.02)*
Employment				
Student	1.7 (0.6–5.1)	1.7 (0.6–4.6)	0.9 (0.3–2.6)	0.8 (0.3–2.0)
Homemaker	0.9 (0.5–1.7)	1.2 (0.6–2.5)	1.2 (0.6–2.6)	0.6 (0.3–1.4)
Retired	0.4* (0.1–1.0)	1.2 (0.3–4.5)	1.5 (0.3–7.1)	0.0* (0.0–0.5)
Other	1.0 (0.5–1.9)	1.7* (1.0–2.8)	0.8 (0.5–1.5)	0.7 (0.4–1.4)
Working				
χ^2_4 (p-value)	5.8 (0.22)	4.6 (0.33)	0.9 (0.93)	8.3 (0.08)
Severity of 12-month suicidal behavior				
Suicide plan	1.3 (0.8–2.1)	1.1 (0.7–1.9)	1.0 (0.5–1.7)	1.1 (0.6–2.1)
Unplanned suicide attempt	1.7 (0.8–3.8)	1.3 (0.6–3.2)	1.3 (0.5–3.5)	0.6 (0.2–1.7)
Planned suicide attempt	1.6 (0.8–3.3)	1.8 (0.9–3.6)	0.7 (0.3–1.4)	1.6 (0.8–3.2)
Ideation only				
χ^2_3 (p-value)	3.6 (0.31)	3.3 (0.34)	1.9 (0.59)	3.7 (0.29)

Appendix Table 14.8. (cont.)

| Category/
sub-category | Among 12-month respondents
with any suicidal behavior (n=972) | Among respondents with any suicidal behavior
who received treatment (n=582) | | |
| | Any 12-month treatment | Any mental
healthcare | General
medical
healthcare | Any non-
healthcare |
	OR (95% CI)	OR (95% CI)	OR (95% CI)	OR (95% CI)
Time since ideation				
Continuous (divided by 10)	0.8* (0.7–1.0)	1.0 (0.8–1.3)	0.9 (0.7–1.2)	1.0 (0.8–1.2)
χ^2_1 (p-value)	4.0 (0.05)*	0.1 (0.76)	0.6 (0.46)	0.0 (0.85)
History of treatment				
Yes	5.0* (3.2–8.0)	1.1 (0.5–2.2)	1.1 (0.5–2.1)	2.0 (0.9–4.4)
χ^2_1 (p-value)	47.0 (<0.001)*	0.1 (0.78)	0.0 (0.84)	2.9 (0.09)
Lifetime disorder				
Any anxiety	2.6* (1.7–3.8)	1.2 (0.7–2.2)	1.6 (0.9–2.9)	0.9 (0.5–1.6)
Any mood	2.0* (1.3–3.0)	1.4 (0.8–2.3)	0.9 (0.6–1.5)	0.8 (0.5–1.4)
Any impulse	1.1 (0.6–2.0)	0.9 (0.4–2.2)	0.9 (0.5–1.9)	0.8 (0.4–1.5)
Any substance	0.7 (0.5–1.1)	1.4 (0.9–2.2)	1.2 (0.8–2.0)	1.3 (0.8–2.3)
χ^2_4 (p-value)	39.5 (<0.001)*	4.9 (0.30)	3.8 (0.43)	1.7 (0.79)
χ^2_{19} (p-value)	133.9 (<0.001)*	30.7 (0.04)*	43.7 (0.001)*	44.2 (0.001)*

* Significant at the 0.05 level, two-sided test.
[a] Results are based on multivariate logistic regression models controlling for country.

Appendix Table 14.9. Multivariate predictors of the treatment of people with suicidal behavior[a] (middle-income countries)

Category/ sub-category	Among 12-month respondents with any suicidal behavior (n=508)	Among respondents with any suicidal behavior who received treatment (n=145)		
	Any 12-month treatment	Any mental healthcare	General medical healthcare	Any non-healthcare
	OR (95% CI)	OR (95% CI)	OR (95% CI)	OR (95% CI)
Age				
Continuous (divided by 10)	1.2 (0.9–1.6)	1.3 (0.7–2.5)	1.4 (0.9–2.2)	0.9 (0.4–2.1)
χ^2_1 (p-value)	2.5 (0.12)	0.7 (0.39)	1.7 (0.19)	0.0 (0.84)
Gender				
Female	0.8 (0.4–1.5)	0.4 (0.1–1.6)	1.7 (0.4–6.3)	0.1* (0.0–0.7)
Male				
χ^2_1 (p-value)	0.5 (0.48)	1.7 (0.19)	0.5 (0.46)	5.4 (0.02)*
Education				
Continuous	1.4 (0.9–2.0)	4.2* (1.9–8.9)	1.1 (0.6–2.1)	0.6 (0.2–1.4)
χ^2_1 (p-value)	2.8 (0.09)	13.7 (<0.001)*	0.2 (0.65)	1.5 (0.22)
Marital status				
Never married	1.1 (0.5–2.4)	0.9 (0.2–5.4)	0.6 (0.2–2.4)	9.9* (1.7–55.9)
Previously married	1.2 (0.5–2.9)	0.3 (0.1–1.3)	1.8 (0.5–6.1)	1.8 (0.2–13.2)
Married/ cohabiting				
χ^2_2 (p-value)	0.3 (0.87)	2.5 (0.29)	1.9 (0.39)	7.1 (0.03)*
Income				
Continuous	1.0 (1.0–1.1)	1.1 (1.0–1.4)	1.0 (0.9–1.0)	0.9 (0.6–1.3)
χ^2_1 (p-value)	2.0 (0.16)	2.5 (0.12)	1.4 (0.23)	0.5 (0.48)
Employment				
Student	1.0 (0.2–6.4)	43.6 (0.0–140000)	0.6 (0.0–33.1)	0.0* (0.0–0.0)
Homemaker	3.6* (1.4–9.2)	2.8 (0.6–13.9)	0.5 (0.1–2.9)	2.4 (0.5–12.8)
Retired	0.9 (0.3–3.0)	3.2 (0.2–61.9)	0.3 (0.0–2.2)	0.1 (0.0–8.7)
Other	1.5 (0.7–3.1)	3.4* (1.0–11.8)	0.6 (0.1–2.2)	1.4 (0.2–7.6)
Working				
χ^2_4 (p-value)	7.7 (0.10)	4.6 (0.33)	1.8 (0.77)	35.2 (<0.001)*
Severity of 12-month suicidal behavior				
Suicide plan	1.5 (0.7–3.2)	0.5 (0.1–2.1)	0.9 (0.3–3.0)	5.6 (0.9–35.9)
Unplanned suicide attempt	4.6* (1.7–13.0)	10.7 (0.8–143.6)	2.5 (0.4–17.2)	0.8 (0.1–7.3)
Planned suicide attempt	3.9* (2.0–7.7)	1.1 (0.3–3.9)	0.4 (0.1–1.2)	13.6* (1.7–110.3)
Ideation only				
χ^2_3 (p-value)	22.2 (<0.001)*	5.1 (0.16)	5.0 (0.17)	7.3 (0.06)

Appendix Table 14.9. (cont.)

Category/ sub-category	Among 12-month respondents with any suicidal behavior (n=508)	Among respondents with any suicidal behavior who received treatment (n=145)		
	Any 12-month treatment	Any mental healthcare	General medical healthcare	Any non-healthcare
	OR (95% CI)	OR (95% CI)	OR (95% CI)	OR (95% CI)
Time since ideation				
Continuous (divided by 10)	1.0 (0.6–1.4)	1.3 (0.6–2.5)	0.8 (0.5–1.2)	0.8 (0.5–1.5)
χ^2_1 (p-value)	0.1 (0.80)	0.5 (0.49)	1.2 (0.27)	0.5 (0.50)
History of treatment				
Yes	10.1* (5.3–19.2)	1.8 (0.6–6.1)	0.7 (0.2–1.9)	1.5 (0.3–8.4)
χ^2_1 (p-value)	50.1 (<0.001)*	1.0 (0.32)	0.6 (0.45)	0.3 (0.61)
Lifetime disorder				
Any anxiety	1.2 (0.6–2.2)	2.3 (0.7–7.0)	0.9 (0.3–2.2)	1.0 (0.2–3.9)
Any mood	1.4 (0.7–2.7)	1.6 (0.4–5.9)	0.6 (0.2–1.8)	16.3* (2.3–113.4)
Any impulse	0.6 (0.3–1.4)	0.8 (0.2–4.1)	2.3 (0.6–8.4)	0.3 (0.0–3.5)
Any substance	1.6 (0.8–3.2)	0.5 (0.1–1.9)	0.7 (0.2–2.4)	0.9 (0.2–5.1)
χ^2_4 (p-value)	3.8 (0.44)	4.0 (0.40)	3.6 (0.46)	8.9 (0.06)
χ^2_{19} (p-value)	130.1 (<0.001)*	35.3 (0.01)*	31.3 (0.04)*	94.2 (<0.001)*

* Significant at the 0.05 level, two-sided test.
− Not included due to small cell size.
[a] Results are based on multivariate logistic regression models controlling for country.

Appendix Table 14.10. Multivariate predictors of the treatment of people with suicidal behavior[a] (low-income countries)

Category/ sub-category	Among 12-month respondents with any suicidal behavior (n=530)	Among respondents with any suicidal behavior who received treatment (n=96)		
	Any 12-month treatment	Any mental healthcare	General medical healthcare	Any non-healthcare
	OR (95% CI)	OR (95% CI)	OR (95% CI)	OR (95% CI)
Age				
Continuous (divided by 10)	1.3 (0.9–1.8)	1.2 (0.6–2.2)	1.6 (0.8–3.3)	0.3* (0.1–1.0)
χ^2_1 (p-value)	2.5 (0.11)	0.3 (0.56)	1.6 (0.21)	4.1 (0.04)*
Gender				
Female	0.7 (0.3–1.5)	0.2 (0.0–1.0)	0.4 (0.1–2.4)	19.4* (1.4–261.8)
Male				
χ^2_1 (p-value)	0.8 (0.38)	3.8 (0.05)	0.9 (0.34)	5.0 (0.03)*
Education				
Continuous	1.6* (1.1–2.5)	1.0 (0.4–2.5)	0.5 (0.2–1.0)	3.1 (1.0–10.0)
χ^2_1 (p-value)	5.8 (0.02)*	0.0 (0.94)	3.7 (0.06)	3.7 (0.05)
Marital status				
Never married	0.9 (0.4–2.0)	6.8* (1.2–37.0)	0.1* (0.0–0.7)	0.0* (0.0–0.7)
Previously married	0.5 (0.1–1.7)	0.5 (0.1–4.8)	1.4 (0.2–10.4)	1.0 (0.1–8.5)
Married/ cohabiting				
χ^2_2 (p-value)	1.4 (0.51)	7.1 (0.03)*	5.7 (0.06)	4.8 (0.09)
Income				
Continuous	1.1 (1.0–1.1)	1.5 (0.8–3.0)	0.7 (0.5–1.2)	0.6 (0.3–1.0)
χ^2_1 (p-value)	2.3 (0.13)	1.6 (0.21)	1.5 (0.21)	3.5 (0.06)
Employment				
Student	1.8 (0.5–7.5)	2.2 (0.1–38.2)	0.6 (0.0–7.0)	566.2* (3.0–110000)
Homemaker	2.3* (1.0–5.3)	6.3 (0.9–45.7)	0.1* (0.0–0.7)	3.6 (0.3–42.1)
Retired	0.5 (0.1–2.2)	7.5 (0.3–204.1)	0.3 (0.0–24.0)	3.6 (0.0–1707.8)
Other	0.3* (0.1–1.0)	3.2 (0.2–59.3)	0.1 (0.0–2.5)	0.3 (0.0–9.7)
Working				
χ^2_4 (p-value)	12.3 (0.02)*	5.7 (0.23)	7.3 (0.12)	7.4 (0.12)
Severity of 12-month suicidal behavior				
Suicide plan	1.3 (0.7–2.6)	1.5 (0.2–11.9)	1.4 (0.2–11.0)	0.0* (0.0–0.5)
Unplanned suicide attempt	5.6* (1.6–19.6)	7.0 (0.6–75.4)	0.6 (0.1–6.0)	0.1 (0.0–3.4)
Planned suicide attempt	1.1 (0.4–2.9)	20.9 (0.4–1121.7)	1.2 (0.0–31.9)	0.3 (0.0–3.1)
Ideation only				
χ^2_3 (p-value)	7.7 (0.05)	4.9 (0.18)	0.6 (0.90)	6.7 (0.08)

Appendix Table 14.10. (cont.)

Category/ sub-category	Among 12-month respondents with any suicidal behavior (n=530)	Among respondents with any suicidal behavior who received treatment (n=96)		
	Any 12-month treatment	Any mental healthcare	General medical healthcare	Any non-healthcare
	OR (95% CI)	OR (95% CI)	OR (95% CI)	OR (95% CI)
Time since ideation				
Continuous (divided by 10)	0.8 (0.6–1.2)	0.9 (0.5–1.7)	0.6 (0.3–1.1)	0.8 (0.3–2.1)
χ^2_1 (p-value)	1.1 (0.29)	0.1 (0.71)	3.0 (0.08)	0.2 (0.66)
History of treatment				
Yes	5.0* (2.5–9.9)	1.1 (0.2–6.2)	0.4 (0.1–2.2)	10.2 (0.5–198.4)
χ^2_1 (p-value)	21.0 (<0.001)*	0.0 (0.93)	1.0 (0.32)	2.4 (0.12)
Lifetime disorder				
Any anxiety	1.6 (0.8–3.2)	0.6 (0.1–2.6)	0.4 (0.1–2.1)	3.5 (0.7–18.2)
Any mood	2.1 (1.0–4.5)	1.6 (0.4–6.2)	2.6 (0.7–9.2)	1.0 (0.1–7.3)
Any impulse	0.6 (0.3–1.2)	0.9 (0.1–6.2)	2.1 (0.4–10.5)	3.6 (0.4–36.2)
Any substance	0.9 (0.3–2.5)	0.3 (0.0–2.7)	0.7 (0.1–5.4)	15.8* (1.2–212.3)
χ^2_4 (p-value)	11.2 (0.03)*	2.2 (0.70)	4.0 (0.41)	8.3 (0.08)
χ^2_{19} (p-value)	109.0 (<0.001)*	77.8 (<0.001)*	41.4 (0.002)*	36.6 (0.01)*

* Significant at the 0.05 level, two-sided test.
⁻ Not included due to small cell size.
[a] Results are based on multivariate logistic regression models controlling for country.

Appendix Table 14.11. Barriers to the treatment of people with suicidal behavior (high-income countries)

Reasons for not seeking 12-month treatment	Ideation only (n=267)			Suicide plan (n=78)			Unplanned suicide attempt (n=18)			Planned suicide attempt (n=23)			Any suicidal behavior (n=386)		
	%	SE	n	%	SE	n	%	SE	n	%	SE	n	%	SE	n
Low perceived need for treatment	47.6	4.6	121	39.7	7.3	33	25.2	11.9	6	40.5	14.4	10	44.8	3.8	170
Any structural barrier	14.3	2.5	47	10.8	3.7	11	21.6	13.0	3	20.2	9.8	6	14.4	2.0	67
Financial	9.1	2.0	32	8.8	3.4	9	13.8	12.4	1	20.2	9.8	6	10.0	1.7	48
Availability	7.9	1.8	28	5.6	2.9	5	7.9	6.2	2	14.1	8.8	3	7.9	1.5	38
Transportation	5.1	1.6	16	5.1	3.0	3	0.0	0.0	0	2.3	2.3	1	4.7	1.3	20
Inconvenient	3.9	1.2	13	3.3	1.7	5	0.0	0.0	0	3.4	3.4	1	3.6	1.0	19
Any attitudinal barrier	50.8	4.6	144	58.9	7.4	44	74.8	11.9	12	56.2	14.6	12	53.5	3.8	212
Wanted to handle on own	33.1	3.7	93	38.2	7.0	30	59.4	14.1	9	48.4	15.4	9	36.0	3.3	141
Perceived ineffectiveness	11.3	2.1	43	17.0	5.3	11	20.5	12.6	4	2.8	2.4	2	12.1	1.9	60
Stigma	5.6	1.4	21	5.5	2.9	5	7.9	6.2	2	16.9	9.2	5	6.4	1.3	33
Thought would get better	11.5	2.6	33	5.2	2.6	5	7.9	6.2	2	10.9	8.1	3	10.2	2.0	43
Problem was not severe	12.5	2.7	33	11.2	4.2	9	10.7	9.9	1	22.0	10.1	6	12.8	2.2	49

Appendix Table 14.12. Barriers to the treatment of people with suicidal behavior (middle-income countries)

Reasons for not seeking 12-month treatment	Ideation only (n=212)			Suicide plan (n=77)			Unplanned suicide attempt (n=14)			Planned suicide attempt (n=51)			Any suicidal behavior (n=354)		
	%	SE	n	%	SE	n	%	SE	n	%	SE	n	%	SE	n
Low perceived need for treatment	61.6	5.6	119	64.4	6.0	41	44.7	13.4	6	67.8	7.5	30	62.3	4.1	196
Any structural barrier	19.2	6.1	42	20.1	4.5	20	16.2	10.6	2	16.6	5.3	13	19.0	4.3	77
Financial	16.2	6.3	32	14.6	4.3	13	6.0	5.9	1	11.5	4.7	9	15.0	4.3	55
Availability	14.4	6.2	29	16.7	4.2	16	16.2	10.6	2	16.3	5.3	12	15.1	4.3	59
Transportation	4.0	1.1	17	10.4	3.4	9	0.0	0.0	0	4.5	2.4	5	5.1	1.1	31
Inconvenient	3.6	1.1	13	3.3	1.9	4	10.2	9.5	1	4.9	3.3	4	3.9	1.0	22
Any attitudinal barrier	36.9	5.7	86	29.6	6.1	29	45.1	13.2	7	27.2	7.2	16	34.6	4.2	138
Wanted to handle on own	21.8	3.2	58	19.2	4.9	20	42.7	13.0	6	16.1	6.6	8	21.3	2.6	92
Perceived ineffectiveness	5.6	1.8	21	9.0	3.8	7	6.0	5.9	1	9.6	4.1	7	6.8	1.5	36
Stigma	6.2	1.9	18	7.3	2.3	7	6.0	5.9	1	4.1	2.4	4	6.2	1.3	30
Thought would get better	18.1	5.8	31	16.4	5.0	11	6.0	5.9	1	5.9	3.4	5	15.9	4.1	48
Problem was not severe	4.6	1.5	13	12.2	4.0	11	2.4	2.5	1	3.1	2.5	2	5.8	1.3	27

Appendix Table 14.13. Barriers to the treatment of people with suicidal behavior (low-income countries)

Reasons for not seeking 12-month treatment	Ideation only (n=244)			Suicide plan (n=98)			Unplanned suicide attempt (n=20)			Planned suicide attempt (n=68)			Any suicidal behavior (n=430)		
	%	SE	n	%	SE	n	%	SE	n	%	SE	n	%	SE	n
Low perceived need for treatment	66.0	4.8	163	83.7	4.2	81	50.4	16.5	14	55.2	7.1	37	67.3	3.8	295
Any structural barrier	12.7	3.8	25	4.5	1.9	7	12.5	10.6	2	22.1	6.5	15	12.3	3.1	49
Financial	10.8	3.8	18	2.9	1.5	5	12.5	10.6	2	17.8	5.9	12	10.2	3.1	37
Availability	9.7	3.3	20	2.0	1.1	3	11.2	10.6	1	20.4	6.4	13	9.6	2.7	37
Transportation	1.1	0.7	3	2.4	1.4	3	0.0	0.0	0	8.3	4.4	5	2.2	0.9	11
Inconvenient	3.5	2.0	7	0.7	0.7	1	0.0	0.0	0	5.8	3.9	4	3.1	1.3	12
Any attitudinal barrier	33.4	4.8	80	14.3	4.1	14	49.6	16.5	6	43.1	7.0	30	31.7	3.8	130
Wanted to handle on own	25.3	4.9	51	8.5	3.2	9	24.0	13.1	4	26.9	6.9	20	22.2	3.8	84
Perceived ineffectiveness	4.8	1.3	21	2.1	1.2	3	1.3	1.3	1	15.5	5.4	10	5.4	1.2	35
Stigma	7.9	3.3	16	2.1	1.2	3	0.0	0.0	0	17.3	4.1	12	7.6	2.1	31
Thought would get better	8.5	2.9	19	4.7	2.7	4	11.2	10.6	1	10.9	4.1	10	8.2	2.4	34
Problem was not severe	6.4	2.3	15	6.5	3.1	6	25.6	19.0	2	3.2	1.8	3	6.9	2.0	26

Appendix Table 14.14. Multivariate predictors of barriers to the treatment of people with suicidal behavior[a] (high-income countries)

Category/subcategory	Among respondents with any suicidal behavior who did not receive treatment (n=386)		
	Low perceived need for treatment	Any structural barrier	Any attitudinal barrier
	OR (95% CI)	OR (95% CI)	OR (95% CI)
Age			
Continuous (divided by 10)	0.9 (0.6–1.1)	0.9 (0.6–1.3)	1.2 (0.9–1.6)
χ^2_1 (p-value)	1.1 (0.28)	0.3 (0.61)	1.2 (0.28)
Gender			
Female	1.6 (0.8–3.1)	0.8 (0.4–1.8)	0.7 (0.3–1.3)
Male			
χ^2_1 (p-value)	1.6 (0.21)	0.3 (0.58)	1.5 (0.22)
Education			
Continuous	0.9 (0.6–1.2)	0.8 (0.5–1.2)	1.2 (0.9–1.6)
χ^2_1 (p-value)	0.9 (0.33)	1.6 (0.21)	1.4 (0.24)
Marital status			
Never married	0.6 (0.3–1.3)	0.6 (0.2–1.6)	1.7 (0.8–3.5)
Previously married	0.7 (0.3–1.6)	0.9 (0.3–2.2)	1.7 (0.7–3.9)
Married/cohabiting			
χ^2_2 (p-value)	1.9 (0.38)	1.2 (0.54)	2.9 (0.24)
Income			
Continuous	0.9 (0.6–1.2)	1.3 (1.0–1.8)	1.2 (0.9–1.6)
χ^2_1 (p-value)	0.8 (0.36)	3.6 (0.06)	1.2 (0.28)
Employment			
Student	3.1 (0.7–13.3)	0.5 (0.0–8.8)	0.4 (0.1–1.4)
Homemaker	0.6 (0.2–1.7)	2.5 (0.8–8.3)	1.8 (0.6–5.0)
Retired	1.6 (0.4–6.0)	1.8 (0.3–9.6)	0.4 (0.1–1.6)
Other	0.5 (0.2–1.3)	2.0 (0.8–4.9)	2.0 (0.8–4.8)
Working			
χ^2_4 (p-value)	6.8 (0.15)	5.2 (0.27)	8.5 (0.08)
Severity of 12-month suicidal behavior			
Suicide plan	1.4 (0.7–3.0)	0.4 (0.2–1.2)	0.7 (0.4–1.5)
Unplanned suicide attempt	0.5 (0.1–2.6)	2.2 (0.4–13.3)	2.1 (0.4–10.7)
Planned suicide attempt	1.2 (0.3–4.3)	0.8 (0.1–5.8)	0.8 (0.2–2.7)
Ideation only			
χ^2_3 (p-value)	1.8 (0.61)	4.1 (0.25)	1.8 (0.61)
Time since ideation			
Continuous (divided by 10)	1.3 (0.9–1.7)	0.9 (0.6–1.2)	0.9 (0.6–1.2)
χ^2_1 (p-value)	2.0 (0.16)	0.8 (0.36)	0.8 (0.37)
History of treatment			
Yes	0.6 (0.3–1.1)	2.7* (1.2–6.1)	1.4 (0.7–2.7)

Appendix Table 14.14. (cont.)

Category/subcategory	Among respondents with any suicidal behavior who did not receive treatment (n=386)		
	Low perceived need for treatment	Any structural barrier	Any attitudinal barrier
	OR (95% CI)	OR (95% CI)	OR (95% CI)
χ^2_1 (p-value)	2.6 (0.11)	5.7 (0.02)*	1.0 (0.33)
Lifetime disorder			
Any anxiety	0.5* (0.2–0.9)	4.1* (1.6–10.5)	1.4 (0.7–2.8)
Any mood	1.0 (0.5–1.9)	1.1 (0.4–2.8)	1.3 (0.7–2.3)
Any impulse	1.0 (0.3–3.7)	1.2 (0.3–4.1)	1.0 (0.3–3.6)
Any substance	1.1 (0.5–2.4)	1.2 (0.5–2.9)	1.0 (0.5–2.1)
χ^2_4 (p-value)	4.7 (0.32)	14.7 (0.01)*	1.8 (0.77)
χ^2_{19} (p-value)	18.8 (0.47)	41.1 (0.002)*	19.1 (0.45)

* Significant at the 0.05 level, two-sided test.
[a] Results are based on multivariate logistic regression models controlling for country.

Appendix Table 14.15. Multivariate predictors of barriers to the treatment of people with suicidal behavior[a] (middle-income countries)

Category/subcategory	Among respondents with any suicidal behavior who did not receive treatment (n=354)		
	Low perceived need for treatment	Any structural barrier	Any attitudinal barrier
	OR (95% CI)	OR (95% CI)	OR (95% CI)
Age			
Continuous (divided by 10)	1.2 (0.8–1.9)	0.7 (0.4–1.1)	0.8 (0.5–1.2)
χ^2_1 (p-value)	0.6 (0.44)	2.6 (0.11)	1.4 (0.23)
Gender			
Female	0.4* (0.1–0.9)	3.1 (1.0–10.1)	2.2 (0.9–5.2)
Male			
χ^2_1 (p-value)	4.7 (0.03)*	3.7 (0.06)	3.0 (0.08)
Education			
Continuous	0.7 (0.4–1.1)	1.0 (0.6–1.6)	1.2 (0.8–1.9)
χ^2_1 (p-value)	3.0 (0.09)	0.0 (0.96)	0.9 (0.33)
Marital status			
Never married	3.9* (1.2–12.4)	0.6 (0.2–1.5)	0.3* (0.1–0.7)
Previously married	1.8 (0.7–4.6)	0.4 (0.1–1.4)	0.6 (0.3–1.7)
Married/cohabiting			
χ^2_2 (p-value)	7.3 (0.03)*	3.6 (0.17)	7.1 (0.03)*
Income			
Continuous	1.0 (0.9–1.1)	1.0 (0.9–1.2)	1.0 (0.9–1.2)
χ^2_1 (p-value)	0.3 (0.60)	0.4 (0.51)	0.3 (0.56)
Employment			
Student	0.4 (0.1–1.8)	2.2 (0.3–16.2)	3.5 (0.8–14.8)
Homemaker	0.9 (0.3–2.5)	1.3 (0.5–3.7)	0.9 (0.4–2.2)
Retired	1.9 (0.3–10.6)	3.2 (0.8–13.0)	0.6 (0.1–3.2)
Other	0.5 (0.2–1.2)	1.1 (0.3–4.3)	1.9 (0.8–4.6)
Working			
χ^2_4 (p-value)	5.1 (0.28)	3.7 (0.45)	6.1 (0.20)
Severity of 12-month suicidal behavior			
Suicide plan	1.2 (0.4–3.5)	1.1 (0.4–2.7)	0.6 (0.2–1.5)
Unplanned suicide attempt	0.3 (0.1–1.0)	0.6 (0.1–2.8)	1.8 (0.6–5.5)
Planned suicide attempt	1.8 (0.6–5.3)	0.8 (0.3–2.1)	0.4 (0.2–1.3)
Ideation only			
χ^2_3 (p-value)	6.9 (0.08)	0.8 (0.86)	5.4 (0.15)
Time since ideation			
Continuous (divided by 10)	1.0 (0.6–1.5)	1.0 (0.6–1.5)	0.9 (0.6–1.3)
χ^2_1 (p-value)	0.0 (0.83)	0.0 (0.90)	0.2 (0.68)

Appendix Table 14.15. (cont.)

	Among respondents with any suicidal behavior who did not receive treatment (n=354)		
	Low perceived need for treatment	**Any structural barrier**	**Any attitudinal barrier**
Category/subcategory	OR (95% CI)	OR (95% CI)	OR (95% CI)
History of treatment			
Yes	0.2* (0.1–0.5)	3.0* (1.2–7.5)	3.4* (1.5–7.7)
χ^2_1 (p-value)	11.8 (0.001)*	5.8 (0.02)*	8.4 (0.004)*
Lifetime disorder			
Any anxiety	1.1 (0.5–2.7)	0.7 (0.3–1.7)	1.2 (0.5–2.5)
Any mood	0.8 (0.3–1.7)	1.8 (0.7–4.2)	1.1 (0.5–2.4)
Any impulse	1.2 (0.5–3.0)	0.9 (0.3–2.3)	0.6 (0.3–1.5)
Any substance	1.2 (0.4–3.4)	1.0 (0.3–2.8)	1.0 (0.4–2.5)
χ^2_4 (p-value)	0.7 (0.95)	2.4 (0.67)	1.3 (0.87)
χ^2_{19} (p-value)	55.2 (<0.001)*	35.9 (0.01)*	45.7 (0.001)*

*Significant at the 0.05 level, two-sided test.
[a] Results are based on multivariate logistic regression models controlling for country.

Appendix Table 14.16. Multivariate predictors of barriers to the treatment of people with suicidal behavior[a] (low-income countries)

Category/subcategory	Among respondents with any suicidal behavior who did not receive treatment (n=430)		
	Low perceived need for treatment	Any structural barrier	Any attitudinal barrier
	OR (95% CI)	OR (95% CI)	OR (95% CI)
Age			
Continuous (divided by 10)	1.1 (0.6–2.1)	0.4* (0.2–0.8)	0.9 (0.5–1.7)
χ^2_1 (p-value)	0.2 (0.69)	8.0 (0.01)*	0.1 (0.72)
Gender			
Female	0.4 (0.2–1.0)	2.0 (0.6–5.9)	1.9 (0.8–4.8)
Male			
χ^2_1 (p-value)	3.7 (0.06)	1.4 (0.24)	1.9 (0.17)
Education			
Continuous	1.2 (0.7–1.9)	0.6* (0.3–1.0)	0.9 (0.6–1.4)
χ^2_1 (p-value)	0.5 (0.49)	4.4 (0.04)*	0.3 (0.58)
Marital status			
Never married	0.8 (0.3–2.2)	1.2 (0.4–3.4)	1.1 (0.4–3.1)
Previously married	0.4 (0.1–1.5)	6.6* (1.5–28.4)	1.7 (0.5–5.3)
Married/cohabiting			
χ^2_2 (p-value)	1.9 (0.39)	6.4 (0.04)*	0.8 (0.66)
Income			
Continuous	1.1 (1.0–1.3)	1.0 (0.9–1.2)	0.9 (0.8–1.0)
χ^2_1 (p-value)	2.1 (0.15)	0.2 (0.68)	2.1 (0.15)
Employment			
Student	0.2 (0.0–3.0)	0.9 (0.1–9.1)	6.3 (0.4–96.5)
Homemaker	4.0* (1.0–15.5)	1.2 (0.3–5.3)	0.4 (0.1–1.3)
Retired	0.9 (0.1–9.7)	2.9 (0.3–33.2)	0.7 (0.0–10.6)
Other	0.5 (0.2–1.7)	1.1 (0.3–3.6)	2.0 (0.6–6.2)
Working			
χ^2_4 (p-value)	6.0 (0.20)	1.0 (0.91)	5.3 (0.25)
Severity of 12-month suicidal behavior			
Suicide plan	0.6 (0.2–1.9)	0.8 (0.2–3.0)	1.0 (0.4–3.1)
Unplanned suicide attempt	0.3 (0.1–1.2)	1.7 (0.1–22.7)	3.0 (0.8–11.7)
Planned suicide attempt	0.2* (0.1–0.7)	2.1 (0.9–5.2)	4.0* (1.1–14.6)
Ideation only			
χ^2_3 (p-value)	8.3 (0.04)*	3.0 (0.39)	6.6 (0.09)
Time since ideation			
Continuous (divided by 10)	0.9 (0.6–1.4)	1.0 (0.6–1.6)	1.1 (0.7–1.7)
χ^2_1 (p-value)	0.1 (0.76)	0.0 (0.97)	0.2 (0.67)

Appendix Table 14.16. (cont.)

Category/subcategory	Among respondents with any suicidal behavior who did not receive treatment (n=430)		
	Low perceived need for treatment	Any structural barrier	Any attitudinal barrier
	OR (95% CI)	OR (95% CI)	OR (95% CI)
History of treatment			
Yes	1.1 (0.4–3.3)	1.6 (0.7–3.7)	1.1 (0.4–3.0)
χ^2_1 (p-value)	0.0 (0.90)	1.2 (0.27)	0.0 (0.93)
Lifetime disorder			
Any anxiety	0.9 (0.4–1.9)	0.7 (0.3–1.6)	1.5 (0.7–3.3)
Any mood	0.6 (0.2–1.5)	1.8 (0.6–5.3)	1.7 (0.6–4.4)
Any impulse	0.8 (0.3–2.2)	0.9 (0.3–2.7)	1.5 (0.5–4.1)
Any substance	0.3* (0.1–0.9)	4.3* (1.3–14.4)	4.1* (1.2–13.5)
χ^2_4 (p-value)	7.6 (0.11)	6.6 (0.16)	10.0 (0.04)*
χ^2_{19} (p-value)	42.1 (0.002)*	32.3 (0.03)*	38.0 (0.01)*

* Significant at the 0.05 level, two-sided test.
a Results are based on multivariate logistic regression models controlling for country.

Index